Anesthesiology Updates for Postgraduates

DISCLAIMER

The markings of *Must Know, Good to Know* and *Nice to Know* are as per Editor thoughts and may not collaborate at all with view of other experts in this field.

These reviews have not undergone peer review or editorial review. The contribution of individual Contributors are based on current knowledge and evidence, and authenticity of their content have been acknowledged.

Anesthesiology Updates for Postgraduates

4th Edition

Editor

Sampa Dutta Gupta

MBBS DMCW MD(Anes) DCC(Cardiac Anes) MAMS

Associate Professor
Department of Anesthesiology
Institute of Postgraduate Medical Education and
Research and Seth Sukhlal Karnani Memorial (SSKM) Hospital
Kolkata, West Bengal, India

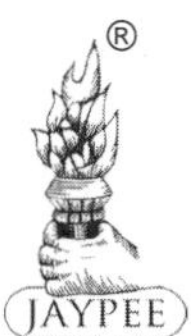

JAYPEE BROTHERS MEDICAL PUBLISHERS (P) LTD

New Delhi • London • Philadelphia • Panama

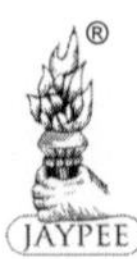

Jaypee Brothers Medical Publishers (P) Ltd.

Headquarters
Jaypee Brothers Medical Publishers (P) Ltd.
4838/24, Ansari Road, Daryaganj
New Delhi 110 002, India
Phone: +91-11-43574357
Fax: +91-11-43574314
Email: jaypee@jaypeebrothers.com

Overseas Offices

J.P. Medical Ltd.
83, Victoria Street, London
SW1H 0HW (UK)
Phone: +44-2031708910
Fax: +02-03-0086180
Email: info@jpmedpub.com

Jaypee-Highlights Medical Publishers Inc.
City of Knowledge, Bld. 237, Clayton
Panama City, Panama
Phone: +1 507-301-0496
Fax: +1 507-301-0499
Email: cservice@jphmedical.com

Jaypee Medical Inc.
The Bourse
111, South Independence Mall East
Suite 835, Philadelphia, PA 19106, USA
Phone: +1 267-519-9789
Email: joe.rusko@jaypeebrothers.com

Jaypee Brothers Medical Publishers (P) Ltd.
17/1-B, Babar Road, Block-B, Shaymali
Mohammadpur, Dhaka-1207
Bangladesh
Mobile: +08801912003485
Email: jaypeedhaka@gmail.com

Jaypee Brothers Medical Publishers (P) Ltd.
Bhotahity, Kathmandu, Nepal
Phone: +977-9741283608
Email: kathmandu@jaypeebrothers.com

Website: www.jaypeebrothers.com
Website: www.jaypeedigital.com

Inquiries for bulk sales may be solicited at: jaypee@jaypeebrothers.com

Anesthesiology Updates for Postgraduates

First Edition: 2010
Second Edition: 2011
Third Edition: 2012
Fourth Edition: **2014**

ISBN: 978-93-5152-096-2

Printed at Rajkamal Electric Press, Plot No. 2, Phase-IV, Kundli, Haryana.

Dedicated to

All the Postgraduate (PG) students of anesthesiology

Contributors

Anil Agarwal MD
Professor and Head
Department of Anesthesiology
Sanjay Gandhi Postgraduate
Institute of Medical Sciences
Lucknow, Uttar Pradesh, India

Anupam Goswami MD
Professor and Head
Department of Cardiac Anesthesiology
Institute of Postgraduate Medical Education and Research (IPGMER) and Seth Sukhlal Karnani Memorial (SSKM) Hospital
Kolkata, West Bengal, India

Arif Ahmed MD
Clinical Fellow
Singapore General Hospital
Singapore

Ashok Kumar Saxena MD FAMS
Professor and Ex-Head
Department of Anesthesiology
University College of Medical Sciences
New Delhi, India

Baljit Singh MD
Director and Professor
Department of Anesthesiology
GB Pant Hospital
New Delhi, India

Bibhukalyani Das MD
Former Professor and Head
Department of Anesthesiology
Nil Ratan Sarkar (NRS)
Medical College and Hospital
Kolkata, West Bengal, India

Chandan Kumar Mandal DNB
Post-Doctoral Fellow
Rabindranath Tagore International
Institute of Cardiac Sciences (RTIICS)
Kolkata, West Bengal, India

Chiranjib Bhattacharyya MD
Associate Professor
Institute of Postgraduate
Medical Education and Research (IPGMER) and
Seth Sukhlal Karnani Memorial (SSKM) Hospital
Kolkata, West Bengal, India

Dalim Kumar Baidya MD
Assistant Professor
Department of Anesthesiology and Intensive care
All India Institute of Medical Sciences
New Delhi, India

Deepak K Tempe MD FRCA FAMS
Dean
Maulana Azad Medical College and
Associated GB Pant, Guru Nanak Eye Center
(GNEC) and Lok Nayak Hospitals
New Delhi, India

Dhanee Majhi MD Student
Department of Anesthesiology
SCB Medical College and Hospital
Cuttack, Odisha, India

Dilip K Pawar MD
Professor
Department of Anesthesiology
All India Institute of Medical Sciences
New Delhi, India

Indira Malik MD
Assistant Professor
Department of Anesthesiology and Intensive Care
GB Pant Hospital
New Delhi, India

Jatisankar Rudra MD
Head
Department of Anesthesiology
Calcutta National Medical College
Kolkata, West Bengal, India

Jayashree Sood MD FFARCS PGDHHM
Chairperson
Department of Anesthesiology
Pain and Perioperative Medicine
Sir Ganga Ram Hospital
New Delhi, India

Jaydeb Prakash Kundu MD FFARCS
Former Professor and Head
Department of Anesthesiology
Nil Ratan Sarkar (NRS) Medical College
Kolkata, West Bengal, India

JV Divatia MD
Professor and Head
Department of Anesthesiology
Critical Care and Pain
Tata Memorial Hospital
Mumbai, Maharashtra, India

Jyotsna Goswami MD
Senior Consultant and Head
Department of Anesthesia and Critical Care
Tata Medical Center
Kolkata, West Bengal, India

Kanak Kanti Kundu DA MD
Professor and Head
Department of Anesthesiology
Institute of Postgraduate
Medical Education and Research (IPGMER)
Kolkata, West Bengal, India

Koel Mitra MD
Assistant Professor
Department of Anesthesiology
Medical College Kolkata
Kolkata, West Bengal, India

LD Mishra MD PhD FICA
Professor and Head
Department of Anesthesiology
Institute of Medical Sciences
Banaras Hindu University
Varanasi, Uttar Pradesh, India

Mahendra Kumar DA MD
Director and Professor
Department of Anesthesia
Guru Teg Bahadur Hospital
New Delhi, India

Maupali Ghosh MBBS MD Student
Department of Anesthesiology
Institute of Postgraduate
Medical Education and Research (IPGMER) and
Seth Sukhlal Karnani Memorial (SSKM) Hospital
Kolkata, West Bengal, India

Minati Choudhury MD
Additional Professor
Department of Cardiac Anesthesia
Cardiothoracic and Neurosciences Center
All India Institute of Medical Sciences
New Delhi, India

Mohona Mukherjee MD
RMO-Cum-Clinical Tutor
Department of Anesthesiology
Institute of Postgraduate
Medical Education and Research (IPGMER) and
Seth Sukhlal Karnani Memorial (SSKM) Hospital
Kolkata, West Bengal, India

Nibedita Pani MD
Professor and Head
Department of Anesthesiology and Critical Care
SCB Medical College and Hospital
Cuttack, Odisha, India

Pooja Banerjee MD Student
Department of Anesthesiology
Institute of Postgraduate Medical
Education and Research and Seth Sukhlal
Karnani Memorial (SSKM) Hospital
Kolkata, West Bengal, India

Prithwis Bhattacharyya MD PDCC
Professor and Head
Department of Anesthesiology
North-Eastern Indira Gandhi
Regional Institute of Health and
Medical Sciences (NEIGRIHMS)
Shillong, Meghalaya, India

Purnima Mukherjee MD
Former Professor and Head
Department of Anesthesiology
Institute of Postgraduate
Medical Education and Research and
Seth Sukhlal Karnani Memorial (SSKM) Hospital
Kolkata, West Bengal, India

Rahul Guha Biswas MD PDCC
Postdoctoral Fellow (Canada)
Senior Consultant
Cardiac Anesthesia and Intensive Care
NH- Rabindranath Tagore International Institute of Cardiac Sciences (RTICCS)
Kolkata, West Bengal, India

Rajan Singh MSc
Clinical Fellow
Department of Gastroenterology
Sanjay Gandhi Postgraduate
Institute of Medical Sciences
Lucknow, Uttar Pradesh, India

Rajat Choudhuri MBBS MD
Assistant Professor
Department of Anesthesiology
Institute of Postgraduate Medical
Education and Research and Seth Sukhlal
Karnani Memorial (SSKM) Hospital
Kolkata, West Bengal, India

Rajib Samal MD
Assistant Professor
Department of Anesthesiology
Institute of Postgraduate Medical
Education and Research and Seth Sukhlal
Karnani Memorial (SSKM) Hospital
Kolkata, West Bengal, India

Ratul Kundu MD
RMO-Cum-Clinical Tutor
Department of Anesthesiology
Institute of Postgraduate Medical
Education and Research and Seth Sukhlal
Karnani Memorial (SSKM) Hospital
Kolkata, West Bengal, India

Sumitra Bakshi MD
Associate Professor
Department of Anesthesiology
Critical Care and Pain
Tata Memorial Hospital
Mumbai, Maharashtra, India

S Parashar MD PDCC (Neuroanesthesia)
Student and Senior Resident
Department of Anesthesiology
Institute of Medical Sciences
Banaras Hindu University
Varanasi, Uttar Pradesh, India

Sabyasachi Das MD
Professor
Department of Anesthesiology
Dean, North Bengal Medical College
Darjeeling, West Bengal, India

Saikat Sengupta MD DNB MNAMS
Professor
Department of Anesthesia
Apollo Hospitals Education and
Research Foundation
Senior Consultant
Apollo Gleneagles Hospitals
Kolkata, West Bengal, India

Samarendra Pal DA MD
Former Professor and Head
Department of Anesthesiology
Institute of Postgraduate Medical
Education and Research and Seth Sukhlal
Karnani Memorial (SSKM) Hospital
Kolkata, West Bengal, India

Samarendra Samui MD
Assistant Professor
Department of Anesthesiology
Institute of Postgraduate Medical
Education and Research and Seth Sukhlal
Karnani Memorial (SSKM) Hospital
Kolkata, West Bengal, India

Sampa Dutta Gupta MBBS DMCW MD(Anes) DCC(Cardiac Anes) MAMS
Associate Professor
Department of Anesthesiology
Institute of Postgraduate
Medical Education and Research and Seth
Sukhlal Karnani Memorial (SSKM) Hospital
Kolkata, West Bengal, India

Sanghamitra Mishra MD
Professor
Department of Anesthesiology
Pain, Palliative and Critical Care
Institute of Medical Sciences and SUM Hospital
Bhubaneswar, Odisha, India

Shalini Chaudhuri MD Student
Department of Anesthesiology
Institute of Postgraduate Medical
Education and Research and Seth Sukhlal
Karnani Memorial (SSKM)Hospital
Kolkata, West Bengal, India

Simantika Ghosh DNB
Fellow
Tata Medical Center
Kolkata, West Bengal, India

Sagarmoy Basu MD (Cal) DA (London) FICA
Professor and Ex-Head
Calcutta National Medical College
Kolkata, West Bengal, India

Soumendu Pal MD DM (Cardiac Anesth)
Associate Consultant
Department of Cardiac Anesthesia
Fortis Memorial Research Institute
Gurgaon, Haryana, India

Souvik Maitra MD
Senior Resident
Department of Anesthesiology and Intensive Care
All India Institute of Medical Sciences (AIIMS)
New Delhi, India

Srabani Basu MD
In-charge
Department of Anesthesiology and
Surgical Intensive Care Unit
BR Singh Hospital
Kolkata, West Bengal, India

Subrata Pahari MD
Professor and Head
Department of Anesthesiology
Medical College Kolkata
Kolkata, West Bengal, India

Sudakshina Mukherji MD
Professor
Bankura Sammilani Medical College
Bankura, West Bengal, India

Sudeshna Bhar (Kundu) MD
Assistant Professor
Department of Anesthesiology
Institute of Postgraduate Medical
Education and Research and Seth Sukhlal
Karnani Memorial (SSKM) Hospital
Kolkata, West Bengal, India

Sujeet Kumar Singh Gautam MD
Assistant Professor
Department of Anesthesiology
Sanjay Gandhi Postgraduate
Institute of Medical Sciences
Lucknow, Uttar Pradesh, India

Sukdev Nayak MD PGDM Dip Pall Med (Wales) LLB
Professor and Head
Department of Anesthesiology
All India Institute of Medical Sciences
Bhubanswar, Odisha, India

Sumanta Dasgupta MD
Additional Chief Health Director
Department of Anesthesiology and
Critical Care Central Hospital
South-Eastern Railway
Kolkata, West Bengal, India

Sushil Kumar MSc
Clinical Fellow
Department of Gastroenterology
Sanjay Gandhi Postgraduate
Institute of Medical Sciences
Lucknow, Uttar Pradesh, India

Sushma Bhatnagar MD
Professor and Head
Anesthesiology, Pain and Palliative Care
Dr Bhim Rao Ambedkar (BRA)
Institute Rotary Cancer Hospital
All India Institute of Medical Sciences
New Delhi, India

Uday C Ghoshal MD DNB DM FACG RFF
Professor
Department of Gastroenterology
Sanjay Gandhi Postgraduate
Institute of Medical Sciences
Lucknow, Uttar Pradesh, India

Preface to the Fourth Edition

Anesthesiology Updates for Postgraduates first published in 2010 has achieved increasing acclaim with each successive two editions. In this edition, some esteemed teachers and examiners across the country have put forth their suggestions on some commonly encountered long and short cases for final MD, DA and DNB practical examination of anesthesiology. This addition has been made with the intention of spreading the mode of discussion of some eloquent teachers of anesthesiology, whose suggestions are worth to include in achieving a good anesthetic management skill for a postgraduate student. Senior esteemed teachers can count on years of experience to direct students for logistic approach of Must Know part during their training period through an easy-to-follow sequence of chapters. No small book can do justice to a large syllabus of anesthesiology for postgraduates, but, chapters of this edition are backed up with an information-packed references which provide succinct and up-to-date advice for practical application along with the new insights into the decision-making process. This book may be used as a learning aid or as a checklist for preparation of postgraduate practical examination of students of anesthesiology.

Sampa Dutta Gupta

Preface to the Third Edition

This book has evolved over last eight years from the interactions between teachers and postgraduate students from eight annual postgraduate assemblies conducted by Department of Anesthesiology of Institute of Postgraduate Medical Education and Research and Seth Sukhlal Karnani Memorial (SSKM) Hospital, Kolkata, West Bengal, India.

The greater part of the book is distilled from the work of eminent and dedicated teachers and their experiences of sharing knowledge with their beloved students. The book is not a substitute for the major anesthetic texts, but concentrates on principles of management of the most challenging anesthetic cases.

The book has resulted in the concept of "Educational spiral", to understand the need to identify what are 'essential' and what are 'not so essential'. Knowledge gathering may spiral out from core knowledge, without which the basic objective of the book would remain unfilled. Must learn area based on the health need of patients, task to be performed by the students for patients and community need depending on the socioeconomic situations, resources available and keeping pace with the scientific advancements.

We have been encouraged by many postgraduate students who have told us that discussions of postgraduate assemblies helped them immensely in preparation for their examination. Topics are chosen for review based on questions and contentions raised by anesthesiology residents. Based on their needs, with an aim to prepare themselves for various postgraduates examinations, we are delighted to have been able to provide this assistance and hope that the book will be even more useful to them.

I like to express my deep gratitude to all those who have nobly contributed to the book, to the reader for their interest and to those who have offered constructive criticism.

Sampa Dutta Gupta

Preface to the Second Edition

The first edition of this book has achieved its purpose in the last one year, having helped our beloved students to prepare their curriculum. We are thankful to all our postgraduate students for their review, criticism, patience and perseverance which have helped us to refine the second edition and screen out certain unintentional errors.

Despite our sincere efforts, the first edition of the book was printed with some technical errors. Therefore, in this edition, the entire book has been revised, with a view to eliminate errors and to incorporate valuable suggestions from the readers. With an aim to update the topics in tune to the recent trends of MD, DA or DNB examination, we have added some new chapters to the book. However, in the interest of the readers, in order to limit the number of pages for ease of reading, we have been unable to include certain previous chapters. This edition will act as a supplement to the previous edition. It is our firm conviction that the book will be of substantial help to all postgraduate students.

The inspiration, encouragement, inputs and moral support we have received from all the students and teachers are commendable. We express immense gratitude to all our students and teachers for their inspiration and incredible support.

Sampa Dutta Gupta
Sudeshna Bhar (Kundu)

Preface to the First Edition

Reading of leading anesthetic texts is essential for success in clinical anesthesiology, but memorization and subsequent recall of important points may be difficult. This book aims to provide guidance to the postgraduate students of anesthesiology to provide safe anesthesia practice in the perioperative period in line with modern concepts with safety.

The greater part of this book is distilled from the work of eminent and dedicated teachers and their experiences of sharing knowledge with their beloved students. The book is not a substitute for the major anesthetic texts, but concentrates on principles of management of the most challenging anesthetic cases.

The book has evolved over last six years from the interactions between teachers and postgraduate students from six annual postgraduate assemblies conducted by Department of Anesthesiology of Institute of Postgraduate Medical Education and Research and SSKM Hospital, Kolkata, West Bengal, India.

We have been encouraged by many postgraduate students who have told us that discussions of postgraduate assemblies helped them immensely in preparation for their examination. Topics are chosen for review based on questions and contentions raised by anesthesiology residents. Based on their needs, with an aim to prepare themselves for various postgraduates examinations, we are delighted to have been able to provide this assistance and hope that the book will be even more useful to them.

We would like to express our deep gratitude to all those who have nobly contributed to the book, to the reader for their interest and to those who have offered constructive criticism.

Sampa Dutta Gupta
Sudeshna Kundu

Acknowledgments

I would like to extend my sincere gratitude to Professor Pradip Kumar Mitra, Director, Institute of Postgraduate Medical Education and Research and Seth Sukhlal Karnani Memorial (SSKM) Hospital, Kolkata, West Bengal, India, for this constant encouragement and inspiration.

My sincere thanks to Sagarmoy Basu, DA (London) MD, Professor and Ex-Head, Calcutta National Medical College (CNMC), Kolkata, West Bengal; Purnima Mukherjee, DA MD, Professor and Ex-Head, Institute of Postgraduate Medical Education and Research and Seth Sukhlal Karnani Memorial (SSKM) Hospital, Kolkata, West Bengal; Amitava Rudra, MD FAMS, Professor and Ex-Head, Calcutta National Medical College, Kolkata, West Bengal; Samarendra Pal, DA MD, Professor and Ex-Head, Institute of Postgraduate Medical Education and Research and Seth Sukhlal Karnani Memorial (SSKM) Hospital, Kolkata, West Bengal; and Nitish Kumar Gazi, DA MD, Professor and Ex-Head, Institute of Postgraduate Medical Education and Research and Seth Sukhlal Karnani Memorial (SSKM) Hospital, Kolkata, West Bengal, India, for their whole-hearted support and encouragement for this difficult task.

I thank Shri Jitendar P Vij (Group Chairman), Mr Ankit Vij (Managing Director), Mr Tarun Duneja (Director-Publishing), Mr KK Raman (Production Manager), Mr Sunil Kumar Dogra (Production Executive), Mr Neelambar Pant (Production Coodinator), Mr Akhilesh Kumar Dubey, Mr Chandra Dutt (Typesetter), Mr Hazra (Kolkata Branch) and the entire team of M/s Jaypee Brothers Medical Publishers (P) Ltd, New Delhi, India, for their help in bringing out the book.

Contents

SECTION 1: SPECIAL TOPICS

SECTION 2: LONG CASES

SECTION 3: SHORT CASES

Plate 1

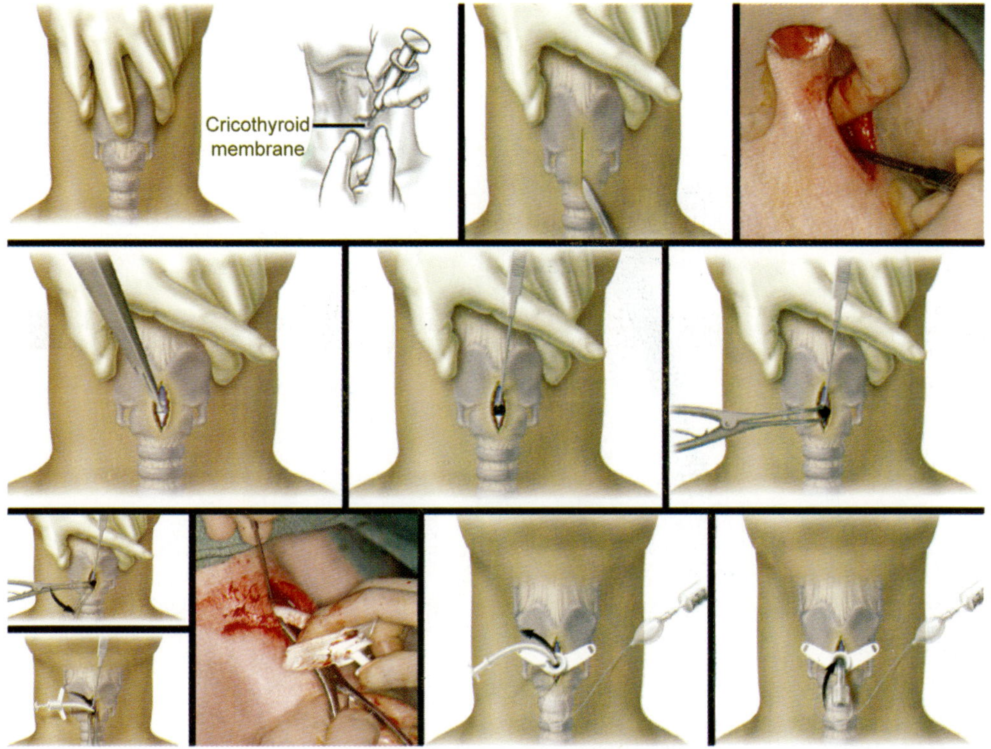

Fig. 2 Techniques of surgical cricothyrotomy

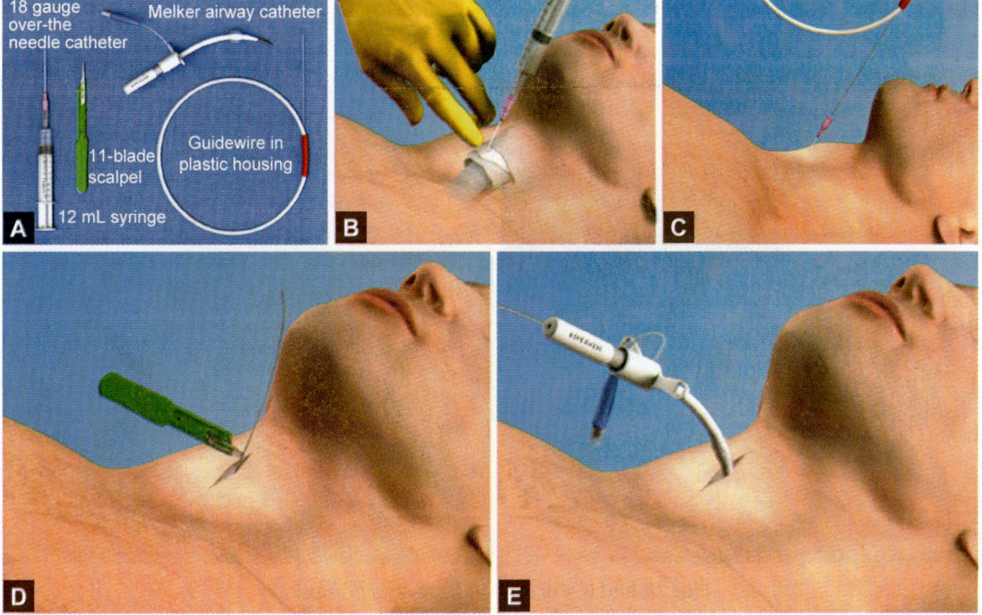

Figs 4A to E Cook Melker cricothyrotomy

Plate 2

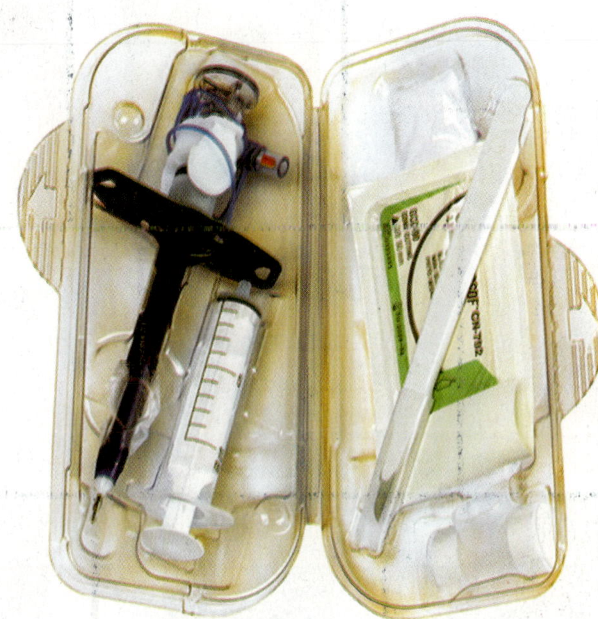

Fig. 5 Portex cricothyrotomy kit

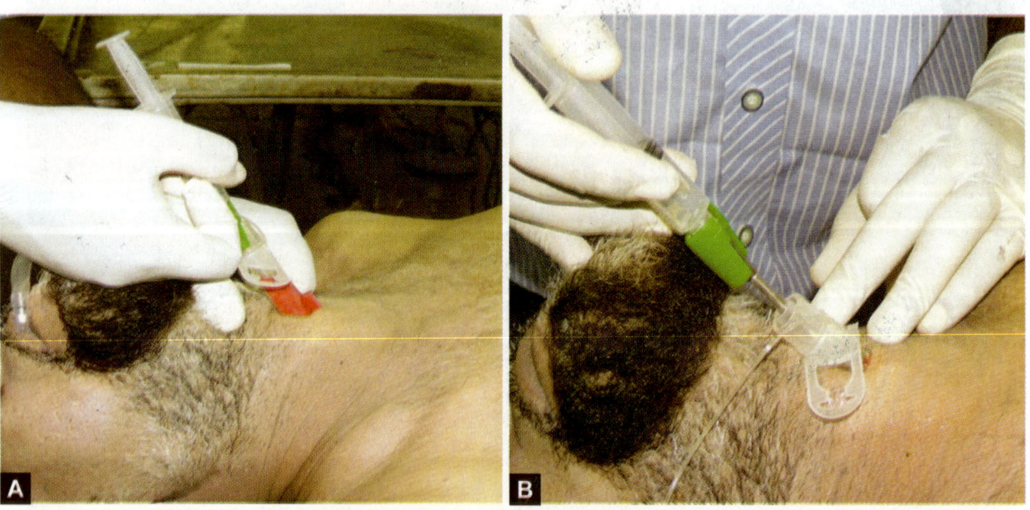

Figs 7A and B Cricothyrotomy using portex kit

Plate 3

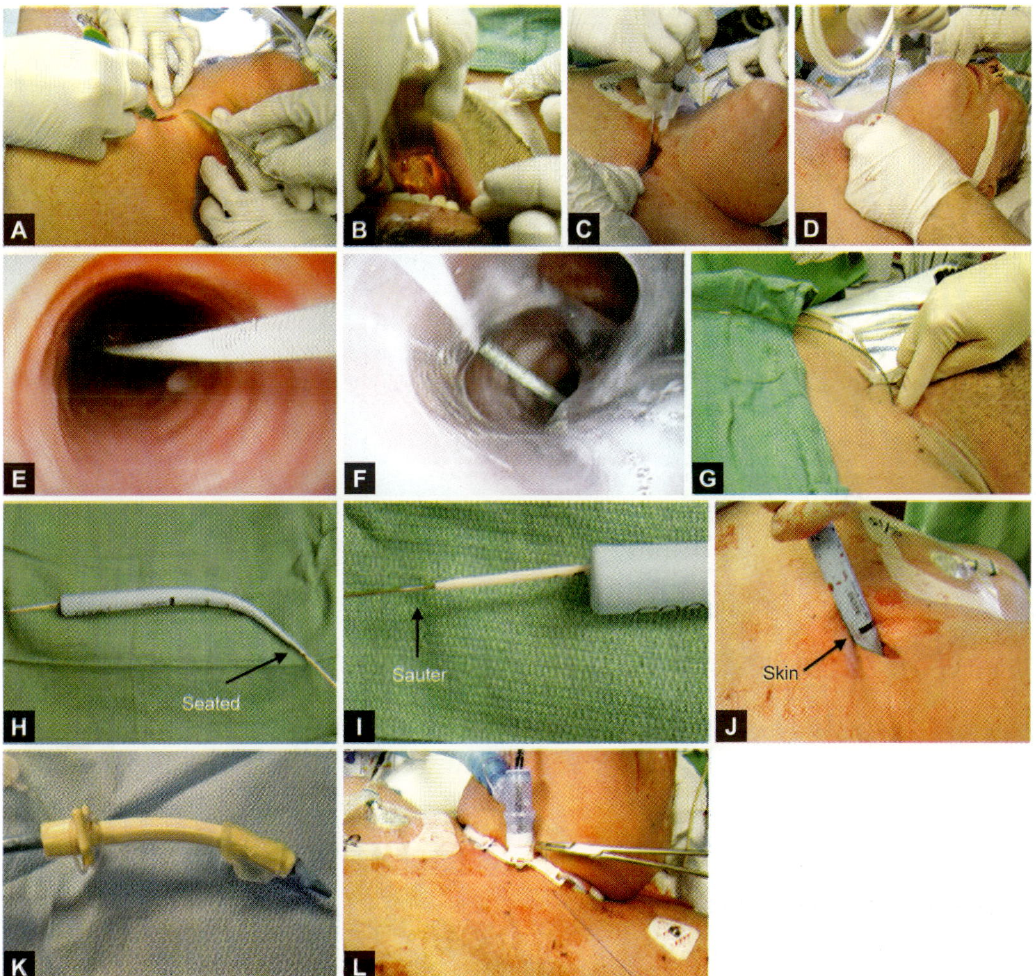

Figs 9A and L Techniques of percutaneous tracheostomy

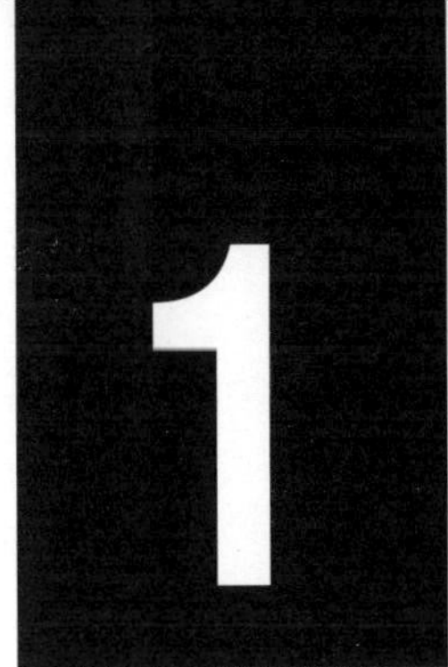

SPECIAL TOPICS

CHAPTERS

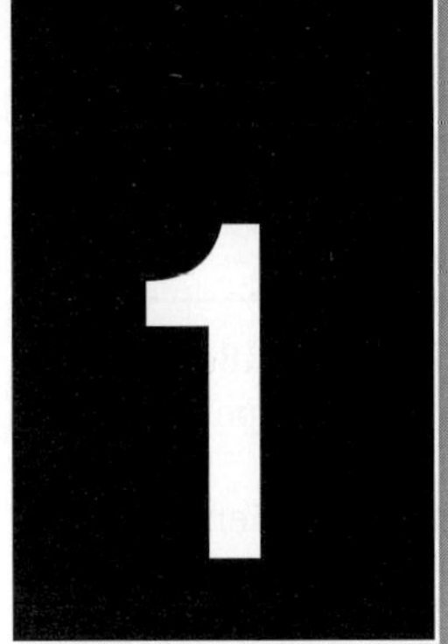

Development of General Anesthesia

Jaydeb Prakash Kundu

INTRODUCTION

Present day anesthesia is a culmination of many earlier efforts, discoveries and failures through ages.

Surgery is known from prehistoric days and there has been a continuous search for some satisfactory methods of pain relief during surgery, ever since.

Attempts at producing a state of anesthesia go back to many recorded history. From many ancient books we come to know that Egyptians used poppy seeds during operation. Romans used extracts of 'Mandragora' plants. Greek used 'Hemp'. Indians and Chinese used cannabis incense and aconitum, before the entry of opium, to alleviate pain of surgery.

Although surgery is being practice from prehistoric days, the first documented mention of surgery and anesthesia is seen in Old Testament 4004 BC 'And The God caused a deep sleep to fall on ADAM and he took one of his ribs'.

In India *Sushruta Samhita* performed surgery using wine and incense of cannabis; exsanguination and nerve compression were other methods used for producing numbness and analgesia (*Sushruta Samhita* 400 BC).

In 5th century AD Chinese surgeons performed surgery using wine and a herbal extract 'Mafeisan' which probably caused unconsciousness with partial neuromuscular block.

In India Raja Bhoj had a cranial surgery done on him where a plant (Sammohani) was used to put him to sleep and another plant '*Sanjivani*' was used to bring him back to senses. (Raj Prabandh:527 AD)

It was in the 8th century the Arab traders brought 'Opium' to India and China. Thereafter opium played an important role in the surgical practice. Hypnosis and mesmerism were often tried here and there. In most cases however when traditional method failed, patient were tied up to poles for given heavy blows on head to make them unconscious thus renders him surgery to almost a butchery.

TENTH CENTURY DOWNWARDS UP TO EIGHTEENTH CENTURY

This was the golden era, particularly for the Muslims world. A combined oral and inhalation method of pain relief was known to Persians. This was reference in the poem of the Persian poet Ferdous. May be this was the first hint of general anesthesia by inhalation.

The mysteries of anesthesia gradually opened up particularly during 15th–18th century. Diethylether was discovered by Roman Llull; Paracelsus described its analgesic properties (1525) and Valerius Cordus synthesized it in 1540.

18th century was the period of Renaissance both in Europe and in America. Science and Art developed. Better knowledge of anatomy and physiology led to expansion of surgical field and a safe and acceptable method for pain relief during surgery was being increasingly felt. Joseph Priestley born near Leeds, amongst many of his achievements', the Unitarian Minister and scientist discovered oxygen (1771) and nitrous oxide (1772).

Humphrey Davy experimented with nitrous oxide. In 1778 he became the superintendent of Thomas Beddoes's Pneumatic Institute, a center for the treatment of Asthma and Tuberculosis in Bristol.

In the following year he published his book 'Researches: chemical and philosophical: chiefly concerning N_2O'. In this book he suggested 'nitrous oxide can be used to relieve pain of surgical operations'.

NINETEENTH CENTURY

In 1804 Friedrich Sertürner isolated morphine from opium and named it after the Greek name of God, 'MORPHOS'. Until 1840, in most industrial areas of Europe and America only two anesthetic agents, morphine and wine were mainly used. Addiction, violence and vomiting were the mainly drawbacks. Neither this ensured satisfactory pain free surgery. At this time hypnotism and mesmerism were also used for surgical pain relief. In India also, besides traditional methods, mesmerism was being practiced by James Esdaile at Hooghly Imambara Hospital, Bengal (1843). He claimed to have operated upon 226 patients with questionable result.

The first description of inhalational anesthesia by using carbone dioxide was reported by Henry Hill Hickman. He made animals to inhale CO_2 to the point of asphyxia and unconsciousness when surgery could be performed on them painlessly. Perhaps this was the first official description of anesthesia by inhalation method. By late 1830's Humphrey Davy's experiments got wide publicity. Wandering lectures started organizing public gatherings where participants used to inhale ether/nitrous oxide as tools of entertainment. Many participants while inhaling ether/nitrous oxide (Ether frolics) injured themselves but nobody complained of pain. The five stalwarts GQ Colton, Horace wells, Edward Clarke, Crawford Long and WTG Morton happened to be present in those gathering. They become curious about the hypnotic and analgesic effects of ether and nitrous oxide.

In January 1842 WE Clarke administered ether to Miss Hobbie, (one of his friend's sisters) for extracting one of her tooth. And she did not fell pain. This was the first successful anesthesia in the world. But Clarke never published this due some confusion.

In March 1842, Crawford Long used Ether anesthesia for the removal of a neck tumor of James Venable. He also did not publish this work until 1849.

In 1844 GQ Colton and Horace wells while participating in a public gathering (Ether frolic) noticed one Solmon Colley who under the influence of nitrous oxide, banged his shine bone and broke it. He never felt pain. Seeing this idea of N_2O being used for extraction of tooth cropped up in the friend of Horace wells. Next day he got of his own teeth pulled out. GQ Colton gave him N_2O for inhalation. He did not feel any pain. Inspired by this Horace wells was tried dental extraction under N_2O anesthesia on several patients. His business partner, WT Green Morton advised him to demonstrate this technique at Massachusetts General Hospital. Wells staged a demonstration on 20 January 1845 with the assistance of surgeon John Collin Warren. The attempt was unsuccessful; the patients complain of pain. Horace Wells was pooh-pooled out of the theater. WTG Morton, who also noticed the effects of ether frolic, became then interested, in ether. At this time one of his teachers Charles T Jackson suggested 'ether can be used as surface analgesic in dentistry'. Morton after some experiments on animals tried this for dental extraction of a patient named Ebon frost. Immediately after this Morton used ether on several patients of Henry Jacob Bigelow. Supported by Henry J Bigelow, Morton later fixed up a public demonstration at Massachusetts General Hospital on 16 October 1846. Morton successfully administered ether for the removal of a jaw tumor from the patient 'Gilbert Abott'. The operation was a grand success. Thus a public demonstration of ether anesthesia; a sentinel event in the history took place at Massachusetts General Hospital. Dr Wassen the surgeon exclaimed, 'Gentlemen, this no humbug'. Anesthesia was born and news spread all over the world. Morton became famous overnight. But Morton never got the official recognition as pioneer in his life time. The dispute arose when his teacher CT Jackson claimed that 'the idea of ether as anesthesia was his'. However Morton still continued to enjoy this reputation until there was another claimed in favor of Crawford Long put forward late in 1849. In despair he started farming. Morton died of cerebral hemorrhage in 1868 when he was absolutely penniless.

News of discovery reached London in 1846. Robert Liston was the first surgeon to operate under ether anesthesia at University College Hospital on 21 December 1846, operation was 'amputation of leg'. And the end of operation Liston shouted, 'This Yankee dodge beats mesmerism hollow'.

Before this use of ether, only lifesaving operations used to be done in England. Surgery comprised mainly, of surface surgery, amputation, fungating cancers and stone removal. Chest, abdomen and skull were 'no go areas'.

The news of ether anesthesia reached India in the 2nd week of March 1847. At that time surgery in India was being done using only contemporary methods, including physical force. Mesmerism was popular at Hooghly Imambara Hospital (Bengal).

Within two weeks after the arrival of the news of ether anesthesia, Dr Saughnessy first performed surgery at Prince of Wales Hospital Calcutta on 22nd March 1847.

CHLOROFORM

Technical difficulty associated with ether anesthesia was partly overcome with the introduction of $CHCl_3$. James Young Simpson; Professor of Midwifery at Edinburgh University initially tried ether for obstetrical surgery but was on the lookout for a better anesthesia agent. Chloroform was discovered by Liebig. In 1847, Flourens showed that it has anesthetic properties (from animal experiment). David Waldie, a Liverpool chemist suggested Simpson to try chloroform on human beings. Having this clue and advice, Simpson along with his three assistants inhaled $CHCl_3$, to try its effect. All of them become unconscious. The milkmaid next morning discovered them lying senseless in the drawing room of Simpson. They had no idea as to what happened to them. Four days later Simpson tried chloroform in clinical obstetric practice. The report was read out at 'Edinburgh Medical and Chirurgical society' on 10 November 1847. An alternative to ether was thus introduced. Simpson was the first to used chloroform for (obstetrical analgesia) relieving pain of labor. This was strongly protested by the clergy. The final seal of acceptance of obstetrical analgesia was however ensured when John Snow administered chloroform to Queen Victoria at the time of birth of Prince Leopold (1853). The use of chloroform gradually spread to most of the countries of the world. In India chloroform become so popular that people used the term 'Chloroform' as a synonymous of anesthesia. It is a coincidence that David Waldie, the chemist who suggested Simpson to use chloroform on man, settled in India in his later life and is still lying in the Park Street Cemetery of Calcutta.

The use of chloroform as an anesthetic in the USA initially replaced ether, but soon it was abandoned in favor of ether when its hepatic and cardiovascular toxicity especially its tendency to ventricular fibrillation becomes apparent.

First report of anesthetic death from chloroform was reported from St Thomas Hospital London on 10 October 1849. Frayed reported first case of death from hepatic failure following $CHCl_3$ anesthesia in India (Ind. Med Gaz. 1869 Vol 4 P 240). During the first 16 years of chloroform anesthesia there were 393 deaths, of which only 48 deaths were attributed to ether. Controversy arose with regard to cause of death. Three commissions were set-up to investigate it. First commission was set by British Medical Association at Glasgow. This Glasgow commission suggested that chloroform was more injurious to heart than ether. Second commission was held at Hyderabad (India) under the captaining of Dr Edward Lawrie who claimed to have administered chloroform anesthesia to 40,000 patients without any fatality (1888). He conducted a trial on 141 animals and concluded 'chloroform can be safely administered without any fear of accidents. This was not accepted in England. Nizam of Hyderabad then sponsored a 2nd commission with Dr Lawrie at helm with representatives from England (1889). The commission conducted this investigation at Afzalganj Hospital (now Osmania Medical College). It was interesting that the world's first qualified lady anesthetist, Dr Rupabai Furdonji from Hyderabad was a member of this team. Second Hyderabad commission corroborated the finding of Glasgow Commission. Gradually become very unpopular and finally become a forgotten name in clinical anesthesia. Curiously enough chloroform continued to be used in India well beyond independence.

Mahatma Gandhi was in Poona Jail when he had an attack of acute appendicitis (1925). He was operated at Sasoon General Hospital Poona on 25 January 1925 under chloroform anesthesia. The lighting arrangement was a kerosene lamp and a hand held torch. The popularity of chloroform, despite its toxicity, continued because of the rough induction process of ether anesthesia, its bad smell, hazards of open flame and fear of ether convulsion in hot and humid weather. Dr MC Ganguli and Dr Jyoti Prasad, in Jodhpur conference (1928) however assured that ether can be used safely in hot weather.

Endotracheal Anesthesia

German surgeon Friedrich Trendlenburgh (1871) described that general anesthesia can be safely administer through tracheostomy.

Macewen of Glasgow passed a tube from the mouth to trachea using finger a guide (1878). Mcreddie, in India, introduced a catheter using Macewen's technique for insufflation anesthesia (1880) (Ind Med Gaz. 443 V 16 P 13). All this attempts of intubation were made through indirect laryngoscopy. Direct vision laryngoscopy was first done by Kirstein of Germany using his 'autoscope'. During 1st world war, Sir Ivan Magill and Elgar Stanley working in a plastic surgery unit at Sidcup introduce inhalation anesthesia through endotracheal tube. Initialy he tried blind nasal method; subsequently he developed his own modification of laryngoscope blade. Magill's endotracheal tube with design curvature, connection, breathing circuit and curved forceps are some of his many contributions to present day anesthesia. Sir Robert Macintosh (1943) made further improvement in the technique of direct vision laryngoscopy. Macintosh's blade is the mostly wide use laryngoscope blade today. His design of Gum elastic catheter as introducer of endotracheal tube in case of difficult intubation is worth mentioning (1949).

In 20th century (1967) fiber optic endoscope was introduce by Peter Murphy, for direct vision intubation.

Intravenous Anesthesia

Thiopentone was synthesized in 1932 by Volwiler and Tabern. It was introduced into clinical practice by Ralth Water and Lundy of Mayo clinic 1934. Jarmen and Abel used it in England (1935), it was initially being used as a 'total anesthetic' which caused many deaths in Perl Harbour (1941).

Later it's used as a part of balanced technique of anesthesia is still in vogue. In India thiopentone was introduced into anesthetic practice in 1940 (Desai & Sarkar). Many new intravenous anesthetics and inhalation anesthetics have been invented in later part of 20th century. These include butyrophenons, haloperidol (1958), doperidol (1961), fentanyl (a piperidinone derivative of opioid—1960). This was followed by sufentanil, alfentanil (1976), carfentanil (1976), lofentanyl (1980). A potent IV anesthetic agent (induction agent) Etomidate was introduced in 1964. Similarly a number of newer anesthetic agent (inhalational agent) have appear in the market and have made anesthesia very safe and patient friendly.

Halothane, synthesized by Suckling in Manchester 1951 was first used clinically by M Johnston at Manchest Royal Hospital and Bryce Smith in Liverpool (1956). Enflurane: Ross Ferrel in USA (1963) and isoflurane tried clinically by Alen B Dobkin (1971).

Premedication

In preanesthetic days both wine and opium was given to alloy apprehension of surgery. This technique was not followed immediately after the discovery of Ether and Chloroform. It was first recommended by Belamy Gardener of University College Hospital London for the first time in the world. Alexander Crombie used hypodermic morphine at Presidency General Hospital, Calcutta (Ind Med Gaz. 1888 Vol. 23) for smoothening the induction of ether anesthesia. While searching for a synthetic substitute for atropine, Meperidine, an opioid with a structural difference from morphine was discovered in 1939. Methadone followed this in 1947.

Muscle Relaxants

Sir Walter Raleigh mentioned about the arrow poison (1596). Benjan Brody first described that artificial respiration could save curarized animals (1812).

King in London isolated d-tubocurarine from *Chondrodendron tomentosum* (1935) for the first time in the world.

Harold Griffith and Enid Johnson from Canada used Curare in anesthesia to produce muscular relaxation on 23rd January 1942. Subsequently Ceil Gray and Halton in Liverpool established its position in England (1946).

Ralph Waters were first person to use curare in general anesthesia using only N_2O and oxygen and IPPV for abdominal surgery.

Gallamine Triethiodide was first used by Boue and Huguenard (1948) and WW Mustin in England (1949). Pancurorium was used for the first time by Burkitt et al (1968), Vecurorium (1979), Durant et al. Atracurium was described by Hughes and Payne 1981.

ANESTHETIC MACHINE

History of anesthesia will remain incomplete until a description of the development of anesthesia is presented.

After the unsuccessful demonstration of Horace Walls and appearance of Ether in the market there was a silent period for nitrous oxide until it was re-introduced by GQ Cotton in 1867–1868. Nitrous oxide was however being used singly and as such it could not be used for a prolonged period. Edmond Andrews, in Chicago added oxygen to N_2O to ensure a longer period of anesthesia (1868). Compressed gases in cylinders were available by that time. McKesson (1910) and Foregger (1914) and Boyle (1917) designed N_2O and O_2 machines using different types of gas flow pattern (e.g. Intermittent flow with each breath and continuous flow).

Most popular machine used in England and India was Boyle's anesthetic apparatus.

Boyle's anesthetic machine and its evolution:
1917: Boyle's original machine for N_2O and O_2 anesthesia had only two water sight feed.
1920: One vaporizing bottle was added
1920: Water's to and fro absorber for CO_2 was added
1926: Second vaporizing bottle was added
1926: Brian Sword two way circle type of absorber later substituted to and fro system
1927: 3rd water sight feed was added for CO_2.
1930: Plunger device was introduce in vaporizing bottle
1933: Dry Bobbin flow meter displaced water sight feed.
1937: Rota-meters displaced dry bobbins.

India

1935: First Boyle's apparatus arrived in Calcutta.
It had fine adjustment valves (no pressure reducing device).
Two water sight feed with two vaporizer bottle.
Two way stop cock (for breathing and nonbreathing), Shipway CO_2 absorption.
Four cylinders of compressed N_2O and O_2 (each of 100 gallon capacity).

Same year oxygen plant was installed at Calcutta. Nitrous Oxide plant was installed in 1956.

'Indian Oxygen Limited' imported first 'F' type Boyle's apparatus in 1950 and started manufacturing it in India from 1956. During the Indo-Pak war IOL manufactured Porta Boyle for army used in forward area.

21th century is the period of digital revolution. Newer devices of direct vision laryngoscope with digital technology have come to the market. Glidescope Video laryngoscope is an example of this. Xenon as an anesthetic is about to occupy the market. With the advances in recovery and re-cycling, Xenon may be affordable economically soon.

ACKNOWLEDGMENTS

This lecture note for the postgraduate students of anesthesia had to be made very short and concise under compulsion. As a result many important events and names of many great scientists who enriched this specialty could not be included. I sincerely apologized for this.

Almost all the information's in this lecture notes have been collected from internet. I am grateful to the authors.

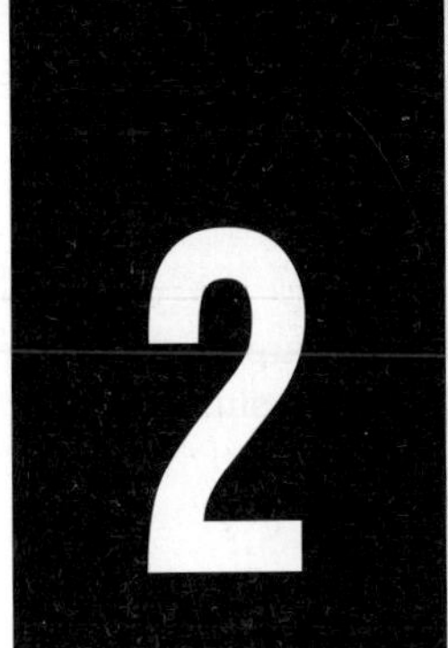

Pediatric Anesthesia: An Overview

Purnima Mukherjee, Shalini Chaudhuri

INTRODUCTION

Pediatric anesthesia has an important role in child health care. Prior to inception of general anesthesia, even a simple operative procedure was a nightmare for both the child and the surgeon. Thus, among the advances in medicine, the introduction of surgical anesthesia must certainly rank with immunization and antibiotics—the anesthesiologists' greatest contribution to humankind, especially the children.[1]

In the mid-1930's, Dr Philip Ayre, a visiting anesthetist at the Babies Hospital, Newcastle-Upon-Tyne (England), developed an especially suitable pediatric anesthesia breathing system for use with tracheal intubation during repair of cleft lip and palate deformities in infants. The key element of the 't' piece through which fresh gases are introduced at a relatively high flow rate forms the basis for modern semi-open pediatric anesthesia systems as well as many infant mechanical ventilator gas circuits. This piece was one of the first important mechanical innovations in anesthetic practice to compensate for the special physiological needs of infants and small children during anesthesia.[2]

Dr G Jackson Rees and his colleagues at the Alder Hey Children's Hospital and the University of Liverpool developed techniques of anesthesia with nitrous oxide-oxygen, muscle relaxants and a minimal concentration of a potent volatile agent, combined with controlled hyperventilation.[3]

Pediatrics and anesthesiology have long been closely allied. Anesthesiologists, such as Dr Virginia Apgar, made valuable contributions to the cause of infants and children.[4]

Neonates and young infants have greater perioperative hazards while undergoing all types of anesthesia and surgery than older children. The anesthesiologist should consider, while administering anesthesia in the neonate, the following:

- The transitional period of the infant.
- The disease process and its anesthetic implication.
- Associated congenital anomalies especially cardiac problems which will increase the risk of anesthesia.
- Maturation of different organs.
- Adequate infrastructure for care of the neonate in the perioperative period.
- Transportation of these critically ill children must be carried out by specialized pediatric transport teams to avoid any complications.
- Hypothermia, hypoglycemia, hypercarbia, hypoxia, hypotension, bradycardia and acidosis may cause transition from neonatal to fetal circulation and must be avoided.

- Risk of anesthesia related cardiac arrest is more in the first year of life compared with older children and adults. This risk may be decreased when anesthetics are given and supervised by experienced pediatric anesthesiologists.[5]

Problems of Anesthesia in Neonates

- Stress is poorly tolerated in premature neonates.
- *Respiratory system:* Ribs are horizontal, intercostal muscles and the diaphragm are poorly developed, attachment of the diaphragm is horizontal. Thus, spontaneous respiration under general anesthesia may lead to respiratory muscle fatigue and even respiratory failure.
- Postoperative apnea, especially in premature infants is more with general anesthesia than with regional anesthesia.
- *Cardiovascular system:* Poor compliance of ventricles leads to hypoxia, acidosis and pulmonary hypertension. Bradycardia and apnea have adverse effects on the neonate. Bradycardia < 80 bpm–cerebral blood flow is diminished. Bradycardia < 60 bpm–cardiac massage is to be started.
- Hypothermia may lead to acidosis, impaired perfusion, decreased platelet function, hypoglycemia, increased oxygen consumption, and even laryngospasm during intubation and after extubation. OT temperature should be kept at 32°C.
- *Intravenous line:* Risk of air embolism and over-transfusion should be kept in mind.
- Increased risk of regurgitation due to distension of the stomach during mask ventilation.
- Fentanyl may cause bradycardia and muscle rigidity.[5]

Preoperative Assessment

During the preoperative visit, the following history should be carefully elicited:

- Problems encountered during previous anesthesia.
- History of previous hospital admission (especially in the ICU) to exclude subglottic stenosis due to prolonged intubation.
- Whether blue or breathless on exercise or during breastfeeding.
- *Respiratory symptoms:* Asthma, frequent cold, chest infection, upper respiratory tract infection.
- *Cardiovascular system:* Congenital anomalies.
- *Drug history:* Allergy to any drug.
- In children with history of upper respiratory tract infection or measles-surgery should be postponed for 4–6 weeks after resolution of all signs and symptoms. This is because, though the child may be afebrile, playful, have a good appetite and no positive chest signs, due to heightened airway edema there is an increased risk of laryngospasm, bronchospasm, increased secretions and alveolar collapse during anesthesia. This risk is more in intubated patients.
- History of immunization must be elicited.
- *In a child with a murmur:* See whether the child desaturates during suckling or exercise. Diastolic and pansystolic murmurs are always pathological.

When a child requires surgery, the stress is borne by the child's entire family. Preoperative visit is the best premedication and reassurance of the parents and the child. Parents must be reassured to allay their anxiety regarding the sick child. Written consent regarding the anesthetic procedure must be taken during the preoperative visit.[5]

FASTING GUIDELINES

Shortening the mandatory fasting interval prior to anesthesia and surgery is one of the most humane advances in the perioperative care of children. Oral fluid therapy is to be continued till two hours before surgery. The advantages of this approach are:

- The child is less thirsty, less hungry and thus less irritable.
- There is less dehydration.
- Increased peristalsis will allow gastric emptying and thereby avoid aspiration.
- Decreased risk of hypotension of during anesthesia.[5]

Fasting guidelines are shown in Table 1.

Table 1 | Fasting guidelines

Types of food	*Minimum fasting time (hrs)*
Clear fluid	2 hrs
Breast milk	4 hrs
Cow's milk	4 hrs
Solid food	6 hrs

Anesthetic Technique

Premedication

Parents are the best premedication. Oral midazolam (0.25–0.33 mg/Kg, maximum 20 mg), triclofos may be used as anxiolytics.

Induction

The child should be induced in mother's lap, while the operating team and anesthesiologists should take off their mask to assure the child that they are living persons and prevent psychotrauma. Prevention of psychotrauma during surgery is very important as some children may develop psychological problems in the future.

The child should be preoxygenated using a transparent face mask, which will enable detection of cyanosis and vomiting, if they occur. During induction, especially with inhalational agents, pulse oximeter may show erroneous reading in an agitated and crying child. There is a caution during anesthesia—it is dangerous to put the child in deeper plane of anesthesia unless the intravenous line has been secured.

Intubation

Before intubation, halothane vaporizers must be switched off. Intubation is done with muscle relaxants. Suxamethonium is avoided. The size of the endotracheal tube must be selected so as to allow a peritubular leak. The ET tube should be fixed to the maxilla. Anesthesia is maintained by controlled ventilation with oxygen, nitrous oxide, muscle relaxant and analgesic. No child should be denied of analgesia due to its age as neuroendocrinal response to pain is more in pediatric patients. During reversal from the effect of muscle relaxant, the child should be warm, well saturated and normocarbic.[5]

REVERSAL CRITERIA

- Child must breathe spontaneously and rhythmically.
- Opens mouth and brings up legs in response to nasopharyngeal suction.
- Moves extremities purposefully.

- Opens eyes
- SpO_2-100%
- Conjugate movement of eyeballs.

These criteria should be ensured before extubation. After extubation, vigorous suction of the throat may initiate laryngospasm, and there may be desaturation, bradycardia and even cardiac arrest, as the airway of the child is physiologically brittle. The decision as to when and whom to extubate requires experience, skill and the technical ability to reintubate should the need arise.[5]

Monitoring

The anesthesiologist's eyes, ears and hands are the best monitor. The standard ASA monitors are to be used. Postoperatively, a dedicated and trained nurse at the bedside is the best monitor.[5]

OPD ANESTHESIA

Exponential expansion of pediatric day care surgery was only possible due to advent of newer, short acting and safe anesthetic drugs and trained and experienced anesthetists. Senior consultant surgeon and anesthesiologist must be present as the child is to be operated and discharged on the same day. Anesthetic agents used are propofol, nerve blocks and caudal epidural. No food should be given immediately after surgery as it causes postoperative nausea and vomiting.

Former preterm infants less than 46 weeks of postconceptual age are at increased-risk of developing postoperative apnea and should not undergo OPD surgery. The incidence of postoperative apnea is inversely related to both postconceptual age and gestational age. These infants should be admitted to the hospital and monitored for apnea and bradycardia for atleast 12–18 hours after surgery using saturation probe, electrocardiography and apnea monitors. Use of intravenous caffeine base 10 mg/Kg is recommended in all infants at risk of postoperative apnea. Regional anesthesia may be beneficial. A former preterm infant with totally unremarkable neonatal history who is currently healthy is deemed fit for day care surgery. In case any child is intubated during an OPD procedure, he should be monitored for atleast 6 hours to exclude any airway edema formation. Local general physicians and pediatricians must be involved in the care of the infant undergoing outpatient surgery to tackle minor problems in the perioperative period. In the postoperative period the child must be pain-free and not have postoperative nausea vomiting.[5,6]

ANESTHETIC DRUGS

Propofol

Propofol can be used as a bolus in infants more than 1-month-old and as an infusion in children more than 3-year-old. It should be avoided in sepsis and respiratory infection.

Ketamine

Increases secretions, laryngeal reflexes are exaggerated. It does not guarantee protection against aspiration. Suctioning may lead to severe spasm. Other undesirable effects include hypertonia causing involuntary muscle movement, emergence delirium, seizures, diplopia and visual disturbances which are distressing in the postoperative period. It causes increase in intraocular, intracranial and intragastric pressures. It causes respiratory depression which may lead to apnea. It causes myocardial depression in patients with depleted catecholamine reserves.[5]

Avoid in Children

- *Awake intubation:* Intubation is very stressful in the awake child, resulting in tachycardia with increase in blood pressure, intracranial pressure, intraocular pressure, and gastric pressure, which may lead to brainstem herniation, intraventricular hemorrhage and aspiration of gastric contents. Thus, awake intubation is only indicated in very sick premature neonates, infant with difficult airway and with full stomach.
- *Hyperextension of neck:* Causes worsening of airway; flexion of neck-causes respiratory obstruction.
- Mask ventilation for prolonged periods—as it causes abdominal distension.
- Do not allow spontaneous respiration under GA for prolonged periods.
- Do not put the mask with force in a panicked child.
- Hypoxia, hyperoxia, hypothermia.
- Blind deep pharyngeal suction.
- Deepening plane of anesthesia before IV line has been secured.[5]

SPECIAL CONSIDERATIONS

Cleft Palate Surgery

During placement of mouth gag by the surgeon, the anesthesiologist must be very careful, as the tube may be displaced, crushed or kinked. The anesthesiologist must constantly monitor saturation, auscultate the chest and keep a finger on the pulse.

Gastroschisis or Exomphalos Surgery

The child should be positioned with head end elevated. Hand ventilation should be done to assess lung compliance and determine how much of abdominal contents can be reduced back into the abdomen. Fluid loss is a major issue.

Hypospadias and Circumcision

Regional anesthesia is beneficial. The child must be pain-free in the postoperative period to prevent erection of the penis and minimize hemorrhage.[5]

CONCLUSION

Always keep in mind the 'Ten Commandments for the Pediatric Anesthesiologist':

1. Let Mum or Dad be there.
2. Take off your mask.
3. Be polite to the child and listen to the child.
4. Peace and quiet in the theater.
5. Be honest. Do not deceive a child, otherwise the next anesthesia will be problematic.
6. Do not use force.
7. Let the child choose his posture for induction.
8. Do not push a mask on to the face of an unprepared child. Prepare the child to accept the mask.
9. Do not bother about the clock. Take your time. Undue haste and premature extubation may lead to fatality.
10. You must have affection and love for the child.

Success should be measured, not only by intact wounds, but also by intact emotions in the child and his family.

REFERENCES

1. Downes J John. Historic origins and role of pediatric anesthesiology in child health care. Paediatric Clinics of North America. Vol. 41, 1994.
2. Ayre P. Endotracheal Anaesthesia for Babies. Curr Res Anesth Analg. 1937;16:330.
3. Rees GJ. Paediatric anaesthesia. Brit J Anaesth. 1960;32:132.
4. Wetzel C Randall. Paediatric Clinics of North America. Vol. 41, 1994.
5. Cote J Charles. Paediatric Anaesthesia, Miller's Anaesthesia, 7th Edition.
6. Cote J Charles. Sedation for the paediatric patient. Paediatric Clinics of North America. Vol. 41, 1994.

3

Neurosurgical Anesthesia: An Overview

Bibhukalyani Das

Neurosurgical anesthesia focuses on patients undergoing brain and spinal cord surgery.

Practice of neuroanesthesia is unique because:

- The target organ of anesthesia is diseased.
- Secondly, the target organ is same for the surgeon and anesthetist. So the anesthetic management has profound impact on surgical goals.

WHAT MAKES NEUROANESTHESIA DIFFERENT?

Neurosurgical anesthetic management is different than usual GA because it can have major effect on the brain and spinal cord through the control of cerebral blood flow (CBF), intracranial pressure (ICP) and cerebral oxygen metabolism ($CMRO_2$).

Anesthesiologists practicing neurosurgical anesthesia required to have special training to understand the inter-relationship of neurophysiology (brain and spinal cord), pathophysiological changes due to disease and trauma and pharmacology related to central nervous system (CNS), special consideration to anesthetics, analgesics, sedatives and other adjuvant drugs.

BASIC PRINCIPLES OF NEUROPHYSIOLOGY

There are six inter-related components that are important to the practice of neuroanesthesia. They are maintenance of cerebral perfusion pressure (CPP), cerebral blood flow (CBF), cerebral blood volume (CBV), intracranial pressure (ICP), CO_2 responsiveness (CO_2R) and cerebral oxygen metabolism ($CMRO_2$).

Management of *cerebral perfusion pressure* ***(CPP)*** *is the most important determinant of* outcome.

CPP is the difference between mean arterial pressure (MAP) and ICP.

$$CPP = MAP - ICP$$

Although in the occasional patient where central venous pressure is higher than ICP, CPP = MAP – CVP. Both intracranial pathology and drugs may compromise CPP through effects on MAP and/or ICP. CPP ideally has to be maintained at >70 mm Hg. An optimal CPP has not been defined but in the context of head trauma, a CPP < 60 is associated with a poorer outcome; a benefit of higher CPP has not been established.

Cerebral Blood Flow

The average CBF is ~40–50 mL/100 gm/min with gray matter having a higher flow than white matter (60 mL/100 gm/min and 20 mL/100 gm/min respectively). CBF is auto regulated over a wide range (~50–150 mm Hg) of perfusion pressures in order to avoid ischemia when MAP reduced and ICP is high due to edema or hemorrhage. *Static autoregulation* refers to changes in flow that occur slowly (minutes) in response to changes in blood pressure and *dynamic autoregulation* is used to describe changes that occur within seconds. The autoregulatory range and the relationship between CBF and perfusion pressure can change rapidly. When sympathetic tone is reduced the entire response can shift to lower pressures and when tone is increased such as during stress, it moves to a higher pressure range. With hyperventilation the response shifts to lower CBF and covers a wider perfusion pressure range while an increased CO_2 results in a narrower range at a higher CBF.

Volatile anesthetics affect CBF both indirectly and directly. The effect of volatile anesthetics on cerebral hemodynamics including CBF and autoregulation has been well reviewed. When cerebral metabolism ($CMRO_2$) is decreased, vasoconstriction occurs to appropriately reduce CBF. However, direct vasodilation also occurs in a dose-dependent fashion but may not manifest as an increased CBF except at higher concentrations. Evidence from both animal and humans suggest that the increase in CBF is more pronounced with desflurane and least with sevoflurane.

Both static and dynamic autoregulations remain essentially intact with both sevoflurane and isoflurane up to 1 MAC but preservation is better and persists to a higher concentration with sevoflurane. Desflurane >1 MAC abolishes autoregulation.

Static autoregulation also appears to be intact in children undergoing non-neurosurgical procedures with doses of sevoflurane up to 1.5 MAC.

Propofol, barbiturates and etomidate are potent cerebral vasoconstrictors reducing CBF secondary to decreasing $CMRO_2$. The effect on CBF is greater with propofol and thiopental than etomidate. Propofol and thiopental do not alter autoregulation. However, the coupling of CBF and $CMRO_2$ is well maintained with thiopentone.

Opioids have minimal effect on CBF.

Cerebral Blood Volume

Approximately 15% of CBV is in the arterial tree and ~15% in the major venous sinuses. The remainder ~70% is in the capillary and venous systems. CBF is often incorrectly used as a surrogate for blood volume, probably because it has been easier to measure. Changes in CBF and CBV are generally proportional to one another but, for instance, changes in head position from standing to supine to head down can increase CBV without changing CBF.

Propofol decreases CBV in humans and sevoflurane increases it but less than isoflurane.

Intracranial Pressure

Maintenance or reduction of ICP (normal value ~10–15 mm Hg) is one of the important aims of neuroanesthesia. ICP is a critical determinant of CPP → CBF and brain function. As ICP increases above ~20 mm Hg, focal reductions in CBF occur and further increases eventually result in global cerebral ischemia. The three major components of the intracranial cavity are brain (~80%), cerebrospinal fluid (CSF) (~10%) and CBV (~10%). If one component increases in its volume, it must be compensated for by a decrease in another to prevent ICP from increasing.

CO_2 Responsiveness

CO_2R of the cerebral arterial tree is important. Hypercarbia results in vasodilation and increased CBV. Conversely, hyperventilation causes cerebral arterial vasoconstriction, decreased CBF and CBV and a decreased ICP. Each 1 mm Hg change in $PaCO_2$ causes 2–4% change in CBF.

While the reduction in ICP is beneficial, the reduced CBF can result in ischemia so that caution must be exercised with the extent and duration of hyperventilation. CO_2 reactivity is maintained with both sevoflurane and isoflurane up to 1.5 MAC in adults and with sevoflurane, isoflurane and halothane up to 1.0 MAC in children. Intravenous anesthetics do not influence CO_2R significantly.

Cerebral Oxygen Metabolism

$CMRO_2$ is a key determinant of the risk of ischemic insult. If metabolic rate is high, then a reduced CBF is more likely to disrupt neuronal function and integrity. This is the rationale behind decreasing $CMRO_2$ in order to prevent ischemia but there are no clinical trials in neuroanesthesia to support such a practice.

Intravenous anesthetics potently reduce $CMRO_2$. As CBF is closely coupled to $CMRO_2$, CBF is reduced in parallel with an associated reduction in CBV and ICP which makes them very useful agents in patients with intracranial hypertension. Volatile anesthetics in contrast reduce $CMRO_2$ but increase CBF through direct effects on the vasculature.

CLINICAL NEUROANESTHESIA

Neurosurgical anesthesia requiring expertise of neuroanesthetists (trained) are:

- Benign and malignant intracranial mass lesions
- Extra and intracranial vascular surgery (Aneurysm; AVM)
- Craniobasal/craniofacial surgery
- Trans-sphenoidal pituitary surgery
- Posterior craniotomies
- Decompressive procedures in major head trauma
- Pediatric neurosurgery
- Stereotactic, endoscopic procedures
- Spinal surgery
- Sitting position neurosurgery
- Functional neurosurgery (Awake craniotomy)
- Intervention NR procedures coiling/stenting/embolization.

The most common of these are intracranial tumor surgery (Supra/Infra-tentorial), decompressive craniectomy and aneurysm/AVM surgery.

PREANESTHETIC EVALUATION AND OPTIMIZATION

Besides the routine assessments the patient should be assessed for signs of elevated ICP (nausea/vomiting, papilledema, headache, visual changes, altered mental status, altered breathing patterns, hypertension, bradycardia) and the neurological deficits documented.

The diagnostic imaging should be seen so as to identify the type of tumor, its location, and vascularity, evidence of midline shift and presence of hydrocephalus. Often, patients are taking steroids and anti-epileptic medications which can have an impact on glucose homeostasis and pharmacodynamics of neuromuscular blockers respectively. Premedication for anxiolysis may be offset by sedation that may hamper neurological assessment and hypercarbia which may increase ICP. In most patients, a carefully titrated dose of intravenous benzodiazepine can safely be given, if needed.

Monitors consist of standard monitors. Continuous intra-arterial blood pressure measurement, preferably via peripheral artery catheter is useful in detecting and treating abrupt hemodynamic changes that might compromise CPP or ICP. Core temperature should be monitored and kept in the normal range. A Foley catheter is important, if diuretics are to be used or the surgery will be long.

BASIC PRINCIPLES

The basic principles of neuroanesthesia are: (i) to provide optimal operating conditions, i.e. brain relaxation, (ii) to maintain adequate cerebral perfusion pressure (CPP), and (iii) cerebral oxygenation.

Most of these patients present with raised ICP due to space occupying lesion (SOL), cerebral edema (peritumor/ischemia) or ventriculomegaly. As CPP = MAP – ICP, management of intracranial hypertension is of prime importance in neurosurgical anesthesia.

Induction of Anesthesia

It is a critical time because of the highly stimulating effects of direct laryngoscopy and intubation which is followed a short time later with pinning the head for optimal positioning which is painful. Excessive increases in blood pressure and coughing should be avoided. The most common induction agents are propofol or thiopental with etomidate or ketamine occasionally used in the hemodynamically unstable patient. These are supplemented with an opioid such as fentanyl 2–3 ug/kg or a remifentanil infusion. In addition 1–1.5 mg/kg lidocaine IV or esmolol 5–10 mg IV may help blunt the hemodynamic effect on ICP but the effect may be incomplete. Either succinylcholine or a nondepolarizing muscle relaxant may be used. There has been controversy about succinylcholine in patients with elevated ICP but the effects are usually of short duration and can be buffered by some additional propofol. The efficacy of lidocaine has not been demonstrated. Level 2 evidence exists to support use of a defasciculating dose of a nondepolarizing relaxant to blunt the increase in ICP with succinylcholine. Expeditious intubation followed by oxygenation and hyperventilation is much preferred to the avoidance of succinylcholine but with a delayed and problematic intubation. Neuromuscular blockade may not be needed during the procedure but should be used during positioning and head pinning.

Maintenance of Anesthesia

There needs to be constant attention to the balance between ICP and CPP together with adequacy of anesthetic depth. Attention to ICP is especially important before the dura is opened; once the dura is open, ICP is effectively zero.

Another important consideration is the need for electrophysiological monitoring, e.g. somatosensory or motor-evoked potentials which are used with increasing frequency during neurosurgical procedures. Good communication between anesthesiologist, neurosurgeon and monitoring technician is essential as local preferences tend to dictate drug choices. This is especially true for direct stimulation of the motor cortex as there is a paucity of clinical studies to support the use of one drug over another. SSEPs are only minimally influenced by total intravenous anesthesia (TIVA) and are suppressed by inhalational agents in a dose-dependent manner although good signals can be obtained with <0.75 MAC vapor.

A typical maintenance anesthetic might consist of a vapor anesthetic at <1 MAC and an opioid (fentanyl, sufentanil or remifentanil) infusion or alternatively a TIVA. The latter is especially appropriate where ICP is markedly elevated or there is acute decompensation.

MANAGEMENT OF INTRACRANIAL PRESSURE

The ICP may be affected by four major variables in the operating room—hyperventilation, anesthetic drugs, diuretics such as mannitol, and head position.

Hyperventilation

Constricts the cerebral arterioles with concomitant decreases in CBF and CBV. The effect takes place rapidly and may be especially useful for decreasing ICP in situations in which ICP is critically elevated or the surgeon is having difficulty with brain bulk. However, cerebral vasoconstriction may lead to critical hypoperfusion and brain ischemia with no improvement or worsened outcomes especially with prolonged use.

Therefore, current recommendations are that hyperventilation:

- Should not be used prophylactically in the traumatically brain injured patient during hypoperfusion phase, i.e. 1st 24 hours of injury.
- Should only be used for brief periods to manage significant increases in ICP not responsive to alternate treatments.
- Unless neurosurgical conditions demand it, ventilation to moderate levels of hypocapnia ($PaCO_2$ 32–35 mm Hg) rather than severe ($PaCO_2$ < 32 mm Hg) should be used.

Anesthetic Drugs

Volatile anesthetics produce direct vasodilatation and thus have the potential to increase ICP. However, the effect on ICP, in both pediatric and adult patients with space occupying lesions is clinically insignificant when anesthetic concentrations are maintained below 1.2 MAC and if the ICP is not critically elevated.

Despite theoretical benefits of IV agents, volatile agents remain popular. Numerous studies have described their differential effects on cerebral hemodynamics and intracranial pressure (ICP). In a study comparing desflurane, isoflurane, and sevoflurane in a porcine model of intracranial hypertension, at the equipotent doses and normocapnia, cerebral blood flow (CBF) and ICP were greatest with desflurane and least with sevoflurane. The authors went on to confirm these findings in clinical studies, demonstrating that sevoflurane caused the least vasodilatation. In two different studies in healthy patients, isoflurane was found to impair autoregulation, while autoregulation was virtually intact with sevoflurane 1–1.2% at normocapnia. Although further large-scale studies are needed, sevoflurane appears to be the most suitable volatile agent for neuroanesthesia.

Propofol, barbiturates (thiopental) and etomidate have minimal effect or decrease ICP. Few randomized controlled trials have compared intravenous and inhalation agents and their effect on ICP. In a trial of 117 patients with supratentorial tumors undergoing elective resection, subjects received propofol or isoflurane or sevoflurane as well as a fentanyl infusion (2–3 µg/kg/hr). ICP was lower, brain swelling less, and CPP better preserved in the propofol group. An earlier trial on 121 patients undergoing elective removal of supratentorial tumors found no difference in mean ICP amongst propofol/fentanyl, fentanyl/nitrous oxide, or isoflurane/nitrous oxide. However, there were significantly more patients in the isoflurane/nitrous oxide group that had an intraoperative ICP > 24 mm Hg.

The benefits of high dose barbiturate coma in the management of elevated ICP have not been demonstrated while deleterious outcomes including increased mortality have been shown.

Opioids do not increase or decrease ICP. However, when blood pressure decreases, the cerebral vasculature dilates to maintain CBF; this dilation may increase ICP.

When comparing the effects of alfentanil, fentanyl and remifentanil on hemodynamics and respiratory variables in patients undergoing craniotomy for tumor, there were no significant differences except a reduced time to eye opening in remifentanil group.

In a separate study, propofol + remifentanil rather than sufentanil was associated with an earlier return of cognitive function.

Systemic hypertension is common during emergence and may contribute to development of hematomas. Increased use of remifentanil may be associated with more postoperative hypertension. The α_2 agonist dexmeditomidine has been shown to provide good hemodynamics stability during IC tumor surgery, attenuating the response to intubation and emergence.

Mannitol

It has become the mainstay of ICP management protocols. An osmotic diuretic, mannitol draws water from the brain and other tissues into the intravascular compartment. Mannitol may also lower ICP by decreasing blood viscosity and expanding plasma volume which increase CBF. When autoregulation is intact this prompts vasoconstriction to restore CBF towards normal (dose 1–1.5 gm/kg bw).

A small, randomized trial concluded that there may be a mortality benefit to using mannitol instead of barbiturate infusion in cases of elevated ICP. Other prospective, randomized studies evaluated long-term outcomes in TBI patients. In each study, one group received early, pre-operative treatment of high-dose mannitol whereas the other group did not. The early, high-dose mannitol groups had clinical reversal of impending signs of brain death, better postoperative control of ICP, and better cerebral perfusion. Thus, current guidelines advocate use of high-dose mannitol boluses for elevated ICP as long as hypovolemia and excessive serum osmolalities (>320 mOsm) are avoided.

The use of mannitol to reduce brain bulk in the OR has not been as well investigated; current practice guidelines are drawn from the head trauma literature. Frusemide, a loop diuretic can be used along with mannitol, but the dose of mannitol has to be reduced. Some centers used mannitol and glycerol combination by IV infusion, but clinical study to support this therapy is lacking.

Hypertonic saline (3%, 5%) is being investigated as an alternative to mannitol. It has been suggested that by using a hypertonic saline solution, a similar ICP lowering effect to mannitol may be achieved with better outcomes, better preservation of MAP and a potentially longer duration of effect.

Steroids

Dexamethasone is prescribed routinely to reduce cerebral edema, but even a single 10 mg dose can significantly increase blood-glucose concentrations in nondiabetic patients. There is an evidence to support tight glycemic control in critically ill, neurologically impaired patients, but whether it improves outcome in elective neurosurgical patients is yet to be established. Nevertheless adverse metabolic and cerebral ischemic effects of high blood-glucose concentrations are well documented.

Head-up Position

It is an effective intervention to reduce ICP although there is concern that MAP and consequently CPP would drop. There have been two cohort craniotomy trials examining 10 degree head-up position. One involved 40 patients, the other 15.

Head-up position of 10 degrees significantly decreased ICP and MAP but left CPP unaffected. Similar results have been found in head trauma patients subjected to 30 degree head up. Current recommendation is 15–30 degree head-up according to the patient's conditions, keeping in mind to avoid hypotension.

Recovery

Emergence and extubation must be smooth, coughing/straining must be avoided. If the patient is to be extubated at the end of surgery, the anesthetic drugs should be appropriately tapered as the scalp is sutured. If fentanyl or sufentanil have been used by infusion, these are usually terminated at dural closure. Remifentanil should be continued till scalp closure and transitional analgesia such as fentanyl 50–100 µg given. The goal is a comfortable patient in whom a neurological examination can be conducted early after the surgery.

Postoperative Care

Depends on preoperative conditions of the patient (raised ICP, brain shift, seizure, GCS, respiration, general condition). Maintenance of cerebral perfusion, control of blood sugar, electrolyte balance, prevention of hyperthermia, prevention of seizure and infection are important. However, management of complications related to particular surgery has to be addressed, e.g. cerebral vasospasm following aneurysm clipping/diabetes inspidus following pituitary surgery.

RECENT ADVANCES IN NEUROSURGERY

Few could have imagined the tremendous growth of endovascular surgery over the last 30 years. With further advances in imaging, computing, and optics the use of minimally invasive and functional procedures will continue to increase. Image-guided navigation (neuronavigation) systems have dramatically improved the ability to treat seemingly inaccessible intracranial lesions.

Endoscopic surgery is now routine for intraventricular pathology but advances in optics and scope design are likely to extend its role into all types of intracranial surgery.

The advantages of minimally invasive surgery include reduced trauma to normal tissue, preservation of function, more rapid recovery, reduced morbidity, and shorter hospital stay. Some procedures can be performed under minimal or local anesthesia. However, anesthetists may be faced with providing care for a newly developed procedure of which there is limited experience. A comprehensive preoperative assessment and management plan is essential. Awareness of potential complications and vigilance enables early identification of airway compromise, seizures, and changes in neurological status.

Awake craniotomy: Awake craniotomy is gaining popularity worldwide. Routine for epilepsy surgery for many years, it is now increasingly used for the removal of intracranial lesions in or adjacent to eloquent brain. Despite the risks in such cases, maximal tumor resection seems to be an important determinant in prognosis, increasing median survival time and time to recurrence. Cortical mapping allows the planning of safe resection margins and, with continuous neurological assessment, maximal resection with minimal postoperative neurological dysfunction can be achieved.

Anesthetic techniques for awake craniotomy have evolved along with the surgical indications, but significant challenges remain. The anesthetist must provide adequate analgesia and sedation, hemodynamic stability, and a safe airway but also an alert, cooperative patient for neurological assessment. Numerous techniques have been described from local anesthesia to conscious sedation to general anesthesia using an asleep-awake-asleep (AAA) technique, with or without airway instrumentation.

SUMMARY AND RECOMMENDATIONS

Management of the patient for neurosurgery requires a good understanding of the interrelationships of neurophysiology, pathophysiology and pharmacology. Good data (mostly level 1) exist to describe the effects of volatile and intravenous anesthetics on cerebral hemodynamics (CBF, autoregulation, CBV, CO_2 reactivity). Based on this data, one would recommend using < 1 MAC sevoflurane or isoflurane over desflurane in adults with elevated ICP with a slight preference for sevoflurane. In children, a similar recommendation can be made. Recent studies indicate use of < 0.5 MAC desflurane reduces postoperative cognitive dysfunction and rapid recovery. For patients with critically elevated ICP, a TIVA anesthetic may be preferred. Most studies, however, have used physiological measurements such as CBF or ICP intraoperatively. No level 1 study exists which measured clinical outcomes.

BIBLIOGRAPHY

1. Cottrell JE and Smith DS. Anesthesia and Neurosurgery, 5th edn, 2004.
2. Lim M, Williams D, Maartens N. Anaesthesia for Pituitary Surgery. J Clin Neurosciences. 2006;13:413.
3. Matta B, Menon DK, Turner JM. Text book of Neuroanesthesia and Critical Care, 2000.
4. Macathur DC, Buxton N. Punt Jloeberghs M. Robertson IJA. The role of Neuroendoscopy in the Management of Brain Tumors. Brit J Neurosurg. 2002:16:465-70.

4

Cardiovascular and Respiratory Physiology

Anupam Goswami

Knowledge of the principles of cardiovascular and respiratory physiology is the foundation for the practice of anesthesia. This chapter reviews few aspects of cardiovascular and respiratory physiology for the understanding of both its scientific significance and its practical applications to patient management.

RESPIRATORY PHYSIOLOGY WITH ANESTHETIC IMPLICATIONS

- Anesthesia causes impairment in pulmonary function, whether the patient is breathing spontaneously or is ventilated mechanically after muscle paralysis
- Impaired oxygenation of blood occurs in most subjects who are anesthetized
- Lung function remains impaired postoperatively, and clinically significant pulmonary complications can be seen in 1–2% after minor surgery in up to 20% after upper abdominal and thoracic surgery.

Lung Volumes during Anesthesia (Fig. 1)

- Functional residual capacity (FRC) is reduced by 0.8–1.0 L by changing body position from upright to supine, and there is another 0.4–0.5 L decrease when anesthesia has been induced
- Anesthesia *per se* causes a fall in FRC despite maintenance of spontaneous breathing

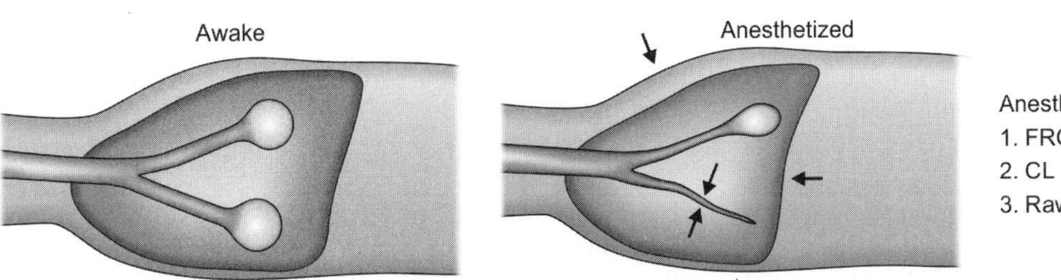

Fig. 1 Airway closure during anesthesia

- End-expiratory lung volume is thus reduced from approximately 3.5–2 L, the latter being close or equal to RV
- The decrease in FRC occurs regardless of whether the anesthetic is inhaled or given intravenously
- Muscle paralysis and mechanical ventilation cause no further decrease in FRC
- The average reduction corresponds to around 20% of awake FRC and may contribute to an altered distribution of ventilation and impaired oxygenation of blood
- The decrease is related to loss of respiratory muscle tone, which shifts the balance between the elastic recoil force of the lung and the outward force of the chest wall to a lower chest and lung volume
- Maintenance of muscle tone, as during ketamine anesthesia, does not reduce FRC
- Magnitude of FRC reduction is related to age and body weight, as obese patients demonstrate a much higher decrease in FRC
- The FRC increases with age if weight and height remain unaltered over the years.

Mechanism of FRC Reduction during Anesthesia

- Atelectasis
- Increased expiratory muscle activity
- Air trapping in distal airway
- Cephalic displacement of diaphragm
- Decreased outward chest wall recoil
- Increasing lung recoil
- Increased thoracic blood volume
- Atelectasis appears in approximately 90% of all patients who are anesthetized
- It is seen during spontaneous breathing and after muscle paralysis and whether intravenous or inhaled anesthetics are used
- 15–20% of the lung is regularly collapsed at the base of the lung during uneventful anesthesia
- It may also be mentioned that after thoracic surgery and cardiopulmonary bypass, more than 50% of the lung can be collapsed even several hours after surgery
- The amount of atelectasis decreases toward the apex, which is mostly spared
- Obese patients showing larger atelectatic areas than lean ones do
- Atelectasis is independent of age, with children and young people showing as much atelectasis as elderly patients
- COPD patients show much less amount of atelectasis
- There is a positive correlation between atelectasis and amount of shunting
- It is likely that it is a focus of infection and can contribute to pulmonary complications.

Prevention of Atelectasis during Anesthesia

Positive End-expiratory Pressure

- The application of 10 cm H_2O positive end-expiratory pressure (PEEP) will consistently reopen collapsed lung tissue
- Shunt is not reduced proportionately, and arterial oxygenation may not improve significantly by PEEP
- The persistence of shunt may be explained by a redistribution of blood flow toward more dependent parts of the lungs when intrathoracic pressure is increased by PEEP
- Increased intrathoracic pressure will impede venous return and decrease cardiac output
- Lung recollapses rapidly after discontinuation of PEEP. Within 1 minute after cessation of PEEP, the collapse is as large as it was before the application of PEEP.

Maintenance of Muscle Tone

- Use of an anesthetic that allows maintenance of respiratory muscle tone will prevent atelectasis from forming
- Ketamine does not impair muscle tone and does not cause atelectasis
- Another technique used in an attempt to restore respiratory muscle tone is pacing of the diaphragm. This was tested by applying phrenic nerve stimulation, which did reduce the atelectatic area.

Recruitment Maneuvers

- The use of a sigh maneuver, or a double Vt, has been advocated to reopen any collapsed lung tissue
- For complete reopening of all collapsed lung tissue, an inflation pressure of 40 cm H_2O is required
- Such a large inflation corresponds to a maximum spontaneous inspiration, and it can thus be called a VC maneuver.

Minimizing Gas Resorption

- Avoidance of the preoxygenation procedure (ventilation with 100% O_2) eliminated atelectasis formation during induction and subsequent anesthesia
- Preoxygenation can also be provided without producing atelectasis if undertaken with continuously increased airway pressure, as with continuous positive airway pressure (CPAP)
- Postoxygenation and airway suctioning at the end of surgery also promote atelectasis.

Compliance and Resistance during Anesthesia

- Static compliance of the total respiratory system (lungs and chest wall) is reduced on an average from 95–60 mL/cm H_2O during anesthesia
- Static lung compliance also decreases during anesthesia
- Resistance to total respiratory system and lung also increases during anesthesia.

Distribution of Ventilation during Anesthesia (Fig. 2)

In the upper part of the lung, the alveoli and airways are open (zone A). In the middle and lower parts of the lung, the airways are intermittently closed and impede ventilation (zone B), and in the bottom of the lung, the alveoli have collapsed (atelectasis, zone C). The corresponding ventilation-perfusion distribution as assessed by the multiple inert gas elimination technique can be seen in the *right panel.* Modes A and B correspond to a well-ventilated and perfused lung region and a region with intermittent airway closure, respectively, and are similar to what was shown in. In addition, there is a shunt that is caused by perfusion of the atelectatic zone (C) in the bottom of the lung.

Regional Blood Flow during Anesthesia

- A successive increase in perfusion down the lung, from the ventral to the dorsal aspect is evident during anesthesia in supine subject, with some reduction in the lowermost region
- PEEP will impede venous return to the right heart and therefore reduce cardiac output
- PEEP causes a redistribution of blood flow toward dependent lung regions.

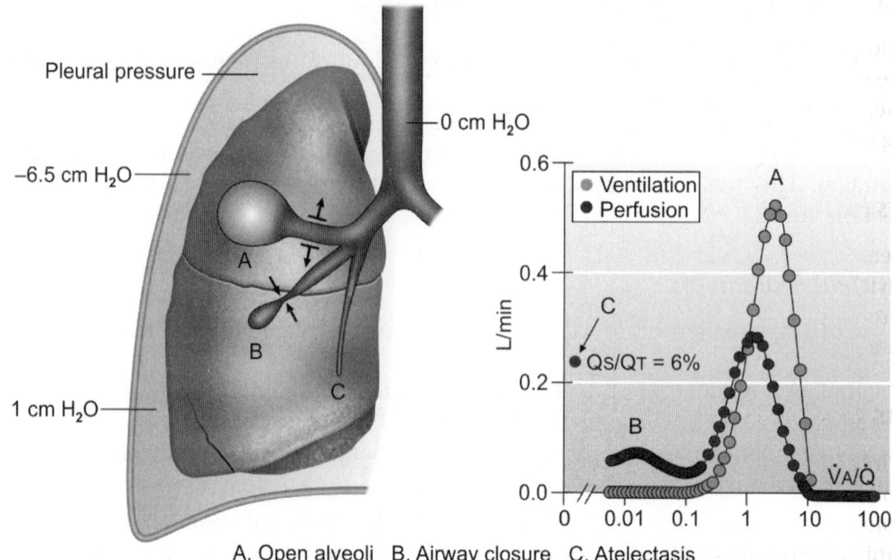

Fig. 2 Distribution of ventilation during anesthesia

Ventilation-perfusion mismatching during Anesthesia

- Both CO_2 elimination and oxygenation of blood are impaired in most patients during anesthesia
- The impeded CO_2 elimination can be attributed to increased dead space ventilation
- Anatomic dead space is unchanged, indicating that the "alveolar" dead space must have increased during anesthesia
- Increased dead space during anesthesia is not really dead space but poorly perfused lung regions that are signified by so-called high V/Q ratio
- Such high V/Q ratio can be explained by the tiny perfusion of corner vessels in interalveolar septa in the upper lung regions (where alveolar pressure may exceed pulmonary vascular pressure [zone I])
- The impaired CO_2 elimination is most easily corrected by increasing the ventilation and is seldom a problem in routine anesthesia with mechanical ventilation
- The impairment in arterial oxygenation during anesthesia is more severe at higher ages, obesity worsens the oxygenation of blood, and smokers show more impairment in gas exchange than nonsmokers do
- Venous admixture, as calculated according to the standard oxygen "shunt" equation, is also increased during anesthesia to approximately 10% of cardiac output.

Hypoxic Pulmonary Vasoconstriction

- Several inhaled anesthetics have been found to inhibit HPV
- No such effect has been seen with intravenous anesthetics
- Nitrous oxide does not have any significant effect upon HPV.

Factors Increasing Pulmonary Vascular Resistance

- Reduction in alveolar PO_2 (HPV)
- A rise in CO_2, acidosis
- Epinephrine, dopamine, histamine, 5-HT
- Lung collapse.

Factors Reducing Pulmonary Vascular Resistance

- Increased cardiac output by recruiting capillaries
- Acetylcholine and cholinergics
- Isoprenaline
- Prostacyclin.

Effects of Anesthetics on Respiratory Drive

- The inhalation anesthetics, opioids and sedative-hypnotics are all respiratory depressant
- Opioids and inhalation agents depress the ventilatory response to hypercarbia
- Opioids decreases respiratory rate and increases tidal volume, but minute ventilation is reduced
- Volatile agents and barbiturates increases respiratory rate but decreases tidal volume
- Anesthesia also reduces the response to hypoxia, but less than hypercarbia
- Attenuation of the hypoxic response may be attributed to an effect on the carotid body chemoreceptor
- The reduced ventilatory response to CO_2 during anesthesia is due to impeded function of the intercostal muscles.

Regional Anesthesia and Lung Function

- The ventilatory effects of regional anesthesia depend on the type and extension of motor blockade
- With extensive blocks that include all of the thoracic and lumbar segments, inspiratory capacity is reduced by 20% and expiratory reserve volume approaches zero
- Diaphragmatic function, however, is often spared, even in cases of inadvertent extension of subarachnoid or epidural sensory block up to the cervical segments
- Arterial oxygenation and carbon dioxide elimination are well maintained during spinal and epidural anesthesia
- Closing capacity (CC) and FRC relationship remain unaltered
- Ventilation-perfusion ratio remains unaltered during epidural anesthesia in all lung regions.

Pneumoperitoneum and Lung Function

- CO_2 pneumoperitoneum may cause hypercapnia and acidosis
- The direct effects of carbon dioxide and acidosis lead to decreased cardiac contractility, sensitization of the myocardium to the arrhythmogenic effects of catecholamine, and systemic vasodilatation
- Pneumoperitoneum causes decreased FRC and VC, formation of atelectasis, reduced respiratory compliance, and increased peak airway pressure
- Shunt is reduced and arterial oxygenation is mostly improved during CO_2 pneumoperitoneum
- CO_2 may enhance HPV, which helps in efficient redistribution of lung blood flow.

CARDIOVASCULAR PHYSIOLOGY WITH ANESTHETIC IMPLICATIONS

Blood Pressure

Blood pressure = Cardiac output × peripheral vascular (arteriolar) Resistance (PVR). Cardiac output = Stroke volume × Heart rate.

So, blood pressure = Stroke volume × heart rate × peripheral arteriolar resistance.

Factors Determining Blood Pressure

- Factors determining stroke volume (stroke volume determines mainly the systolic blood pressure).
- Factors determining heart rate.
- Factors determining peripheral vascular (arteriolar), resistance (PVR determines mainly the diastolic blood pressure).

- *Factors determining stroke volume:*
  - *VEDV (ventricular end-diastolic volume).* Which is dependent on (a) Venous return, which in turn depends on position of body, skeletal muscle pump, and respiratory pump (preload), (b) Blood volume.
  - *Strength of myocardial contraction (inotropicity).*
  - *Ventricular afterload.*
- *Factors determining heart rate*—depends on autonomic nerve stimulation, circulating chemicals, activity and exercise, emotional stress, gender, age, body temperature, and baroreceptor reflex.
- *Factors determining peripheral arteriolar resistance*—constriction and dilatation of the arterioles are the main determinants.

Control of Blood Pressure

The cardiovascular center (CVC) is a collection of interconnected neurones in the medulla and pons.

CVC receives, integrates and coordinates inputs from:

- Baroreceptors (the primary mechanism)
- Chemoreceptors
- Higher centers in the brain.

CVC—via the autonomic nervous system (ANS) to the heart and blood vessels enables rapid response to changes in blood pressure.

Factors Modifying Systolic Blood Pressure

Systolic blood pressure is an interaction between stroke volume and distensibility (compliance) of the arterial system which decreases on ageing resulting in isolated/disproportionate systolic hypertension in the elderly.

The role of baroreceptors and chemoreceptors in the control of arterial blood pressure are shown in Flow charts 1 and 2.

Flow chart 1 The role of baroreceptors in the control of arterial blood pressure

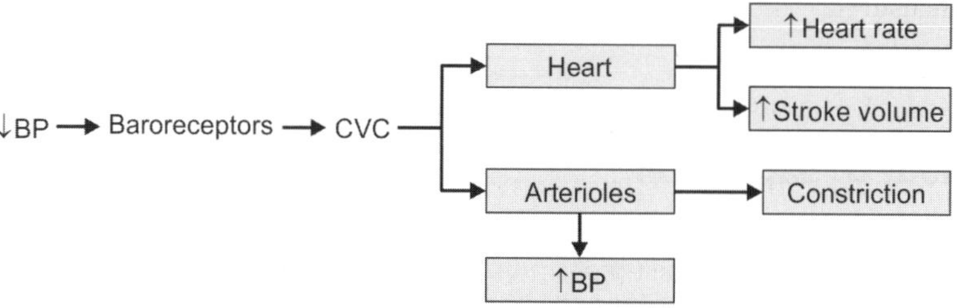

Flow chart 2 The role of chemoreceptors in the control of arterial blood pressure

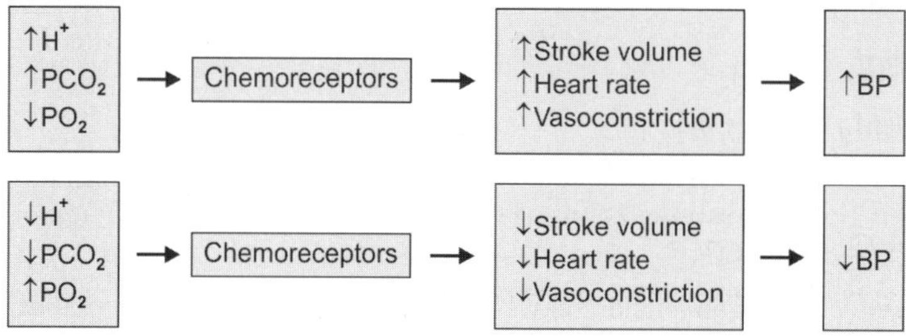

Factors Modifying Diastolic Blood Pressure

Diastolic blood pressure is principally determined by cardiac afterload. SVR is a major contributor to diastolic BP. Diastolic BP itself is a determinant of coronary arterial filling and both duration of diastole and diastolic blood pressure have a bearing on the adequacy of coronary perfusion.

Measurement of Blood Volume

^{51}Cr-radiolabeled red cells are injected into the circulation, and blood volume may be calculated from:

$$\text{Blood volume (mL)} = \frac{\text{Quantity of test substance}^{**}\text{ injected}}{\text{Concentration of test substance}^{**}\text{ observed}}$$

(**Test substance is labeled red cells)

When radiolabeled albumin or Evans blue is injected initially, it will reside in plasma, its volume may be calculated from:

$$\text{Plasma volume (mL)} = \frac{\text{Quantity of test substance}^{**}\text{ injected}}{\text{Concentration of test substance}^{**}\text{ observed in plasma}}$$

(**Test substance is radiolabeled albumin or Evans blue)

$$\text{Blood volume (mL)} = \text{Plasma volume} \times \frac{100}{100 - \text{hematocrit}}$$

Fick Principle

The Fick principle states that the amount of a substance taken up by an organ (or by the whole body) per unit of time is equal to the arterial level of the substance minus the venous level multiplied by the blood flow (Q). It can be employed to calculate blood flow, or to calculate VO_2 (O_2 consumption).

To derive the difference in O_2 content, simultaneous arterial (CaO_2) and mixed venous (CvO_2) samples are measured.

$$Q = \frac{VO_2}{(CaO_2 - CvO_2)}$$

Mixed Venous O_2 Saturation

Mixed venous O_2 saturation (SvO_2) is the percentage of oxygenated mixed venous blood which may be measured photometrically at the tip of a pulmonary artery (PA) catheter.

It is increased in sepsis with peripheral shunting, cyanide toxicity, hypothermia, sampling on wedging of a PA catheter (erroneously collecting pulmonary venous blood).

It is decreased in anemia, low cardiac output, arterial O_2 desaturation, increased O_2 consumption.

O_2 Flux/Content

- Oxygen flux (mL) = CO × CaO_2
- O_2 content (mL/dL blood) = (1.31 × Hb × saturation/100) + 0.02 PO_2

Arteriovenous O_2 Difference

This is the difference in oxygen tension between the arterial and venous circulations, reflecting the oxygen consumption of an organ or of the whole body.

Oxygen Consumption

- O_2 content = 1.31 × (Hb × Sat/100) + 0.02 PO_2
- For CvO_2, pulmonary arterial sample from a PA catheter tip without wedging is required
- For CaO_2 arterial sample is required
- Q (CO) is obtained from calorimetric measurement (PAC)
- VO_2 (O_2 consumption) is calculated from Fick's equation.

$$Q = \frac{VO_2}{(CaO_2 - CvO_2)}$$

Diminished VO_2 is the earliest pathophysiological event in shock, and usually precedes the hypotension.

Ejection Fraction (EF) of Left Ventricle

$$EF = \frac{\text{Stroke volume}}{\text{Left ventricular end-diastolic volume}}$$

Measured by Doppler at echocardiography: Normal > 0.55 or 55%

Starling's law of heart: Stroke volume is proportional to left ventricular end-diastolic volume/ pressure/length of the myofibril (Fig. 3).

Implications: The failing heart will generate less stroke volume for the same end-diastolic volume in comparison with a nonfailing heart. If compliance of the heart is assumed to be constant then stroke volume is proportional to the end-diastolic pressure.

If mitral valve functions normally then: LVEDP = LAP = PCWP . SV ∞ PCWP.

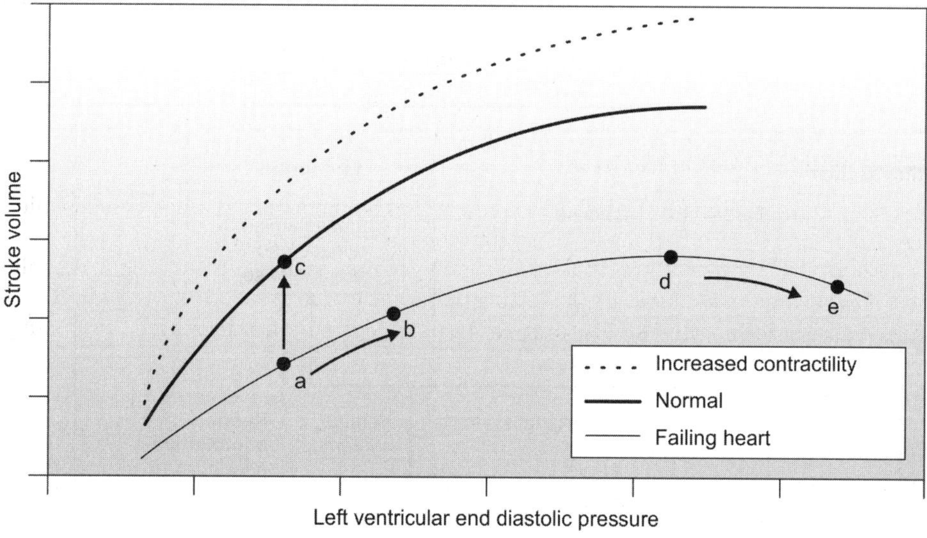

Fig. 3 Starting's law of heart

Starling Forces in Capillaries

P_c = Capillary hydrostatic pressure (varies from artery to vein)

P_{if} = Interstitial hydrostatic pressure (usually 0/constant)

Π_p = Oncotic pressure due to plasma proteins (28 mm Hg/constant)

Π_{if} = Oncotic pressure due to interstitial proteins (3 mm Hg/constant)

Net filtration = $(Pc - P_{if}) - (\Pi_p - \Pi_{if})$

Starling Forces and Blood Loss

If patient loses blood acutely, then the capillary hydrostatic pressure falls especially at the venous end. Balance is no longer maintained, the net pressure into the capillaries increases and fluid is retrieved into the circulation from the interstitium until P_c is restored. Flow chart 3 shows physiology response to hemorrhage.

1. What are the factors that regulate peripheral resistance?

Ans. A fast acting mechanism, controlled by three mechanisms:

(1) Intrinsic, (2) Extrinsic, (3) Paracrine.

Extrinsic mechanism is controlled through several reflex mechanisms, most important is baroreceptors reflex, *chemoreceptors reflex and other vasomotor reflexes.*

Baroreceptors are receptors found in carotid sinus and aortic arch and are stimulated by changes in BP. *Chemoreceptors reflex*: Chemoreceptors are receptors found in carotid and aortic bodies are stimulated by chemical changes in blood mainly hypoxia ($\downarrow O_2$), hypercapnia ($\uparrow CO_2$), and pH changes. *Other vasomotor reflexes* include *atrial stretch receptor reflex where, with increase in* venous return lead to stimulation of atrial stretch receptors cause reflex vasodilatation and lowering of BP.

Thermoreceptors: Present in skin/or hypothalamus when exposure to heat cause vasodilatation, when expose to cold cause vasoconstriction.

Flow chart 3 Physiological response to hemorrhage

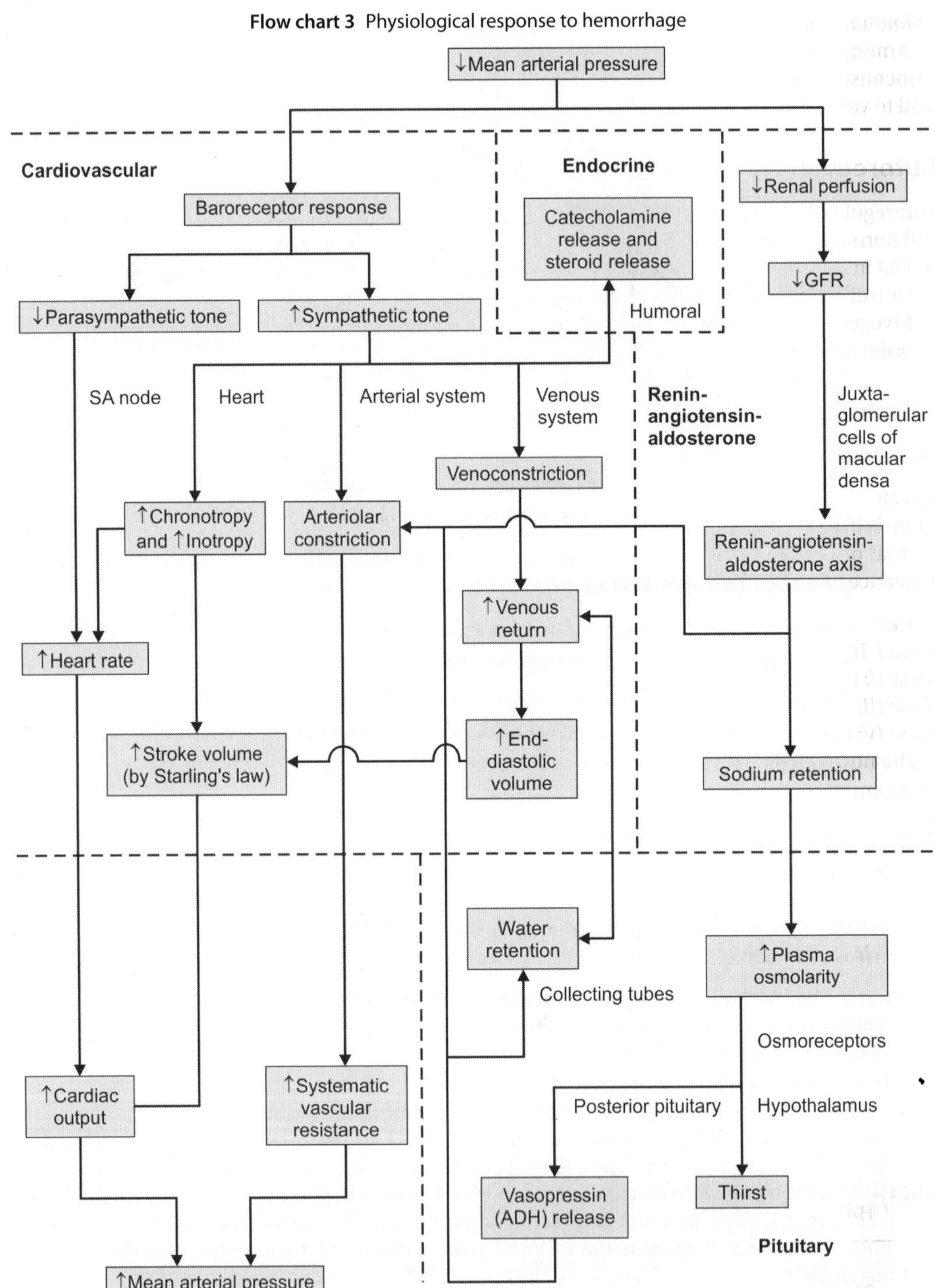

Pulmonary receptor: Vasoconstriction *with* lung inflation

Among hormonal agents, noradrenaline cause vasoconstriction, adrenaline cause vasoconstriction (except in skeletal muscle). Angiotensin II cause vasoconstriction, vasopressin lead to vasoconstriction.

Autoregulation of Blood Flow

Autoregulation is the ability of an organ to control its own blood supply independently of neural and hormonal influences. There are two main mechanisms whereby it is mediated:

- Fall in arterial pressure resulting in a reduction in blood flow, accumulation of metabolites thus causdilates terminal arterioles restoring blood flow.
- Myogenic response involving local neural reflexes in response to stretch at the level of the 1st order arteriole.

Valsalva Maneuver

The valsalva maneuver (Fig. 4) is forced expiration against closed glottis.

Effects:

There is increase in intrathoracic pressure and decrease in venous return.

Normal person maintains mean arterial pressure by increasing heart rate and systemic vascular resistance, and demonstrates on release transient hypertension and bradycardia.

Phases:

Phase I: Increase in intrathoracic pressure and MAP.

Phase II: Decreased venous return and MAP.

Phase III: Overshoot as vasoconstriction and increase in heart rate persists.

Phase IV: Return to normal.

The normal valsalva response is absent or abnormal in autonomic dysfunction, in particular in autonomic neuropathy in DM and after sympathectomy.

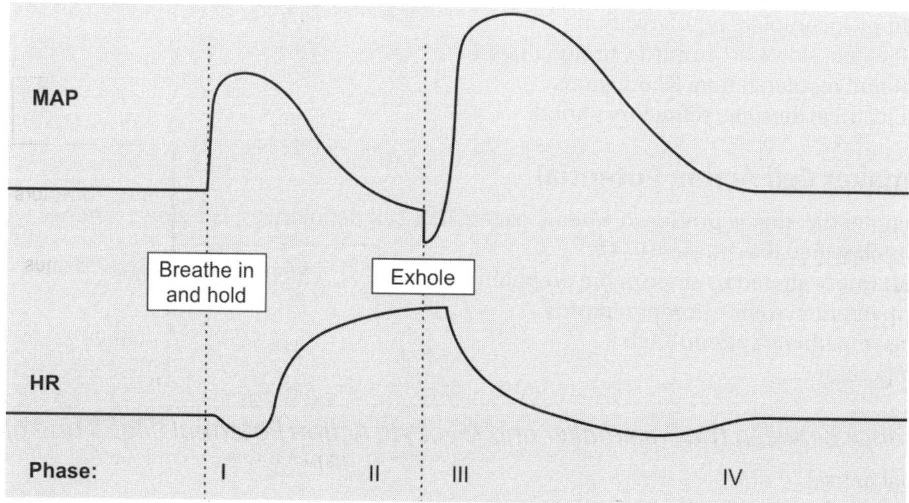

Fig. 4 Valsalva maneuver

Cardiac Action Potential

Specialized cardiac myocytes in the SA node generate cardiac action potential (AP) which is transmitted through the heart via the conducting system causing normal myocytes to contract. The cells of the conducting system are modified myocytes classified as nodal, transitional and Purkinje myocytes and all are capable of spontaneous and rhythmic generation of APs. Any focus generating cardiac action potential at a higher frequency acts as the pacemaker. Normally, in sinus rhythm this is the SA node.

There is an electrical charge difference across the myocardial cell membrane in the resting/polarized state known as resting membrane potential (RMP). Potassium (K^+), sodium (Na^+), calcium (Ca^{2+}) ions are principally responsible for this. Concentration of (K^+) inside the cell is 151 mEq/L and 4 mEq/L outside. For Na^+ these are 144 mEq/L outside and 7 mEq/L inside, and for Ca^{2+} these are 5 mEq/L outside and less than 1 mEq/L inside. In the resting or polarized state the inside of the cell is negatively charged and outside is positive. The Na^+/K^+ pump establishes an increased Na^+ concentration outside and an increased K^+ concentration inside the cell. Both ions diffuse along their concentration gradient, K^+ coming outside while Na^+ diffusing inside the cell. For every 50–75 K^+ ions diffusing out, only one Na^+ diffuses inside, causing a deficiency of positive cations inside the cell creating a RMP of magnitude around -90 mV. As at rest the membrane is more permeable to K^+ than Na^+ the potential difference (Nernst equation) applies more to K^+ (-90 mv) than to Na^+ (+ 60 mv). It is the continuation of depolarization which distinguishes cardiac action potential (AP) from skeletal AP. This is due to the action of slow Ca^{2+} channels, allowing Ca^{2+} entry into the cell, maintaining a balance against K^+ diffusing outwards, causing a prolonged depolarization.

- Ca^{2+} is functionally related to β-receptors
- K^+ is functionally related to M2 receptors and β-receptors
- Changes in external K^+ affect the resting membrane potential level
- Changes in internal Na^+ affect the magnitude of the action potential.

Phases for Depolarization

Depolarization is the trigger for myocardial contraction.

- 0 = Fast depolarization, Na^+ inwards
- 1 = Early incomplete repolarization
- 2 = Plateau, slow Ca^{++} inwards, prolonging AP
- 3 = Rapid repolarization, K^+ outwards
- 4 = Electrical diastole, refractory period.

Pacemaker Cell Action Potential

Action potential, that is produced when a pacemaker cell depolarizes, is a slow response type AP, which is classified into phases (0–4):

Heart rate is altered by slope of the prepotential (phase 4), which is affected by:

- Sympathetic system—norepinephrine
- Parasympathetic system—Ach
- Temperature.

Difference Between the Pacemaker and Myocyte Action Potential (Figs 5 and 6)

Pacemaker has:

- Less negative phase 4 membrane potential
- Less negative threshold potential

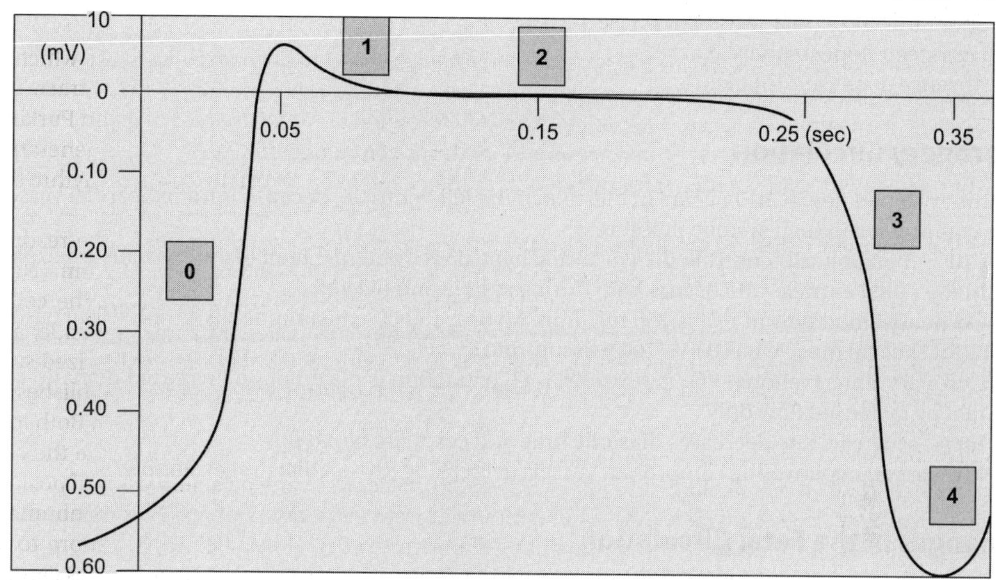

Fig. 5 Myocardial AP

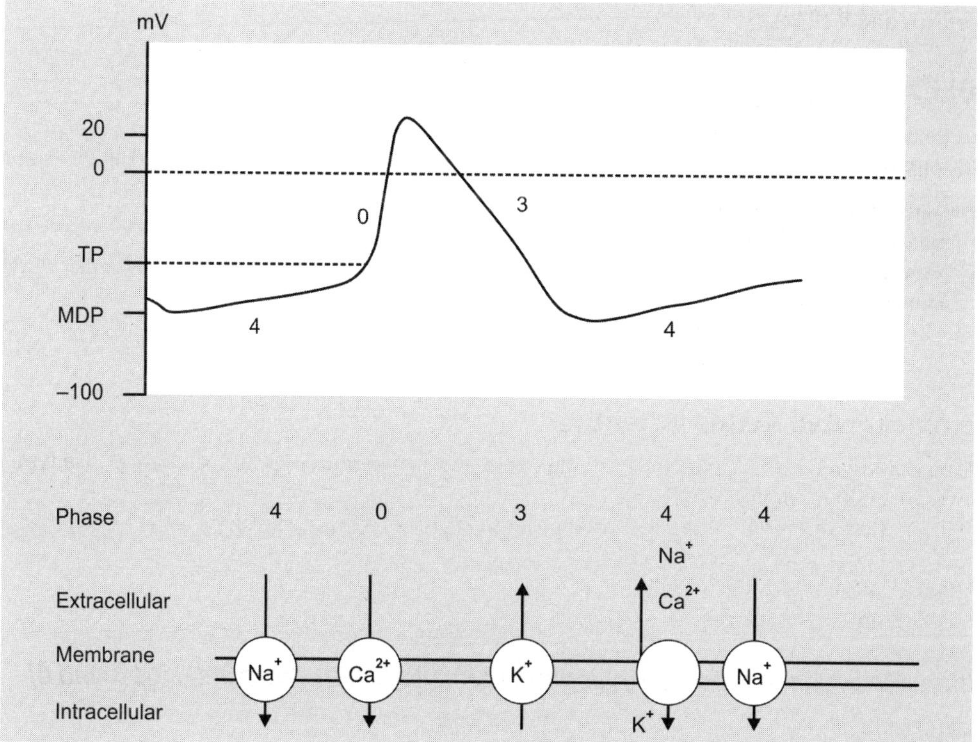

Fig. 6 Pacemaker AP

- Spontaneous depolarization in phase 4
- Less steep slope in phase 0
- Absence of phase 2 (plateau).

Coronary Circulation

Coronary blood flow (CBF) occurs in diastole in the left ventricle, because intramyocardial vessels are compressed in high systolic pressure.

CBF is metabolically controlled, myocardial hypoxia is a potent dilator of the coronary arterioles.

In the right ventricle CBF occurs both during systole and diastole.

Coronary blood flow at rest is 250 mL/min. Myocardial O_2 consumption is 11 mL/100 g tissue/min (for skeletal muscle it is 8 mL/100 g tissue/min).

Coronary sinus (venous) PO_2 is very low as O_2 extraction is maximal, so increased demand can be met by increased flow only.

Increased heart rate decreases diastolic time and coronary blood flow.

Myocardial hypertrophy compresses vessels decreasing myocardial oxygen supply.

Changes in the Fetal Circulation

The key is the change in pressure induced by the sudden fall in pulmonary vascular resistance (PVR). Prior to birth the pulmonary vascular resistance is high, as the lung inflates and PVR falls, there is sudden reduction in right sided pressure, and pressure in left side exceeds that on the right. For this pressure change the foramen ovale closes, oxygenated blood flows retrograde in the ductus arteriosus and it closes.

BIBLIOGRAPHY

1. Braunwald's Heart Disease, 8th edn, Volume 1, 2008.
2. Harrison's Principles of Internal Medicine. 18th edn, Longo DL, Boston MA Mc Graw-Hill Professional, 2011.
3. Joel A Kaplan, Peter D Slinger. Thoracic Anesthesia, 3rd edn.
4. Miller's Anesthesia, 7th edn.
5. Narasimhan Ranganathan, Franklin B Saksena, Vahe Sivaciyan. The Art and Science of Cardiac Physical Examination, 2008.

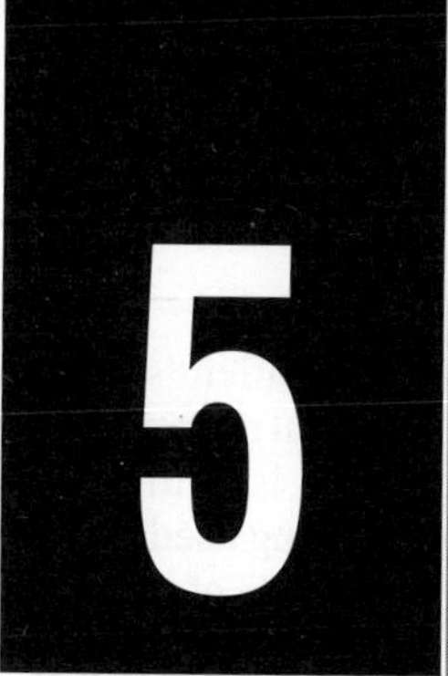

Role of Anesthesiologist in Pain Management in the Preoperative Period

Sushma Bhatnagar, Arif Ahmed

A directed pain history, a directed physical examination, and a pain control plan be included in the anesthetic preoperative evaluation.

Patient preparation for perioperative pain management should include appropriate adjustments or continuation of medications to avert an abstinence syndrome, treatment of pre-existent pain, or preoperative initiation of therapy for postoperative pain management.

Anesthesiologists should provide patient and family education regarding their important roles in achieving comfort, reporting pain, and in proper use of the recommended analgesic methods, removing the misconceptions that overestimate the risk of adverse effects and addiction. Patient education for optimal use of patient-controlled analgesia (PCA) and other sophisticated methods, such as patient-controlled epidural analgesia, might include discussion of these analgesic methods at the time of the preanesthetic evaluation, brochures and video-tapes to educate patients about therapeutic options, and discussion at the bedside during postoperative visits. Such education may also include instruction in behavioral modalities for control of pain and anxiety.

1. Describe multimodal approach to perioperative pain management.

Ans. A multimodal approach to analgesia includes a combination of interventional analgesic techniques (epidural catheter or peripheral nerve catheter analgesia) and a combination of systemic pharmacologic therapies [nonsteroidal anti-inflammatory agents (NSAIDs), α-adrenergic agonists, NMDA receptor antagonists, membrane stabilizers, and opioid administration].

The essential elements of multimodal analgesia are the following:

- Neuronal blockade by local anesthetics that may be administered via epidural anesthesia, spinal anesthesia, peripheral nerve blockade, skin infiltration before surgical incision, or wound infiltration before surgical closure.
- Infusion of opioids via the IV, intrathecal, or epidural route before surgical incision and throughout the perioperative period.
- Administration of NSAIDs before surgical incision, throughout the intraoperative period, and postoperatively.
- Administration of other adjuvant medication.

The principles of a multimodal strategy include a sufficient diminution of the patient's pain to instill a sense of control over their pain, enable early mobilization, allow early enteral nutrition, and attenuate the perioperative stress response. The secondary goal of this approach is to maximize the benefit (analgesia) while minimizing the risk (side effects of the medication being used). These goals are often achieved through regional anesthetic techniques and a combination of analgesic drugs. The utilization of epidural anesthesia and analgesia is an integral part of the multimodal strategy because of the superior analgesia and physiologic benefits conferred by epidural analgesia.

Patients undergoing major abdominal or thoracic procedures and managed with a multimodal strategy have a reduction in hormonal and metabolic stress, preservation of total-body protein, shorter times to tracheal extubation, lower pain scores, earlier return of bowel function, and earlier achievement of criteria for discharge from the intensive care unit.

By integrating the most recent data and techniques for surgery, anesthesiology, and pain treatment, the multimodal approach is an extension of clinical pathways or fast track protocols by revamping traditional care programs into effective postoperative rehabilitation pathways. This approach may potentially decrease perioperative morbidity, decrease the length of hospital stay, and improve patient satisfaction without compromising safety. However, the widespread implementation of these programs requires multidisciplinary collaboration, changes in the traditional principles of postoperative care, additional resources, and expansion of the traditional acute pain service, all of which may be difficult in the current medical-economic climate.

ASA recommendation is for the use multimodal pain management therapy. Central regional blockade with local anesthetics should be considered. Unless contraindicated, patients should receive an around-the-clock regimen of Coxibs, NSAIDs, or acetaminophen. Dosing regimens should be administered to optimize efficacy while minimizing the risk of adverse events. The choice of medication, dose, route, and duration of therapy should be individualized.

2. Define pre-emptive and preventive analgesia. Describe the measures useful for pre-emptive and preventive analgesia.

Ans. Pre-emptive analgesia is the administration of an analgesic agent before the surgical incision to decreases or modulates the perioperative pain and also helps in minimizing central sensitization.

Some analgesic interventions have an effect on postoperative pain and/or analgesic consumption that exceeds the expected duration of action of the drug, defined as preventive analgesia.

Protective analgesia describes a technique that reduces measures of sensitization such as hyperalgesia.

Pre-emptive epidural analgesia results in lowering of pain intensity scores, supplemental analgesic consumption, time to first analgesic. While wound infiltration of local anesthetics and NSAIDs administration has also provided some benefit. Where systemic NMDA antagonist administration is of equivocal effects, and no clear evidence of pre-emptive opioids.

For preventive effects, NMDA antagonist, gabapentin, epidural has shown some benefit. Perioperative epidural analgesia combined with IV ketamine decreases the pain up to 1 year following colonic resection.

3. Outline some practical important measures to reduce pain.

Ans. In surgery, subsequent postoperative pain can be decreased with gentle intubation, careful positioning and transfer of the patient, adequate muscle relaxation, and minimization of surgical trauma.

4. What are the physiological and psychological effects of acute pain?

Ans. Acute pain activates the complex neurohumoral and immune response to injury, and both peripheral and central injury responses have a major influence on acute pain mechanisms. Thus acute pain and injury of various types are inevitably inter-related and if severe and prolonged, the injury response becomes counterproductive and can have adverse effects on outcome.

ADVERSE PHYSIOLOGICAL EFFECTS

Metabolic and endocrine responses to injury are shown in Table 1.

Table 1 | Metabolic and endocrine responses to injury

Endocrine	↑ Catabolic hormones	↑ ACTH, cortisol, ADH, growth hormone, catecholamines, angiotensin II, aldosterone, glucagons, IL-1, TNF, IL-6
	↓ Anabolic hormones	↓ Insulin, testosterone
Metabolic		
Carbohydrate	Hyperglycemia, glucose intolerance, insulin resistance	↑ Glycogenolysis, gluconeogenesis (cortisol, glucagon, growth hormone, adrenaline, free fatty acids) ↓ Insulin secretion/activation
Protein	Muscle protein catabolism, ↑ synthesis of acute phase proteins	↑ Cortisol, adrenaline, glucagons, IL-1, IL-6, TNF
Lipid	↑ Lipolysis and oxidation	↑ Catecholamines, cortisol, glucagon, growth hormone
Water and electrolyte	Retention of water and sodium, ↑ excretion of potassium and ↓ functional ECF with shifts to ICF	↑ Catecholamine, aldosterone, ADH, cortisol, angiotensin II, prostaglandins and other factors

Hyperglycemia

Hyperglycemia is proportional to injury response.

Circulating glucose enters cells that do not require insulin for uptake, resulting in cellular glucose overload and diverse toxic effects. Excess intracellular glucose nonenzymatically glycosylates proteins such as immunoglobulins, rendering them dysfunctional. Alternatively, excess glucose enters glycolysis and oxidative phosphorylation pathways, leading to excess superoxide molecules that bind to nitric oxide (NO), with formation of peroxynitrate, ultimately resulting in mitochondrial dysfunction and death of cells.

Even modest increases in blood glucose can be associated with poor outcome. Tight glycemic control is associated with improved outcomes with coronary artery bypass surgery (CABG), whereas in intensive care the tight glycemic control is still debatable.

Lipotoxicity

High levels of free fatty acids can depress myocardial contractility, increase myocardial oxygen consumption, and impair calcium homeostasis and increase free radical production leading to electrical instability and ventricular arrhythmias.

Protein Catabolism

After injury there is increase in protein catabolism to amino acids and amino acid oxidation, with decreased protein synthesis, this leads to loss of lean tissue. This leads to increased in length of time for normal return of physical function and increased hospital stay.

Protein loss may lead to delayed wound healing, reduced immune function (Chandra, 1983) and diminished muscle strength.

Pain and Analgesia: Effects on Organ Dysfunction

Pain activates the sympathetic nervous system leads to the following:
- Increased heart rate, blood pressure, inotropy
- Increased myocardial oxygen demand, reduced myocardial oxygen demand leading to ischemia, and arrhythmias
- Reduced gastrointestinal motility and ileus.

Pain from upper abdominal and thoracic surgeries leads to decreased cough, reduction of functional capacity, leading to atelectasis, hypoxemia, and pulmonary complications.

The injury response also contributes to suppression of cellular and humoral immune response, and leads to a hypercoagulable state.

Adverse Psychological Effects

Pain leads increasing anxiety, inability to sleep, demoralization, a feeling of helplessness, loss of control, inability to think and interact with others.

5. Describe the tools of pain assessment. Describe each tool in details.

Ans. Pain is a subjective experience modulated by physiological, psychological and environmental factors such as previous events, culture, prognosis, coping strategies, fear and anxiety. Therefore, most measures of pain are based on self-report. These results are influenced by mood, sleep disturbance and medications.

There are some instances when it may not be possible to obtain reliable self-reports of pain (e.g. patients with impaired consciousness or cognitive impairment, young children, elderly patients, or where there are failures of communication due to language difficulties, inability to understand the measures, unwillingness to cooperate or severe anxiety). For them other methods of pain assessment are used.

There are no objective measures of 'pain'. But associated factors such as hyperalgesia, the stress response (e.g. plasma cortisol concentrations), behavioral responses (e.g. facial expression), functional impairment (e.g. coughing, ambulation) or physiological responses (e.g. changes in heart rate) may provide additional information.

Analgesic requirements (e.g. patient-controlled opioid doses delivered) are commonly used as posthoc measures of pain experienced.

Pain intensity should be recorded as a fifth vital sign. Regular and repeated measurement leads to assessment of analgesic efficacy. Both static and dynamic assessment of pain should be made.

Pain can be measured by both unidimensional or multidimensional tools, but unidimensional ones are more useful in the perioperative setting.

UNIDIMENSIONAL TOOLS

Visual Analog Scale

The visual analog scale (VAS) is a straight 100-mm line, without demarcation, that has the words 'no pain' at the left-most end and 'worst pain imaginable' (or something similar) at the right-most end. Patients are instructed to place a mark on the line that indicates the amount of pain that they feel at the time of the evaluation. The distance of this mark from the left end is then measured, and this number is used as a numeric representation of the severity of the patient's pain.

VAS can also be used to measure other aspects of the pain experience (e.g. affective components, patient satisfaction, side effects).

Advantage: Validated, easy to use.

Disadvantage: It attempts to assign a single value to the multidimensional experience of pain, there is no concept of worst imaginable pain as pain experience later may be more worse than present ones but the patient cannot at a later date change his previous score.
Pain assessment after surgery may be difficult due to transient anesthetic-related cognitive impairment and decreases in visual acuity.

Numeric Rating Scale

The numeric rating scale is consists of numbers written from 0–10 from left to right, 0 for 'no pain' and 10 for 'worst pain imaginable'. Patients are instructed to circle the number that represents the amount of pain that they are experiencing at the time of the evaluation. A variation of this scale is the verbal numeric scale (VNS), in which patients are asked to verbally state a number between 0 and 10 that corresponds to their present pain intensity.

Pain relief may be measured in the reverse direction with 0 representing 'no relief' to 10 representing 'complete relief'.

VAS ratings of greater than 70 mm are indicative of 'severe pain' and 0–5 mm 'no pain', 5–44 mm 'mild pain' and 45–74 'moderate pain'. A reduction in pain intensity by 30–35% has been rated as clinically meaningful by patients with postoperative pain, acute pain in the emergency department.

Advantage: Quick, easy to use, validated pain measure.

Disadvantage: It assigns single number to pain, has also a ceiling effect, i.e. if a value of '10' is chosen and the pain worsens, the patient officially has no way to express this change, also, with the VNS, patients often rate their pain as some number higher than 10 (e.g. '15 out of 10') in an attempt to express their extreme level of pain intensity.

Verbal Descriptor Scale

A verbal descriptor scale (VDS) is a list of words, ordered in terms of severity from least to most, that describe the amount of pain that a patient may be experiencing. Patients are asked to either circle or state the word that best describes their pain intensity at that moment in time. These terms can then be converted to numeric scores for charting and easy comparison over time.

Advantage: It is validated, simple and quick. May be useful in the elderly or visually impaired patient and in some children.

Disadvantage: It assigns only one objective to the pain experience, limited choice of 4 to 6 values, forces patient to choose from 4–6 values.

Pain relief may also be graded as none, mild, moderate or complete using a VDS.

Multidimensional Measures of Pain

Multidimensional tools provide information about the characteristics of the pain and its impact on the individual. Among them, most commonly used scales are Brief Pain Inventory, which assesses pain intensity and associated disability and the McGill Pain Questionnaire, which assesses the sensory, affective and evaluative dimensions of pain.

Also for measurement of neuropathic pain, there is DN4, pain detect tools.

FUNCTIONAL MEASUREMENT OF ACUTE PAIN

Most of the unidimensional pain measures only evaluates the pain intensity at rest. The measure of the ability to undertake functional activity measures the functional aspect of pain. This helps to titrate analgesia for optimized recovery.

Measurement of pain intensity scores on movement or with coughing is a useful guide.

The Functional Activity Scale score (FAS score) is a simple three-level ranked categorical score. Its fundamental purpose is to assess whether the patient can undertake appropriate activity at their current level of pain control and to act as a trigger for intervention should this not be the case. The patient is asked to perform the activity, or is taken through the activity in the case of structured physiotherapy (joint mobilization) or nurse-assisted care (e.g. ambulation, turned in bed).

The ability to complete the activity is then assessed using the FAS as:
A—no limitation the patient is able to undertake the activity without limitation due to pain (pain intensity score is typically 0 – 3);
B—mild limitation the patient is able to undertake the activity but experiences moderate to severe pain (pain intensity score is typically 4 – 10); and
C—significant limitation the patient is unable to complete the activity due to pain, or pain treatment-related side effects, independent of pain intensity scores.

This score is then used to track effectiveness of analgesia on function and trigger interventions if required.

Disadvantages of the FAS score are that it has not been independently validated and clinical staff need to be educated in its application.

Outcome Measures of Pain

Pain:

The degree of analgesic effect:

- Difference between the baseline and postintervention score of pain intensity or pain relief (Summed pain intensity difference [SPID]).
- The area under the time-analgesic effect curve for a given time (total pain relief [TOTPAR]).
- Dose of rescue analgesic consumption required in a given time period (e.g. PCA use).

The time to analgesic effect:

- The time to onset of analgesic effect.
- Mean time to maximum reduction in pain intensity or to peak relief.

The duration of effect:

- Time for pain to return to at least 50% of baseline.
- Time for pain intensity to return to baseline or for pain relief to fall to zero.
- Time to remedication/rescue analgesia.

Emotional Functioning

The unpleasantness of the experience and its meaning for the individual may have short-term (anxiety, depression, irritability) and long-term consequences (lost confidence or self-efficacy or post-traumatic stress disorder) for the individual's emotional functioning.

Adverse symptoms and events: If adverse events are sufficiently common (e.g. nausea with opioids) they may be quantifiable in trials of efficacy and specifically measured using dichotomous (present or absent), categorical (none, mild, moderate, severe) or interval (analog or Likert) scales. Analogous to NNTs, the number-needed-to-harm (NNH) may be used to describe the incidence of adverse effects.

PAIN ASSESSMENT IN PEDIATRIC POPULATION

Children's self-report of their pain, where possible, is the preferred approach.

For children who are unable to self-report, an appropriate behavioral or composite tool should be used. If pain is suspected or anticipated, use a validated pain assessment tool is recommended. Assessment, recording, and re-evaluation of pain at regular intervals to be done; the frequency of assessment should be determined according to the individual needs of the child and setting.

The tools useful for assessment of pain in neonates are Comfort scale, Cries scale, Neonatal facial coding system, neonatal infant pain scale, objective pain scale, premature infant pain profile (PIPP), all of them except Comfort scale can be used for premature neonates also.

For children between 3 and 12 years, the tools that can be used are Chedoke-McMaster Pediatric Pain Management Sheet, Children's Hospital of Eastern Ontario Pain Scale (CHEOPS), Faces Pain Scale, Oucher, etc.

For children with cognitive impairment the tools that cab used are Face, Legs, Activity, Cry, Consolability (FLACC) tool (including a revised version of the FLACC tool), Pediatric Pain Profile (PPP), Noncommunicating Children's Pain Checklist, etc.

Pain Assessment in Intubated Postoperative Patients

6. What are the different tools of pain assessment in elderly patients with dementia? Describe one of them.

Ans. Many patients with moderate to severe dementia can report pain reliably at the moment or when prompted, however, pain recall and integration of pain experience over a period of time may be less reliable. Also, the number of pain complaints decreases as dementia progresses.

In older adults with dementia, pain expression sometimes takes on less obvious forms, such as confusion, social withdrawal, aggression, or subtle changes in behavior. So for measurement of pain in these group of patients, various observational scales have been described. These scales are based on the six of the following behavioral patterns:

1. Facial expressions
2. Verbalizations, vocalizations
3. Body movements
4. Changes in interpersonal interactions
5. Changes in activity patterns or routines
6. Mental status changes.

The Abbey tool, the ADD protocol, CNPI, DS-DAT, Doloplus 2, PAINAD, FLACC scale, etc.

The PAINAD Scale75 was developed to provide a clinically relevant and easy to use pain assessment tool for individuals with advanced dementia. It includes five items: breathing, negative vocalization, facial expression, body language, and consolability. Each item is leveled on a 3-point scale from 0 to 2 for intensity.

Pain assessment to be done by using behavioral pain scale (BPS) and the critical-care pain observation tool (CPOT) in postoperative patients who are unable to report pain. In them, using only the vital signs alone is not acceptable.

7. Describe the routes of administration of analgesics.

Ans. *Routes of administration and their uses:*

Oral route: Oral route may not be useful for immediate postoperative patients as most of the patients are not orally allowed. However, they can be used once the pain intensity is decreased. They are also used to decrease opioid requirement and postoperative pain.

The use of an opioid or nonopioid analgesic orally for postoperative pain is governed by the severity of the pain, patient-related factors (comorbidities, allergies, prior experience with analgesics), the risk of postoperative bleeding (for aspirin or NSAIDs), and the plan for home analgesia. If an analgesic has already been chosen as a discharge medication, transition to that medication in the postoperative period is appropriate.

While using oral agents it is advisable to give single agents, rather than the combination to allow more flexibility. The NSAIDs were usually given as standing order, with opioids are used as an rescue analgesics.

Intramuscular Route

Used for moderate to severe pain, produces rapid analgesic effect. But nowadays are replaced by IV or subcutaneous injection. Disadvantages of this route include pain on administration, variable and sometimes slow onset of effect, and peaks and valleys of analgesic effect.

Intravenous Route

Used to treat acute and severe pain and produces rapid relief. Can be used as an continuous infusion or PCA or intermittent boluses.

Disadvantages of bolus IV injection include more pronounced peaks and valleys of analgesic effect and side effects and a relatively short duration of analgesic.

Continuous infusion results in better analgesia by eliminating peaks and valleys, and also provides a good patient satisfaction with less side effects. Continuous infusion results delay in analgesia if a bolus is not given. Also needs more vigilant monitoring.

Subcutaneous Route

Useful for patients without an intravenous access. Used in patients requiring long-term care, e.g. in oncology patients.

Transdermal/Iontophoretic Administration

Transdermal fentanyl is not ideal for acute perioperative pain. However, iontophoretic delivery of fentanyl provides sufficient analgesia in the perioperative period.

Transmucosal Administration

Used by oncology patients for control of breakthrough pain.

Intrathecal Analgesia

Intrathecal opioids provides short or intermediate term analgesia, which can be increased with hydrophilic opioids like morphine providing analgesia up to 12–36 hours. Useful for lower abdominal surgeries with spinal anesthesia.

For hip and knee arthroplasty, cesarean section, intrathecal morphine provided excellent analgesia for 24 hours after surgery with no difference in side effects; with significant reduction in postoperative patient-controlled (PCA) morphine requirements. Intrathecal fentanyl, sufentanil are also used, but they provides shorter analgesia.

Continuous intrathecal administration is not done due to previous reports of cauda equina from intrathecal administration of high concentration of local anesthetics.

Disadvantage: Cannot be repeated.

Intra-articular Administration

Intra-articular injection of opioids may provide analgesia for up to 24 hours postoperatively and prevent the development of chronic postsurgical pain. The analgesic benefit of intra-articular opioids over systemic administration has not been demonstrated, and the systemic analgesic effect of these injections has not been excluded. Glenohumeral intra-articular continuous catheters have been associated with chondrolysis when bupivacaine is used.

Intrapleural Regional Analgesia

Intrapleural regional analgesia is produced by the injection of a local anesthetic solution through a catheter inserted percutaneously into the intrapleural space. The local anesthetic diffuses across the parietal pleura to the intercostal neurovascular bundle and produces a unilateral intercostal nerve block at multiple levels. Effective postoperative pain relief requires intermittent intrapleural injections approximately every 6 hours of large volumes of local anesthetic (20 mL of 0.25 - 0.5% bupivacaine). This large bolus of local anesthetic into the intrapleural space produces significant side effects while providing minimal analgesia. Pleural drainage tubes also causes loss of the local anesthetic solution and, consequently, poor analgesia. This technique is recommended only if all other options have been exhausted.

Paravertebral Blocks

This block is effective for controlling acute pain associated with breast surgery, but has also demonstrated benefit in decreasing the development of chronic postsurgical pain over other analgesic regimens. This technique can be performed as a single-shot technique or as a continuous catheter infusion to provide ongoing perioperative analgesia.

PERIPHERAL NERVE BLOCK

Intermediate-term pain relief (<24 hours) can be achieved with a combination of a local anesthetic and adjuvant drugs in a single injection. Longer-acting pain control may be indicated by the surgical technique, rehabilitation needs, and patient comorbidities; and can be achieved by utilizing perineural catheters for continuous local anesthetic infusions.

Techniques

Nerve blocks can be inserted using anatomic landmarks, nerve stimulation, and ultrasound guidance. The efficacy between ultrasound-guided techniques and nerve stimulation vary, depending on the skill of the provider, primarily resulting in differences in comfort during placement and procedural time of the blockade.

Adjuvant Drugs

Commonly used adjuvant drugs include epinephrine, clonidine, and opioids. Epinephrine for peripheral nerve blockade significantly increases the duration of the blockade, with minimal side effects. Epinephrine can also increase the sensitivity of intravascular injection; concentrations of 2.5 to 5 mg/mL are generally used. Opioid should not be added to a peripheral nerve blockade. Clonidine is beneficial in extending the duration of preoperative blockade, but hypotension, bradycardia, and sedation, are less likely to occur in doses less than 1.5 mg/kg.

Catheter versus Single-shot Techniques

Upper Extremity

Continuous interscalene blockade allows for longer duration of action compared with single-shot techniques, with better pain relief, with minimal opioid supplementation and increased patient satisfaction and sleep quality.

Lower Extremity

Lower extremity perineural catheters are utilized for major joint surgery of the hip, knee, ankle, and foot. Lumbar plexus catheters have been utilized as part of a multimodal regimen that include PCA with or without femoral catheters for unilateral hip repairs.

8. Epidural analgesia, its advantage over other routes. Advantages of thoracic over lumbar epidural. Drugs used and complications. What are adjuvant medication that can be used epidurally?

Ans. Epidural analgesia can be provided with local anesthetics alone or with opioids. It provides superior analgesia in upper abdominal surgeries, thoracotomies, joint replacement surgeries.

As compared to systemic opioids via PCA, epidural analgesia provides better pain relief at rest and with movement after all types of surgery and lower incidence of nausea/vomiting and sedation, pulmonary infections and pulmonary complications but a higher incidence of pruritus, urinary retention and motor block.

Addition of epidural analgesia in addition to general anesthesia resulted in a reduced rate of arrhythmias, earlier extubation, reduced intensive care unit (ICU) stay, reduced stress hormone, cortisol and glucose concentrations as well as reduced incidence of renal failure, when local anesthetics were used.

Usually a continuous infusion is used.

LEVEL OF ADMINISTRATION—THORACIC VS LUMBAR

Thoracic epidural analgesia (TEA) for the treatment of pain after major abdominal and thoracic surgery, resulted in improved bowel recovery after abdominal surgery and also postoperative myocardial infarction, while these benefits were not consistent with lumbar administration.

In patients undergoing gynecological surgery showed that TEA provided better pain relief only when the incision extended above the umbilicus.

Drug used for Epidural Analgesia

Local anesthetics: Infusions of bupivacaine or levobupivacaine at 0.1% or 0.125% with ropivacaine 0.2% are used. Local anesthetics alone results in more motor or sensory blockade, mostly employed to avoid opioid related adverse effects.

Opioids: The actions of epidural opioids is also governed largely by their lipid solubility. Lipophilic opioids (e.g. fentanyl) have a faster onset but shorter duration of action compared with hydrophilic drugs (e.g. morphine).

Morphine has a prolonged analgesic effect and it can be given by intermittent bolus dose or infusion; the risk of respiratory depression may be higher and analgesia less effective with bolus dose regimens. An infusion of epidural fentanyl appears to produce analgesia by uptake into the systemic circulation, whereas a bolus dose of fentanyl produces analgesia by a selective spinal mechanism. There is no evidence of benefit of epidural versus systemic administration of alfentanil or sufentanil.

The addition of butorphanol to epidural bupivacaine resulted in more rapid and prolonged pain relief compared with butorphanol alone.

Neuraxial Drugs and their Doses (Table 2)

Table 2 | Neuraxial drugs and doses

Drugs	*Intrathecal single dose*	*Epidural single dose*	*Epidural infusion*
Fentanyl	5–25 mcg	50–100 mcg	25–100 mcg/hour
Sufentanil	2–10 mcg	10–50 mcg	10–20 mcg/hour
Morphine	0.1–0.3 mg	1–5 mg	0.1–1 mg/hour
Methadone		4–8 mg	0.3–0.5 mg/hour
Alfentanil	0.5–1 mg	0.1–1 mg	
Bupivacaine	5–15 mg	25–150 mg	1–25 mg/hour
Ropivacaine	—	25–200 mg	1–25 mg/hour
Clonidine	—	100–900 mcg	10–50 mcg/hour

Local Anesthetic Agents and Opioids

Combinations of low concentrations of local anesthetic agents and opioids have been shown to provide consistently superior pain relief compared with either of the drugs alone. Addition of fentanyl to a continuous epidural infusion of ropivacaine reduced the rate of regression of sensory block and decreased the discontinuation of postoperative epidural infusion due to lack of efficacy.

Adjuvant Drugs

The efficacy of adding of adjuvant drugs such as adrenaline (epinephrine), clonidine, ketamine, midazolam, neostigmine and magnesium to solutions used for epidural analgesia.

Complications

Permanant neurological injury, epidural hematoma, epidural abscess, respiratory depression, hypotension, postdural puncture headache.

9. What is patient-controlled analgesia? Described the route, drugs and doses used, advantages of PCA. Setting of PCA. Need for background infusion. What are the Complications?

Ans. PCA can be delivered via oral, intravenous, subcutaneous, epidural, and intrathecal routes, as well as by peripheral nerve catheter. There is limitation of the number of doses per unit time and also the time interval between two successive doses. A background continuous infusion is not indicated unless a opioid tolerant patient.

PCA provide better patient satisfaction, safety, better pain relief, less total drug use, less sleep disturbance, less sedation, more rapid return of physical function.

PCA may lead to sedation, so monitoring of respiratory rate and capnography (in critical cases) to be done.

IV PCA Drugs and Dose and Settings (Table 3)

Table 3 | IV PCA drugs and doses

Drug	*Bolus dose*	*Lock out*	*Continuous infusion*
Morphine	0.5–2.5 mg	5–10 min	1–2 mg/hour
Fentanyl	25–50 mcg	5–10 min	10–100 mcg/hour
Alfentanil	0.1–0.2 mg	5–10 min	
Oxymorphone	0.2–0.4 mg	8–10 min	
Sufentanil	2–10 mcg	4–10 min	2–8 mcg/hour
Methadone	0.5–1.5 mg	10–30 min	

While the optimal sized bolus dose should provide good pain relief with minimal side effects. Initial orders for bolus doses should take into account factors such as a history of prior opioid use and patient age. While adjust bolus dose the number of both successful and unsuccessful attempts should be taken into account. The routine use of a background infusion is not recommended, except for opioid-tolerant patients. Patient's pain should be controlled before PCA is started by administration of individually titrated loading doses.

Adjuvent Medications

Adjuvent medications like droperidol, ondansetron reduces nausea, vomitting. Concurrent ketamine infusion leads to decrease in opioid dose. Addition of clonidine, dexmedetomidine, magnesium to PCA leads to better pain relief and less adverse effects.

Equipment

- *Programmable PCA pumps:* Adjustments can be made to the dose delivered and lockout intervals, background infusions can be added, and accurate assessments can be made of the total dose of drug delivered. In addition, access to the syringe (or other drug reservoir) and the microprocessor program is only possible using a key or access code.
- *Disposable PCA devices:* No adjustments can be made and of single use.
- *Parenteral PCA devices:* Advantages include small size and weight, freedom from an external power source, elimination of programming errors, and simplicity of use.

  Disadvantages include an inability to alter the volume of the bolus dose delivered or add a background infusion, difficulties determining the amount of drug the patient has received accurately, the possibility of inaccurate flow rates, and long-term costs
- *Transmucosal PCA devices:* Metered-dose PCINA devices are available. The drugs must be administered in small volumes to avoid significant run-off into the pharynx.
- *Transdermal PCA devices:* The fentanyl PCTS uses a low-intensity electric current to drive the drug from the reservoir through the skin and into the systemic circulation. The Ionsys device, which is applied to the chest or upper outer arm, delivers a fixed dose of 40 mcg fentanyl over a 10 minutes period following a patient demand and allows delivery of up to 6 doses each hour, up to a maximum of 80 doses in 24 hours, to be replaced every 24 hours.

Complications Related to PCA

Complications related to the use of PCA can be divided into:
- Operator or patient-related errors
- Due to the equipment
- The opioid used.

Equipment-related Complications

There may be 'run-away' pumps, where the PCA pump unexpectedly delivers an unprescribed dose of drug due to spontaneous triggering and also uncontrolled syphoning of syringe contents when the PCA machine was above patient level.

Patient and Staff Factors

Education: Education of the patient about the opioid and PCA helps in removing worries about addiction and safety of PCA.

Inappropriate use of PCA occurs when some unauthorized person or family pressing the PCA, patient pressing PCA thinking it to a doorbell.

Nursing and Medical Staff

Wrong concentration of drug. Avoided by standard drug concentration in PCA. Also errors in programming bolus, and other setting can be avoided by using a present standard settings without a continuous infusion.

Other Types of PCA

- Patient-controlled regional analgesia via:
  - Incision (incisional PCRA) with local anesthetics
  - Intra-articular (IA) tissue (IAPCRA) with local anesthetics and opioids
  - Perineural site (perineural PCRA) with local anesthetics.
- Patient-controlled intranasal analgesia (PCINA) with fentanyl
- Patient-controlled transpulmonary analgesia.

It is a novel, proprietary inhalation formulation of free and liposome-encapsulated fentanyl intended to provide rapid, extended, and personalized analgesia for patients experiencing acute pain episodes.

Using this patients can identify and select a personalized dose for each pain episode, achieving both rapid onset and extended duration of analgesia.

10. Describe the various adjuvant medications used in perioperatve pain management.

Ans. *Alpha-2 agonists (Clonidine, Dexmedetomidine)*

The addition of clonidine to epidural, intrathecal, peripheral nerve blocks lead to prolonged analgesia and decreased opioid consumption. But intrathecal clonidine leads to sedation and hypotension.

With IVRA, dexmedetomidine prolongs increased duration and quality of analgesia, whereas clonidine delays the tourniquet pain. Intra-articular use has also resulted in improved pain relief.

Systemic administration (oral, IM, IV) of single doses of the alpha-2 agonists clonidine and dexmedetomidine decreased perioperative opioid requirements in surgical patients.

Additon of clonidine or dexmedetomidine to morphine PCA resulted better pain relief and lesser nausea, but lead to hypotension and sedation. Dexmedetomidine infusion in ventilated patients resulted in 50% decrease of morphine requirement.

Glucocorticoids: Systemic dexamethasone reduces postoperative pain, nausea and vomiting, and fatigue. It also reduces dynamic pain in breast and hip surgeries, reduces radicular pain in lumbar disectomy. Perioperative methylprednisolone resulted in less hyperesthesia.

Adrenaline: In postoperative thoracic epidural infusions, the addition of adrenaline (epinephrine) to fentanyl and ropivacaine or bupivacaine improved analgesia. The addition of adrenaline to intrathecal bupivacaine prolonged motor and sensory block.

NMDA receptor antagonists: The NMDA-receptor antagonists are ketamine, dextromethorphan, amantadine, memantine.

Ketamine: Perioperative low-dose ketamine used in conjunction with patient-controlled analgesia morphine is opioid-sparing and reduces the incidence of nausea and vomiting, but does not produce a clinically significant reduction in pain scores. Ketamine is a safe and effective analgesic for painful procedures in children. Ketamine may improve analgesia in patients with severe acute pain that is poorly responsive to opioids. Ketamine reduces postoperative pain in opioid-tolerant patients.

Amantadine and memantine: Oral amantadine and memantine lead to decreased opioid consumption. Oral amantadine has also reduced the incidence of phantom limb pain.

Neuraxial: Preservative free ketamine when added to intrathecal opioid analgesia results in improved pain relief, less opioid requirements, and less adverse effects. Ketamine and midazolam when added together to the intrathecal local anesthetics leads to better pain relief as compared to local anesthetic (LA) or LA and ketamine. Caudal epidural ketamine (0.25–0.5 mg/kg) resulted in prolonged pain relief with minimal adverse effects. There is no advantage of using ketamine in peripheral blocks, wound infiltration, intra-articular, etc.

A transdermal ketamine patch (delivering 25 mg over 24 hours) reduced analgesic consumption after gynecological surgery, but topical ketamine applied to tonsils has no advantage.

Midazolam

Preservative free midazolam has been proposed as a potential spinal analgesic due to its action on GABA A receptors. Intrathecal midazolam leads to increase in duration of analgesia and less nausea and vomitting. Caudal epidural midazolam in children prolongs the bupivacaine analgesia.

Neostigmine

Neostigmine acts as a spinal analgesic by potentiation of muscarinic cholinergic activity.

Intrathecal neostigmine resulted in higher nausea and vomiting, bradycardia requiring atropine and anxiety, agitation and restlessness; and also the pain relief is minimal.

Epidural neostigmine and resulted in improved analgesia, lesser opioid requirement.

Magnesium

Magnesium acts as an NMDA receptor antagonist. The benefits of using magnesium are:

- Combined intrathecal and epidural in orthopedic surgery leading to decreased opioid requirement

- With lignocaine in IVRA prolongs analgesia and improves tolerance to tourniquet
- Intra-articularly leads to better pain relief
- Magnesium added to morphine for PCA was opioid-sparing and led to better pain relief; added to tramadol, it was opioid-sparing but only provided better.

Membrane Stabilizers

Perioperative IV lignocaine (lidocaine) infusion was opioid-sparing and significantly reduced pain scores, nausea, vomiting and duration of ileus up to 72 hours after abdominal surgery and also reduced length of hospital stay. However addition of lignocaine to morphine PCA has no benefit.

Gabapentin and Pregabalin

Perioperative gabapentinoids improved analgesia (at rest and with movement) and reduced postoperative opioid consumption, decreased opioid induced adverse effects like nausea, vomiting, pruritus, urinary retention, but increased the incidence of sedation. The effects of gabapentin were not dose-dependent in the range of 300–1200 mg. They also reduce the epidural opioid requirement.

Pregabalin reduces opioid requirements, prevents and reduces of opioid tolerance, improves the quality of opioid analgesia, decreases incidence of respiratory depression and relieves anxiety.

Antidepressant Drugs

Amitriptyline is effective in the treatment of neuropathic pain following breast surgery.

Capsaicin

Injectable capsaicin is used for the control of postoperative pain, such as after total knee replacement, total hip replacement, hernia repair, shoulder arthroscopy, and bunionectomy. Preadministration of neural blockade before injection of capsaicin may greatly decrease the burning discomfort.

11. Describe the usefulness of paracetamol in postoperative pain.

Ans. Paracetamol (acetaminophen) is an effective analgesic and antipyretic.

Mechanism of action is still elusive. Suggested mechanisms include the activation of the endocannabinoid system and spinal serotonergic pathways, prevention of prostaglandin production at the cellular transcriptional level, independent of cyclo-oxygenase activity.

Single doses of paracetamol are effective in the treatment of postoperative pain. Paracetamol is also an effective adjunct to opioid analgesia, opioid requirements being reduced by 20–30% when combined with a regular regimen of oral or rectal paracetamol. In the same doses, orally administered paracetamol was less effective and of slower onset than paracetamol given by IV injection, but more effective and of faster onset than paracetamol administered by the rectal route. IV paracetamol was as effective as ketorolac, diclofenac and was equivalent to morphine and better tolerated after dental surgery.

It should be used with caution or in reduced doses in patients with active liver disease, history of heavy alcohol intake and glucose-6-phosphate dehydrogenase deficiency. But there is no evidence that therapeutic doses will lead to hepatic dysfunction in these groups of patients.

NONSELECTIVE NONSTEROIDAL ANTI-INFLAMMATORY DRUGS (nsNSAIDs)

These are of the following classes:
- *Proprionic acid derivatives:* Ibuprofen and naproxen
- *Salicylates:* Aspirin and choline salicylate
- *Anthranilic acid derivatives:* Indomethacin and ketorolac
- *Oxicams:* Piroxicam
- *Cyclo-oxygenase-2 inhibitors:* Celecoxib.

Single doses of nsNSAIDs are effective in the treatment of pain after surgery. nsNSAIDs are integral components of multimodal analgesia. When given in combination with opioids after surgery, nsNSAIDs resulted in better analgesia, reduced opioid consumption and a lower incidence of PONV and sedation, however there was no effect on pruritus, urinary retention and respiratory depression. The combination of paracetamol and nsNSAID was more effective than paracetamol alone.

Guide for Choosing NSAIDs

- Assess patient's renal, cardiac, and gastrointestinal status before starting drug treatment.
- Determine best route of administration.
- Identify drugs that are appropriate for route of administration desired.
- Select familiar agent among the drugs whose time between onset of activity and peak effect is appropriate for pain syndrome being treated.

Guide for Administering NSAIDs

- Review properties of agent selected
- Start at low end of dosing range
- Use loading dose when appropriate
- Do not exceed ceiling dose
- Ensure that equianalgesic doses are given if route of administration is changed.

Adverse Effects

NSAID side effects are more common with long-term use.

Renal function: The risk of adverse renal effects of NSAIDs and coxibs is increased in the presence of factors such as pre-existing renal impairment, hypovolemia, hypotension, use of other nephrotoxic agents and angiotensin-converting enzyme (ACE) inhibitors. With proper selection and monitoring, the incidence of NSAID-induced perioperative renal impairment is low and NSAIDs need not be withheld in patients with normal preoperative renal function.

Platelet function: NSAIDs inhibit platelet function. NSAIDs were found to increase the risk of reoperation for bleeding in tonsillectomy. NSAIDS results in increased bleeding in many surgeries including hip replacement, gynecological, breast surgeries, etc.

Peptic ulceration: Risks were shown to be significantly increased for patients using naproxen, diclofenac, ibuprofen, aspirin and rofecoxib, but not those taking celecoxib. Risk is increased with higher doses, a history of peptic ulceration, use for more than 5 days and in elderly people. Risk is very low with COX 2 inhibitors. Concurrent use of a proton-pump inhibitor (PPI) significantly reduced the incidence of NSAID-related peptic ulcer disease.

Aspirin-exacerbated respiratory disease: Aspirin-exacerbated respiratory disease (AERD) affects 10–15% of people with asthma, can be severe and there is a cross-sensitivity with nsNSAIDs but not coxibs. So, nsNSAIDS are contraindicated in these group of patients.

Cardiovascular events: Adverse cardiovascular events is higher with NSAIDS. Coxibs also causes CV events and are contraindicated in patients after CABG. Risks were significantly increased for patients using rofecoxib, diclofenac and ibuprofen. Naproxen as the preferred NSAID for long-term use in patients with or at high-risk for cardiovascular disease. Ibuprofen abolishes the protective effect of aspirin, and a gap of 8 hours should be there between ibuprofen intake and aspirin dosing.

Cyclo-oxygenase-2 Selective Inhibitors (Coxibs)

The coxibs available at present include celecoxib, etoricoxib and parecoxib.

Coxibs were as effective as NSAIDs in the management of postoperative pain. Preoperative coxibs reduced postoperative pain and opioid consumption and increased patient satisfaction. When given in combination with opioids after surgery, coxibs were opioid-sparing, but both a decrease in the incidence of opioid-related side effects or pain scores were not observed.

Opioids

All full opioid agonists given in appropriate doses produce the same analgesic effect and therapeutic index, although accurate determination of equianalgesic doses is difficult due to interindividual variability in kinetics and dynamics. Equianalgesic conversion dose tables are often used to assist in the change from one opioid to another. However, such tables should be used as a guide only as they are based largely on single-dose studies in opioid-naive subjects and may not be as relevant when conversions are made after repeated doses of an opioid have been given.

Buprenorphine

Buprenorphine is a semisynthetic derivative of thebaine, an alkaloid of opium, and a partial mu-opioid receptor agonist and kappa-opioid receptor antagonist with high receptor affinity and slow dissociation from the mu-receptor. Mean half life is 2–3 hours after parenteral injection; two-thirds of the drug is excreted unchanged, mainly in feces, while the remaining one-third is metabolized predominantly in the liver and gut wall via glucuronidation. There was a ceiling effect found for respiratory depression but not for analgesia. The risk of respiratory depression is low compared with morphine, methadone, hydromorphone and fentanyl. To reverse buprenorphine induced respiratory depression, higher dose and prolong infusion of naloxane is needed. Withdrawal symptoms, which may be seen if the drug is ceased after long-term treatment, are milder and more delayed in onset (72 hours or more) than other opioids. Preoperatively patient may be on buprenorphine for opioid addiction.

Codeine

It is a very weak mu-receptor agonist and its analgesic action depends on the metabolism of about 10% of the dose given to morphine.

In Caucasian populations, 8–10% of people are poor metabolizers; however 3 - 5% are ultrarapid metabolizers. Those who are ultrarapid metabolizers (carriers of the *CYP2D6* gene duplication) have significantly higher levels of morphine and morphine metabolites after the same dose of codeine.

Fentanyl

Fentanyl is a highly potent phenylpiperidine derivative. It is metabolized almost exclusively in the liver to minimally active metabolites. Fentanyl is commonly used in the treatment of acute pain, especially when its lack of active metabolites and fast onset of action may be of clinical benefit.

Hydromorphone

Hydromorphone is a derivative of morphine that is approximately five times as potent as morphine. The main metabolite of hydromorphone is hydromorphone-3-glucuronide (H3G), a structural analog of morphine-3-glucuronide (M3G). Like M3G H3G is dependent on the kidney for excretion, has no analgesic action and can lead to dose-dependent neurotoxic effects.

Methadone

Methadone is a synthetic opioid commonly used for the maintenance treatment of patients with an addiction to opioids and in patients with chronic pain. It is commercially available as a racemic mixture of R- and L-enantiomers, but it is the R-enantiomer that is responsible for most, if not all, its mu-opioid receptor mediated analgesic effects.

It has good oral bioavailability (70–80%), high potency and long duration of action, and a lack of active metabolites. It is also a weak NMDA receptor antagonist and monoamine (serotonin and norepinephrine) reuptake inhibitor and has a long and unpredictable half-life (mean of 22 hours; range 4–190 hours) leading to an increased risk of accumulation. Therefore, it is of limited use for acute pain treatment. Dose conversion is complex and depends on many factors including absolute doses of other opioids and duration of treatment.

High dose methadone has been associated with prolonged QT intervals.

Morphine

Morphine is a naturally occurring opioid with poor lipid solubility. After oral administration, plasma levels of morphine peak at 30–90 minutes. Bioavailiability is low via oral route, usually 20–30%. Protein binding is 45%. Mean elimination half life is 1.5–3.5 hours. Morphine is rapidly distributed to highly perfused tissues like kidney, lungs, liver, spleen. It is metabolized in liver to morphine-3-glucoronide, morphine-6-glucoronide and morphine-3, 6-glucoronide. Morphine-3-glucoronide is inactive and responsible for the development of tolerence. Morphine-6-glucoronide is active and accumulates in renal failure leading to toxixcity.

12. Describe the changes in drugs metabolism in hepatic and renal failure, and the dose adjustments of the drugs.

Ans. *Hepatic impairment*

- While there are limited data, dose adjustments are usually not required for alfentanil, buprenorphine, fentanyl, morphine, oxycodone and sufentanil
- Tramadol may need to be given at lower doses
- Methadone should be used with caution in the presence of severe liver disease because of the potential for greatly prolonged clearance
- The clearance of local anesthetics may be significantly impaired; doses may need to be decreased if use is prolonged
- Carbamazepine and valproate should be avoided in patients with severe hepatic impairment

- It may be wise to reduce the dose of paracetamol in patients with significant degrees of hepatic impairment.

Renal impairment:

- Analgesics that exhibit the safest pharmacological profile in patients with renal impairment are alfentanil, buprenorphine, fentanyl, ketamine, paracetamol (except with compound analgesics) and sufentanil. None of these drugs delivers a high active metabolite load or has a significantly prolonged clearance
- Oxycodone can usually be used without any dose adjustment in patients with renal impairment. Its metabolites do not appear to contribute to any clinical effect in patients with normal renal function
- Amitriptyline, bupivacaine, levobupivacaine, lignocaine, ropivacaine, clonidine, gabapentin, codeine, hydromorphone, methadone, morphine and tramadol have been used in patients with renal disease but depending on the degree of impairment and, in the case of local anesthetics, whether or not administration is prolonged, may require a reduction in dose
- Levobupivacaine, with similar clearance mechanisms, and ropivacaine may be safer than bupivacaine because of a higher therapeutic ratio
- NSAIDs (both nsNSAIDs and coxibs), dextropropoxyphene and pethidine should not be used in the presence of significant renal impairment.

Analgesic Drugs in Patients with Renal Impairment (Tables 4 and 5)

Table 4 | Analgesic drugs with renal impairment

Drug	*Pharmacokinetics and pharmacodynamics*	*Recommendations*
Alfentanil	• No active metabolites • 92% protein bound; increases in free fraction may result from alterations in protein binding	No dose adjustment required unless renal failure is severe
Buprenorphine	• Pharmacokinetics unchanged; predominantly biliary excretion of metabolites • Pharmacokinetics also unchanged with dialysis	No dose adjustment required
Codeine	• Accumulation of active metabolites can occur; prolonged sedation and respiratory arrest have been reported in patients with renal impairment • No good data on removal by dialysis	Dose adjustment recommended or use an alternative opioid
Dihydrocodeine	• Metabolic pathway probably similar to codeine	*Insufficient evidence:* Use not recommended
Fentanyl	• No active metabolites • Not removed to any significant degree by dialysis	No dose adjustment required; may be used in patients with severe renal impairment
Hydromorphone	• Neurotoxicity from accumulation of H3G possible • H3G is effectively removed during dialysis	Dose adjustment recommended or use alternative opioid

Contd...

Contd...

Drug	*Pharmacokinetics and pharmacodynamics*	*Recommendations*
Methadone	• Methadone and its metabolites are excreted in urine and feces; in anuric patients it may be mostly in feces • High protein binding, high volume of distribution and moderate water solubility would suggest that it is likely to be poorly removed by dialysis	Dose adjustment may be required in severe renal impairment
Morphine	• Major metabolites M3G and M6G excreted via kidney and accumulate in renal impairment • M6G is an opioid agonist that crosses the blood-brain barrier slowly; delayed sedation from M6G has been reported in renal failure • Neurotoxicity from accumulation of M3G possible • Oral administration results in proportionally higher metabolite load • Morphine and its metabolites are cleared by most hemodialysis procedures but may not be significantly affected by peritoneal dialysis • M6G also removed but slow diffusion from CNS delays response	Dose adjustment recommended or use alternative opioid
Oxycodone	• The metabolite oxymorphone is active but plasma levels are normally negligible and therefore it has an insignificant clinical effect in patients with normal renal function. • Higher blood concentrations of oxycodone and metabolites with moderate to severe renal impairment; half life significantly increased in endstage renal disease • Oxycodone and its metabolites are dialyzable	No dose adjustment required in most patients
Pethidine	• Norpethidine is the only active metabolite and is renally excreted; it is dialyzable • Accumulation of norpethidine can lead to neuroexcitation including seizures	Use of alternative agent recommended
Sufentanil	Minimally active metabolite	No dose adjustment required
Tramadol	• Increased tramadol-like effects from active metabolite • O-desmethyltramadol (M1) • Tramadol is removed by dialysis	Dose adjustment recommended Use of alternative agent recommended with significant renal impairment

Contd...

Contd...

Drug	*Pharmacokinetics and pharmacodynamics*	*Recommendations*
Local anesthetics	• There may be no significant difference in plasma concentration of levobupivacaine, bupivacaine or ropivacaine in patients with chronic renal failure unless renal failure is severe, continuous infusions are used or repeated doses are used • Risk of toxicity may be affected by abnormalities in acid-base balance and/or potassium levels	Doses may need to be reduced if prolonged or repeated administration, e.g. continuous infusions
Paracetamol	• Terminal elimination half-life may be prolonged and is dialysable	• May need to increase dose interval if renal impairment is severe • Weak evidence that it may increase the rate of progression to chronic renal failure
nsNSAIDs and coxibs	• Can affect renal function • Behavior during dialysis not clearly elucidated for most	• Use with caution in patients with mild renal impairment and avoid in patients with severe renal impairment
Clonidine	• Half-life is increased in severe renal failure 50% metabolized by the liver; remained excreted unchanged by the kidney	• Limited data; dose adjustment has been recommended
Tricyclic antidepressants	• Amitriptyline is metabolized in the liver to nortriptyline, the active agent • Not significantly removed by dialysis	• Limited data; metabolite accumulation may occur and increase the risk of side effects but little evidence to indicate need for dose reduction
Ketamine	• Dehydronorketamine levels are increased but it has only 1% of potency of ketamine • Ketamine is not removed well by dialysis	• Limited data; probable that no dose adjustment is required
Gabapentin	• Impaired renal function results in reduced clearance in direct proportion to creatinine clearance; about 35% cleared by dialysis	• Dose adjustment recommended on basis of creatinine clearance
Pregabalin	• Impaired renal function results in reduced clearance in direct proportion to creatinine clearance; highly cleared by dialysis	• Dose adjustment recommended on basis of creatinine clearance

Table 5 | Analgesic drugs in patients with hepatic impairment		
Alfentanil	• No significant difference in half-life found in children undergoing liver transplant	*Limited data:* No dose adjustment required
Buprenorphine	• Buprenorphine • Lower blood concentrations of buprenorphine and norbuprenorphine • Limited	*Limited data:* No dose adjustment required
Fentanyl	• Disposition appears to be unaffected	*Limited data:* No dose adjustment required
Methadone	• Increased half-life but limited significance	*Limited data:* No dose adjustment required in chronic stable liver disease
Morphine	• Hepatic impairment does not appear to have a significant effect on morphine pharmacokinetics; even in patients with cirrhosis there is a large hepatic reserve for glucuronidation • Blood concentrations of morphine but not morphine metabolites higher after liver resection; blood concentrations also higher in patients with liver cancer Increased oral bioavailability of morphine due to its normal high first pass metabolism when given via this route	In most patients no dose adjustment required
Oxycodone	Decreased oxycodone clearance with mild to moderate hepatic impairment	*Limited data:* No dose adjustment required in most patients
Pethidine	Reduced clearance	*Limited data:* Dose adjustment may be required; use not recommended
Sufentanil	No difference in clearance or elimination	No dose adjustment required
Tramadol	Reduced clearance	*Limited data:* Dose adjustment may be required if impairment is severe
Local anesthetics	• Amide-type local anesthetics undergo hepatic metabolism and clearance may be reduced in hepatic disease • Increased plasma concentrations of ropivacaine after continuous infusion but not single dose	*Limited data:* Dose adjustment may be required with prolonged or repeated use
Paracetamol	• Metabolized in the liver; small proportion metabolized to the potentially hepatotoxic metabolite • N-acetyl-p-benzoquinone imine • This is normally inactivated by hepatic glutathione • Clearance is reduced	• Used with caution or in reduced doses or frequency with active liver disease, alcohol-related liver disease and glucose-6-phosphate dehydrogenase deficiency. However, others report that it can be used safely in patients with liver disease and is preferred to NSAIDs, and that therapeutic doses of paracetamol, at least for short-term use, are an unlikely cause of hepatotoxicity in patients who ingest moderate to large amounts of alcohol
Tricyclic antidepressants	Amitriptyline is metabolized in the liver to nortriptyline, the active agent	Reduce dose if hepatic impairment is severe

Pharmacogenetics and its Influence on Pain Sensitivity and Drug Metabolism

With time an increasing number of genetic variants modulating nociception, susceptibility to pain conditions, as well as response to pharmacotherapy have been discovered.

Pharmacogenomics deals with the influence of genetic variation on drug response in patients. By correlating gene expression or single-nucleotide polymorphisms with a drug's efficacy or toxicity, the aim is to develop rational means to optimize drug therapy with respect to the patient's genotype and ensure maximum efficacy with minimal adverse effects.

Loss of Pain Sensation

Loss of pain sensations occurs in some recognized hereditary syndromes that include:
- Channelopathy-associated insensitivity to pain'caused by variants in the *SCN9A* gene
- Hereditary sensory and autonomic neuropathy (HSAN) I-V syndromes.

Reduced Sensitivity to Pain

Reduced pain sensitivity has been associated with variants in genes encoding the mu-opioid receptor (OPRM1), catechol-O-methyltransferase (COMT), guanosine triphosphate cyclohydrolase 1/dopa-responsive dystonia (GCH1), transient receptor potential (TRPV 1), and the melanocortin-1 receptor (MC1R).

Drug Metabolism

Most of the drugs are metabolized by the polymorphic cytochrome P450 enzymes and they show interindividual variability in their catalytic activity.

Codeine

In children and adults receiving codeine for postoperative pain, very low or undetectable levels of plasma morphine have been noted in those with poor metabolizer or intermediate metabolizer genotypes, but with variable impact on analgesia.

With ultrarapid metabolizers, there is more than 50% increase in morphine concentration in the plasma, this along with concurrent renal failure may cause toxicity.

Tramadol

Poor metabolizers have low concentration of its metabolite and poor analgesic efficacy. Whereas ultrarapid metabolizers have higher concentration of the metabolite, and it may result in respiratory depression with concurrent renal failure.

Methadone

Genetic polymorphisms in genes coding for methadone-metabolizing enzymes, transporter proteins (p-glycoprotein), and mu-opioid receptors may explain part of the observed inter-individual variation in the pharmacokinetics and pharmacodynamics of methadone; blood concentrations may vary up to 20-fold for a given dose.

NSAIDs

NSAIDs like ibuprofen, naproxen and piroxicam are metabolized by CYP2C9. Between 1 and 3% of Caucasians are poor metabolizers. Homozygous carriers of the CYP2D9* 3 allele may accumulate celecoxib and ibuprofen in blood and tissues and be at risk of increased adverse effects.

13. Define tolerance, addiction, pseudoaddiction.

Ans. *Tolerance:* A predictable physiological decrease in the effect of a drug over time so that a progressive increase in the amount of that drug is required to achieve the same effect. Tolerance develops to desired (e.g. analgesia) and undesired (e.g. euphoria, opioid-related sedation, nausea or constipation) effects at different rates.

Physical dependence: A physiological adaptation to a drug whereby abrupt discontinuation or reversal of that drug, or a sudden reduction in its dose, leads to a withdrawal (abstinence) syndrome.

Withdrawal can be terminated by administration of the same or similar drug.

Addiction: A disease that is characterized by aberrant drug-seeking and maladaptive drug-taking behaviors that may include cravings, compulsive drug use and loss of control over drug use, despite the risk of physical, social and psychological harm.

While psychoactive drugs have an addiction liability, psychological, social, environmental and genetic factors play an important role in the development of addiction.

Unlike tolerance and physical dependence, addiction is not a predictable effect of a drug.

Pseudoaddiction: Behaviors that may seem inappropriately drug seeking but are a result of under treatment of pain and resolve when pain relief is adequate.

Clinical Implications of Opioid Tolerance and Opioid-induced Hyperalgesia and Plan of Acute Pain Management in these Groups of Patients

Both tolerance and opioid induced hyperalgesia (OIH) may contribute to increased pain.

If inadequate pain relief is due to OIH, a reduction in opioid dose may help; if it is due to opioid tolerance, increased doses may provide better pain relief.

Other reasons for increased pain and/or increased opioid requirements should also be considered. These include acute neuropathic pain, pain due to other causes including postoperative complications, major psychological distress, and aberrant drug-seeking behaviors.

Three main groups of opioid-tolerant patients/patients with OIH are encountered in acute pain settings:

1. Patients with chronic cancer or noncancer pain being treated with opioids, some of whom may exhibit features opioid addiction.
2. Patients with a substance abuse disorder either using illicit opioids or on an opioid maintenance treatment program.
3. Patients who have developed acute opioid tolerance or OIH due to perioperative opioid administration, particularly opioids of high potency.

MANAGEMENT OF ACUTE PAIN

Management of these patients should focus on:

- Effective analgesia
- Use of strategies that may help to attenuate tolerance or OIH
- Prevention of withdrawal
- Close liaison with other treating clinicians and specialist teams as required and appropriate discharge planning.

Effective Analgesia

Opioid requirements are usually significantly higher in opioid-tolerant compared with opioid-naive patients. Opioid-tolerant patients using PCA or epidural analgesia may require approximately three times the dose than their opioid-naive counterparts. Opioid-tolerant patients with chronic pain also reported higher pain scores after surgery and their pain resolved more slowly compared with opioid-naive patients, which may even higher in patients with opioid tolerant noncancer chronic pain.

The incidence of opioid-induced nausea and vomiting may be lower in opioid-tolerant patients although the risk of excessive sedation/respiratory depression may be higher.

IV PCA is a useful modality for pain relief in opioid-tolerant patients provided that pain intensity and opioid consumption are carefully monitored and background requirements are provided if the patient cannot take their usual opioid; larger bolus doses will often be needed. Regardless of the initial dose prescribed, subsequent doses will need to be titrated to effect for each patient.

Neuraxial opioids have been used effectively in opioid-tolerant patients; although higher doses may be required and may not result in an increase in adverse effects. Effective analgesia using intrathecal or epidural opioids will not necessarily prevent symptoms of opioid withdrawal.

Attenuation of Tolerance and Opioid-induced Hyperalgesia

There are a number of strategies that may help attenuate opioid tolerance and OIH, at least to a certain degree. These include:

- Use of NMDA- or opioid-receptor antagonists
- Opioid rotation
- Other adjuvant drugs.

NMDA and opioid-receptor antagonists: In patients taking opioids on a long-term basis, the administration of ketamine has been reported to lead to improved pain relief and reduced opioid requirements.

Opioid rotation: Opioid rotation is commonly used in the treatment of chronic noncancer and cancer pain when a change to another opioid can improve analgesia and reduce side effects. Opioid rotation (e.g. using an opioid that is different from the preadmission opioid) may also be of use in the acute pain setting. The concept is based on the rationale that the different opioids do not act to the same degree on different opioid receptor subtypes and are metabolized differently, and also takes advantage of the fact that cross-tolerance is likely to be incomplete and that the degree of OIH and tolerance appears to vary between opioids.

Prevention of withdrawal: Withdrawal from opioids is characterized by excitatory and autonomic symptoms including abdominal cramping, muscle aches and pain, insomnia, dysphoria, anxiety, restlessness, nausea and vomiting, diarrhea, rhinorrhea and sneezing, trembling, yawning, runny eyes and piloerection or 'gooseflesh'. The time of onset of withdrawal symptoms after cessation of the drug will depend on the duration of action of the opioid.

It should be prevented by maintenance of normal preadmission opioid regimens where possible or appropriate substitutions with another opioid or the same opioid via another route.

While multimodal analgesic regimens (e.g. nsNSAIDs, paracetamol, ketamine, tramadol, regional analgesia) are of analgesic benefit, opioid-tolerant patients are at risk of opioid withdrawal if a purely nonopioid analgesic regimen or tramadol is used. For this reason opioid antagonists (naloxone, naltrexone) or mixed agonist-antagonists (e.g. buprenorphine, pentazocine) should be also avoided (unless the former are needed to treat respiratory depression) as their use may precipitate acute withdrawal reactions.

Use of intrathecal or epidural opioids will not necessarily prevent symptoms of opioid withdrawal and additional systemic opioids may be required.

Clonidine, administered orally or parenterally, will aid in the symptomatic management of opioid withdrawal symptoms.

14. Describe the pain management in patients with addiction disorder.

Ans. Effective management of perioperative pain in patients with an addiction disorder may be complex due to:

- Psychological and behavioral characteristics associated with that disorder
- Presence of the drug (or drugs) of abuse
- Medications used to assist with drug withdrawal and/or rehabilitation
- Complications related to drug abuse including organ impairment and infectious diseases
- Presence of tolerance, physical dependence and the risk of withdrawal.

Effective analgesia may be difficult, may be required for longer periods than in other patients and often requires significant deviations from 'standard' treatment protocols.

Management of pain in patients with an addiction disorder should focus on:

- Effective analgesia
- Use of strategies that may attenuate tolerance, and prevention of withdrawal
- Symptomatic treatment of affective disorders and behavioral disturbances
- The use of secure drug administration procedures.

Not all aberrant drug behaviors indicate opioid addiction. Those that may include unsanctioned dose escalations, 'lost' or 'stolen' medications, obtaining the drugs from a number of different prescribers, polysubstance abuse, use of opioids obtained illicitly, and forging prescriptions.

In general, when opioids are used in the short-term to treat acute pain, they are usually effective and the risk of abuse is considered to be very small. This may not be the case when these drugs are used in the management of chronic noncancer pain, where long-term use of opioids may not provide as effective pain relief and the risk of abuse of the drugs may be higher. Both patients with chronic pain and those with an addiction disorder have a high rate of psychiatric comorbidities (such as anxiety, depression and personality disorders) and patients with chronic pain may therefore be more at risk of developing behavioral problems associated with opioid use.

The prevalence of addiction in chronic pain patients prescribed opioids is reported to range from 0–50%.

Alcohol and benzodiazepines: There is no cross-tolerance between opioids and alcohol or benzodiazepines and there is therefore no pharmacological reason to use higher than 'standard' initial opioid doses in patients with an alcohol or benzodiazepine addiction.

Alcohol and/or benzodiazepine abuse is relatively common and prevention of withdrawal should be a clinical priority in all patients. If benzodiazepines are administered for the treatment of withdrawal signs and symptoms, patient sedation levels must be monitored, especially if they are receiving concurrent opioids. Excessive sedation will limit the amount of opioid than can safely be given.

Cannabinoids: Anecdotal reports suggest higher opioid doses may be required for the management of acute pain in patients who are heavy users of cannabinoids, there is no published information to support this.

Drugs used in the treatment of addiction disorders.

Methadone: Methadone is a long-acting opioid agonist used in the management of patients with an opioid addiction. It is usually given once a day, which is often enough to suppress symptoms of opioid withdrawal; the duration of any analgesic effect from the dose is likely to be much shorter. In the acute pain setting methadone should be continued, where possible, as usual at the same dose. If the patient is unable to take methadone by mouth, substitution with parenteral methadone or other opioids will be required in the short-term. Parenteral methadone doses should be based on half to two-thirds of the oral maintenance dose by IM or SC in 2–4 times.

Buprenorphine: Buprenorphine is a partial opioid agonist used in the treatment of opioid addiction. It is usually given once everyday or two, which again is often enough to suppress symptoms of opioid withdrawal; like methadone the duration of any analgesic effect from the dose is likely to be much shorter. Preparations that combine buprenorphine and naloxone are available to reduce potential parenteral abuse of the drug.

If shorter-acting opioid agonists will be required, a decision needs be made whether or not to continue buprenorphine. Suggestions for management vary from withholding the buprenorphine and substituting an alternative opioid (e.g. methadone), to continuing the buprenorphine as usual. However, in practice, there appears to be little problem if the buprenorphine is continued and acute pain managed with the combination of a short-acting pure opioid agonist as well as other multimodal analgesic strategies. As with methadone, dividing the daily doses on a temporary basis may take advantage of the analgesic properties of the buprenorphine.

Naltrexone: Naltrexone is a pure opioid antagonist used in the management of patients with opioid or alcohol addiction. The usual oral maintenance dose is up to 25–50 mg daily. Orally administered, naltrexone has an apparent half-life of about 14 hours and binds to opioid receptors for over 24 hours following a single dose.

It has been recommended that, where possible, naltrexone be stopped for at least 24 hours before surgery. In these patients and in patients requiring surgery within this 24-hour period, multimodal analgesic regimens (e.g. NSAIDs, paracetamol, ketamine, tramadol and regional analgesia) should also be employed.

There is experimental evidence of μ (mu)-opioid receptor upregulation following antagonist withdrawal and abrupt discontinuation of naltrexone, leading to a period of increased opioid sensitivity, so the amount of opioid required to maintain analgesia may also need to be decreased in order to avoid signs of excessive opioid dose (in particular, respiratory depression).

Recovering Patients

Patients in drug treatment programs or in drug-free recovery may be concerned about the risk of relapse if they are given opioids for the management of their acute pain.

However, there is no evidence that the use of opioids to treat acute pain increases the rate of relapse. Effective communication and planning, the use of multimodal analgesic strategies, reassurance that the risk of reversion to an active addiction disorder is small, and information that ineffective analgesia can paradoxically lead to relapses in recovering patients, will help to prevent undertreatment.

15. Pain management in elderly patients. What are the clinical implications of the changes in the elderly population?

Ans. *Clinical implications:* Pain intensity after surgery may also be less. Older patients, matched for surgical procedure, reported less pain in the postoperative period: pain intensity decreased by 10–20% each decade after 60 years of age.

Nonselective nonsteroidal anti-inflammatory drugs, coxibs and paracetamol: Older patients are more likely to suffer adverse gastric and renal side effects following administration of nsNSAIDs and may also be more likely to develop cognitive dysfunction.

Coxibs have a significantly lower incidence of upper gastrointestinal complications and have no antiplatelet effects, which might be of some advantage in the older patient; the risk of other adverse effects, including effects on renal function and exacerbation of cardiac failure, are similar to nsNSAIDs.

Opioid Dose

Older patients require less opioid than younger patients to achieve the same degree of pain relief. In the clinical setting there is evidence of an age-related 2- to 4-fold decrease in morphine and fentanyl requirements. It has been suggested that doses of fentanyl, sufentanil and alfentanil should all be reduced by up to 50% in older patients; reductions in the doses of other opioids is also advised.

In patients over 75 years the elimination half-life of tramadol was slightly prolonged. Lower daily doses have been suggested.

Side Effects of Opioids

The incidence of nausea/vomiting and pruritus in the postoperative period lessens with increasing age. In older people, fentanyl may cause less postoperative cognitive dysfunction than morphine and less confusion, although administration of an appropriate opioid medication is often associated with higher levels of cognitive function compared with cognitive function if postoperative pain is undertreated.

Local Anesthetics

Older patients are more sensitive to the effects of local anesthetic agents because of a slowing of conduction velocity in peripheral nerves and a decrease in the number of neurons in the spinal cord.

Ketamine

There are no good data on the need or otherwise to alter ketamine doses in the older patient.

Tricyclic Antidepressants

Clearance of tricyclic antidepressant (TCA) drugs may decrease with increasing patient age and lower initial doses are recommended in older people and are more prone to the adverse effects.

In addition, clinical conditions that may require TCAs to be administered with caution are more common in older people and include prostatic hypertrophy, narrow angle glaucoma, CV disease and impaired liver function.

Anticonvulsants

Initial doses of anticonvulsant agents should be lower than for younger patients and any increases in dose should be titrated slowly. The side effects such as somnolence and dizziness with pregabalin may be more common. However, other features of gabapentin and pregabalin, such as a lower risk of drug—drug interactions, lower (less than 3%) protein binding, no hepatic metabolism and the lack of any need to monitor liver function and blood count on a regular basis, means that these drugs may be well-suited to the older patient population.

Patient-controlled Analgesia

Patient-controlled analgesia (PCA) is an effective method of pain relief in older people. They require less opioid, but pain relief, adverse effects, risks of addiction is similar to young ones. Compared to IM morphine PCA morphine provides better analgesia with fewer pull complications.

Epidural Analgesia

Older patients given PCEA had lower pain scores at rest and movement, higher satisfaction scores, improved mental status and more rapid recovery of bowel function compared with those using IV PCA. Epidural morphine requirements decrease as patient age increases. Older patients require less volume and are more susceptible to adverse effects like hypotension.

Intrathecal Opioid Analgesia

Intrathecal morphine using a variety of doses provided more effective pain relief after major surgery compared with other opioid analgesia, although the risk of respiratory depression and pruritus was greater.

Intrathecal morphine 100 mcg dose provided the best balance between good pain relief and pruritus.

Other Regional Analgesia

Possible advantages include a reduction in the incidence of side effects compared with central neuraxial blockade. The duration of action of sciatic nerve and brachial plexus blocks is prolonged in the older patient. In older patients regional blocks like femoral, paravertebral are useful.

16. Implication of pregnancy in pain management (Describe the precautions in using the drugs and the analgesic techniques).

Ans. *Paracetamol:* Paracetamol is regarded as the analgesic of choice during pregnancy, although it has been suggested that prostaglandin actions may have adverse effects in women at high-risk of pre-eclampsia such as preterm birth, increase incidence of asthma in infants.

Nonselective nonsteroidal anti-inflammatory drugs: Use of nsNSAIDs during pregnancy was associated with increased risk of miscarriage. While relatively safe in early and mid pregnancy, they can precipitate fetal cardiac and renal complications in late pregnancy, as well as interfere with fetal brain development and the production of amniotic fluid; they should be discontinued in the 32nd gestational week. Fetal exposure to nsNSAIDs has been associated with persistent pulmonary hypertension in the neonate and an increased risk of premature closure of the ductus arteriosus.

Opioids: Much of the information about the effects of opioids on neonates comes from pregnant patients who abuse opioids or who are on maintenance programs for drug dependence. Maternal long term opioid use can have significant developmental effects in the fetus, although social and environmental factors may also have an impact.

Neonatal abstinence syndrome (NAS) requiring treatment occurs in over 60–90% of infants exposed to opioids *in utero*. Outcomes tend to be better in mothers on maintenance therapy rather than heroin, even better with mothers receiving it for pain than addiction.

Overall, the short-term use of opioids to treat pain in pregnancy appears safe.

Risk Factors for Progression from Acute Postoperative Pain to Chronic Pain

Risk factors for chronic postsurgical pain:
- Preoperative factors
  - Pain, moderate to severe, lasting more than 1 month
  - Repeat surgery
  - Psychological vulnerability (e.g. catastrophizing)
  - Preoperative anxiety
  - Female gender
  - Younger age (adults)
  - Workers' compensation
  - Genetic predisposition
  - Inefficient diffuse noxious inhibitory control (DNIC)
- Intraoperative factors: Surgical approach with risk of nerve damage.
- Postoperative factors
  - Pain (acute, moderate to severe) and radiation area pain
  - Neurotoxic chemotherapy pain
  - Depression
  - Anxiety.

17. Describe the preventive approaches for the chronic postsurgical pain syndromes.
Ans. *Acute postamputation pain syndromes:* Following amputation of a limb, and also breast, tongue, teeth, genitalia and even inner organs such as the rectum, or a deafferentation injury such as brachial plexus avulsion a number of phantom phenomena can develop.

Prevention: Perioperative (pre, intra and postoperative) epidural analgesia has reduced the incidence of severe phantom limb pain. Perioperative ketamine, preoperative gabapentin, local anesthetic infusion via peripheral nerve catheters are not effective in preventing phantom pain.

Treatment: Medications such as opioids, gabapentin, ketamine, TCA are effective in treatment of phantom pain. IV or locally injected local anesthetics are also useful. Nonpharmacological measures such as sensory discrimination training, mental imagery of limb movement and motor imagery, consisting of 2 weeks each of limb laterality recognition, imagined movements and mirror movements.

Post-thoracotomy Pain Syndrome

Post-thoracotomy pain syndrome is one of the most common chronic pain states. It is thought to be caused primarily by trauma to intercostal nerves and most patients relate their pain directly to the site of surgery.

The preventive measures includes:
- Epidural analgesia initiated prior to thoracotomy and continued into the postoperative period.
- The addition of low-dose IV ketamine to thoracic epidural analgesia
- Cryoanalgesia.

Postmastectomy Pain Syndrome

Measures to prevent it includes:
- Preincisional paravertebral block
- Perioperative use of gabapentin or mexiletine
- The use of a eutectic mixture of local anesthetics alone or in combination with gabapentin.

Posthysterectomy Pain Syndrome

Spinal anesthesia in comparison with general anesthesia reduced the risk of chronic postsurgical pain after hysterectomy.

18. What are the various nonopioid infusions that are used in perioperative period?
Ans. Infusions of ketamine, lidocaine, and naloxone and wound infusion of local anesthetics (Table 6).

Table 6 | Doses of ketamine and lignocanine

Drugs	*Bolus dose*	*Infusion dose*
Ketamine	0.5–1 mg/kg	40–100 mcg/hour
Lignocaine	1–1.5 mg/kg	2–3 mg/minute

Lignocaine and ketamine infusion is useful in abdominal and gynecological surgeries.

Ketamine is not useful when the total analgesia is given via the IV route.

IV ketamine may find its use as an adjunct in opioid-tolerant patients, or in patients with a higher incidence of chronic postsurgical pain such as thoracotomy, inguinal herniorrhaphies, limb amputation procedures, or even mastectomies. Most of the studies on perioperative IV lidocaine infusion showed salutary effects especially in abdominal surgery. The infusion appears to be less effective in total hip surgery and coronary artery bypass surgery.

The efficacy of perioperative IV lidocaine infusion may be related to the degree of trauma, it may not be as effective when the surgical trauma is greater.

IV naloxone infusion is used to control the side effects of neuraxial opioids.

A **local anesthetic wound infusion** is an effective and simple technique to decrease postoperative pain. Side effects are minimal and blood levels of the local anesthetic after 48–55 hours of infusion are below toxic levels. Infusion dose is 0.25–0.5% bupivacaine at rate of 2–10 mL per hour. Local anesthetic wound infiltration resulted in improved analgesia across a range of procedures, a very low technical failure rate, and zero reported toxicity, with no increase in wound infection. Found useful in cesarean section, hystectomy, laparotomy, thoracotomy, etc.

Nonpharmacological Techniques for Postoperative Pain

Accupunture: Perioperative accupuncture might be a useful adjunct for acute postoperative pain management.

TENS—may be useful in a few conditions like herniorrhaphy, thoracotomy.

Psychological interventions:
- Relaxation techniques are useful in management of postoperative pain, especially in cancer patients, in whom it also helped in improving nausea, blood pressure, pulse rate, and also helped in reducing anxiety and depression
- Hypnosis may be useful for the management, but evidence is limited
- Attention techniques may be useful, but limited evidence
- Listening to music leads to decreased postoperative pain and opioid requirement
- Distraction is useful in children for procedure related pain.

Physical Therapy

- *Massage therapy:* There is little inconsistent evidence in the use of massage therapy
- *Heat or cold therapy:* The evidence is mixed with few good results from orthopedic surgery, while few others reported no benefit.

Issues in the Pain Management in Children

Pain assessment in children is more difficult than in adults. Children are not malingerers; they are very open about expressing their feelings. But many a times it may not be easy to differentiate between pain and distress.

As the emotional component of pain is very strong in children, psychological support is very important. Minimal separation from parents, holding, nurturing, and distraction are all important modalities.

Nonopioid analgesics such as acetaminophen or nonsteroidal anti-inflammatory agents are useful for mild pain control and as an opiate-sparing measure. Oral, rectal, or intravenous routes are the preferred methods of administration of analgesics—and avoid intramuscular injections. Intravenous fentanyl, morphine are the most popular opiates. Patient-controlled analgesia has been used successfully even with very young children. Regional analgesia performed while the patient is under general anesthesia can provide excellent early postoperative pain relief.

BIBLIOGRAPHY

1. Acute pain management: Scientific evidence. Australia and New Zeland College of Anaesthesiologist and Faculty of Pain Medicine. 3rd edn, 2010.
2. Clinical Practice Guidelines for the Management of Pain, Agitation, and Delirium in Adult Patients in the Intensive Care Unit. Critical Care Medicine. 2013;41(1):263-306.
3. Honorio T Benzon. Perioperative Nonopioid Infusions for Postoperative Pain Management.
4. Joel Katz, Hance Clarke, Ze'ev Seltzer. Preventive Analgesia: Quo Vadimus?. Anesthesia-analgesia. 2011;113(5):1242-53.
5. Micheal AE. Ramsay. Acute postoperative pain management. BUMC Proceedings. 2000;13:244.24.
6. Mitchell Jay Cohen William P. Schecter. Perioperative Pain Control: A Strategy for Management. Surg Clin N Am. 2005;85:1243-57.
7. Nalini Vadivelu, Sukanya Mitra Deepak Narayan. Recent Advances in Postoperative Pain Management. Yale journal of biology and medicine. 2010;83:11-25.
8. Practice Guidelines for Acute Pain Management in the Perioperative Setting. An Updated Report by the American Society of Anesthesiologists Task Force on Acute Pain Management. Anesthesiology. 2012;116(2):248-73.
9. Robert Hallivis, Todd A Derksen, Andrew J Meyr. Peri-Operative Pain Management. Clin Podiatr Med Sur. 2008;25:443-63.
10. Robert W. Hurley, Meredith CB. Adams. Perioperative Pain Management. Miller's Anaesthesia. 7th edn. Chapter 40. pp. 650-62.
11. Steven D Waldman. Management of Acute and Postoperative Pain. 2011.pp. 216-27.
12. The recognition and assessment of acute pain in children. Clinical practice guidelines. British pain society. September 2009.

6

How to Write a Thesis?

Uday C Ghoshal, Rajan Singh, Sushil Kumar

INTRODUCTION

Thesis is an important and essential component of postgraduate training in various disciplines of medical sciences. Unfortunately, many students consider this as a burden to them. However, since this is a necessity in many of the curriculum, it is better to do it well so that the efforts do not go in vain. The following monograph presents some guidelines to write a thesis of reasonable standard.

WHAT IS THESIS?

A systematically written document on a research work in complete form is known as a thesis. Whereas a research paper published in a journal is written in concise form, the thesis is written in more elaborate form. While writing both the documents, one should keep in mind that each of these must communicate the research works effectively to the readers. Thesis is a work supervised by experts and completed within a defined time period. Thesis is generally required in graduation and postgraduation in the form of a 'Dissertations'. However, it is almost always necessary for the higher degrees like Master or Doctor of Philosophy.

In medical sciences, it promotes academia and contributes to growth of the existing scientific knowledge. A well-conducted thesis that explored a new idea may change current practices and even change people's viewpoint. The purpose of thesis writing is to effectively communicate new scientific findings, thus it has to be clear, simple and well-ordered communication to transmit new scientific findings. As in journal articles, thesis may be written under the following broad headings, which is also known as IMRAD format.

I = Introduction; why a particular question (problem) was studied?
M = Methods; how was the problem studied?
R = Results; what was/were found?
A = And
D = Discussion; what do these findings mean?

Essential Parts of a Thesis

The thesis may be divided into the following subheadings:

- *Title:* Describe concisely the core contents of the subject.
- *Acknowledgment:* Give credit to those who helped in the research work.
- *Abstract/summary of thesis:* Summarize the major elements of the paper and the findings.
- *Table of contents:* List of all the section of the thesis and their page ranges.
- *Introduction:* Provide context and rationale for the study.
- *Review of literature:* Provide all the previous data in relation to subject of the study.
- *Aims and objectives:* This section should clearly list the major aims of the study. A good study should have limited number of aims.
- *Materials and methods:* Describe the experimental design and procedures clearly. It should be so clearly written so that another investigator should be able to reproduce similar result if he or she follows the methods described. Statistical analysis should also be clearly mentioned at the end of this section.
- *Results:* Summarize the findings without interpretation.
- *Discussion:* Interpret the findings of the study.
- *Conclusion:* Presents the major conclusions of the study.
- *References:* List all scientific papers, books and websites that should be cited.
- *Appendices:* Obviously, the sections listed above constitute an outline the generally accepted parts of the thesis. However, depending upon the type of the study, these may be modified. General principles of writing these sections are described below:

Title

A good title should contain fewest possible words that adequately describe the contents. It should be attractive and catch the attention of the readers. It should briefly mention the result of the study. It should not end with a note of interrogation. It is extremely important and must be chosen with great care as it will be read by thousands, whereas a few will read the entire thesis. Indexing and abstracting of the paper depends on the accuracy of the title. An improperly titled thesis will get lost. It should neither be too short nor too long as to be meaningless. It should be concise, specific and informative.

Acknowledgments

It is important to acknowledge supervisors, statistical advisers and others who have helped or offered support in any form. These include help in the form of technical support from any individual or laboratory within the same institution or outside it, special equipment, cultures, or any other material, financial assistance such as grants contracts or fellowships. One should show the proposed wording of the acknowledgment to the person whose help is being acknowledged.

Abstract

The abstract is a high-level overall summary of the thesis. The abstract should include a brief introduction and statement of the problem, as well as a summary of the methodology, findings and conclusions. A structured abstract should be preferred. It is good to present the essential data in the abstract on which conclusions are based.

Table of Contents

Conventionally, there should be a table of contents, followed by a list of tables and a list of figures. The table of contents includes all the major divisions of the thesis, including subsections. The relationship between major divisions and minor subdivisions should be shown by an appropriate use of capitals and indentations. The preliminary pages (Abstract, Acknowledgments and Contents) are numbered using roman numerals (i, ii, iii . . . .) and the remainder of the thesis is numbered using Arabic numerals (1, 2, 3 . . .). The title page is not numbered.

HOW TO WRITE THE INTRODUCTION AND BACKGROUND?

Introduction briefly presents why a particular research question has been addressed? The Introduction should state the purpose of the work and provide a pertinent summary of the rationale for the study. It should present the nature and scope of the problem investigated. It draws attention of the readers at the beginning so that he/she develops interest to read the rest of the thesis. Therefore, it should be interesting to motivate the readers to read the thesis with interest. It should focus on important scientific problem that the thesis either solves or addresses. This section should also focus on the previous relevant researches done in this area. It is good idea to state the hypothesis at the end of the introduction section.

Some of the tips to write the Introduction section of the thesis are given below:

Points one must know:
- One should give statement(s) reflecting the goal(s) of the thesis: why a particular study has been undertaken, or why the thesis has been written?
- It must contain sufficient background information so that the readers can understand the context and significance of the question.
- The authors should explain the scope of the work.
- It is good to break-up the introduction section into logical segments by using subheadings.

Points which are worth knowing:
- Introduction provides the rationale for the thesis.
- Authors should not tend to repeat the Abstract in the Introduction section.
- Authors should cite the previous works on which the current thesis built. Sufficient number of references should be cited in the Introduction section so that the readers could, by going to the library, achieve a sophisticated understanding of the context and significance of the question.

Points which are nice to know:
- Use the active voice as much as possible.
- Avoid lengthy or unfocused reviews of previous research.
- Cite peer-reviewed scientific literature or scholarly reviews. Avoid general reference works such as textbooks.
- Avoid using studies which are very old.

HOW TO WRITE AIMS?

In this section, clearly stated aims should be provided. If possible, they should be numbered. Generally speaking, while formulating aims for a thesis, the following points should be taken into consideration:
- Research question should be limited to one or two original questions answer to which is not available in the existing literature

- If one attempts to answer multiple questions in one thesis, this is unlikely to result in a good thesis
- One should creatively use theoretical insights relevant to the problem at hand while formulating the research questions
- When writing up the results and discussion, it is important to make sure that this hypothesis is actually answered.

HOW TO WRITE A REVIEW OF LITERATURE?

Review of literature describes the results, relevant methods and limitations of the previous studies in the area. This section may include the following issues: who conducted these studies and who were the participants, what protocols were followed and what were the findings and conclusions? It should be informative, evaluative and integrative. It is one of the areas of the thesis in which many students struggle for proper and sufficient amount of literature. The meticulousness with which the literature review is performed, is important to have complete coverage in this section. A literature review has several functions. The most important of these are:

Points one must know:

- The writer should present the current knowledge in the field relevant to the thesis
- Meta-analysis and systemic review should be preferred over poor quality studies. However, many times an original question related to a unique population or geographical area might be lost in a meta-analysis. In such situation, relevant original study must be cited.
- Compare and contrast the relevant studies and findings according to the thesis subject in question.
- Keep the literature search under control of Boolean search (A type of search allowing users to combine keywords with operators) tools like 'AND', 'OR' and 'NOT' in Pubmed (www.ncbi.nlm.nih.gov/pubmed). This would limit the search results to only those documents containing the two keywords.
- In this section, the writer is presenting a scholarly conversation already in progress. Therefore, after assessing the literature in the field, one should be able to answer the following questions:
  - Where did the problem come from?
  - What is already known about this problem?
  - What other methods have been tried to solve it?
  - What are the limitations in the existing literature?
  - How could limitation be solved in the current study to perform a better study?
- At the end of the Review of Literature section, readers should be able to find the following points:
  - The review is appropriate for the degree for which the thesis is being written.
  - The writer has reviewed the sources relevant to the research topic.
  - There has been full critical engagement with the literature.
  - It is clear how the current research objectives/questions/hypotheses fit in with previous scholarly work.

Points which are worth knowing:

- Comment on the strengths and limitations of the relevant previous studies and findings.
- Identify any gap in knowledge pertinent to the research questions to be addressed in the thesis.
- Selection of the literature for inclusion in the review is the ability to make connections between relevant materials and to choose which information to include and which information to omit.
- Reading other literature reviews in the same area is a useful guide to these decisions.

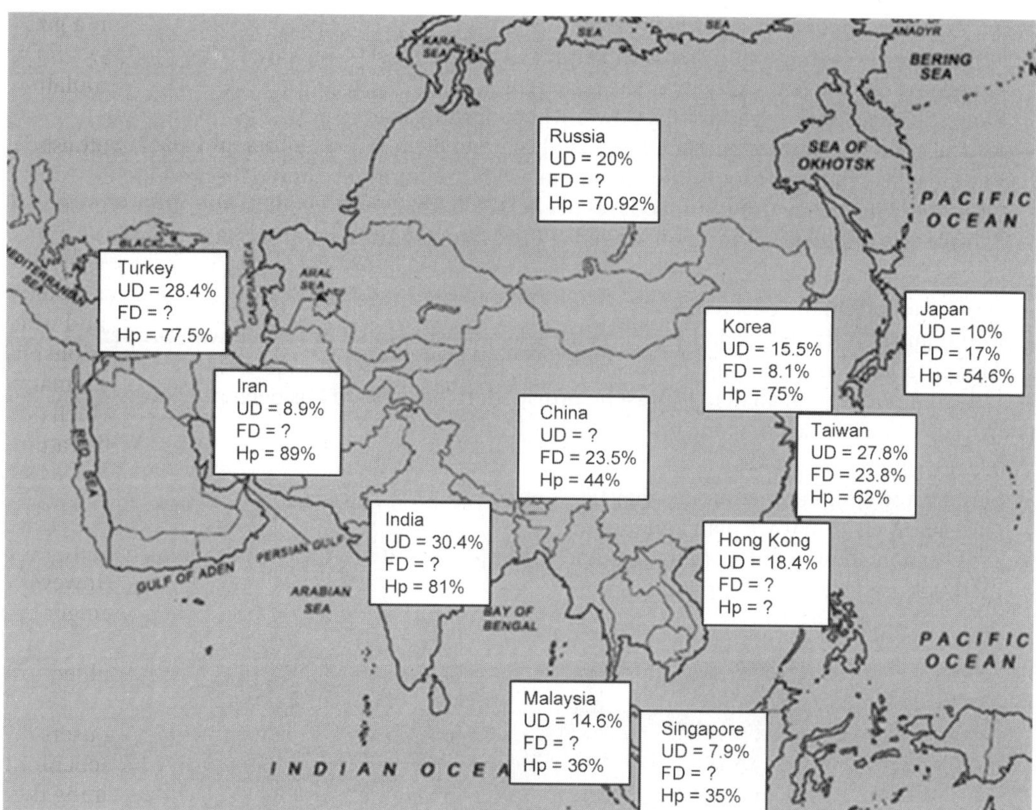

Fig. 1 Prevalence of uninvestigated **dyspepsia**, functional **dyspepsia** and seroprevalence of *Helicobacter pylori* infection of different Asian countries. Both population-based studies and institutional studies were included. *Abbreviations:* UD, uninvestigated dyspepsia; FD, functional dyspepsia; Hp, *Helicobacter pylori*
Source: Reproduced with permission from Ghoshal UC, et al. J Neurogastroenterol Motil. 2011;17:235-44

Points which are nice to know:

- Authors should first write the details of the studies to be reviewed in a neutral way.
- Subsequently, he/she should add critical (this does not always mean negative) analysis of the existing literature.
- Finally, he/she should integrate the various studies to compare and contrast their findings.
- Geographical distribution may be indicated by map (Fig. 1). One should remember that "a picture is more than 1000 words".
- Authors should ideally compose original figures himself/herself. However, if figures from other sources are used, one should mention the source and take necessary permission.

HOW TO WRITE METHOD SECTION?

Full details (observational or experimental subjects) should be described in the materials and methods. The methods should be stated in sufficient detail to allow other workers to reproduce the results. The statistical methods used should be outlined with enough detail to enable knowledgeable readers with access to the original data to verify the reported results.

Points one must know:

- Settings, types of study, study tools and ethics clearance must be included in methods section by which one can judge the quality of the research.
- State statistical analyses and study power where appropriate.
- Ethical guidelines for human or animal study should be described and approval of institutional human research review committee or animal welfare committee should be cited.
- Describe in detail hazardous procedures or chemicals involved, including precautions observed.
- Sample size calculation (how you arrived at the estimated number of subjects/samples, etc.)

Points which are worth knowing:

- Write methods in the past tense.
- If human subjects are used, the criteria for selection should be described with proper consent. Also criteria for inclusion and exclusion should be given.
- If the method is new, all details must be provided. If the method has been previously published in a scientific journal, only the reference should be given.

Points which are nice to know:

- Some of the complex techniques may be given in Figures 2 and 3.
- Give a flow chart of work plan and method
- This section allows readers to understand the objectives of the study and to judge whether the methods used were appropriate.

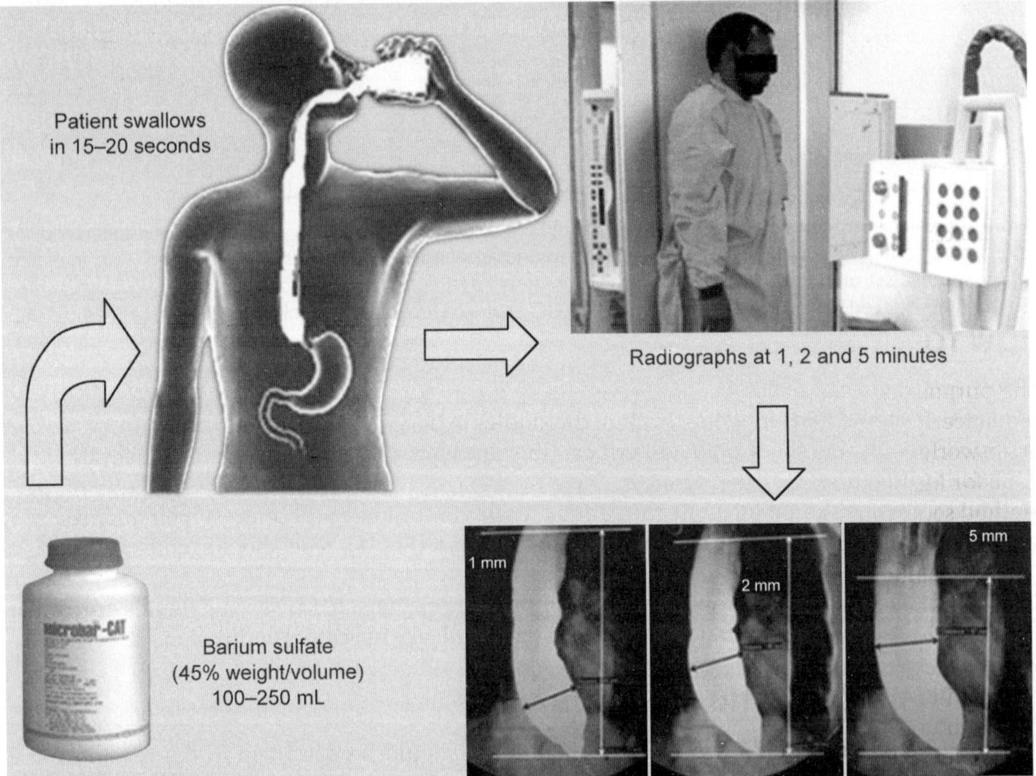

Fig. 2 Technique of timed barium esophagogram. Barium sulfate suspension (45% weight/volume) is swallowed by patient in standing position. Three radiographs are taken 1, 2 and 5 minutes later in left posterior oblique position

Source: Reproduced with permission from Neyaz Z, et al. J Neurogastroenterol Motil. 2013;19:251-6

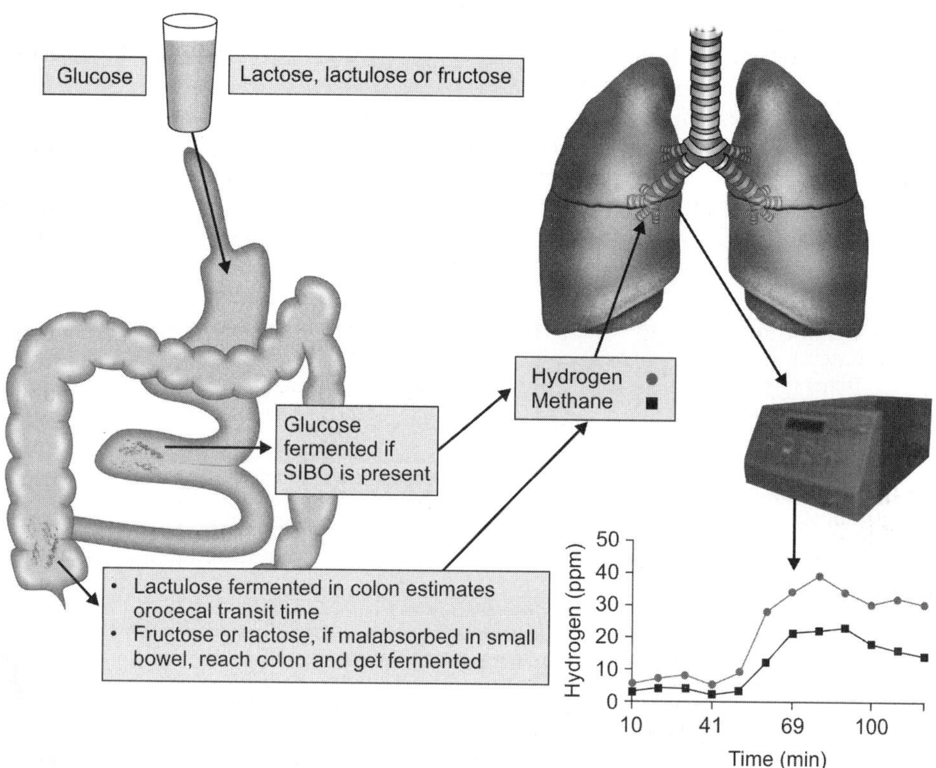

Fig. 3 A schematic diagram that shows principle of hydrogen breath test.
Abbreviations: SIBO, small intestinal bacterial overgrowth; ppm, parts per million
Source: Reproduced with permission from Ghoshal UC, et al. J Neurogastroenterol Motil. 2011;17:312-7

HOW TO WRITE RESULTS?

The purpose of this section is to summarize and illustrate the findings in an orderly and logical sequence. It needs to be clearly and simply stated since it constitutes the new knowledge contributed to the world. It is a good practice to sub-divide result section into multiple sub-sections as has been done for Method section. Even the chronology of different sub-headings should be similar to the Method section.

Points one must know:
- Results section must be written in past tense.
- One must not describe the methods that have already been described.

Points which are worth knowing:
- Repetitive presentation of the same data in different forms should be avoided.
- It is good to present complex data in the form of tables.
- Simple data should better be presented in the text rather than in the form of tables.
- Figures should be used to present some of the data (Fig. 4). Some of the complex data should be presented as graphs (Fig. 5). It is worth reiterating that "a picture is more than 1000 words".
- One should not present the same data in the text as well as in the tables and figures.

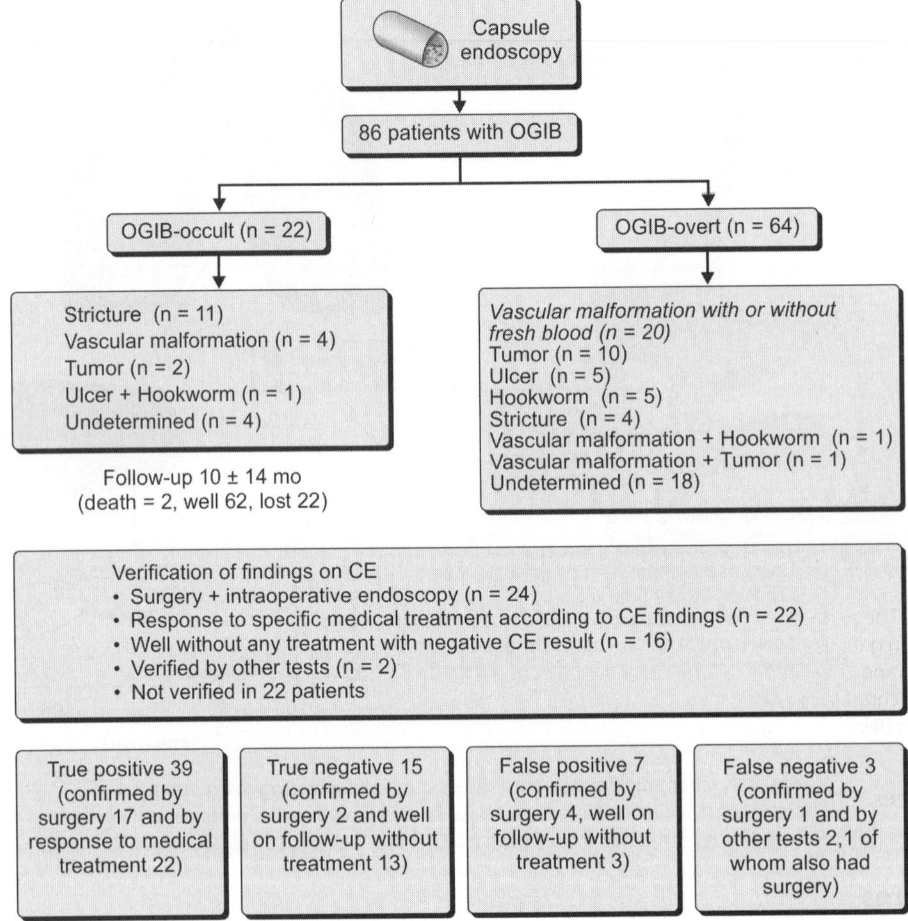

Fig. 4 Graphical presentation of data to interpret results

Source: Reproduced with permission from Ghoshal UC, et al. Digestive Endoscopy. 2011;23:17-23

Points which are nice to know:

- Results should be presented in logical sequence in the text, tables and illustrations.
- All figures and tables must be accompanied by a textual presentation of the key findings.
- All the figures should be accompanied by appropriate legends to figures.
- There should not be any table or figure that is not mentioned in the text.

Tables

Tables should be self-contained and complement, but not duplicate, information contained in the text. Tables should be numbered consecutively in Arabic numerals. Tables should be double-spaced and vertical lines should not be used to separate columns. Column headings should be brief, with units of measurement in parentheses; all abbreviations should be defined in footnotes. Footnote symbols: †, ‡, §, ¶, should be used (in that order) and *, **, *** should be reserved for

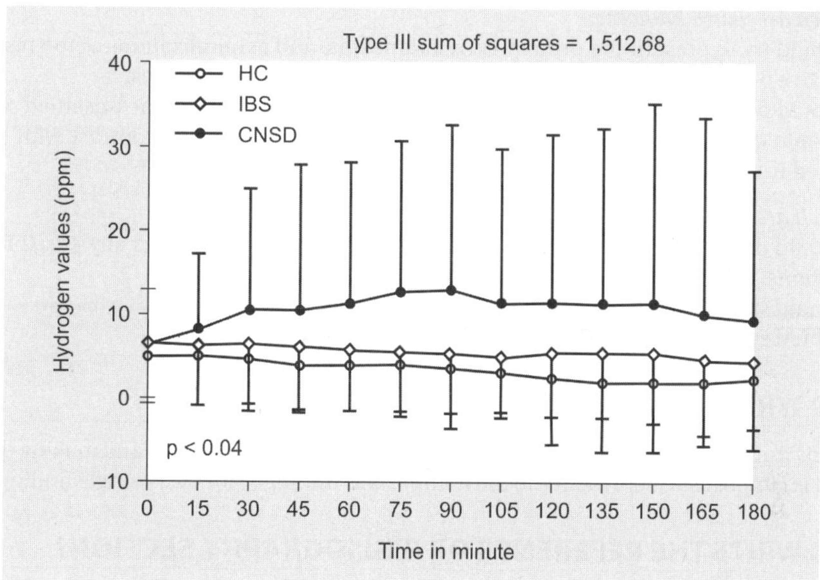

Fig. 5 The time by group interaction showing the correlation of hydrogen excretion at different time interval on CHBT in patients with IBS, CNSD, and HC. The data was analyzed using repeated measures ANOVA using general linear model for the time by group interaction in both the analysis. *Abbreviations:* IBS, irritable bowel syndrome; CNSD, chronic nonspecific diarrhea; HC, healthy control.
Source: Reproduced with permission from Ghoshal UC, et al. J Neurogastroenterol Motil. 2010;16:40-6.

P-values. The table and its legend/footnotes should be understandable without reference to the text.

Figures

Figures are appropriate for data sets that exhibit trends, patterns, or relationships that are best conveyed visually. Figure must be sufficiently described by its title and caption or legend, to be understandable without reading the main text of the results section.

HOW TO WRITE DISCUSSION?

Discussion section generally presents what do the findings presented in the study mean? It should present the strengths and weaknesses of the study, strengths and weaknesses of the present data in relation to other studies, a consideration of important differences in results, the meaning of the study, including possible explanations and implications for clinicians and policymakers, and a commentary considering unanswered questions and future research. Discussion considers the results in relation to the hypotheses proposed in the introduction section. This may include an evaluation of the methodology and of the relationship of new information to the existing corpus of knowledge in that field. Data given in the results section should not be reiterated here.

Points one must know:
- Most students feel that this is the most difficult section to write.
- Its primary purpose is to show the relationships among observed facts.
- It should end with a short summary or conclusion regarding the significance of the work.

Points which are worth knowing:

- One should try to present the principles, relationships, and generalizations of the results in the perspective of previous studies, clinical or social or patients' perspectives.
- One should point out any exceptions or any lack of correlation and define unsettled points.
- One should be show how these results and interpretations agree or contrast with previously published work.

Points which are nice to know:

- One should discuss the theoretical implications of the present work, and any possible practical applications.
- One should state the conclusions as clearly as possible.
- One should summarize the evidences for each conclusion.

HOW TO WRITE CONCLUSION?

Conclusions from your work should be summarized. Try to avoid repetition and making this section too long; it is supposed to represent the most important findings; not every single finding.

HOW TO WRITE THE REFERENCE OR BIBLIOGRAPHY SECTION?

Reference section is a standardized way of presenting the sources of information and ideas that have been used in the thesis. References refer to details of those works cited in the text. However, a bibliography also includes sources, which have not been cited in the text but was relevant to the subject and found useful in the formulation of the thesis. The main purpose of citing the references is to allow the readers to locate and read these documents, if they wish to do so. Referencing tools, like the use of the internet, can save a lot of time and deliver a higher quality outcome than manual methods. One may like to use referencing softwares like End-Note, Pro-Cite and Reference Manager. One should follow the same pattern for citing the references and outlined below:

Author-Date System

- This is a Harvard system. According to this system, the references are cited in the text by giving the author's surname and the year of publications and the papers are listed in a bibliography at the end of the text. If there are two authors, the last names of both the authors are written. If there are more than two authors, only the last name of the first author is written followed by the abbreviation 'et al.'. If a single statement requires more than one citation then the references are arranged chronologically from oldest to more recent, separated by semicolons. For example, e.g. "Gastric cancer (GC) is the world's second most common malignancy, which carries a poor prognosis (Parkin et al. 2001; Dikshit et al. 2012)".

Dikshit R, Gupta PC, et al. "Cancer mortality in India: a nationally representative survey." Lancet. 2012;379(9828):1807-16.

Parkin DM, Bray F, et al. "Estimating the world cancer burden: Globocan 2000." Int J Cancer. 2001;94(2):153-6.

Citation Order System

The references are numbered in the order they are mentioned in the text.

Points one must know:

- A list of all references used in the text must be written.
- One should use either 'Vancouver style' or 'author-date' style depending upon the preference of the Institution in which thesis is being submitted.
- One must follow the same pattern for adding the references.

APPENDICES

This section provides space for presenting the data on supportive materials used in the work. The thesis might, e.g. present machine learning models for automatically recognizing 500 different concepts. Rather than listing all 500 concepts in a table, one could choose 20 representative concepts for a table and mention the complete list of concepts in an appendix. Many organizations have regulation that limits the number of words in a thesis, but typically the material in the appendix does not count towards this word limit. Also, the examiners are not regularly expected to read or examine on the material in the appendix, but they can pick-up some observations from it.

General Points to be Followed while Writing the Thesis

- Present your ideas clearly. Identify the ideas you want to communicate and explain their relevance or significance.
- Present your ideas logically. Organize your ideas so that you lead your readers down your line of reasoning and, ultimately, to the same conclusion as you.
- Writing can be one of the most difficult aspects of the thesis because it requires you to organize many thoughts and express these in words.
- Writing a thesis is like writing any academic paper. If you take time to think about what you want to say and to plan out the different sections and their key ideas, it is much easier to put your thoughts into sentences.
- Begin planning and writing as soon as possible and do not feel obligated to start with the introduction. For example, you know you will have a section on your methodology; if you are already familiar with your methodology, you can start that section first.
- Do not worry about having everything planned out exactly from the very beginning. Your main ideas will stay the same even if your sections and their order may change.
- Do not feel pressurized to write a section perfectly the first time. It is more important to get words onto paper-even if they are half-formed phrases, than to write a perfect sentence on the first attempt. Do not spend too much time revising a section either. Save major revisions for the next step.

Points to be Remembered while Revising the Thesis

- It is important to plan time for revising after the bulk of your text is written. Ideally, you should put your work aside for a significant amount of time and then come back to revise.
- Setting aside your work allows you to return to it with a fresh perspective.
- Remember to leave plenty of time for your supervisor to provide feedback as well as for further revisions.
- Revision should be done with the readers in mind. Your goal is to communicate your research so that others can easily understand your ideas and argument(s).

Checklist for Revision

Ask the following questions on three aspects of your thesis while revising:

1. **Organization**
   - Do the introduction and conclusion present the same argument?
   - Are the chapters and sections in a logical order?
   - Are the ideas within sections and paragraphs in a logical order?
2. **Communication**
   - Do the section-titles adequately portray their contents?
   - Are main ideas in sections and paragraphs clearly stated?
   - Are the links between sections, paragraphs, and sentences made clear?
   - Do the paragraphs and sentences flow well?
   - Are figures and other images explained in the text?
   - Is your work free from grammatical errors (spelling, punctuation, etc.)?
   - Have you correctly referenced all borrowed material?
   - Is there plagiarism? (copying some other authors sentences in your thesis, which must be avoided)
3. **Presentation**
   - Are figures and other images easy-to-read and understand?
   - Are section headers clearly distinguishable?
   - Are your table of contents and title page accurate and free from errors?
   - Does the format (font, numbers, sections, page numbers, etc.) meet the requirements of your department or supervisor? Is it consistent?

SOME IMPORTANT LANGUAGE POINTS

Avoid complex sentence structure. Use simple and clear English. Use active voice. Always keep in mind that the paragraph is the essential unit of thought. It should start with an aim, briefly described in the mid and end with conclusion. Redundancy, plagiarism should be avoided. Syntax must be very carefully considered.

BIBLIOGRAPHY

1. American Psychological Association. Electronic references. Retrieved April 2006. http://www.apastyle.org/elecsource.html.
2. Judith Bell. Doing your research project. A guide for first-time researchers in education, health and social sciences. Maidenhead, Berkshire: Open University Press, 2005.
3. Guidelines for the preparation and submission of theses and written creative works. San Francisco State University, Graduate studies, USA, 2003.
4. Literature Reviews. The Writing Center, University of North Carolina-Chapel Hill, NC. 2005. http://www.unc.edu/depts/wcweb/handouts/literature_review.html.
5. Shane A Thomas. How to write health sciences papers, dissertations and theses. Churchill Livingstone, Harcourt Publishers Limited, first published 2000. p. 140.

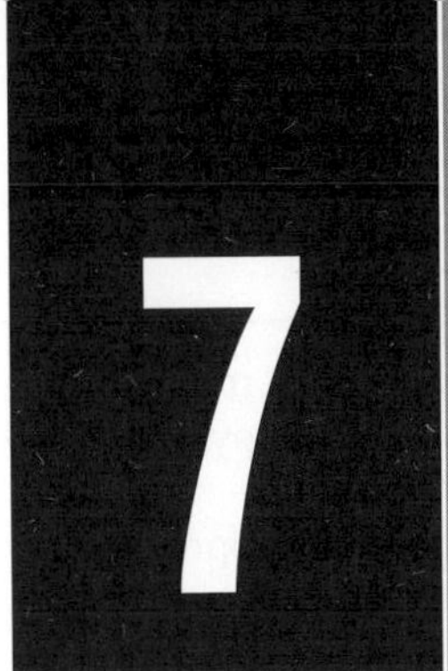

Renal Physiology and Anesthetic Implications: An Overview

Srabani Basu

ANATOMY OF THE KIDNEY

There are two separate kidneys each with its own fibrous capsule. They are located retroperitoneally in the upper abdomen, one in each paravertebral gutter adjacent to T12 to L3. They are approximately 12 cm long and weigh about 150 gm each. The right kidney is slightly lower than the left due to the presence of the liver in the right upper abdomen (Figs 1A and B).

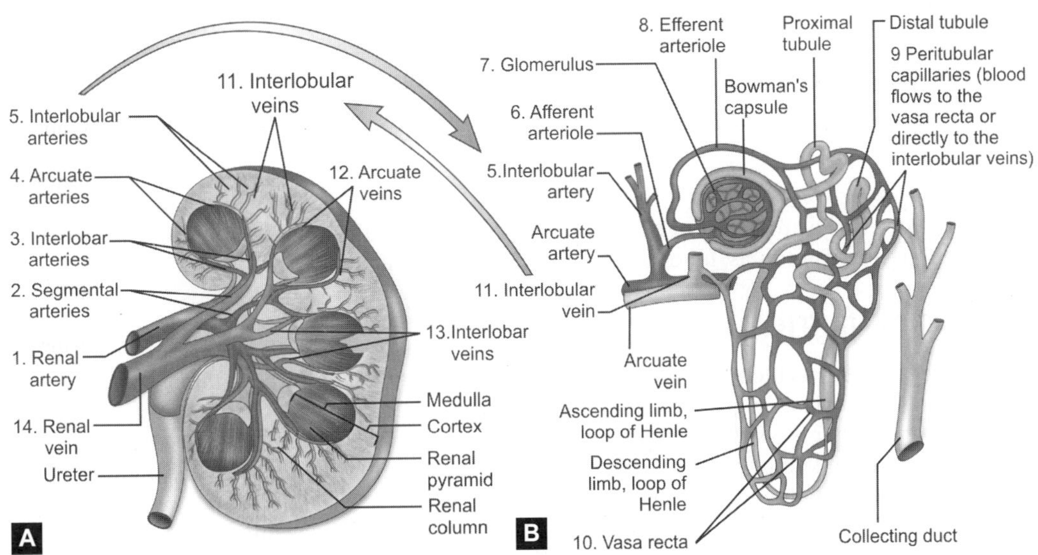

Figs 1A and B Normal anatomy of the kidney

The kidney has two distinct regions, a cortex around the outer edge and an inner medulla. The medulla is composed of numerous renal pyramids. At the innermost ends of the pyramids are calyces which receive urine, which then drain to the renal pelvis and the ureter.

The basic functional unit of the kidney is the nephron. Each kidney contains approximately 1–1.5 million nephrons. The kidney cannot regenerate new nephrons. Therefore, with renal injury, disease, or normal aging, there is a gradual decrease in nephron number.

Each nephron is basically a folded up tube which has a complex capillary network and capsule (the glomerulus and Bowman's capsule) situated proximally where plasma is filtered. Situated distally are the collecting ducts from which urine drains. Between Bowman's capsule and the collecting duct is the proximal convoluted tubule (PCT), the loop of Henle and the distal tubule, each of which serve specific functions. The nephrons are all oriented such that the glomerulus and Bowman's capsule lie in the cortex with their loop of Henle and collecting duct pointing towards and entering the medulla.

The final part of the ascending limb of the loop of Henle is located in the cortex of the kidney immediately adjacent to the afferent and efferent arterioles of its own glomerulus. This region contains the juxtaglomerular apparatus which consists of: (i) Macula densa, which are specialized cells in the wall of the tubule that are capable of sensing and responding to the composition of tubular fluid, (ii) Afferent arteriole granular cells which are specialized cells in the wall of the afferent arterioles that secrete renin.

FUNCTIONS OF THE KIDNEY

The kidneys are not just excretory organs that produce urine to remove waste products from the body, but are much more complex, performing many functions which have a wide range of physiological effects. The main functions of the kidney are:

To regulate:

- Extracellular fluid volume
- Extracellular fluid electrolyte composition
- Total body water volume
- The body's acid–base balance

To produce:

- The active form of vitamin D (1, 25-dihydroxycholecalciferol)
- Renin
- Erythropoietin
- Glucose

To excrete:

- Endogenous waste products; for example, urea, creatinine, uric acid, and bilirubin
- Exogenous waste products; for example, drugs and drug metabolites.

RENAL CIRCULATION

Each kidney receives its blood via the renal artery, a direct branch of the abdominal aorta. Venous drainage is usually via a single renal vein into the inferior vena cava (IVC). These vessels, (along with the ureter) enter the kidney via an indentation in its medial surface called the hilum. Due to the location of each kidney relative to the aorta and the IVC, the right kidney has a longer renal artery, whilst the left kidney has a longer renal vein.

Once the renal artery has entered the hilum of the kidney it divides into numerous interlobar arteries which radiate out towards the cortex. The interlobar arteries divide into arcuate arteries which arc around, following the line of the corticomedullary junction. The arcuate arteries give

Flow chart 1 Renal circulation system

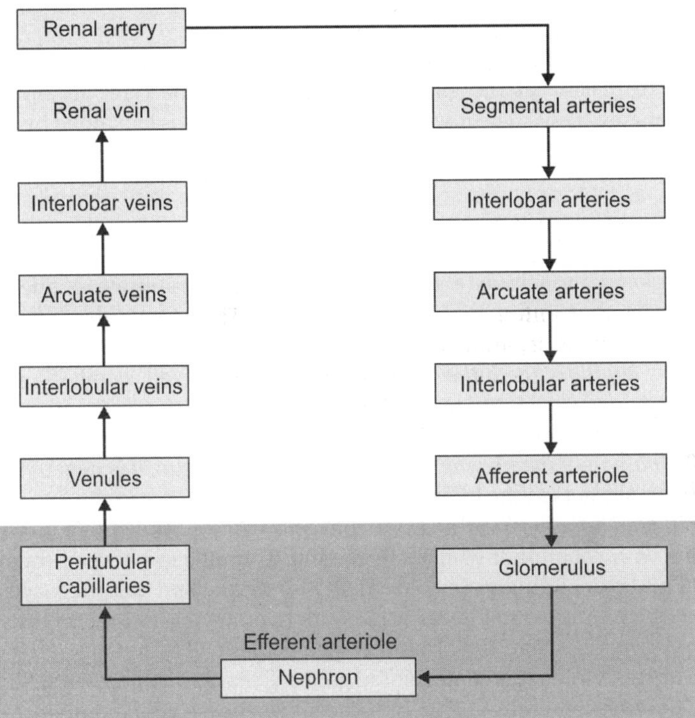

rise to several interlobular arteries which extend outwards towards the outer edge of the cortex. The afferent arterioles arise from the interlobular arteries, which supply blood to the glomerular capillaries. The glomerular capillaries are followed by the efferent arterioles and then the peritubular capillaries. There is a careful arrangement so that each set of glomerular capillaries and peritubular capillaries are associated with the same nephron.

The renal circulation is unique in having a capillary bed (glomerular capillaries) with arterioles at both ends. The tone of both the afferent and efferent arterioles can be varied to influence blood flow and pressure within the glomerulus. The venous system follows a similar pattern in reverse; blood flows from the peritubular capillaries into interlobular veins, arcuate veins, interlobar veins and then the renal vein (Flow chart 1).

RENAL BLOOD FLOW

The kidneys receive a total blood flow of approximately 1000 mL minute (20% of the cardiac output). This equates to 300–400 mL minute per 100 gm of tissue which is approximately six times that of the brain and five times that of the heart, weight for weight. The blood flow is not evenly distributed throughout the kidney and is not related to the level of metabolic activity. The cortex receives 90% of blood flow, which is the least metabolically active, while only 10% goes to the more metabolically active medulla. Consequently, the cortex has "luxury perfusion" with blood flow equating to ten times what is needed for oxygen delivery, whilst flow to the inner medulla is barely adequate to meet the oxygen demands.

- *Cortex blood flow:* 500 mL/min/100 gm
- *Outer medulla blood flow:* 100 mL/min/100 gm
- *Inner medulla blood flow:* 20 mL/min/100 gm.

The reason for such a seemingly excessive blood flow to the cortex, is that this is what is required to drive filtration of plasma at the glomerulus at an adequate rate, i.e. provide an adequate glomerular filtration rate (GFR). The lower blood flow of medulla is explained by the fact that higher flows would wash out solutes which are responsible for high tonicity of inner medulla.

GLOMERULUS AND ITS FUNCTION

The glomerulus essentially acts as a filter, producing an ultrafiltrate of the plasma from the glomerular capillaries that enters the Bowman's space. The glomerular filter is made of three distinct layers, each fulfilling separate functions:

1. *The glomerular capillary endothelium:* A highly specialized capillary endothelium with fenestrations (windows) to minimize the filter thickness. This layer prevents cellular components of blood coming into contact with the basement membrane.
2. *The glomerular basement membrane:* Made of connective tissue, it is negatively charged. This is the layer that actually acts as the filter.
3. *Bowman's epithelial cells (podocytes):* Epithelial cells with multiple projections (foot processes) which interlink with each other whilst still keeping a small gap between them creating a large surface area. This layer maintains the basement membrane and has phagocytic functions.

The degree to which solutes are filtered is dependent on two physical properties:

1. *Molecular weight:* Less than 7000 Daltons—molecules will be freely filtered
2. *Electrical charge:* A lower percentage of negatively charged molecules will be filtered. This is due to the basement membrane having a negative charge which therefore repels negatively charged molecules like albumin.

Normal Glomerular Filtration Rate (GFR)

Glomerular filtration rate (GFR) in an average-sized normal man is approximately 125 mL/min. Its magnitude correlates fairly well with surface area, but values in women are 10% lower than those in men even after correction for surface area. A rate of 125 mL/min is 7.5 L/hour, or 180 L/day, whereas the normal urine volume is about 1 L/day. Thus, 99% or more of the filtrate is normally reabsorbed. At the rate of 125 mL/min, the kidneys filter in 1 day an amount of fluid equal to 4 times the total body water, 15 times the ECF volume, and 60 times the plasma volume.

Control of GFR

The factors governing filtration across the glomerular capillaries are the same as those governing filtration across all other capillaries, i.e. the size of the capillary bed, the permeability of the capillaries, and the hydrostatic and osmotic pressure gradients across the capillary wall. For each nephron, K_f, the glomerular ultrafiltration coefficient, is the product of the glomerular capillary wall hydraulic conductivity (i.e. its permeability) and the effective filtration surface area. Permeability of glomerular capillaries (PGC) is the mean hydrostatic pressure in the glomerular capillaries, PT the mean hydrostatic pressure in the tubule, π_{GC} the osmotic pressure of the plasma in the glomerular capillaries, and π_T the osmotic pressure of the filtrate in the tubule.

Permeability of Glomerular Capillaries

The permeability of the glomerular capillaries is about 50 times that of the capillaries in skeletal muscle. Neutral substances with effective molecular diameters of less than 4 nm are freely filtered, and the filtration of neutral substances with diameters of more than 8 nm approaches zero. Between these values, filtration is inversely proportionate to diameter. Sialoproteins in the glomerular capillary wall are negatively charged. The amount of protein in the urine is normally less than 100 mg/day, and most of this is not filtered but comes from shed tubular cells. The presence of significant amounts of albumin in the urine is called albuminuria. In nephritis, the negative charges in the glomerular wall are dissipated, and albuminuria can occur for this reason without an increase in the size of the "pores" in the membrane.

Hydrostatic and Osmotic Pressure

The pressure in the glomerular capillaries is higher than that in other capillary beds because the afferent arterioles are short, straight branches of the interlobular arteries. The vessels "downstream" from the glomeruli, the efferent arterioles, have a relatively high resistance. The capillary hydrostatic pressure is opposed by the hydrostatic pressure in Bowman's capsule. It is also opposed by the osmotic pressure gradient across the glomerular capillaries and the gradient is equal to the oncotic pressure of the plasma proteins. The net filtration pressure is 15 mm Hg at the afferent end of the glomerular capillaries, but it falls to zero, i.e. filtration equilibrium is reached—proximal to the efferent end of the glomerular capillaries. This is because fluid leaves the plasma and the oncotic pressure rises as blood passes through the glomerular capillaries.

Factors Affecting the GFR

- Changes in renal blood flow
- Changes in glomerular capillary hydrostatic pressure
- Changes in systemic blood pressure
- Afferent or efferent arteriolar constriction
- Changes in hydrostatic pressure in Bowman's capsule
- Ureteral obstruction
- Edema of kidney inside tight renal capsule
- *Changes in concentration of plasma proteins:* Dehydration, hypoproteinemia, etc. (minor factors)
- Changes in K_f
- Changes in glomerular capillary permeability
- Changes in effective filtration surface area.

Changes in renal vascular resistance as a result of autoregulation tend to stabilize filtration pressure, but when the mean systemic arterial pressure drops below 90 mm Hg, there is a sharp drop in GFR. The GFR tends to be maintained when efferent arteriolar constriction is greater than afferent constriction, but either type of constriction decreases blood flow to the tubules.

Filtration Fraction

The ratio of the GFR to the renal plasma flow (RPF) is called the filtration fraction. Normally, 0.16–0.20. The GFR varies less than the RPF. When there is a fall in systemic blood pressure, the GFR falls less than the RPF because of efferent arteriolar constriction, and consequently the filtration fraction rises.

TUBULAR FUNCTION

General Considerations

The amount of any substance (X) that is filtered is the product of the GFR and the plasma level of the substance ($C_{In}P_X$). The tubular cells may add more of the substance to the filtrate (tubular secretion), may remove some or all of the substance from the filtrate (tubular reabsorption), or may do both. The amount of the substance excreted per unit time (U_XV) equals the amount filtered plus the net amount transferred by the tubules (TX). The clearance of the substance equals the GFR, if there is no net tubular secretion or reabsorption, exceeds the GFR, if there is net tubular secretion, and is less than the GFR, if there is net tubular reabsorption.

Mechanisms of Tubular Reabsorption and Secretion

Small proteins and some peptide hormones are reabsorbed in the proximal tubules by endocytosis. Other substances are secreted or reabsorbed in the tubules by passive diffusion between cells and through cells by facilitated diffusion down chemical or electrical gradients or active transport against such gradients. Movement is by way of ion channels, exchangers, cotransporters, and pumps.

Renal active transport systems have a maximal rate, or transport maximum (Tm), at which they can transport a particular solute. Thus, the amount of a particular solute transported is proportionate to the amount present up to the Tm for the solute, but at higher concentrations, the transport mechanism is saturated and there is no appreciable increment in the amount transported.

Tubular epithelium is a leaky epithelium in the tight junctions between cells permit the passage of some water and electrolytes. Paracellin-1, a protein localized to tight junctions, is related to Mg^{2+} reabsorption, and a loss-of-function mutation of its gene causes severe Mg^{2+} and Ca^{2+} loss in the urine.

Na^+ Reabsorption

The reabsorption of Na^+ and Cl^- plays a major role in body electrolyte and water metabolism. In addition, Na^+ transport is coupled to the movement of H^+, other electrolytes, glucose, amino acids, organic acids, phosphate, and other substances across the tubule walls. Na^+ is actively transported out of all parts of the renal tubule except the thin portions of the loop of Henle. Na^+ is pumped into the interstitium by Na^+-K^+-ATPase. Three Na^+ extrudes out in exchange for two K^+ that are pumped into the cell. The tubular cells are connected by tight junctions at their luminal edges. There is space between the cells along the rest of their lateral borders. Much of the Na^+ is actively transported into these extensions of the interstitial space called the lateral intercellular spaces. Proximal tubular reabsorbed fluid is slightly hypertonic, and water moves passively along the osmotic gradient created by its absorption into tubular epithelial cells. From the cells, the water moves into the lateral intercellular spaces. The rate at which solutes and water move into the capillaries from the lateral intercellular spaces and the rest of the interstitium is determined by the Starling forces determining movement across the walls of all capillaries, i.e. the hydrostatic and osmotic pressures in the interstitium and the capillaries Na^+ and H_2O leak back to the tubular lumen via the intercellular junctions, when the lateral intercellular spaces are distended.

Glucose Reabsorption

Glucose, amino acids, and bicarbonate are reabsorbed along with Na^+ in the early portion of the proximal tubule, Na^+ is reabsorbed with Cl^-. Glucose is typical of substances removed from the urine by secondary active transport. It is filtered at a rate of approximately 100 mg/min (80 mg/dL of plasma × 125 mL/min). Essentially, all of the glucose is reabsorbed, and no more than a few milligrams appear in the urine per 24 hours. The amount reabsorbed is proportionate to the amount filtered and hence to the plasma glucose level (PG) times the GFR up to the transport maximum (Tm_G); but when the Tm_G is exceeded, the amount of glucose in the urine rises. The Tm_G is about 375 mg/min in men and 300 mg/min in women. The renal threshold for glucose is the plasma level at which the glucose first appears in the urine in more than the normal minute amounts. One would predict that the renal threshold would be about 300 mg/dL, i.e. 375 mg/min (Tm_G) divided by 125 mL/min (GFR). However, the actual renal threshold is about 200 mg/dL of arterial plasma, which corresponds to a venous level of about 180 mg/dL. The actual renal threshold is less than the predicted threshold.

Glucose Transport Mechanism

Glucose reabsorption in the kidneys is similar to glucose reabsorption in the intestine. Glucose and Na^+ bind to the common carrier SGLT 2 in the luminal membrane, and glucose is carried into the cell as Na^+ moves down its electrical and chemical gradient. The Na^+ is then pumped out of the cell into the lateral intercellular spaces, and the glucose is transported by GLUT 2 into the interstitial fluid. Thus, glucose transport in the kidneys as well as in the intestine is an example of secondary active transport. The common carrier specifically binds the d-isomer of glucose, and the rate of transport of d-glucose is many times greater than that of l-glucose.

Other Secondary Active Transport

Symport is the transport of some amino acids, lactate, inorganic phosphate (Pi), H^+, and Cl^-. Secondary to the energy provided by active transport of Na^+ out of the renal tubular cells.

Like glucose reabsorption, amino acid reabsorption is most marked in the early portion of the proximal convoluted tubule. The main carriers in the luminal membrane cotransport Na^+, whereas the carriers in the basolateral membranes are not Na^+-dependent. Na^+ is pumped out of the cells by Na^+-K^+ ATPase and the amino acids leave by passive or facilitated diffusion to the interstitial fluid. Some Cl^- is reabsorbed with Na^+ and K^+ in the thick ascending limb of the loop of Henle.

REGULATION OF GLOMERULAR BLOOD FLOW

Autoregulation

Systemic blood pressure and the relative distribution of cardiac output continuously vary under the control of the autonomic nervous system. If these were allowed to cause alterations in renal blood flow (RBF), then the glomerular filtration rate (GFR) would be unpredictable. In order to prevent this, renal blood flow is kept constant across a wide range of perfusing pressures, i.e. RBF is autoregulated, and the GFR kept almost constant. Autoregulation aims to ensure that changes in blood pressure do not alter renal blood flow or GFR. Autoregulation of renal blood flow normally occurs between MAP of 80–180 mm Hg. There are also a number of other factors that affect renal blood flow and GFR.

Sympathetic Nervous System

Sympathetic nervous system (SNS) activation causes widespread vasoconstriction mediated by noradrenaline acting on α_1-adrenoreceptors on blood vessel smooth muscle cells. The afferent and efferent arterioles receive sympathetic innervation, and both constrict in response to increased SNS activity. This results in a significantly reduced renal blood flow. However, glomerular perfusion pressure is maintained due to greater constriction of the efferent arterioles. Overall the GFR only drops a little.

Renin-Angiotensin- Aldosterone System

The afferent arteriole wall contains some specialized 'granular' cells which secrete the proteolytic hormone renin. Renin release is stimulated by decreased afferent arteriole wall tension and decreased sodium and chloride delivery to the macula densa. Renin converts angiotensinogen to angiotensin 1 in the liver which is subsequently converted to angiotensin 2 in the lung by angiotensin converting enzyme (ACE). Angiotensin 2 causes greater constriction of efferent than afferent arterioles. Overall the GFR is maintained through an increase in filtration fraction.

Renal Prostaglandins

Prostaglandins are produced from arachidonic acid within the kidney when renal blood flow is compromized, for example, during increased SNS activity. Prostacyclin (PGI2) acts to cause afferent arteriole vasodilatation to maintain glomerular blood flow and GFR.

Atrial Natriuretic Peptide

Atrial natriuretic peptide (ANP) is stored in cardiac atrial cells and released in response to increased atrial stretch, i.e. an expansion in circulating volume. One of the actions of ANP is to cause vasodilatation of the afferent arterioles and increase GFR.

FORMATION OF URINE

The nephrons modify the 180 L/day of glomerular filtrate in order to maintain total body water and electrolyte homeostasis, and produce the usual 1–1.5 L/day of urine that allows excretion of waste products. The transformation of glomerular filtrate into urine through reabsorption of electrolytes and water by the nephrons relies on several distinct transport processes.

PROXIMAL TUBULE AND PERITUBULAR CAPILLARIES

The proximal tubule continues from Bowman's capsule and receives the glomerular filtrate. The role of the proximal tubule is to reabsorb most of the electrolytes and water it receives. The proximal tubules receive 180 L/day of glomerular filtrate and reabsorbs approximately 70% of this (127 L/day). The most important substances to be reabsorbed in the proximal tubules are sodium (Na^+), bicarbonate (HCO_3^-), chloride (Cl^-), glucose and water. The proximal tubule is also able to secrete certain substances into the lumen for excretion in the urine.

The peritubular capillaries are continuations of the efferent arterioles from the same nephron's glomerulus. These capillaries have a very low hydrostatic pressure and a high plasma oncotic pressure. The low hydrostatic pressure and high oncotic pressure favors reabsorption of the water and electrolytes that accumulate in the lateral spaces back into the plasma.

LOOP OF HENLE AND VASA RECTA

The main role of the loop of Henle is to produce a hypertonic environment within the renal medulla to allow the reabsorption of water by osmosis from the collecting tubules in order to retain water within the body and produce concentrated urine. Paradoxically, as part of this process the loop of Henle also alters the tubular fluid osmolality from being isotonic to plasma (290 mOsm/kg H_2O) to being hypotonic to plasma. The descending limb of the loop of Henle is permeable to water, and a further 30 L/day of the glomerular filtrate is reabsorbed here. The ascending limb of the loop of Henle is impermeable to water. The mechanism that allows the loop of Henle to establish this large osmotic gradient between the tubular lumen and the medullary interstitium is known as 'counter current multiplication'.

Counter Current Multiplication

The tubular cells of the thick part of the ascending limb of the loop of Henle contain Na^+/K^+ ATPases which actively pump Na^+ ions out of the cell and into the medullary interstitium. This sets up a concentration gradient from the tubular lumen into the cell for the reabsorption of other ions. In this case it leads to the reabsorption of one Na^+, one K^+ and two Cl^- ions via a specific co-transporter. However, as is seen elsewhere in the nephron the K^+ readily diffuses back out of the cells meaning that it is only really Na^+ and Cl that are reabsorbed. Also, the ascending limb of the loop of Henle is impermeable to water. The result is to deplete the tubular fluid of its osmotically active particles rendering it hypotonic, while increasing the concentration of osmotically active particles in the medullary interstitium making it hypertonic. The descending limb of the loop of Henle is permeable to water and ions and so readily equilibrates with the interstitium. The Na^+ and Cl^- reabsorbed from the ascending limb diffuse into the descending limb. Therefore, in effect, an osmotic gradient is established between the descending and ascending limbs of the loop of Henle. A difference in osmolality between the ascending and descending limbs at any given level within the medulla of around 200 mOsm/kg H_2O can be achieved. The absolute values of osmolality in the lumen and interstitium vary hugely up and down the medulla. The constant addition of Na^+ and Cl^- to the fluid of the descending limb of the loop of Henle leads to a progressive increase in its tonicity until it reaches the tip of the loop of Henle. In the ascending limb the tonicity of the fluid decreases as the Na^+ and Cl^- ions are reabsorbed as described earlier, 'trapping' a very high solute concentration within the medulla. By the time, the fluid leaves the loop of Henle and its tonicity has fallen to around 90 mOsm/kg H_2O.

Urea from the interstitium diffuses down its concentration gradient into the descending loop of Henle, resulting in a high urea concentration in the tubular fluid. The tubular fluid retains the high urea concentration all the way to the medullary part of the collecting ducts, where it is reabsorbed under the control of antidiuretic hormone. Through this mechanism the urea is recycled and can help make the medullary interstitium even more hypertonic than the counter-current multiplication mechanism could alone.

Counter Current Exchange

There is also a specialized network of blood vessels that mirrors the arrangement of the loops of Henle. These looped blood vessels are called the 'vasa recta' and are necessary in order to supply blood to the renal medulla and still maintain the osmotic gradients established in the medulla by the loop of Henle. If blood was supplied to the medulla and loop of Henle by a simple straight capillary, the hypertonic interstitium deep in the medulla would draw water out of the capillary by osmosis and ruin the work of the loop of Henle by reducing the osmotic gradient. In the descending limb of the vasa recta, water is drawn out of the capillaries and solutes enter to maintain osmotic equilibrium as the medullary interstitium becomes increasingly hypertonic. This process is then reversed in the ascending limb of the vasa recta with the water re-entering the capillary and solutes leaving—this is the 'counter-current exchange'. At the same time, the blood flowing in the vasa recta delivers nutrients (oxygen, glucose) to, and removes waste products (carbon dioxide) from the renal medulla. The net result of the process is to allow blood to flow through the medulla without altering the osmotic gradients that are present.

DISTAL TUBULE AND COLLECTING DUCTS

Of the original 180 L/day of glomerular filtrate, 127 L is reabsorbed in the proximal tubules and a further 30 L is reabsorbed in the descending limb of the loop of Henle leaving 23 L/day to enter the distal tubules and collecting ducts. Reabsorption of this part of the glomerular filtrate can be varied depending upon extracellular fluid volume and osmolality (Fig. 2). Clearly, this is still a very large volume and the vast majority of this must be reabsorbed every day to prevent rapid dehydration. In healthy adults, the concentration and volume of urine produced can vary enormously. The range is from about 90 mOsmol/kg H_2O and 23 L/day at its most dilute (if no water is reabsorbed in the collecting ducts) to 1400 mOsmol/kg H_2O and 400 mL/day (if the maximum amount of water is reabsorbed in the collecting ducts). The distal tubule is impermeable to water, but some Na^+ and Cl^- is reabsorbed here. The collecting duct is responsible for controlling what happens to this final 23 L/day of fluid. The collecting ducts can be divided into two regions; that part in the cortex of the kidney and the part in the medulla. There are several hormones that act on the collecting ducts, but the two most important are antidiuretic hormone (ADH) and aldosterone.

In their natural state, the collecting ducts are not permeable to water even though there is a huge osmotic gradient between the lumen and the surrounding medullary interstitium. Collecting ducts only become permeable to water under the influence of ADH. ADH controls the retention or loss

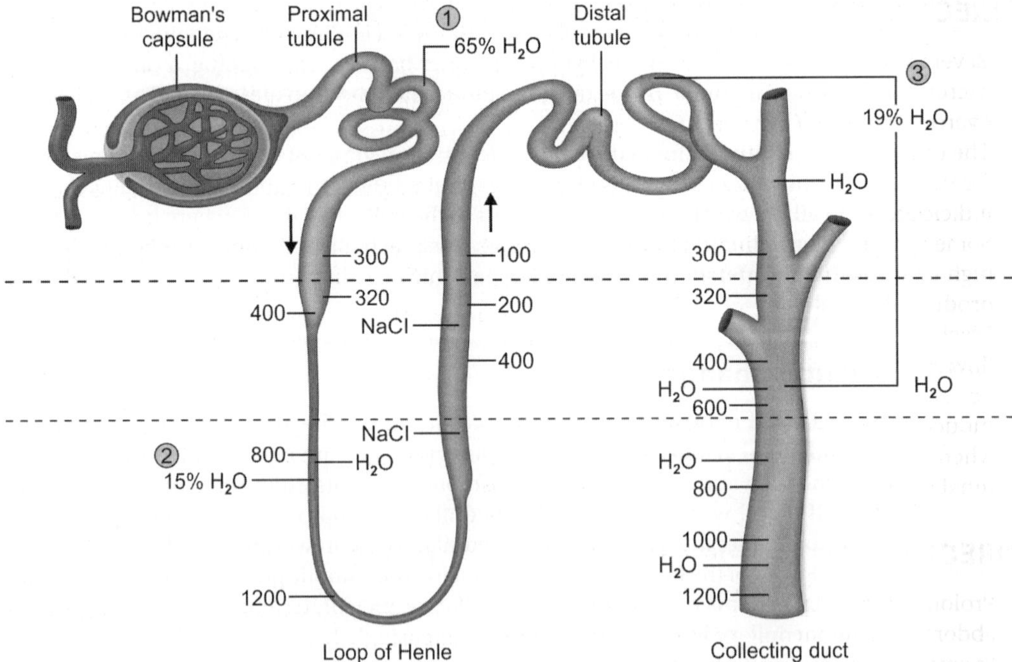

Fig. 2 Absorption and secretion of water electrolyte from different part of nephron

of water without any electrolytes, so called 'free' water. At all other points in the nephron water, reabsorption occurs with solute reabsorption so osmolality does not vary. By being able to retain or lose free water in this way ADH controls the ECF osmolality. If ECF osmolality increases, e.g. due to dehydration, an increase in ADH secretion will occur. If ECF osmolality decreases, e.g. after ingestion of water, there will be a decrease in ADH secretion.

Aldosterone is synthesized in the zona glomerulosa of the adrenal glands, and acts on the cortical part of the collecting duct. Its release is stimulated by a rise in plasma K^+ concentration and also by angiotensin II, if there is a reduction in the extracellular fluid (ECF) volume. A reduction in ECF volume, e.g. hemorrhage, leads to sympathetic nervous system (SNS) activation, a decreased blood flow through renal afferent arterioles and a reduced GFR and nephron tubular fluid flow. These three effects stimulate renin release and hence increase angiotensin II concentration. Aldosterone increases Na^+ reabsorption from the tubular fluid in exchange for K^+ and H^+ ions. The Na^+ that is reabsorbed in this way returns to the ECF and does not lead to water reabsorption as the cortical collecting ducts are impermeable to water. Therefore, aldosterone acts to increase ECF Na^+ content, which then via ADH dependent osmoregulatory mechanisms will lead to retention of water and restoration of ECF volume.

PERIOPERATIVE RENAL FUNCTION AND ANESTHETIC IMPLICATIONS

Several perioperative agents and events may disrupt renal physiology. If the disruption is severe enough or occurs in susceptible individuals it may induce ischemic or nephrotoxic acute tubular necrosis, the most common form of perioperative acute kidney injury. The risk factors for perioperative renal dysfunction include hypovolemia, hypotension, shock, congestive heart failure, diabetes, advanced age, pre-existing renal insufficiency and sepsis.

DIRECT ANESTHETIC EFFECTS ON RENAL FUNCTION

- Reversible decreases in renal blood flow, glomerular filtration rate, urinary flow and sodium excretion occur during both regional and general anesthesia. These effects can partly be overcome by maintenance of adequate intravascular volume and a normal blood pressure.
- The endocrine response to surgery and anesthesia is a stress response and is partly responsible for transient postoperative fluid retention and therefore perioperative fluid therapy should be judicious.
- Some volatile anesthetic agents may be nephrotoxic because of the release of fluoride ions in high concentration in blood, e.g. methoxyflurane, enflurane. Also compound A, a breakdown product of sevoflurane formed at low flows, is nephrotoxic in lab animals.
- Mechanical ventilation and PEEP may cause decreased RBF, GFR, sodium excretion and urine flow rate in susceptible individuals. Lung protective strategy of mechanical ventilation should be used.
- Induced hypotension during anesthesia, substantially reduces GFR and urine flow rate. However, when the duration of hypotension is kept less than two hours, no permanent impairment of renal function occurs.

DIRECT SURGICAL EFFECTS ON RENAL FUNCTION

- Prolonged pneumoperitoneum, produced in laparoscopic procedures, may produce an abdominal compartment like syndrome leading to oliguria.
- In aortic cross clamping, acute injury to the tubular epithelium and vascular endothelium causes decrease in RBF, rapid decline in GFR and tubular functions. But urine flow can be maintained

with early detection in reduction of GFR and prompt therapeutic interventions with mannitol, fenoldopam, etc.

- During cardiopulmonary bypass, hypotension promotes renal vasoconstriction and decreases RBF but the incidence ARF is usually low after uncomplicated surgery.

NEPHROTOXIC INSULTS IN THE PERIOPERATIVE PERIOD

- Drug-induced nephrotoxicity is usually seen in susceptible individuals with pre-existing risk factors. Aminoglycosides are the most common nephrotoxic drugs as they are polycationic and bind to the anionic brush border. Adequate hydration, avoidance of risk factors and once daily dose may reduce the incidence of nephrotoxicity. Some NSAIDs inhibit cyclo-oxygenase 1, and therefore the renal protective action of prostaglandins is lost. Nephrotoxicity of NSAIDs is increased in presence of other nephrotoxins and cardiovascular instability.
- The nephrotoxicity of radiocontrast dyes is probably due to microvascular obstruction and the risk is increased in diabetes, hypovolemia and CHF. Prevention of toxicity depends on adequate hydration and use of nonionic, low or isoosmolar radiocontrast media.
- *Sepsis:* Sepsis is the most common cause of new onset acute renal failure in the perioperative period. Renal autoregulation is impaired in sepsis. Renal dysfunction in sepsis is characterized as a vasomotor nephropathy. Renal vasoconstriction, decreased ultrafiltration and decreased GFR are induced by endotoxin.

CONCLUSION

Good perioperative care and attention to details will be the best chance of avoiding deterioration in renal function and development of renal failure in the perioperative period. These include:

- Judicious fluid therapy
- Proper oxygen transport
- Short crossclamp time in aortic surgery
- Short bypass time in cardiac surgery
- Appropriate use of drugs like frusemide, mannitol, fenoldopam, etc.
- Avoidance of nephrotoxic drugs.

BIBLIOGRAPHY

1. Matthew Gwinnutt, Mersey Deanery, Jennifer Gwinnutt, Mersey Deanery. Renal physiology, Part 1. Anaesthesia Tutorial, 2012.
2. Matthew Gwinnutt, Mersey Deanery, Jennifer Gwinnutt, Mersey Deanery. Renal physiology, Part 2. Anaesthesia Tutorial, 2012.
3. Miller R. Millers Anesthesia, Renal physiology, 7th edn. Churchill Livingstone: Elsevier; 2010.pp.441-79. (2010 Chapter 18.pp.441-79.)
4. Morgan Michael's Clinical Anesthesiology, Renal Physiology and Anesthesia, 4th edn, Chapter 31.

8

Anesthetic Considerations in Pregnant Patients with Cardiac Disease

Sampa Dutta Gupta

INTRODUCTION

The prevalence of cardiac disease in pregnancy has fallen over the last three decades to less than 1%.[1] Rheumatic heart disease is still a major heart problem associated with pregnancy in India, despite its declining trend.[2,3]

1. What are the physiological considerations in pregnancy and puerperium? (Must know)

Ans. Table 1 shows cardiovascular changes during pregnancy and Tables 2 and 3 show hemodynamics during labor and puerperium.

Table 1 | Cardiovascular changes during pregnancy

Parameter	*Percentage of change*
Cardiac output	40–50% increase
Stroke volume	30% increase
Heart rate	15–25% increase
Intravascular volume	45% increase
Systemic vascular resistance	20% decrease
Systolic BP	Minimal change
Diastolic BP	20% decrease at mid-pregnancy Pre-pregnant values at term
CVP	Unchanged
O_2 consumption	30–40% increase

Table 2 | Hemodynamics during labor

Parameter	*Stage of labor*	*Percentage of change*
Cardiac output	Latent phase	10% increase
	Active phase	25% increase
	Expulsive phase	40% increase
	Immediate postpartum	75–80% increase
Heart rate	All stages	Increase
CVP	All stages	Increase

Table 3 | Hemodynamics during puerperium

Parameter	*Postpartum*	*Percentage of change*
Cardiac output	Within 1 hour	30% above pre-labor values
	24–48 hours	Just below pre-labor values
	2 weeks	10% above pre-pregnant values
	12–24 weeks	Baseline pre-pregnancy values
Heart rate	Immediate	Decrease
	2 weeks	Pre-pregnant values
Stroke volume	48 hours	Remains above prelabor values
	24 weeks	10% above pre-pregnant values

VALVULAR HEART DISEASE

Management of valvular heart disease during pregnancy must be multidisciplinary. The following need to be addressed:

- Accurate diagnosis as to which valves are involved
- Assessment of the severity of the lesion
- Degree of impairment resulting from the lesion and concomitant therapy.

Rheumatic mitral stenosis forms 88% of the heart diseases complicating pregnancy in the tertiary referral center in India.[4] The mortality and morbidity are considerably reduced[5] by better perinatal care.

2. What are the risk factors for pregnant women with cardiac disease?

Ans. Risk assessment

- NYHA 111 or 1V or cyanosis
- Left ventricular systolic dysfunction (ejection fraction <.40)
- Left heart obstruction (mitral valve area <2.0 cm^2, aortic valve area <1.5 cm^2 or left ventricular outflow gradient >30 mm Hg)
- A cardiac event like arrhythmia, stroke, transient ischemic attack, pulmonary edema before pregnancy.

Siu and colleagues, developed a risk index incorporating these factors.

In a woman with heart disease and with no other risk factors, the incidence of a cardiac event during pregnancy is about 5%, increasing to 25% with one risk factor and 75% with more than one risk factor.

Ref:[9] Data taken from Siu SC, Sermer M, Colman JM, et al. Retrospective multicenter study of pregnancy outcomes in women with heart disease. Circulation 2001;104:515-21.

Table 4 | The New York Heart Association (NYHA) Functional Classification in a patient with heart disease

Class	*Symptoms with physical activity*	*Limitations of physical activity*	*Findings at rest*
I	None	None	Comfortable at rest
II	Symptomatic with greater than ordinary activities	Slight	Comfortable at rest
III	Symptomatic with ordinary activities	Marked	Comfortable at rest
IV	Symptomatic at less than ordinary levels of activity	Any activity	May or may not be symptomatic at rest

Symptoms include fatigue, dyspnea, palpitations, heart failure.

Ref:[10] Data taken from The Criteria Committee of the New York Heart Association Nomenclature and Criteria for Diagnosis of Diseases of the Heart and Great vessels Ninth edition. Little Brown and Company; 1994. pp.253-5.

3. What are the clinical features in a normal pregnancy that can mimic a cardiac lesion?

Ans.

- Dyspnea
- Pedal edema
- Cardiac impulse
- Jugular vein becomes distended and JVP is raised
- Systolic ejection murmur along the left sternal border occur in 96% women.

Nevertheless, in the developed world, rheumatic disease has become uncommon and complex congenital heart disease is increasing in the recent decades. With the advent of intensive obstetric and anesthetic care, the death rate of pregnant women with heart disease is lower in mitral stenosis compared with other congenital heart diseases like Eisenmenger's syndrome.[6] Although mitral stenosis is often associated with mitral regurgitation, morbidity is usually related to mitral stenosis.[7] Regurgitant valvular lesions are well tolerated in pregnancy in comparison to stenotic lesions which have a greater potential for decompensation.

MITRAL STENOSIS

4. What is the pathophysiology of mitral stenosis?

Ans. When the normal mitral valve orifice area of 4–6 cm^2 is progressively reduced to 2 cm^2, the classical symptoms of mitral heart disease start appearing. Consequent to the fixed cardiac output state, the heart cannot cope up with situations warranting increased metabolic demand or increased blood volume. When the stenosis progresses, the left atrium dilates and the left atrial pressure increases. A pressure gradient develops during diastole between the left atrium and the left ventricle. This pressure gradient is the hemodynamic hallmark of mitral stenosis. Hence, the back pressure on the pulmonary vessels leads to pulmonary congestion and, in severe cases, pulmonary edema and if longstanding pulmonary hypertension develops during pregnancy.

5. What are the effects of mitral stenosis on pregnancy?

Ans. Women with severe mitral stenosis (Table 5) often do not tolerate the cardiovascular demands of pregnancy. The increased volume load and tachycardia of pregnancy together cause the patients to deteriorate and advance from one New York Heart Association (NYHA) class to another.

- The physiologic tachycardia of pregnancy limits the time available for left ventricular filling and increased left atrial and pulmonary arterial pressures.

Table 5 | Severity grading of mitral stenosis

Measurement	*Normal*	*Mild*	*Moderate*	*Severe*
Mitral valve area (cm^2)	4.0–6.0	1.5–2.5	1.0–1.5	<1.0
Mean pressure gradient (mm Hg)	<2	2–6	6–12	>12
Pulmonary artery mean pressure (mm Hg)	10–20	<30	30–50	>50

- The expanded blood volume results in pulmonary congestion and edema.
- Atrial fibrillation worsens this scenario and about 80% of the cases of systemic emboli occur in patients with atrial fibrillation.

6. When is the risk of maternal death highest and why?

Ans. The risk of maternal death is greatest during labor and during the immediate post-partum period. The sudden increase in the preload immediately after delivery, due to autotransfusion from the uterus, may flood the central circulation, resulting in severe pulmonary edema. In addition, there continues to be autotransfusion of blood for 24–72 hours after delivery. Thus, the risk of pulmonary edema extends for several days after delivery.[8] Therefore, it is prudent to continue hemodynamic monitoring for up to 24 hours after delivery.

7. How do you predict maternal morbidity and mortality in a parturient with mitral stenosis?

Ans. The maternal outcome correlates well with the New York Heart Association (NYHA) functional classification.[10] Maternal cardiac complications, such as pulmonary edema and arrhythmias, occurred in 35% of the pregnancies. The incidence of maternal cardiac complications correlates with the severity of the mitral stenosis (67% for severe, 38% for moderate and 26% for mild disease).[11] Mortality rates for class I and II amount to <1%, whereas they range between 5 and 15% for class III and IV. The perinatal mortality rate for class III and IV is as high as 20–30%.

8. How do you evaluate a pregnant patient with symptomatic mitral stenosis?

Ans. The evaluation includes:

- History
- Physical examination
- ECG in 12 leads
- 2D echocardiography (diagnostic tool of choice) to evaluate the mitral valve morphology, mitral valve hemodynamics and pulmonary artery pressure.
- Diagnostic cardiac catheterization when echocardiography is nondiagnostic or results are discordant with clinical findings.[12]

9. How do you manage a patient with mitral stenosis?

Ans. *Medical:* In symptomatic patients, medical treatment should be the first line of management. Treatment involves bed rest, oxygen therapy and diuretics. Beta-adrenergic receptor blockade is useful to prevent tachycardia during pregnancy. Propranolol or atenolol decreases the incidence of maternal pulmonary edema without adverse effects on the fetus or neonate.[13] Recent trials conclude that digoxin has no role in prevention and in the treatment of cardiac failure.[14] Salt restriction and administration of a diuretic if there is evidence of pulmonary vascular congestion are advocated.

Atrial fibrillation requires aggressive treatment with digoxin and beta blockers to revert it to sinus rhythm and anticoagulation to prevent systemic embolization. Cardioversion should be performed if pharmacologic therapy fails to control the ventricular response. Anticoagulation, even in the absence of atrial fibrillation, is beneficial.[15,16]

Warfarin is not used during 12–36 weeks of gestation due to the risks of fetal embryopathy[44,45] and bleeding during parturition. One of the standard regimens followed during pregnancy is

- SC/IV heparin up to 12 weeks gestation (aPTT 1.5–2.5 times normal)
- Warfarin from 12–36 weeks gestation (maintain INR 2.0–3.0)
- SC/IV heparin after 36 weeks gestation.[48]
- Antibiotic coverage for infective endocarditis is reserved only for patients with previous history of infective endocarditis or presence of established infection.[43]

Surgical: If mitral stenosis is diagnosed before pregnancy, mitral commissurotomy is preferred. During pregnancy, the second trimester is the preferred period for any invasive procedure. Percutaneous valvuloplasty using the Inoue balloon technique has become the accepted treatment for patients with severe symptomatic mitral stenosis. Percutaneous balloon mitral valvuloplasty provides palliation for pregnant women with mitral stenosis, and the reported success rate is nearly 100%. Successful balloon valvuloplasty increases the valve area to >1.5 cm^2 without a substantial increase in mitral regurgitation.[17] Although the maternal outcome in percutaneous balloon mitral valvuloplasty and open commissurotomy are the same, the fetal loss is high in open commissurotomy, at a ratio of 1:8.[18] Valve replacement is reserved for severe cases with calcified valve and in mural thrombus where the maternal mortality is 1.5–5% and the fetal loss is 16–33%.[19]

10. What is the scope of epidural labor analgesia in patients with mitral stenosis?

Ans. Most reports have recommended vaginal delivery under epidural labor analgesia, unless obstetrically contraindicated. Tachycardia, secondary to labor pain, increases flow across the mitral valve, producing sudden rises in left atrial pressure, leading to acute pulmonary edema. This tachycardia is averted by epidural analgesia without significantly altering the patient hemodynamics.[20] Invasive cardiac monitoring like radial artery cannulation and pulmonary catheter are beneficial in assessing the cardiac output, pulmonary artery pressure and for guiding fluid and drug therapy, especially in the high risk patients.[21,22] Sudden drops in systemic vascular resistance (SVR) in the presence of a fixed cardiac output can be prevented by small bolus doses of phenylephrine, with volume expansion when necessary.

11. What are the anesthetic considerations while administering neuraxial blockade to parturients with mitral stenosis when vaginal delivery is contemplated?

Ans. Combined spinal-epidural analgesia during labor using intrathecal fentanyl 25 µg produces good analgesia without major hemodynamic changes during the first stage of labor.

During the second stage of labor, only the uterine contractile force should be allowed rather than the maternal expulsive effort that is always associated with the Valsalva maneuver and hence instrumentation is indicated.

Supplementary analgesia for instrumentation with slow epidural boluses of fentanyl and a low concentration of bupivacaine reduces SVR and the cardiac preload.[23] Low spinal anesthesia for vaginal instrumental delivery has also given good results.[24]

12. What are the goals anesthetic management for ceserean delivery?

Ans. The goals for the anesthetic management of patients with mitral stenosis are:

- Maintenance of an acceptable slow heart rate in sinus rhythm
- Immediate treatment of acute atrial fibrillation and reversion to sinus rhythm
- Avoidance of aortocaval compression
- Maintenance of adequate venous return
- Maintenance of adequate SVR
- Prevention of pain, hypoxemia, hypercarbia and acidosis, which may increase pulmonary vascular resistance.

13. How do you plan the anesthetic technique for cesarean section in a parturient with mitral stenosis?

Ans. Epidural and continuous spinal anesthetic techniques are attractive options.

One of the major advantages of epidural analgesia is that it can be administered in incremental doses and that the total dose could be titrated to the desired sensory level. This, coupled with the slower onset of anesthesia, allows the maternal cardiovascular system to compensate for the occurrence of sympathetic blockade, resulting in a lower risk of hypotension and decreased uteroplacental perfusion. Moreover, the segmental blockade spares the lower extremity 'muscle pump,' aiding in venous return, and also decreases the incidence of thromboembolic events. Invasive hemodynamic monitoring, judicious intravenous administration of crystalloid and administration of small bolus doses of phenylephrine maintain maternal hemodynamic stability.[24]

Continuous spinal anesthesia, although infrequently practiced, could be a better option in some rare situations like accidental dural puncture.

14. What are the disadvantages of administering general anesthesia in parturients with cesarean section?

Ans. General anesthesia has the disadvantage of increased pulmonary arterial pressure and tachycardia during laryngoscopy and tracheal intubation. Moreover, the adverse effects of positive-pressure ventilation on the venous return may ultimately lead to cardiac failure.[25]

Despite these disadvantages, if general anesthesia is contemplated, tachycardia, inducing drugs like atropine, ketamine, pancuronium and meperidine, should be totally avoided. A beta-adrenergic receptor antagonist and an adequate dose of opioid like fentanyl should be used.

MITRAL REGURGITATION

15. What are the most common causes of mitral regurgitation in pregnancy?

Ans. The most common causes of mitral regurgitation are myxomatous degeneration, ischemic papillary muscle disease, rheumatic fever and endocarditis. During pregnancy, the usual causes are rheumatic valvular disease and mitral valve prolapse.[1]

16. How does mitral regurgitation affect a pregnant patient?

Ans. The hemodynamic changes of pregnancy are beneficial to patients with mitral regurgitation. The greater volume of blood and lower SVR promote forward flow across the incompetent valve.

- Pulmonary congestion can be treated with a diuretic and a vasodilator if there is associated systemic hypertension.
- There is a higher risk of atrial fibrillation during pregnancy in women with mitral regurgitation.
- The hypercoagulability of pregnancy increases the risk of systemic embolization. Anticoagulation may be indicated if:
  - Cardioversion is planned
  - There is a history of embolic phenomenon
  - A new onset of atrial fibrillation occurs.

17. What are the goals of anesthetic management for patients with mitral regurgitation?

Ans.

- Prevention of increases in SVR.
- Maintenance of a normal to slightly increased heart rate in sinus rhythm
- Aggressive treatment of acute atrial fibrillation
- Avoidance of aortocaval compression
- Maintenance of venous return
- Prevention of increases in central blood volume

- Avoidance of myocardial depression during general anesthesia
- Prevention of pain, hypoxemia, hypercarbia and acidosis which can increase pulmonary vascular resistance.

18. What is the anesthesia of choice for management of vaginal/cesarean delivery?

Ans.

- Continuous epidural anesthesia is preferred.
- Pain provokes an increase in SVR which is minimized by epidural anesthesia and may in fact lead to a modest decrease in SVR, which promotes forward flow of blood and minimizes pulmonary congestion.
- The hypotension with epidural anesthesia should be managed with:
  - The careful administration of a crystalloid
  - Left uterine displacement
  - Ephedrine (chronotropic agent is desirable)

19. What are the preferred drugs if general anesthesia is administered?

Ans. Keeping in mind the hemodynamic goals discussed earlier, the anesthesiologist should try to maintain a heart rate slightly on the higher side and decreased SVR. Ketamine and pancuronium may be useful in parturients with mitral regurgitation.

AORTIC STENOSIS

20. What is the most common cause of aortic stenosis in pregnancy?

Ans. Congenital bicuspid aortic valve is the most common cause of AS in pregnancy. Rheumatic aortic disease is less common and occurs with mitral valve disease in approximately 5% of women with rheumatic valvular disease.

21. When does aortic stenosis become severe or critical?

Ans. Normal valve area is 2.6–3.5 cm^2. Severe aortic stenosis is defined as a valve area less than 0.8–1.0 cm^2 and a peak gradient of greater than 40–50 mm Hg.[1]

22. What is the impact of aortic stenosis on pregnancy?

Ans.

- The greater blood volume of pregnancy allows women with mild disease to tolerate pregnancy well. Management is conservative. Prophylactic antibiotics may be administered to decrease the risk of infective endocarditis in patients with suspected bacteremia.[52]
- Women with severe aortic stenosis are advised to undergo corrective surgery before conception. They are unable to meet the greater demands of pregnancy and present with dyspnea, angina or syncope. Symptoms early in gestation may warrant termination of pregnancy to save the life of the mother.

23. What are the goals of anesthetic management in a parturient with aortic stenosis?

Ans.

- Maintenance of a normal heart rate in sinus rhythm
- Maintenance of adequate SVR
- Maintenance of intravascular volume
- Avoidance of aortocaval compression
- Avoidance of myocardial depression during general anesthesia.

24. How do you evaluate a patient with aortic stenosis?

Ans. Next to the physical examination and ECG, echocardiography is used to assess the anatomy of the aortic valve, grade the stenosis severity and assess left ventricular function.[26]

25. What is the anesthetic technique of choice in vaginal/cesarean delivery in a parturient with aortic stenosis?

Ans. Moderate to severe aortic stenosis remains a relative contraindication for single shot spinal anesthesia.

Numerous reports have described the safe use of continuous epidural or continuous spinal anesthesia for vaginal or cesarean delivery.

Epidural anesthesia can be administered in incremental doses of a local anesthetic and fentanyl to achieve a desired sensory level. Hypotension can be tackled with careful titration of small volumes of a crystalloid.

Typically, local anesthetic solutions containing epinephrine should be avoided in patients with moderate to severe stenosis, because 1) unintentional intravascular injection of epinephrine can precipitate tachycardia, 2) systemic absorption of epinephrine from the epidural space can diminish SVR and lower venous return.

26. What anesthetic agent will you prefer and why, if general anesthesia is required?

Ans. A combination of etomidate and a modest dose of an opioid are the induction agents of choice and preferred to sodium thiopental and/or propofol which causes myocardial depression and/or vasodilatation and ketamine that causes tachycardia.

However, a combination of low dose thiopental and ketamine may be suitable induction agents if etomidate is not available.

AORTIC REGURGITATION

27. What are the causes of aortic regurgitation ?

Ans. Aortic regurgitation occurs more frequently than aortic stenosis in women of child bearing age. Aortic regurgitation in young women may be due to congenital bicuspid valve, rheumatic heart disease, endocarditis or a dilated aortic annulus.[1]

Rheumatic heart disease accounts approximately 75% of affected patients.

28. What are the hemodynamic effects of aortic regurgitation on pregnancy?

Ans. Aortic regurgitation is often well tolerated in pregnancy for at least three reasons:

1. The physiologic tachycardia of pregnancy results in a decrease in time for the regurgitant blood flow during systole.
2. Pregnancy results in decreased SVR and this favors a forward flow of blood and decreases the amount of regurgitant blood flow.
3. The expanded blood volume of pregnancy helps to maintain adequate filling pressures.

29. What are the goals of anesthetic management in a parturient with aortic regurgitation?

Ans.

- Maintenance of a normal or slightly elevated heart rate
- Avoidance of increases in SVR
- Avoidance of aortocaval compression
- Avoidance of myocardial depression in general anesthesia.

30. What is the anesthetic technique of choice for vaginal/cesarean section in a parturient with mitral regurgitation?

Ans. Epidural anesthesia is preferred as it decreases afterload (Increased SVR can precipitate acute left ventricular volume overload in patients with aortic regurgitation).

CONGENITAL HEART DISEASE

With the advent of pediatric cardiac surgeries, 85% of children with congenital heart disease can be expected to live into adulthood. This dramatic success has created an ever-increasing population of young adults with "grown-up congenital heart disease" (GUCHD).[27,28]

GUCHD patients can broadly be divided into three categories:

1. Those who have undergone some sort of reparative operations.
2. Those who have undergone a palliative procedure.
3. Those who have not previously undergone a corrective or palliative procedures.

There are five major maternal risk factors for maternal and fetal complications of pregnancy.

1. Pulmonary hypertension
2. Cyanosis
3. Maternal functional class
4. Arrhythmias
5. Cardiac disease in pregnancy (CARPREG) risk index.[29-31]

The CARPREG risk index was developed based upon the collection of retrospective data from women with heart disease who become pregnant. Eisenmenger's syndrome is excluded.

A patient is assigned one point for each of the criteria that they meet from the list below:

- Left ventricular systolic dysfunction (EF<40%)
- Previous cardiac event (heart failure, stroke, transient ischemic attack) or arrhythmia.
- Poor functional class (NYHA class III or IV) or cyanosis.
- Left heart obstruction (Mitral valve area <2 cm^2, or aortic valve area <1.5 cm^2, Peak left ventricular outflow gradient >30 mm Hg)

The rates of pulmonary edema, arrhythmia requiring treatment, stroke, cardiac arrest or death were:

0 points; 5%
1 points; 27%
>2 points; 75%
Reference[31]

The risk of adverse outcomes goes up even further in patients with score of 1 if they have subpulmonary ventricular dysfunction and/or severe pulmonary regurgitation.

The Zahara risk score[31] incorporates a number of new variables

1. Prior arrhythmia
2. NYHA III or IV
3. Left heart obstruction (Mitral valve area <2 cm^2, or aortic valve area <1.5 cm^2, Peak left ventricular outflow gradient >30 mm Hg)
4. Mechanical valve prosthesis
5. Systemic AV valve regurgitation (moderate/severe)
6. Pulmonary AV valve regurgitation (moderate/severe)
7. Cardiac medications before pregnancy
8. Cyanotic heart disease (corrected or uncorrected)

Left-to-Right Shunts

31. What are the most common left-to-right shunts encountered in pregnancy?

Ans. *Atrial septal defects:*

- Remains asymptomatic till the reproductive years
- Coexisting mitral valve prolapse may be present

- Complications include arrhythmias, pulmonary hypertension, right ventricular failure (usually develop after the age of 40 years)

  Ventricular septal defect:
- Infrequently diagnosed in pregnancy
- Close spontaneously or are repaired in childhood
- Membranous ventricular septal defects are the most common type and can be associated with atrial regurgitation

  Patent ductus arteriosus:
- Uncommonly diagnosed in pregnancy as it either closes spontaneously or is surgically corrected in childhood.

32. What is the anesthetic technique of choice in parturients with left-to-right shunts presenting for labor and cesarean section?

Ans. Early administration of epidural labor analgesia is preferred to avoid pain associated increase in SVR. Loss of resistance to saline rather than air should be used to identify the epidural space.[32] The anesthesiologist should always bear in mind to maintain a balance between SVR and PVR.

- A slow onset of epidural analgesia is preferred, as rapid decrease in systemic vascular resistance (SVR) could result in reversal of shunt with maternal hypoxemia.
- Supplemental O_2 should be given to the patient throughout the procedure if regional technique is used.
- It is advisable to monitor O_2 saturation as mild hypoxemia may result in increased pulmonary vascular resistance (PVR) and reversal of shunt flow.
- Hypercarbia and acidosis should be avoided, as it may result in increased PVR and reversal of shunt flow. In patients who had successful surgery in infancy or childhood, no special treatment is required.

Tetralogy of Fallot

33. What is the incidence of TOF in pregnant women?

Ans. Tetralogy of Fallot (TOF)—constitutes 5% of all congenital cardiac defects (CCD) in pregnant women.[1] It is the most common congenital heart lesion associated with a right-to-left shunt.

34. What are the components of TOF?

Ans. TOF is the most common etiologic factor in the right-to-left shunt.[33] TOF consists of 4 structural abnormalities, i.e. ventricular septal defect (VSD), right ventricular hypertrophy (RVH), pulmonic stenosis, right ventricular outflow obstruction and over-riding of the aorta.

35. What are the detrimental effects of reoccurrence of VSD in parturients with TOF on pregnancy?

Ans. Most pregnant women will have had corrective surgery, which consists of closure of the VSD and widening of the pulmonary tract. This surgery is usually successful but in some patients, a small VSD may reoccur, or progressive hypertrophy of the pulmonary outflow tract may occur slowly over the years.[34] Patients with history of syncope, polycythemia, decreased arterial O_2 saturation, right ventricular hypertension and congestive cardiac failure (CCF) are particularly at risk.

36. What are the factors that affect PVR?

Ans. *Decrease in PVR:* Increasing PaO_2, hypocarbia, alkalemia, minimizing intrathoracic pressure, spontaneous ventilation, avoidance of sympathetic stimulation, deep anesthesia, pharmacological methods, e.g. isoprenaline, phosphodiesterase inhibitors, prostaglandin infusion (PGE1 and PGE2), inhaled nitric oxide.

Increase in PVR: Sympathetic stimulation, academia, hypoxia, hypercarbia, hypothermia, increased intrathoracic pressure, e.g. controlled ventilation, PEEP, atelactasis.

37. What are the salient anesthetic considerations that should be kept in mind while evaluating a parturient with TOF?

Ans. In patients with uncorrected lesion or corrected Tetralogy of Fallot with residua, anesthetic considerations must focus on minimizing the hemodynamic changes that would increase right to left shunting. Strict avoidance of:

- Decrease in SVR
- Decrease in venous return
- Hypoxemia
- Myocardial depression is advocated.

38. What would be the considerations if neuraxial blockade is planned for labor and cesarean section?

Ans. Administration of epidural labor analgesia minimizes pain and limits increases in PVR and hence decreases right to left shunting. Slow induction of epidural is advisable for cesarean section.[35] Single shot spinal anesthesia is a poor choice as it can cause abrupt reduction of SVR with reversal of shunt flow and hypoxemia.

39. What would be the considerations for administering general anesthesia for cesarean section?

Ans. When general anesthesia is planned, induction agents of choice should be those agents which would cause least hemodynamic disturbance, i.e. narcotic induction with etomidate. Neonatal depression as a result of narcotic induction can be easily treated with endotracheal intubation (ET) tube and no further medical treatment is required.

EISENMENGER'S SYNDROME

40. What is the effect of Eisenmenger's syndrome on pregnancy?

Ans. Eisenmenger syndrome is a complex combination of cardiovascular abnormalities. It consists of pulmonary hypertension, a right to left extra cardiac shunt and arterial hypoxemia.[36] Pregnancy is not well tolerated by patients with this condition. When pregnancy occurs in women with Eisenmenger's syndrome, medical termination is considered safer than any mode of delivery.[35] Acute arrhythmias are particularly dangerous as these patients have little or no cardiac reserve and need a normal sinus rhythm to keep up with the increased workload. Maternal mortality rate is estimated at 30–50%.

41. What is the pathophysiology of Eisenmenger's syndrome?

Ans. Pathophysiology of Eisenmenger syndrome is described as a chronic, uncorrected right to left shunt, right ventricular hypertrophy (RVH), elevated pulmonary artery pressure, and right ventricular (RV) dysfunction. The primary lesion may be either an ASD, VSD or PDA.[37] The pulmonary and the RV musculature undergoes remodelling in response to the chronic pulmonary volume overload, the high fixed pulmonary artery pressure limits flow through the pulmonary vasculature and when pulmonary artery pressure exceeds the level of systemic pressure, reversal of shunt flow occurs. The initial left to right shunt becomes a right to left shunt, ultimately leading to the Eisenmenger syndrome, which includes the sequelae of arterial hypoxemia, and RV failure. Clinical manifestations include dyspnea, clubbing of nails, polycythemia and peripheral edema and cyanosis. In an established case of Eisenmenger syndrome pulmonary hypertension when permanent, surgical correction of the defect at this stage is unhelpful and may increase mortality.[38]

42. What are the salient points to be kept in mind for the administration of safe anesthesia for cesarean section?

Ans. Anesthetic management of patients with Eisenmenger's syndrome is challenging. If the patient does reach full term, a multidisciplinary approach with close communication between obstetrician, cardiologist and anesthesiologist is essential. Anesthetic consideration centers on the avoidance of any decrease in the SVR.

Hypotension from any cause can progress to insufficient RV pressure required to perfuse the hypertensive pulmonary arterial bed and may result in sudden death of the patient. The anesthetist must be aware of the maternal anticoagulation. If there are no contraindications to regional block, a titrated epidural anesthesia is probably the technique of choice.[35] A slow induction of epidural allows compensation for sympathectomy below the level of block, a dilute solution of phenylephrine may be given as needed to maintain maternal SVR. O_2 should be administered to all patients undergoing surgery under regional anesthesia, as O_2 reduces pulmonary vascular resistance, which benefits the patient with Eisenmenger.[39] The blood loss should be promptly replaced by crystalloids, colloids, or packed cells. Postpartum autotransfusion may cause intravascular volume overload in these patients. Regional anesthesia may reduce the risk of postoperative deep vein thrombosis.[40]

43. What are the drawbacks of administering general anesthesia to parturients with Eisenmenger's syndrome?

Ans. Cesarean section can also be conducted under general anesthesia, but there several disadvantages associated with general anesthesia,[35] e.g. effects of IPPV on venous return, ventilation/perfusion mismatch, high pulmonary artery pressure, increased shunt through the anatomic defect and myocardial depression by halogenated agents. If slow induction of anesthesia is used, there is a risk of maternal aspiration. Monitoring includes invasive blood pressure monitoring (A-line), and central venous pressure (CVP) monitoring. Pulmonary artery (PA) catheter use is controversial.[41] It is difficult to position the balloon tipped flow directed catheter into the pulmonary artery and risk of pulmonary artery rupture is always present.

COARCTATION OF THE AORTA

Coarctation of aorta is a congenital lesion consisting of discrete narrowing of the descending aorta, most common distal to the subclavian artery, with proximal hypertension and distal hypoperfusion.

44. How many cases go undiagnosed to pregnancy?

Ans. 80% of cases are detected in childhood, although occasionally the initial diagnosis is made during pregnancy.

45. How do you assess good pregnancy outcomes?

Ans.

- A maternal arm-to-leg blood pressure gradient of less than 20 mm Hg
- Patients who have normal arm and leg pressures after successful corrective surgery.[1]

46. What are complications encountered in pregnant women with uncorrected lesions or residual disease?

Ans.

- Left ventricular failure
- Aortic rupture or dissection
- Endocarditis
- Reduced uteroplacental perfusion (fetal mortality may approach 20%).

47. When is elective cesarean section preferred?

Ans. Patients with coarctation of aorta are more likely to have a bicuspid aortic valve or an aneurysm in the Circle of Willis. As wide fluctuations in blood pressure during labor increase the risk of intracranial aneurysm rupture or aortic dissection, elective cesarean section is preferred by some obstetricians, especially if there is gross widening of the ascending aorta.

48. How is labor and delivery managed in patients who have undergone corrective surgery?

Ans. Parturients who have an arm-to-leg blood pressure gradient less than 20 mm Hg or have undergone corrective surgery, vaginal delivery is preferred. Epidual labor analgesia is advocated to minimize the hemodynamic consequences of maternal expulsive efforts and pain.

Prior Prosthetic Valve Surgery

49. What are the complications encountered in a parturient with prior prosthetic valve surgery?

Ans.

- Thromboembolic phenomenon
- Valve failure
- Infective endocarditis

Though endocarditis is a grave risk, antibiotic prophylaxis for vaginal delivery is not recommended unless bacteremia is suspected.[42,43]

50. How do you choose an anticoagulant for parturients?

Ans. Pregnant women are hypercoagulable and require anticoagulation particularly if they have mechanical heart valves.

- Unfractionated heparin is a large, water soluble molecule which does not cross the placental barrier and hence its administration avoids the risk of fetal embryopathy.
- Warfarin is probably safe in the first 6 weeks of pregnancy. But it crosses the placental barrier and is associated with the risk of fetal embryopathy (4–10%),[44,45] when used between 6 and 12 weeks of gestation.
- It is relatively safe and can be used during the second and third trimesters but should be replaced by heparin at 36 weeks of gestation which allows easier reversal of anticoagulation before delivery and reduces blood loss during parturition.

51. What is the anticoagulation regimen for a pregnant women with a mechanical prosthetic valve?

Ans. The anticoagulation regimen for a pregnant women with a mechanical prosthetic valve is given in the following box

- All pregnant patients with mechanical prosthetic valves must receive continuous therapeutic anticoagulation with frequent monitoring.
- For women requiring long term anticoagulant warfarin therapy who are attempting pregnancy, pregnancy test results should be monitored with discussions about subsequent anticoagulation therapy, so that anticoagulation can be continued uninterrupted when pregnancy is achieved. The decision about anticoagulant management during pregnancy should include an assessment of additional risk factors for thromboembolism, including valve type, valve position, and the decision should also be influenced strongly by patient references.
- For patient with mechanical heart valves, one of the following anticoagulant regimens should be used:
  - Adjusted-dose, twice daily LMWH throughout pregnancy. Doses should be adjusted to achieve the manufacturer's recommended peak anti-factor Xa level four hrs after subcutaneous injection.

- Adjusted dose UFH throughout pregnancy, administered subcutaneously q12 in doses adjusted to keep the mid-interval aPTT value at least twice the control, to attain an anti-factor Xa heparin level of 0.35–0.7 U/mL.
- Adjusted dose UFH or LMWH (as above) until the 13th week of gestation, with warfarin substitution until close to delivery, when either UFH or LMWH is resumed.

- In women judged to be at very high risk of thromboembolism in whom concerns exist about the efficacy and safety of UFH or LMWH administered as above (e.g. older generation prosthesis in the mitral position or history of thromboembolism), vitamin K antagonists should be administered throughout pregnancy, with replacement by UFH or LMWH (as above) close to delivery, after a thorough discussion of the potential risks and benefits of the approach.
  - If warfarin is used, the dose should be adjusted to a target INR of 3.0 (range 2.5–3.5); a lower therapeutic range, 2.0–3.0, can be used in patients with bileaflet aortic valves, provided they do not have atrial fibrillation or left ventricular dysfunction.
  - If subcutaneous UFH is used, it should be initiated in high doses (17,500–20,000 U q12h) and adjusted to prolong a 6 hr post injection aPTT into the therapeutic range.
  - For pregnant women with prosthetic valves at high risk of thromboembolism, low-dose aspirin (75–100 mg/day) should also be administered.

Abbreviations: UFH, unfractionated heparin; LMWH, low-molecular-weight-heparin; aPTT, activated partial thromboplastin time; INR, international normalized ratio.

Ref:[48] Data taken from Bates SM, Greer IA, Pabinger I, et al. Venous thromboembolism, thrombophilia, antithrombotic therapy, and pregnancy: American College of Chest Physicians Evidence Based Clinical Practice Guidelines (8th edn). Chest. 2008;133:844S-86S.

52. What are the anesthetic implications in a parturient with prior prosthetic valve surgery?

Ans. The Second American Society of Regional Anesthesia and Pain Medicine (ASRA) Consensus Conference on Neuraxial Anesthesia and Anticoagulation published a risk assessment with clinical guidelines in 2003.

- UFH is discontinued with the onset of active labor. Neuraxial analgesia is withheld until the aPTT value is near normal or the blood heparin concentration is near zero. Till then, the parturient is given intravenous opioid for labor analgesia.
- LMWH thromboprophylaxis precludes the use of of neuraxial techniques until at least 10–12 hours have elapsed from the time of the last prophylactic dose. When therapeutic anticoagulation with high dose LMWH is planned, the use of neuraxial techniques should be started 24 hours since the time of the last dose.[46] Standard UFH may be substituted for LMWH by 38 weeks gestation to allow:
  - Faster resolution of anticoagulant activity
  - The ability to monitor anticoagulation activity by monitoring aPTT.[47]
- Protamine reversal of heparin therapy is not advocated.[47]
- For patients on long term warfarin therapy, the presence of a normal or near normal prothrombin time (PT) and INR is mandatory before the administration of neuraxial anesthesia.[46]
- General anesthesia should be considered in patients with abnormal coagulation activity.
- For postpartum thromboprophylaxis with once daily dosing regimen of LMWH, it is preferable to start the first dose of LMWH 6–8 hours after operative therapy. The second dose should be given 24 hours after the first dose. For patients receiving therapeutic, i.e. twice daily dosing of LMWH, 24 hours should elapse after the operative delivery before giving the first dose. In case of a bloody tap, 24 hours should elapse before the needle and catheter placement and initiation of LMWH therapy.[46]

- The ASRA guidelines state that neuraxial catheters may be safely maintained in patients receiving single daily dose of LMWH postoperatively. The catheter should be removed 10–12 hours after the last dose of LMWH and subsequent doses of LMWH should be administered at least 2 hours after catheter removal. For patients receiving twice daily dosing of LMWH, catheters should removed before starting LMWH thromboprophylaxis. The first dose of LMWH should be administered at least 2 hours after catheter removal.[46]
- Parturients in whom warfarin has been started after delivery, it is necessary that an INR less than1.5 be achieved before catheter removal.[46]

INFECTIVE ENDOCARDITIS

53. What is the incidence of infective endocarditis in the obstetric population?

Ans. The incidence of infective endocarditis appears to be diminishing in the obstetric population due to:

- A diminishing prevalence of rheumatic heart disease
- Increase in aseptic procedures in obstetrics
- Increasing practice of early treatment of obstetric infections
- Diminishing incidence of illegal abortion

However, intravenous drug abuse has now become a major cause of infective endocarditis in women of child bearing age.[49]

54. What are the risks factors of infective endocarditis in pregnant women?

Ans. Typically infective endocarditis occurs in hearts with a pre-existing lesion, however normal heart valves may also be affected.[50]

Risk factors for the infection of pre-existing cardiac lesions include:

- Dental and urologic procedures
- Prolonged intravenous therapy
- Intravenous drug abuse

Risk factors for infection of normal cardiac tissue include:

- Prolonged intravenous therapy
- Intravenous drug abuse
- Infection of an arteriovenous shunt
- Renal dialysis.[50]

55. What organism is most commonly associated with the risk of infective endocarditis?

Ans. Streptococci is the most predominant pathogen causing 74% of infective endocarditis. While *Streptococcus viridans* is associated with obstetetric and gynecologic procedures, enterococci and group B streptococci are the common pathogens after an abortion.[51]

56. How do you diagnose a case of subacute infective endocarditis?

Ans. Subacute infective endocarditis is characterized by:

- A gradual onset of fever, malaise
- Blood cultures are positive in 90% cases
- Murmurs may be present
- Systemic embolism result in splinter hemorrhages and mucosal petechia
- Septic abscesses lead to atrioventricular nodal dysfunction, conduction block.
- Splenomegaly
- Nephritis
- Major causes of death include congestive cardiac failure, cerebral infarction, arrhythmias and renal failure.

57. How do you diagnose a case of acute infective endocarditis?

Ans. Acute infective endocarditis is characterized by:

- Abrupt onset of shaking chills and fever
- Systemic embolism result in skin and mucosal petechiae
- Cardiac decompensation may occur suddenly with erosion of a valve or rupture of chorda tendineae
- Murmurs occur in patients with vegetations
- Aortic ring abscesses produce conduction disturbances or ventricular septal defects.

Major causes of death include congestive cardiac failure, arrhythmias, uncontrolled sepsis, septic emboli and mycotic aneurysm formation with rupture.

58. What are the high risk cardiac conditions in which antibiotic prophylaxis is indicated?

Ans. High-risk cardiac conditions associated with the highest risk of adverse outcome from endocarditis, for which antibiotic prophylaxis for deliveries associated with infection, or certain dental procedures, is reasonable:

- Prosthetic cardiac valve or prosthetic material used for cardiac valve repair
- Previous infective endocarditis
- Complex congenital heart disease
  - Unrepaired cyanotic heart disease, including palliative shunts and conduits
  - Completely repaired congenital heart defect with prosthetic material or device (during the first 6 months after the procedure)
  - Repaired congenital heart disease with residual defects at the site or adjacent to the site of the prosthetic patch or device
- Cardiac transplantation recipients who develop cardiac valvulopathy.

Ref:[52] Data taken from (1) American Heart Association Rheumatic Fever, Endocarditis, Kawasaki Disease Committee, Council on Cardiovascular Disease in the Young, and the Council on Clinical Cardiology, Council on Cardiovascular Surgery and Anesthesia, and the Quality of Care and Outcomes Research Interdisciplinary Working Group. Prevention of Infective Endocarditis: Guidelines from the American Heart Association. Circulation 2007;116:1736-54.

59. What is the antibiotic prophylaxis for parturients with infective endocarditis?

Ans.

- Cephalosporins should not be used in patients with a significant sensitivity to penicillins.
- This regimen does not cover enterococcus. Vancomycin (1 gm IV) can be used if enterococcus is of concern.

Ref:[43] Data taken from American College of Obstetricians and Gynecologists Committee on Obstetric Practice. Antibiotic prophylaxis for infective endocarditis. ACOG Committee Opinion No. 421. Washington DC, November 2008. (Obstet Gynecol. 2008;112:1193-4)

Infective endocarditis prophylaxis is no longer recommended for vaginal or cesarean delivery in the absence of infection, regardless of the type of maternal cardiac lesion. Mitral valve prolapse is no longer considered a lesion that needs infective endocarditis prophylaxis. Only cardiac conditions associated with the highest risk of adverse outcome from endocarditis are appropriate for any infective endocarditis prophylaxis (in the Q6). In patients with one of the above conditions and who have an established infection that would cause bacteremia, such as chorioamnionitis or pyelonephritis, the underlying infection should be treated in the usual fashion and the treatment should include a regimen effective for infective endocarditis prophylaxis (Table 6). Prophylaxis should be given intravenously.[1]

Table 6 | Antibiotic prophylaxis appropriate for infective endocarditis

Treatment	*Antibiotic*	*Regimen (preferably 30–60 mins before procedure)*
Intravenous therapy	Ampicillin or cephazolin	2 gm intravenously
	Or ceftriaxone	1gm intravenously
Allergic to penicillin	Cephazolin or ceftriaxone	1gm intravenously
Or ampicillin	Or clindamycin	600 mg intravenously
Oral	Amoxicillin	2 gm

REFERENCES

1. Chestnut DH. 4th edn. Philadelphia: Mosby Elsevier. Obstetric anesthesia: Principles and practice; 2009. pp. 881–907.
2. Jose VJ, Gomathi M. Declining prevalence of rheumatic heart disease in rural school children in India: 2001-2002. Indian Heart J. 2003;55:158–60.
3. Misra M, Mittal M, Singh R, Verma A, Rai R, Chandra G, et al. Prevalence of rheumatic heart disease in school-going children of Eastern Uttar Pradesh. Indian Heart J. 2007;59:42–3.
4. Bhatla N, Lal S, Behera G, Kriplani A, Mittal S, Agarwal N, et al. Cardiac disease in pregnancy. Int J Gynaecol Obstet. 2003;82:153–9.
5. Malhotra M, Sharma JB, Tripathii R, Arora P, Arora R. Maternal and fetal outcome in valvular heart disease. Int J Gynaecol Obstet. 2004;84:11–6.
6. Sawhney H, Aggarwal N, Suri V, Vasishta K, Sharma Y, Grover A. Maternal and perinatal outcome in rheumatic heart disease. Int J Gynaecol Obstet. 2003;80:9–14.
7. Elkayam U, Bitar F. Valvular heart disease and pregnancy. J Am Coll Cardiol. 2005;46:223–30.
8. Warnes CA. Pregnancy and heart disease. In: Libby P, Bonow RO, Mann DL, Zipes DP, editors. Braunwald's Heart Disease: A Textbook of Cardiovascular Medicine. 8th ed. Philadelphia PA: WB Saunders. 2007. pp. 1967–82.
9. Siu SC , Sermer M, Colman JM, et al. Retrospective multicenter study of pregnancy outcomes in women with heart disease. Circulation 2001;104:515-21.
10. The Criteria Committee of the New York Heart Association Nomenclature and Criteria for Diagnosis of Diseases of the Heart and Great vessels Ninth edition. Little Brown and Company.1994. pp. 253-5.
11. Silversides CK, Colman JM, Sermer M, Siu SC. Cardiac risk in pregnant women with rheumatic mitral stenosis. Am J Cardiol. 2003;91:1382–5.
12. ACC/AHA Practice Guidelines for the management of patients with valvular heart disease. Executive Summary Report of the American College of Cardiology/American Heart Association Task Force on Practice Guidelines (Ccommittee on management of patients with valvular heart disease) Circulation. 1998;98:1949-84.
13. Al Kasab SM, Sabag T, al Zaibag M, Awaad M, al Bitar I, Halim MA, et al. Beta-adrenergic blockade in the management of pregnant women with mitral stenosis. Am J Obstet Gynecol. 1990;165:37–40.
14. The effect of digoxin on the mortality and morbidity in patients with heart failure. The Digitalis Investigation Group. N Engl J Med. 1997;336:525–33.
15. Reimold SC, Rutherford JD. Valvular heart disease in pregnancy. N Engl J Med. 2003;349:52–9.
16. Hameed A, Akhter MW, Bitar F, Khan SA, Sarma R, Goodwin TM, et al. Left atrial thrombosis in pregnant women with mitral stenosis and sinus rhythm. Am J Obstet Gynecol. 2005;193:501–4.
17. Fawzy ME, Kinsara AJ, Stefadouros M, Hegazy H, Kattan H, Chaudhary A, et al. Long-term outcome of mitral balloon valvotomy in pregnant women. J Heart Valve Dis. 2001;10:153–7.
18. De Souza JA, Martinez EE, Jr, Ambrose JA, Alves CM, Born D, Buffolo E, et al. Percutaneous balloon mitral valvuloplasty in comparison with open mitral valve commissurotomy for mitral stenosis during pregnancy. J Am Coll Cardiol. 2001;37:900–3.

19. Sutton SW, Duncan MA, Chase VA, Marce RJ, Meyers TP, Wood RE. Cardiopulmonary bypass and mitral valve replacement during pregnancy. Perfusion. 2005;20:359–68.
20. Sharma SK, Gambling DR, Gajraj NM, Truong C, Sidawi EJ. Anesthetic management of a parturient with mixed mitral valve disease and uncontrolled atrial fibrillation. Int J Obstet Anesth. 1994;3:157–62.
21. Stout KK, Otto CM. Pregnancy in women with valvular heart disease. Heart. 2007;93:552–8.
22. Hermmings GT, Whalley DG, O'Connor PH. Invasive monitoring and anesthesia management of patients with mitral stenosis. Can J Anaesth. 1987;34:182–5.
23. Ngan Kee WD, Shen J, Chiu AT, Lok I, Khaw KS. Combined spinal-epidural analgesia in the management of labouring parturients with mitral stenosis. Anaesth Intensive Care. 1999;27:523–6.
24. Langesaeter E, Dragsund M, Rosseland LA. Regional anaesthesia for a Caesarean section in women with cardiac disease: A prospective study. Acta Anaesthesiol Scand. 2010;54:46–54.
25. Blaise G, Langleben D, Hubert B. Pulmonary arterial hypertension: Pathophysiology and anesthetic approach. Anesthesiology. 2003;99:1415–32.
26. Otto CM. Valvular stenosis:diagnosis, quantitation and clinical approach. In Otto CM Text Book of Clinical Echocardiography, 2nd edn. Philadelphia: WB Saunders Company; 2000.pp.229-64.
27. ACC/AHA guidelines break new ground in adult congenital heart disease; American college of cardiology 7 Nov, 2008.
28. Pregnancy and Heart disease; Congenital heart disease-wikidoc.
29. Predictors of pregnancy complications in women with congenital heart disease. Eur Heart J. 2010;31(17): 2124-32.
30. AHA. Cardiovascular Disease in Women. Pregnancy outcomes in women with congenital heart disease. Circulation. 2006;113:517-24.
31. Pieper PH. Department of cardiology, University Medical Centre Groningen, University of Groningen. Pre-pregnancy risk assessment and counselling of the cardiac patient. Neth Heart J. 2011;11:477-81.
32. Naulty JS, Ostheimer GW, Datta S, Knapp R, Weiss JB. Incidence of venous air embolism during epidural catheter insertion. Anaesthesiology. 1982;57:410-2.
33. Lewis NL, Dob DP, Yentis SM. UK registry of high risk obstetric anaesthesia: arrythmias, cardio-myopathy, aortic stenosis, transposition of great arteries and mairfare syndrome. IJOA 2003;12:28-34.
34. Kirklin JW, Blackstone EH, Kirklin JK, et al. Surgical results and protocols in the spectrum of tetralogy of fallot. Ann Surg 1983;198:251-65.
35. Ghai B, Mohan V, Khetarpal M, Malhotra N. Epidural anaesthesia for C Section patients with Eisenmenger syndrome. Int J Obstet Anaesthesia 2002;11:44-7.
36. Kuczhowski KM. Labour analgesia for parturient with cardiac disease – what does an obstetrician need to know? Acta Obstet Gynecol Scand 2004;83:223-33.
37. Laura L, Klein MD, Henry L, Galar MD. Cardiac diseases in pregnancy. Clin Obstet Gynecol N Am. 2004; 58:588-90.
38. Blanchard DG, Shabetai R. Cardiac diseases. In: Cer asy RK, Resnik R, lams JD (Eds). Maternal-fetal medicine. 5th edn. Philadelphia: Saunders; 2004.pp.823-4.
39. Marshall HW, Swan HJC, Burchell HB, Wood EH. Effect of breathing oxygen on pulmonary arterial pressure and pulmonary vascular resistance in patients with ventricular septal defect. Circulation. 1961; 23:241-52.
40. Tuman KJ, McCarthy RJ, March RJ, DeLaria GA, Patel RV, Ivankovich AD. Effects of epidural anaesthesia and analgesia on coagulation and outcome after major vascular surgery. Anesth analg. 1989;62:243-7.
41. Robinbson S. Pulmonary artery catheters in Eisenmenger's syndrome: Many risks few benefits (letter). Anaesthesiology. 1983;58:588-90.
42. American College of Cardiology/American Heart Association Task Force on Practice Guidelines, 2006 Guidelines for the management of patients with valvular heart disease Circulation. 2006;114:e84-231.
43. American College of Obstetricians and Gynecologists Committee on Obstetric Practice. Antibiotic prophylaxis for infective endocarditis. ACOG Committee Opinion No. 421. Washington DC, November 2008. (Obstet Gynecol. 2008;112:1193-4).
44. Hirsh J, Fuster V. Guide to anticoagulant therapy. Part 2: Oral anticongulants, Circulation 1994;89:1469-80.

45. Salazar E, Izaguirre R, Verdejo J, Mutchinick O. Failure of adjusted does of subcutaneous heparin to prevent thromboembolic phenomena in pregnant patient with mechanical cardiac valve prostheses. J Am Coll Cardiol. 1996;27:1698-703.
46. Horlocker TT, Wedel DJ, Benzon H, et al. Regional anesthesia in the anticogulated patient. Defining the risks. (The Second ASRA Consensus Conference on Neuraxial Anesthesia and Antico-agulation.) Reg Anesth Pain Med. 2003;28:172-97.
47. Harnett MJ, Walsh ME, McElrath TF, Tsen LC. The use of central hexaxial techniques in parturients with factor V Leiden mutation. Anesth Analg. 2005;101:1821-3.
48. Bates SM, Greer IA, Pabinger I, et al. Venous thromboembolism, thrombophilia, antithrombotic therapy, and pregnancy: American College of Chest Physicians Evidence Based Clinical Practice Guidelines (8th edn). Chest. 2008;133:844S-86S.
49. Cox SM, Leveno KJ. Pregnancy complicagted by bacterial endocarditis. Clin Obstet Gynecol. 1989;32:48-53.
50. Karchmer AW. Infective endocarditis. In: Braunwaid E, Zipe DP, Libby P (Eds). Heart Disease 6th edn. Philadelphia, WB Saunders; 2001.pp.1723-47.
51. Seaworth BJ, Durack DT. Infective endocarditis in obstetric and gynaecologic practice. Am J Obstet Gynecol. 1986;154:180-8.
52. American Heart Association Rheumatic Fever, Endocarditis, Kawasaki Disease Committee, Council on Cardiovascular Disease in the Young, and the Council on Clinical Cardiology, Council on Cardiovascular Surgery and Anesthesia, and the Quality of Care and Outcomes Research Interdisciplinary Working Group. Prevention of Infective Endocarditis: Guidelines from the American Heart Association. Circulation. 2007;116:1736-54.

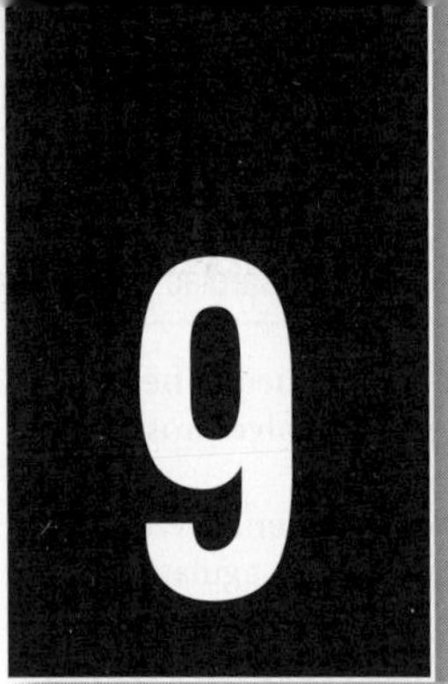

Anesthetic Considerations for Liver Transplantation

Jyotsna Goswami

Liver transplantation (LT) is the replacement of unhealthy liver with a new liver allograft and is the treatment of choice for end-stage liver disease. Liver transplantation has undergone continual improvement since it was first performed by Starzl in 1963.[1] The continued advances in perioperative care, anesthetic management, surgical technique and immunosuppressive agents helped into significant reduction in morbidity and mortality.

1. What are the different types of liver transplantation?

Ans. Three different types of LT are practiced, i.e. DDLT (deceased donor liver transplant or cadaveric), LDLT (live donor liver transplant) and split-liver or reduced-sized liver transplant.

Deceased donor liver transplant (DDLT): When liver is harvested from a deceased donor, it is known as DDLT or cadaveric transplant (Figs 1A and B). These livers come from brain dead organ

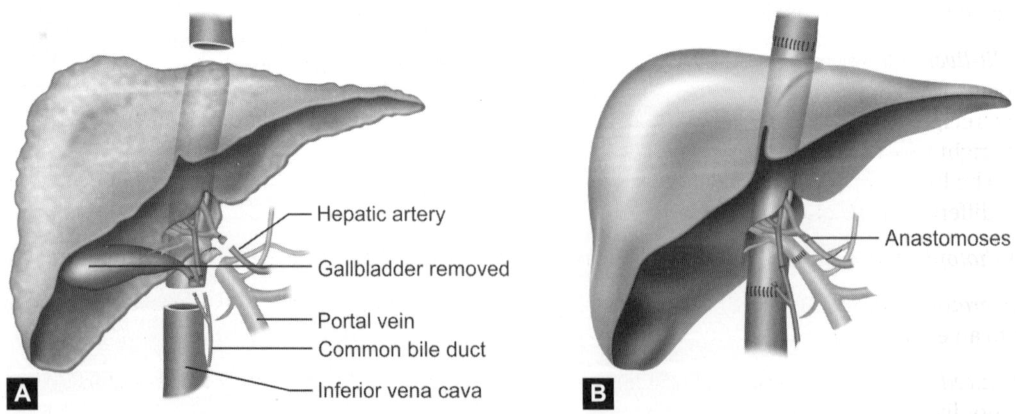

Figs 1A and B Orthotopic approach of liver: (A) Diseased liver removed; (B) Donor liver transplanted

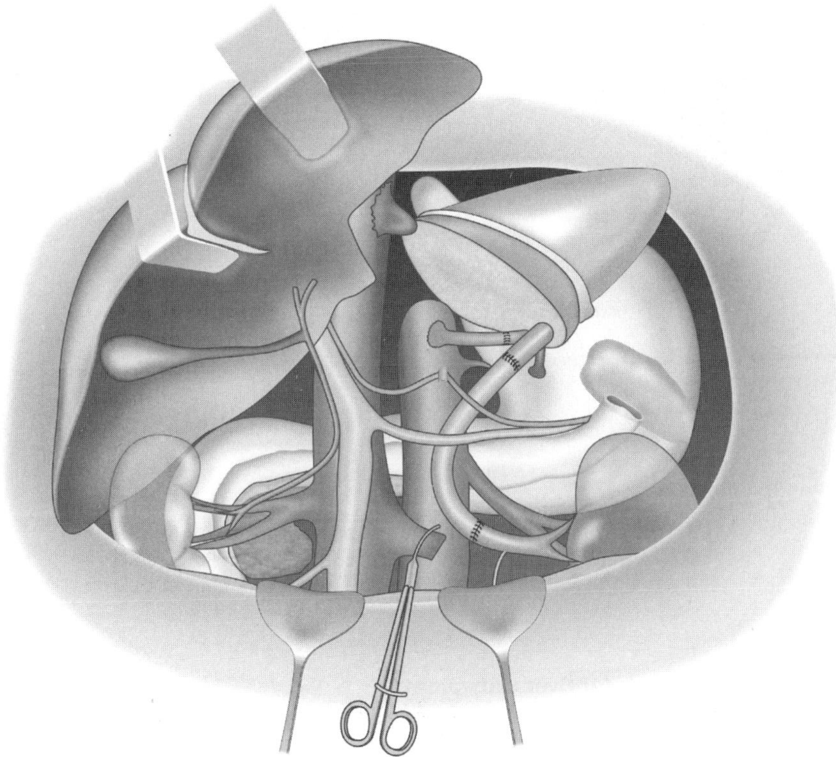

Fig. 2 Heterotopic approach of liver transplant

donors where consent is available and need to be transplanted within 12–24 hours after the liver is removed from the donor.

Live donor liver transplantation (LDLT): In this procedure, part of the liver is harvested from a compatible donor. The most important disadvantage of LDLT is the potential for complications or even death of a healthy donor.

Split-liver transplantation: Because of the unique anatomical organization of the liver, donor organs from deceased donor can be divided into two separate parts which are transplanted into two recipients. Usually, the left lobe of an adult donor organ can be transplanted into a child and the right lobe into an adult.[2]

The liver transplant may also be described as orthotopic, heterotopic and auxiliary depending on different surgical approaches.

Orthotopic approach (OLT): It is the replacement of a whole diseased liver with a healthy liver.

Heterotopic approach (Fig. 2): When the recipient's liver is left *in situ* and the donor liver is placed into an ectopic site.

Reduced-size liver transplant: Replacement of a whole diseased liver with a portion of a healthy donor liver (Fig. 3).

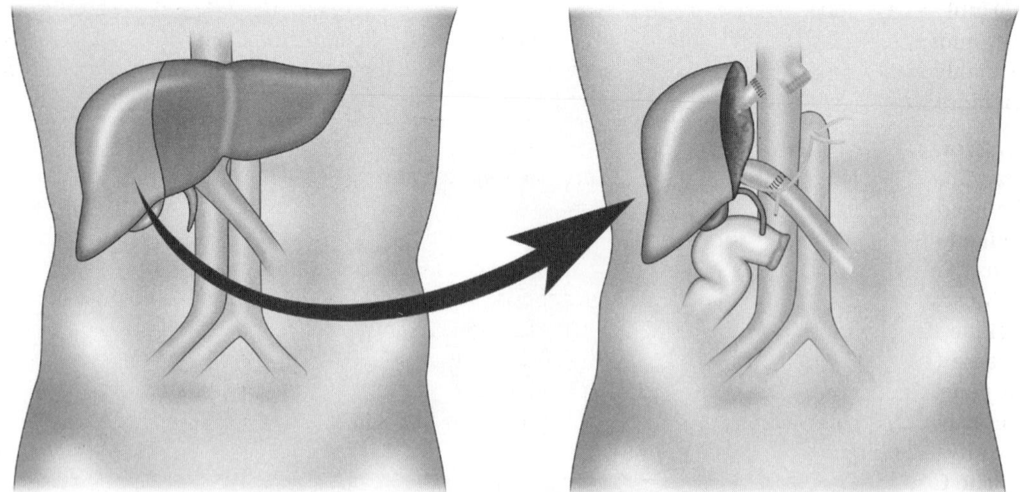

Fig. 3 Portion of donor liver is removed and transplanted to recipient
Source: Mayo Foundation for Medical Education and Research

2. What are the indications for liver transplant?

Ans. Liver transplant is indicated for acute or chronic liver failure of any cause. Common indications are:

- *Cholestatic liver disorders:* Primary biliary cirrhosis, primary sclerosing cholangitis, secondary biliary cirrhosis, biliary atresia, cystic fibrosis
- *Chronic hepatitis:* Hepatitis B, hepatitis C, hepatitis D, autoimmune chronic active hepatitis, cryptogenic cirrhosis, chronic drug toxicity or toxin exposure
- *Alcoholic cirrhosis:* Patients with alcoholic cirrhosis are considered for transplant, if they meet criteria for abstinence for six months and rehabilitation.
- *Metabolic diseases:* Hemochromatosis, Wilson's disease, alpha-1-antitrypsin deficiency, glycogen storage disease, tyrosinemia, familial amyloidotic polyneuropathy, other metabolic disorders treatable by liver replacement.
- *Fulminant acute hepatic necrosis:* Viral hepatitis, drug toxicity, toxin, Wilson's disease.
- *Primary hepatic tumors:* Selected patients with hepatocellular carcinoma.
- *Miscellaneous conditions:* Budd-Chiari syndrome, metastatic neuroendocrine tumors, polycystic disease
- Retransplantation.

3. What are the contraindications to liver transplantation?

Ans. While each patient is evaluated on an individual basis, the presence of one or more of the following will frequently preclude acceptance as a candidate for liver transplantation:

- Active alcohol or substance abuse
- Systemic infections
- Life-limiting coexisting medical conditions—advanced heart, lung or neurologic conditions.
- Uncontrolled psychiatric disorder
- Inability to comply with pre- and post-transplant regimens

Until early 2000, HIV infection was a contraindication for LT due to concerns of immunosuppressive-related opportunistic infections and increased mortality. But with advent of highly active antiretroviral therapy (HAART), HIV infection is no longer a contraindication anymore.[3-5]

4. How are the transplant candidates selected?

Ans. Growing need for liver transplantation and a nonexpanding cadaveric donor pool mandated the need for an improved graft allocation system. In 1998, the principles of organ allocation was defined to minimize waiting time in favor of allocation based on medical urgency, to avoid futile transplantations and to promote the efficient use of scarce donor organs.[1]

Most widely used clinical tools to determine prognosis in patients with chronic liver diseases include the Child-Turcotte-Pugh (CTP) classification, the prognostic model for end-stage liver disease (MELD), disease-specific indices and the impact of specific complications of cirrhosis on patient survival.[2] The CTP classification, which was originally designed to assess the risk of portacaval shunt in patients with ESLD, is still used as a simple prognostic tool to assess the disease severity (Table 1).

The CTP strongly correlates with mortality. More than one-third of patients with CTP class C, waiting for transplantation, can be expected to die within 1 year. In contrast, 5-year survival for CTP class B patients is 80% and CTP class A is 90% without transplantation.[2] The model for end-stage liver disease (MELD) and pediatric end-stage liver disease (PELD) models were adopted in February 2002 to allocate organs based on medical urgency and to decrease the number of waiting list patient deaths. The MELD score is based on three laboratory results: bilirubin, creatinine, and the international normalized ratio (INR). MELD calculation is as follows: MELD = [0.957 (logs-creatinine) + 0.378 (logs-bilirubin) + 1.120 (log INR) + 0.643] × 10.

The MELD predicts 3-month waiting list mortality. Using the MELD model, patients are assigned a score in a continuous scale from 6–40, which equates to estimated 3-month survival rates from 90–7%, respectively. A modification of this model is now used to prioritize patients for donor allocation which has been shown useful both in predicting short-term survival in patients on the waiting list as well as the risk of postoperative mortality.

The PELD uses a similar model in which variables are age younger than 1 year, serum albumin, serum bilirubin, INR and growth failure (2 SD below the age-based mean). The higher the PELD score, the lower the likelihood of 3-month survival without transplantation. It is recommended that patients with cirrhosis should be referred for transplantation when they develop evidence of hepatic dysfunction (CTP > 7 and MELD > 10) or when they experience their first major complication (ascites, variceal bleeding, or hepatic encephalopathy).

Table 1 | Child-Turcotte-Pugh (CTP) scoring system

Variables	*Points scored*		
	1	*2*	*3*
Encephalopathy	None	1–2	3–4
Ascites	Absent	Slight	Moderate
Prothrombin time	<4	4–6	>6
Albumin (g/dL)	>3.5	2.8–3.5	<2.8
Bilirubin (mg/dL)	<4	4–10	>10
Child-Turcotte-Pugh	**Class A**	**Class B**	**Class C**
	5–6	7–9	10–15

Children with chronic liver disease should be referred when they deviate from normal growth curves or develop evidence of hepatic dysfunction or portal hypertension. Patients with type I hepatorenal syndrome should have an expedited referral for liver transplantation.[2]

5. How will you evaluate and optimize LT recipient?

Ans. The ESLD affects almost all organ systems and warrants thorough understanding to guide meticulous anesthetic management.

Cardiovascular system (CVS): The ESLD is associated with hyperdynamic circulatory state[1] characterized by high cardiac output (CO) and low systemic vascular resistance (SVR). This occurs due to increased level of circulating inflammatory mediators as a result of either excess endogenous production or decreased hepatic clearance. There is splanchnic vasodilatation and neovascularization leading to increased venous capacitance.[6,7] Cardiomyopathy is commonly associated with alcoholic cirrhosis, amyloidosis and hemochromatosis. Significant arrhythmia has been reported in about 27% cases [6] which may be due to acid-base or electrolyte disturbances. With the expansion of transplantation criteria, more elderly patients are now included with coronary artery disease (CAD), a frequent coexisting condition. The American Association for the Study of Liver Diseases (AASLD) recommends dobutamine stress echocardiography (DSE) followed by coronary angiography when appropriate in addition to ECG and echocardiogram. These guidelines recommend an evaluation for CAD in LT candidates who are chronic smokers with personal or family history of CAD or DM.[2,7] Coronary revascularization should be considered in LT candidates, if the extent of CAD contraindicates transplantation. For patients undergoing percutaneous coronary intervention (PCI), bare-metal stents are preferred because of the increased risk of bleeding from the prolonged duration of dual antiplatelet therapy required for drug-eluting stents.

Renal

Splanchnic vasodilatation and raised intra-abdominal pressure due to ascites result into renal hypoperfusion which activates the renin-angiotensin-aldosterone (RAA) axis. Stress events like sepsis, gastrointestinal (GI) bleeding, use of diuretics, vasodilators or nephrotoxic drugs easily tip the fine balance between circulatory performance and adequacy of renal perfusion resulting in renal ischemia.[8]

Hepatorenal syndrome (HRS) is a form of prerenal acute kidney injury that occurs in decompensated cirrhosis. The diagnosis is based on the exclusion of other causes of renal injury. Criteria for the diagnosis of HRS in cirrhosis were updated in 2007 (Table 2).[9] The syndrome is classified into two types: Type 1 is characterized by doubling of the serum creatinine level to greater than 2.5 mg/dL (221 μmol/L) in less than 2 weeks while type 2 is characterized by a stable or slower progressive course of renal failure.[10] Patients with type 1 HRS have an extremely poor prognosis

Table 2 | Diagnostic criteria for hepatorenal syndrome[9]

- Cirrhosis with ascites
- Serum creatinine >1.5 mg/dL (133 μmol/L)
- No improvement of serum creatinine (decrease to a level of 1.5 mg/dL or less) after at least 2 days with diuretic withdrawal and volume expansion with albumin (recommended dose of 1 gm/kg body weight/day up to a maximum of 100 gm/day)
- Absence of shock
- No current or recent treatment with nephrotoxic drugs
- Absence of parenchymal kidney disease as indicated by proteinuria > 500 mg/day, microhematuria (>50 RBCs/high power field), and/or abnormal renal ultrasonography

with a median survival of two to four weeks compared with type 2 HRS, where the median survival is approximately 6 months.[10]

To estimate renal function, serum creatinine, creatinine clearance, GFR, serum electrolytes and renal ultrasonography helps to rule out any structural abnormality. Treatment includes the use of loop diuretics and aldosterone antagonists, but the application of vasoconstrictors seems most effective. Vasopressin analogs, e.g. terlipressin, have been suggested as first line therapy.[10,11] As type 1 HRS have an extremely poor prognosis with a median survival of only 2–4 weeks, patients with this syndrome should have an expedited referral for evaluation and selected patients with chronic renal and liver disease should be considered for combined liver-kidney transplantation.[2]

Pulmonary

The ESLD may be associated with multiple pulmonary complications which include restrictive lung disease and two other very distinct syndromes, i.e. hepatopulmonary syndrome (HPS) and portopulmonary hypertension (POPH). Restrictive lung disease frequently results from ascites or pleural effusion which can be drained to give temporary symptomatic relief. Apart from chest radiograph, sonography is a very helpful tool to diagnose pleural effusion. Clinical triad of chronic liver disease, decreased arterial oxygenation ($PaO_2 < 80$ mm Hg and alveolar-arterial O_2 gradient >15 mm Hg on room air) and widespread intrapulmonary vasodilation are the hallmark of HPS leading to physiologic shunting, ventilation-perfusion mismatch, and hypoxemia. It should be suspected, if there is orthodeoxia (SpO_2 decreases in sitting position and improves in lying down posture). ABG in room air and with O_2 supplementation, contrast (bubble) echocardiogram and MAA scan (Macroaggregate albumin scan) confirm the diagnosis of HPS. Bubble-contrast echocardiogram helps to distinguish HPS from intracardiac shunt. LT is a curative treatment. POPH is a form of pulmonary arterial hypertension with increased pulmonary vascular resistance due to vasoconstriction and progressive pulmonary vascular remodeling with incidence of approximately 5–10% of LT candidates.[7] It is characterized by raised mean pulmonary artery pressure (mPAP) more than 25 mm Hg at rest, elevated pulmonary vascular resistance more than 120 dyne/s/cm^{-5} and normal or decreased pulmonary artery wedge pressure less than 15 mm Hg. It can be mild (mPAP 25–35 mm Hg), moderate (mPAP 35–45 mm Hg) or severe (>45 mm Hg) depending on mPAP. The OLT in presence of uncontrolled POPH is associated with increased mortality due to right heart failure and hepatic failure. The AASLD guidelines[2] recommended that all patients scheduled for OLT should undergo screening for pulmonary hypertension. Doppler echocardiography is an excellent screening test in this setting. If right ventricular systolic pressure (RVSP) > 50 mm Hg, right heart catheterization should be done to rule out other causes of pulmonary hypertension.[12] However, long-term vasodilator treatment with epoprostenol helps to reduce PAP and improves post-OLT mortality rate. Patients with severe pulmonary hypertension should be considered for liver transplantation only, if the condition can be effectively controlled with medical therapy.

Hematological

During preoperative evaluation for OLT, commonly encountered hematological problems are anemia, thrombocytopenia, coagulopathy, etc. It is evident that patients with liver disease may experience both bleeding complications as well as thrombotic episodes. The occurrence of bleeding complications has been explained by the reduced platelet count, the decreased plasma levels of coagulation factors, and the decreased plasma levels of inhibitors of fibrinolysis. Thrombotic disease has been attributed to decreased plasma levels of the natural anticoagulants protein C and S and antithrombin. As fibrinogen and factor VIII are not synthesized in liver, decreasing levels of these factors indicate primary fibrinolysis or DIC, not liver disorders. Some consider the coagulopathy of liver failure to be a balanced coagulopathy having an equal decrease in pro and anticoagulant factors.[13] Prolonged prothrombin time (PT) correlates with the severity of liver disease and is one of the variables commonly used as a prognostic marker.[1]

Central nervous system (CNS): Up to 80% of patients with acute liver failure develop cerebral edema and increased intracranial pressure. Decreased liver clearance leads to accumulation of neurotoxins like ammonia, manganese, etc. and also imbalance of neurotransmitters like γ-aminobutyric acid (GABA), glutamate and nitric oxide resulting into cerebral symptoms. Clinical signs range from a mild form with behavioral changes to the most severe form including decerebrate posturing and coma. It is important to avoid factors that might precipitate hepatic encephalopathy. Therefore, correction of reversible factors, e.g. hypokalemia, alkalemia, hypoglycemia, hypovolemia, and a very restrictive use of benzodiazepines must be considered.[11]

Gastrointestinal (GI): Esophageal varices, portal hypertension, and ascites are common manifestation in ESLD. Gastric emptying is delayed and drug metabolism is affected. Preoperative optimization may include sclerotherapy, portosystemic shunts and treatment of ascites with diuretics, paracentesis, and albumin administration.[1]

6. What should be the anesthetic preparation and induction?

Ans. Although transplant recipients are already evaluated and optimized, they should be reassessed after admission for surgery with recent investigations. Sedative-anxiolytics and proton pump inhibitors used as premedication.

Rapid sequence induction should be planned because of the emergent nature of the surgery and presence of ascites. Two large-bore intravenous access is obtained. An arterial catheter is placed either before induction or shortly thereafter. The 9 Fr. cannula with port for pulmonary catheter insertion may be used as central access. Some anesthesiologists use two different access for central and pulmonary catheter. Although many centres in Western countries stopped using pulmonary artery catheter except for specific indications, it is still being used routinely in most of the Indian centres. Sites designated for venovenous bypass are avoided. A rapid infusion system capable of high transfusion flow rates (500–1500 mL/min) is a must-have tool to combat massive bleeding. Such systems incorporate a reservoir, pump, filters, heat exchanger, and safety features designed to avoid and monitor for the presence of blood or air embolism, hypothermia, and line occlusion.

7. How should you maintain the patient intraoperatively?

Ans. Usually, a balanced anesthetic technique is used consisting of volatile agent in low to moderate concentrations (0.5–1.0 MAC), an opioid, usually fentanyl (Remifentanil is better choice) and neuromuscular blocking agent (NMBA) which is independent of liver metabolism. However, some investigators have suggested the use of rocuronium because the duration of the neuromuscular block appears to be a useful predictor of primary allograft function. All patients whose recovery time was >150 minutes experienced primary graft dysfunction.[1] The volatile agent of choice is isoflurane, which preserves splanchnic blood flow better than other volatile drugs. N_2O is avoided as it is detrimental in cases of air embolism, causes bowel inflation and has bone marrow suppressant effect.

8. What parameters to be monitored?

Ans. The recipients should be extensively monitored:

- *Cardiovascular:* ECG, invasive BP, CVP, PAP, PAOP, CO, SVR, PVR, TEE.
- *Respiratory:* SaO_2, $ETCO_2$ and ABG.
- *Renal:* urine output
- Temperature
- *Hematological:* Hb/PCV, platelet count
- *Coagulation profile:* PT/PTT/INR, serum fibrinogen, thromboelastograph (TEG)
- *Biochemical:* *Electrolytes:* Na, K, iCa, Mg, lactate, glucose

All investigations should be done at regular intervals preferably at induction and at 1 hour interval in preanhepatic phase. Then it should be repeated 5 minutes before and 10 minutes into anhepatic phase. Thereafter, it should be done 5 minutes before and 10 minutes into reperfusion phase.

9. What are the different phases of surgery?

Ans. Liver transplant surgery can be divided into the preanhepatic phase, the anhepatic phase, and the reperfusion or neohepatic phase with important anesthetic considerations at each phase. The preanhepatic stage begins with surgical incision and ends with cross-clamping of the portal vein, the suprahepatic inferior vena cava, the infrahepatic inferior vena cava, and the hepatic artery. This phase involves dissection and mobilization of the liver and identification of the porta hepatis.

The anhepatic stage begins with the occlusion of vascular inflow to the liver and ends with graft reperfusion.

Neohepatic stage starts with reperfusion of the new liver following unclamping of all three vessels: suprahepatic, infrahepatic vena cava and portal vein after completion of vascular anastomosis. After successful reperfusion, hepatic artery and biliary anastomosis are completed followed by hemostasis and closure.

10. What are the problems in the preanhepatic phase and how will you manage?

Ans. After abdominal incision, drainage of ascitic fluid leads to hypovolemia which should be anticipated and treated with colloid-containing fluid. There is risk of excessive bleeding due to pre-existing coagulopathy, portal hypertension, adhesion and bleeding from venous collaterals. Transfusion of blood and products may be necessary with the aim to maintain Hb% of 7–9 gm/dL, INR between 1.5–2.5 and platelet count ≥ 50,000/cmm. Thromboelastography, ROTEM or standard laboratory tests (prothrombin time, fibrinogen and platelet count) are used to guide the correction of coagulopathy. Many centers avoid giving any procoagulant unless the diagnosis of coagulopathy is supported by both laboratory evidence (usually TEG or platelet count) and clinical evidence (e.g. diffuse oozing and lack of clot in the field).[14] Use of cell-saver in selected cases reduce transfusion requirement. As fibrinolysis is rare during this phase administration of cryoprecipitate and antifibrinolytics is usually not necessary. Prophylactic antifibrinolytic agents may be used in case of portal hypertension. Recent trial showed that a policy of restrictive transfusions and low CVP during LT leads to a significant reduction in intraoperative blood loss and transfusion requirement, especially during the preanhepatic phase.[13] Citrate-induced ionized hypocalcemia resulting from the transfusion of blood products in the absence of hepatic function, is avoided by the administration of calcium gluconate/chloride. Ionized hypomagnesemia also results from citrate infusion, but magnesium level gradually return to normal after graft reperfusion. The clinical significance of this remains speculative, but cardiovascular function may be affected. Aggressive treatment of hypokalemia is avoided, as serum potassium usually increases after reperfusion. Hyponatremia should not be corrected rapidly. Supplemental glucose is usually not required except in pediatric patients or those with fulminant hepatic failure. Metabolic acidosis should be corrected. Temperature and urine output should be maintained. However, there is no role of low-dose dopamine for this reason. The use of heated venovenous bypass during the anhepatic phase permits core temperature control.

11. What are the problems in the anhepatic phase and how will you manage?

Ans. Cross-clamping of the suprahepatic and infrahepatic vena cava (IVC) decreases venous return by as much as 50%. Venovenous bypass (VVB), which diverts blood flow from inferior vena cava and portal vein to the axillary vein, attenuates the decrease in preload, improves renal perfusion pressure, lessens splanchnic congestion, and delays the development of metabolic acidosis. The risk of VVB is multifold like airembolism, thromboembolism, and inadvertent decannulation which may be fatal or result in significant morbidity. The VVB is now being used in selected cases as in patients with severe pulmonary hypertension, with difficult surgical dissection, preoperative severe renal or cardiac disease, signs of inadequate systemic perfusion and hypotension on trial clamping.[15,16] The use of 'piggyback' technique, with inferior vena caval preservation, decreases the need for VVB. Usually, fibrinolysis may begin during this stage, caused by an absence of liver-produced plasminogen activator inhibitor, which results in the unopposed action of tissue plasminogen activator. The use of antifibrinolytics varies among centers. Reduction in intraoperative bleeding and transfusion requirement with aprotinin and tranexamic acid has been well established in patients undergoing OLT. However, patient selection should be on an individual basis to avoid complications.[17]

12. What are the problems in the neohepatic phase and how will you manage?

Ans. Reperfusion of the new liver through the portal vein begins the neohepatic stage. With reperfusion, cold, acidotic and hyperkalemic blood enters the circulation resulting into an increase in preload, decrease in SVR and blood pressure. Hypothermia, monitored through a centrally placed catheter, is a marker for the presence of graft outflow into the central circulation. Life-threatening hyperkalemia, clinically detectable by changes in the ECG, requires prompt treatment with calcium gluconate/chloride and sodium bicarbonate. If time permits, albuterol and insulin are also effective. Intraoperative dialysis or continuous renal replacement therapy (CRRT) should be considered early in the procedure for oliguric patients with elevated potassium levels.[18] The hallmark of the postreperfusion syndrome (PRS) is systemic hypotension and pulmonary hypertension occurring within the first 5 minutes after reperfusion of the graft and persisting for at least 1 minute and associated with bradycardia. Approximately, one in three patients undergoing OLT has profound hypotension after reperfusion. The cause is uncertain, but a number of factors, such as hyperkalemia, acidosis, hypothermia, emboli (air or thrombotic), and vasoactive substances, have been implicated. One common predictor appears to be cold ischemic time. It was observed that prolonged cold ischemia time contributed to a higher incidence of PRS in cadaveric liver transplantation.[19] If it should occur, PRS should be treated with boluses and infusion vasopressors and inotropes. Acidosis, hyperkalemia and hypocalcemia should be corrected prior to reperfusion to reduce the impact of PRS. Hepatic arterial anastomosis and biliary reconstruction are generally performed after venous reperfusion. Signs of graft function that may be observed in the operating room include decreased calcium requirements, improvement in acidosis, increased urine output, rise in core temperature and bile production from the graft.

13. How are transplant recipients managed postoperatively?

Ans. Postoperatively, the recipient is managed in the intensive care unit. The decision to extubate the patient in the operating theater will depend on the patient's preoperative condition and intraoperative events, i.e. lesser disease severity, absence of encephalopathy or co-existing disease, age <50 years, good graft function, RBC transfusion <10 U, alveolar-arterial oxygen gradient <150 mm Hg and no vasoactive support at end of surgery.[14] The recipients are monitored closely for bleeding, hepatic artery thrombosis, portal vein thrombosis and early graft rejection. Systemic opioids are administered for postoperative analgesia. Extubated patients should be carefully observed for sedation and respiratory depression.

REFERENCES

1. Steadman RH. Anesthesia for liver transplant surgery. Anesthesiology Clin N Am. 2004:22;687-711.
2. Murray KF, Carithers RL Jr. AASLD Practice Guidelines: Evaluation of the Patient for Liver Transplantation. Hepatology. 2005;41:1407-32.

3. Terrault NA, Roland ME, Schiano T, Dove L, Wong MT, Poordad F, et al. Outcomes of Liver Transplantation in HCV-HIV Coinfected Recipients. Liver Transpl. 2012;18(6):716-26.
4. Baccarani U, Scudeller L, Adani GL. Is liver transplantation feasible in patients coinfected with human immunodeficiency virus and hepatitis C virus? Liver Transplantation. 2012;18:744-5.
5. Groszmann RJ, Iwakiri Y, Taddei TH. Liver Transplantation in the human immunodeficiency virus-hepatitis C virus coinfected patient: Time to Sum-up. Hepatology. 2013;57(1):409-11.
6. Mandell SM, Tsou MY. Cardiovascular dysfunction in patients with end-stage liver disease. J Chin Med Assoc. 2008;71:331-5.
7. Raval Z, Harinstein ME, Skaro AI, Erdogan A, DeWolf AM, Shah SJ, et al. Cardiovascular risk assessment of the liver transplant candidate. Journal of American College of Cardiology. 2011;58(3):223-31.
8. Slack A, Yeoman A, Wendon J. Renal dysfunction in chronic liver disease. Critical Care. 2010;14:214-24.
9. Salerno F, Gerbes A, Gines P, et al. Diagnosis, prevention and treatment of hepatorenal syndrome in cirrhosis. Gut. 2007;56:1310-18.
10. Gines P, Schrier RW. Renal failure in cirrhosis. N Engl J Med. 2009;361:1279-90.
11. Hoetzel A, Ryan H, Schmidt R. Anesthetic considerations for the patient with liver disease. Curr Opin Anesthesiol. 2012,25:340-7.
12. Nandhakumar A, McCluskey SA, Srinivas C, Chandy TT. Liver transplantation: advances and perioperative care. IJA. 2012;56:326-35 (accessed on Sept 10, 2013).
13. Lisman T, Porte RJ. Rebalanced hemostasis in patients with liver disease: evidence and clinical consequences. Blood. 2010;116:878-85.
14. Manley JL, Plotkin JS, Yosaitis J, Plevak DJ. Controversies in anesthetic management of liver transplantation. HPB. 2005;7:183-5.
15. Fonouni H, Mehrabi A, Soleimani M, Muller SA, Buchler MW, Schmidt J. The need for venovenous bypass in liver transplantation. HPB. 2008;10:196-203.
16. Ozier Y, Klinck JR. Anesthetic management of hepatic transplantation. Current Opinion in Anaesthesiology. 2008;21:391-400.
17. Makwana J, Paranjape S, Goswami J. Antifibrinolytics in liver surgery. Indian J Anaesth. 2010;54:489-95.
18. Hall TH, Dhir A. Anesthesia for liver transplantation. Semin Cardiothorac Vasc Anesth. 2013;17:180-94.
19. Xu ZD, Xu HT, Yuan HB, Zhang H, Ji RH, Zou Z, et al. Postreperfusion syndrome during orthotopic liver transplantation: a single-center experience. Hepatobiliary Pancreat Dis Int. 2012;11:34-9.

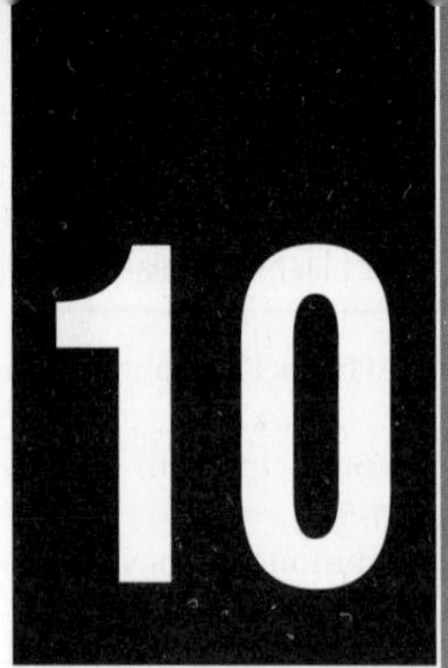

Preanesthetic Evaluation

Dalim Kumar Baidya, Souvik Maitra

Preanesthetic evaluation is the process of clinical assessment that precedes the delivery of anesthesia care for surgery and nonsurgical procedures. It includes clinical evaluation, necessary preoperative optimization and formulation of proper anesthetic plan. During preanesthetic evaluation the anesthesiologist may choose to consult with other healthcare experts regarding patient's coexisting medical conditions which are relevant to perioperative anesthetic care.

APPROACH TO A PATIENT IN PREANESTHETIC CLINIC

- History taking
- Physical examination
- Review of previous anesthetic records
- Review of diagnostic records (e.g. laboratory investigations, ECG, etc.)
- Assignment of ASA physical status score
- Formulation and discussion of anesthetic plan with patient
- Obtaining proper informed consent.

History Taking

Single most important step in preanesthetic evaluation is history taking. The following issues must be kept in mind during history taking for preanesthetic evaluation:

- Identification of the patient
- History of the present illness for which posted for surgery
- History of any comorbid diseases (e.g. HTN/DM/COPD, etc.)
- History of any medication
- Past history of surgery and anesthesia related complications, if any (e.g. history of PONV, awareness, postoperative jaundice, difficult airway, etc. during previous surgery)
- History of any major illness or hospital admission in the past
- Personal history (e.g. menstrual history in females, history of addiction to nicotine or alcohol, etc.)
- History of allergy to any drugs, food or natural rubber (latex).

A computer generated preformed questionnaire may be used for this purpose. Although it may be desirable, there is little evidence to suggest that the anesthesiologist who is evaluating a patient should also provide anesthesia care for that very patient.

In family history all patients should be enquired about:

- Inherited conditions in the family
- History of prolonged apnea
- Unexplained death
- Malignant hyperpyrexia
- Surgery postponed
- Conditions are identified
- Patient investigated appropriately
- Emergency situation, anesthesia adjusted accordingly.

Physical Examinations

- General survey (includes vitals, height and weight, anemia, jaundice, cyanosis, clubbing, edema, etc.)
- Airway assessment
- Cardiovascular system
- Pulmonary system
- Nervous system.

Till today no clinical trial has been performed to assess the utility of preoperative history taking and clinical evaluation on anesthetic management. Observational studies have found that perioperative complications (e.g. cardiac, respiratory, renal, hemorrhagic) are associated with specific pre-existing conditions (e.g. diabetes, pulmonary disease, chronic hypertension, previous myocardial infarction, history of smoking, high body mass index, extremes of age). At minimum, an airway evaluation and examination of pulmonary and cardiovascular system and documentation of vital parameters must be done during preoperative visit.

The timing of preoperative evaluation is also debatable. For patients undergoing surgeries of high invasiveness, preanesthetic evaluation should be done at least one day before surgery and for surgeries of low invasiveness, evaluation can be done either on the day before or on the day of surgery.

Airway Assessment

Purpose of the airway assessment is to identify the patients who are likely to have a difficult airway in terms of mask ventilation and/or laryngoscopy and intubation. However, no single test alone is capable of identifying these patients with certainty. A battery of clinical tests are recommended for these purposes. The following criteria may be used to identify the patients who are at risk of potential difficult mask ventilation:

- Bearded individual
- Obesity (BMI >26 kg/m^2)
- No teeth
- Elderly (Age >55 yrs)
- Snoring history.

The components of airway assessment includes but not limited to:

- Assessment of neck movements
  - Ask the patient to touch his manubrium with chin followed by asking him to look at the ceiling without raising eyebrow.
  - Normal neck flexion is 25–35° and atlanto-occipital joint extension 85°.

- Assessment of temporomandibular joint function
  - Mouth opening > 5 cm or three finger breadth of the patient
  - Sliding function of the mandible
- Assessment of mandibular space.

Thyromental distance

- Distance between thyroid notch and mentum when neck is fully extended
- *>6.5 cm:* No problem in laryngoscopy and intubation
- *6.0–6.5 cm:* Laryngoscopy and intubation difficult but possible
- *<6.0 cm:* Laryngoscopy may be impossible
- Assessment of adequacy of oropharynx.

Narrowness of palate: A narrow and high arched palate is often associated with difficult intubation.

Mallampati grading: Most commonly done tests in PAC clinic. This is performed by having the patient open the mouth as wide as possible and protrude the tongue without phonation.
Grade I: Faucial pillars, uvula, soft and hard palate is visible
Grade II: Uvula, soft and hard palate is visible
Grade III: Base of uvula or none, soft and hard palate is visible
Grade IV: Only hard palate is visible.

Sternomental distance

- Measured in head extension with mouth closed
- <12.5 cm predicts difficult laryngoscopy and intubation
- It has highest sensitivity and specificity as a single most test.

Evaluation of the Cardiovascular System

Cardiovascular complications are the most serious perioperative adverse events. Cardiac morbidity occurs in 1–5% unselected patients undergoing noncardiac surgery.

Goals of preoperative cardiac evaluation

- Identify the risk for heart disease based on risk factors
- Identify the presence and severity of heart disease from symptoms, physical findings or diagnostic tests
- Determine the need for preoperative interventions
- Modify the risk for perioperative adverse events.

History taking for cardiovascular evaluation: The history should be aimed to identify cardiac conditions those require optimum management before elective surgery, such as unstable coronary syndromes, prior angina, recent or past MI, decompensated HF, significant arrhythmias, and severe valvular disease. It should also determine whether the patient has a prior history of a pacemaker or implantable cardioverter defibrillator (ICD) or a history of orthostatic intolerance. Modifiable risk factors for coronary artery disease (CAD) should be recorded, along with evidence of associated diseases, such as peripheral vascular disease, cerebrovascular disease, diabetes mellitus, renal impairment, and chronic pulmonary disease. In patients with established cardiac disease, any recent change in symptoms must be ascertained. Accurate recording of current medications used, including herbal and other nutritional supplements, and dosages is essential. Use of alcohol, tobacco, over-the-counter and illicit drugs should be documented.

The history should also be aimed to determine the patient's functional capacity (Table 1). An assessment of an individual's functional capacity correlates well with maximum oxygen uptake by treadmill testing.

Table 1 | Patient functionial capacity

1 MET	Can you ... take care of yourself?	4 METs	Can you... climb a flight of stairs or walk up a hill?	
	Eat, dress, or use the toilet?		Walk on level ground at 4 mph (6.4 kph)?	
	Walk indoors around the house?		Run a short distance?	
	Walk a block or 2 on level ground at 2–3 mph (3.2–4.8 kph)?		Do heavy work around the house like scrubbing floors or lifting or moving heavy furniture?	
	4 METs		Do light work around the house like dusting or washing dishes?	Participate in moderate recreational activities like golf, bowling, dancing, doubles tennis, or throwing a baseball or football?
			Greater than 10 METs	Participate in strenuous sports like swimming, singles tennis, football, basketball, or skiing?

Physical examination for cardiovascular evaluation

Vital signs

- *Pulse:* Regularity, radial, carotid, femoral
- Blood pressure
- Pulse pressure
- Respiration.

Cardiac examination

- Jugular venous pressure (JVP)
- Peripheral edema
- Displaced apical impulse—cardiomegaly
- S3 gallop (increased LVEDP)
- S4 (decreased compliance)
- Apical systolic murmur (papillary muscle dysfunction)
- Pulmonary edema
- Murmurs.

Active cardiac conditions (Table 2) for which the patient should undergo evaluation and treatment before noncardiac surgery.

Table 2 | Evaluation and treatment for cardiac condition

Condition	*Examples*
Unstable coronary syndromes	Unstable or severe angina* (CCS class III or IV)†
	Recent MI‡
Decompensated HF (NYHA functional class IV; worsening or new-onset HF)	
Significant arrhythmias	High-grade atrioventricular block
	Mobitz II atrioventricular block
	Third-degree atrioventricular heart block
	Symptomatic ventricular arrhythmias
	Supraventricular arrhythmias (including atrial fibrillation) with uncontrolled ventricular rate (HR greater than 100 bpm at rest)
	Symptomatic bradycardia
	Newly recognized ventricular tachycardia
Severe valvular disease	Severe aortic stenosis (mean pressure gradient greater than 40 mm Hg, aortic valve area less than 1.0 cm^2, or symptomatic)
	Symptomatic mitral stenosis (progressive dyspnea on exertion, exertional presyncope, or HF)

CCS indicates Canadian Cardiovascular Society; HF, heart failure; HR, heart rate; MI, myocardial infarction; NYHA, New York Heart Association.
*According to Campeau.
†May include 'stable' angina in patients who are unusually sedentary.
‡The American College of Cardiology National Database Library defines recent MI as more than 7 days but less than or equal to 1 month (within 30 days).

Composite risk index for cardiac complications: The revised cardiac risk index

Lee et al formulated an index for the prediction of cardiac risk for stable patients undergoing nonurgent major noncardiac surgery. Six independent risk correlates were identified:

1. *Ischemic heart disease* (defined as history of MI, history of positive treadmill test, use of nitroglycerin, current complaints of chest pain thought to be secondary to coronary ischemia, or ECG with abnormal Q waves).
2. *Congestive HF* (defined as history of HF, pulmonary edema, paroxysmal nocturnal dyspnea, peripheral edema, bilateral rales, S3, or X-ray with pulmonary vascular redistribution).
3. *Cerebral vascular disease* (history of transient ischemic attack or stroke).
4. *High-risk surgery* (abdominal aortic aneurysm or other vascular, thoracic, abdominal, or orthopedic surgery).
5. *Preoperative insulin treatment for diabetes mellitus.*
6. *Preoperative creatinine greater than 2 mg per dL.*

Increasing numbers of risk factors correlated with increased risk, yet the risk was substantially lower than described in many of the original indices.

Flow chart 1 shows step-wise approach for cardiac evaluations.

Flow chart 1 Step-wise approach for cardiac evaluations

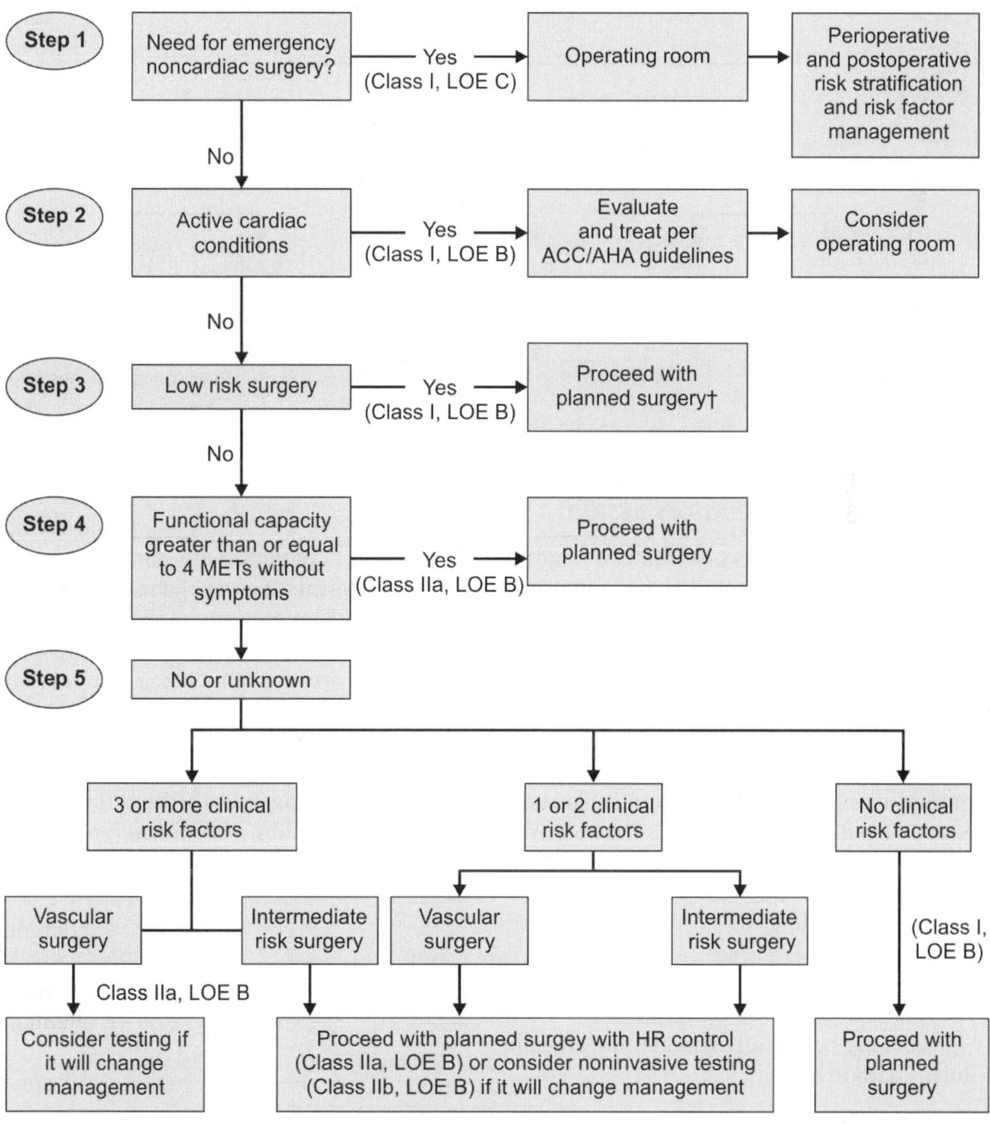

A patient with history of PCI/Balloon angioplasty: ACC/AHA has formulated guideline (Flow chart 2) for such patients with the emphasis to continue at least one antiplatelet drug in the perioperative period.

Flow chart 2 ACC/AHA guidelines

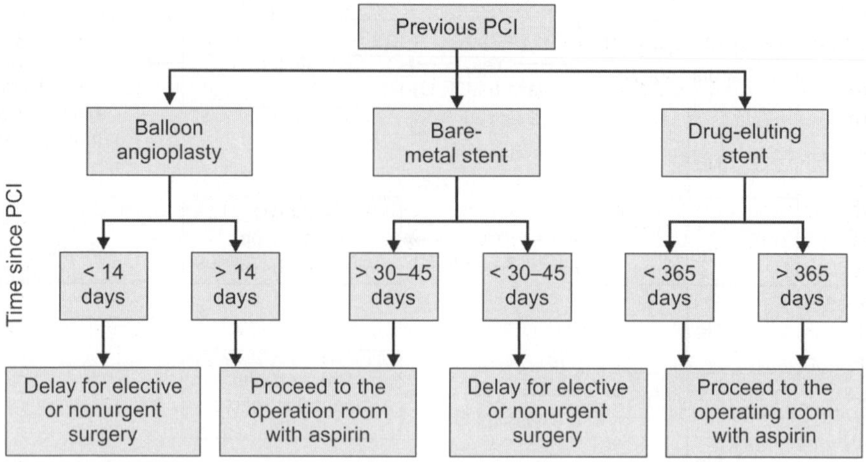

Previous PCI

- Balloon angioplasty
  - < 14 days → Delay for elective or nonurgent surgery
  - > 14 days → Proceed to the operation room with aspirin
- Bare-metal stent
  - > 30–45 days → Proceed to the operation room with aspirin
  - < 30–45 days → Delay for elective or nonurgent surgery
- Drug-eluting stent
  - < 365 days → Delay for elective or nonurgent surgery
  - > 365 days → Proceed to the operating room with aspirin

Time since PCI

Evaluation of the Respiratory System

Respiratory complications occur in two major patient groups: (1) patients with normal lungs who develop respiratory abnormalities secondary to surgery and anesthesia and (2) patients with overt chronic lung disease in whom the problems of anesthesia and the operation are superimposed on intrinsically diseased pulmonary tissue.

The respiratory system can be afflicted with a vast number of disorders, but asthma and diseases that contribute to chronic obstructive pulmonary disease are most prevalent. Furthermore, these particular disorders have the most significant impact on patient management.

The aim of evaluation of respiratory system is to identify the risk factors of postoperative pulmonary complications (POPC) and ensure optimum medical management of the patients having pre-existing pulmonary diseases. The following points must be addressed during preoperative evaluation:

- Cyanosis
- Pattern of breathing
- Respiratory rate
- Dyspnea
- Wheeze
- Signs of lung collapse/consolidation/effusion
- Pulsus paradoxus.

Risk factors of postoperative pulmonary complication: Established risk factors are *age* [odds ratio for postoperative pulmonary complications 2.09 (confidence interval, CI 1.70–2.58) for patients aged 60–69 years and 3.04 (CI 2.11–4.39) for ages 70–79, both compared with patients younger than 60 years of age]; *chronic obstructive lung disease* (odds ratio 1.79, CI 1.44–2.22); *cigarette use* (odds ratio 1.26, CI 1.01–1.56); *congestive heart failure* (odds ratio 2.93, CI 1.02–8.43); *functional dependence* [for total functional dependence, odds ratio 2.51 (CI 1.99–3.15) and for partial dependence, odds ratio 1.64 (CI 1.36–2.01)]; and a *higher ASA classification* and *prolonged duration of surgery* (odds ratio 2.14, CI 1.33–3.46).

Additional risk factors (type of surgery, weight loss, cerebral vascular disease, long-term steroid use as well as alcohol use) have been identified and included in a risk index for predicting postoperative pneumonia after major noncardiac surgery.

Preoperative investigations: Preoperative investigations have very limited role in evaluation of respiratory system before non-thoracic surgery. Spirometry has value in diagnosing obstructive lung disease, but it has not been shown to translate into effective risk prediction for individual patients. In addition, there are no data indicating a prohibitive threshold for spirometric values below which the risk for surgery would be unacceptable. Changes in clinical management due to findings from preoperative spirometry were also not reported.

Though chest X-rays are frequently advised routinely, they are not predictive of postoperative pulmonary complications. A change in management or cancellation of elective surgery was reported in only a fraction of patients on the basis of abnormal chest X-ray. However, possibility of abnormal X-ray finding increases in the extreme age groups.

Scope of optimization: Preoperative incentive spirometry and deep breathing exercises before major upper abdominal surgery, smoking cessation even for a short period and improvement of nutritional status may have beneficial role in preventing postoperative pulmonary complications.

Evaluation of Renal System

Perioperative acute renal failure has a very high morbidity and mortality rate; hence identification of patients who are at risk of acute kidney injury is highly desirable. Chronic renal disease also affects multiple organ system and affects perioperative care to a significant extent. Even a moderate preoperative elevation of serum creatinine is associated with adverse outcomes such as complications and death in patients undergoing general surgery. Kheterpal et al identified risk factors of postoperative renal dysfunction and these are: *intraperitoneal surgery* (relative risk 3.3, 95% CI 2.4–4.7); *moderate renal insufficiency* (relative risk 3.2, 95% CI 2.8–3.7); *mild renal insufficiency* (relative risk 3.1, 95% CI 2.5–3.9); *ascites* (relative risk 3.0, 95% CI 2.2–4.0); *active congestive heart failure* (relative risk 2.0, 95% CI 1.4–3.0); *emergency surgery* (relative risk 1.9, 95% CI 1.5–2.3), *age of at least 56 years* (relative risk 1.7, 95% CI 1.4–2.2); *diabetes requiring insulin therapy* (relative risk 1.7, 95% CI 1.3–2.3); *hypertension* (relative risk 1.5, 95% CI 1.2–1.9); *male sex* (relative risk 1.4, 95% CI 1.2–1.7); and *diabetes requiring oral medication* (relative risk 1.3, 95% CI 1.0–1.7).

Preoperative evaluation of a chronic kidney disease (CKD) patient

Hematological: Identify and treat anemia, coagulation abnormality and platelet function abnormalities.

Cardiovascular: Identify coexisting cardiac problems like hypertension, left ventricular hypertrophy, coronary artery disease, atherosclerosis and volume overload.

Metabolic: Metabolic acidosis, hyperkalemia, hypocalcemia and hypermagnesemia, etc. should be detected and optimized.

Need for renal replacement therapy (RRT): Ensure hemodialysis of the patients, who are already on RRT, 24–48 hours before surgery and assess the volume status pre and postdialysis period.

Evaluation of Hepatic System

A thorough preoperative history usually detects overt liver dysfunction. However, in early stages of chronic liver diseases or with mild hepatitis, patients may be asymptomatic. The aim of history and physical examination is to identify the degree of liver dysfunction and identify the complications of chronic liver failure. Patients, when symptomatic, usually presents with the complaints of fatigue, weight loss, dark urine, pale stools, pruritus, right upper quadrant pain, bloating, and jaundice. Physical examination may reveal jaundice, bruising, ascites, pleural effusions, peripheral edema, or hypoxia. The presence of encephalopathy, coagulopathy, ascites, volume overload, pulmonary dysfunction and cardiac dysfunction such as pulmonary hypertension, etc. need to be assessed preoperatively.

The Child-Turcotte-Pugh (CTP) classification (Table 3) and model for end-stage liver disease (MELD) formula, which factors bilirubin, the international normalized ratio (INR), creatinine, and the cause of the liver disease, can predict perioperative morbidity and mortality in chronic liver disease patients and may be better than the CTP.

Table 3 | Child-Turcotte-Pugh classification

Parameter	*Points*		
	1	2	3
Ascites	Absent	Slight	Moderate
Bilirubin (mg/dL)	<2	2–3	>3
Albumin (g/dL)	>3.5	2.8–3.5	<2.8
Prothrombin time (seconds over control)	<4	4–6	>6
Encephalopathy	None	Grade 1–2	Grade 3–4

Class A: <7 points; Class B: 7–9 points; Class C: >9 points.

For cholestatic diseases (e.g. primarily biliary cirrhosis), the bilirubin level is disproportionate to the impairment in hepatic function and an allowance should be made. For these conditions, assign 1 point for a bilirubin level less than 4 mg/dL, 2 points for a bilirubin level of 4 to 10 mg/dL, and 3 points for a bilirubin level over 10 mg/dL

The CTP classification correlates well with the perioperative mortality after major abdominal surgery in these patients and mortality may be as high as up to 80% in CTP- class–C patients particularly during emergency surgery. Ziser and coworkers identified male gender, CTP class C, ascites, azotemia, perioperative infection, higher American Society of Anesthesiologists (ASA) physical classification, a diagnosis of cryptogenic cirrhosis, and surgery on the respiratory system as risk factors independently associated with mortality.

Patients of both acute hepatitis and chronic liver dieses are at risk of perioperative complications. Elective surgery in the presence of acute hepatitis should be delayed till liver enzymes becomes normal. However, isolated liver enzyme elevation up to two times of normal are common and may be present in 4% normal individuals and poses no special anesthetic concerns. In a patient with elevated liver enzyme following protocol may be followed (Flow chart 3) (Mayo ClinProc 1999;74;593-9).

Patients of obstructive jaundice are also at increased risk of perioperative mortality and morbidity. Predictors of surgical mortality are a preoperative hematocrit <30%, serum bilirubin > 11 mg/dL, and malignancy; and mortality may be as high as 60% if all three are present. Acute renal failure may occur in up to 8% cases postoperatively.

Flow chart 3 Patient with elevated liver ensyme protocol

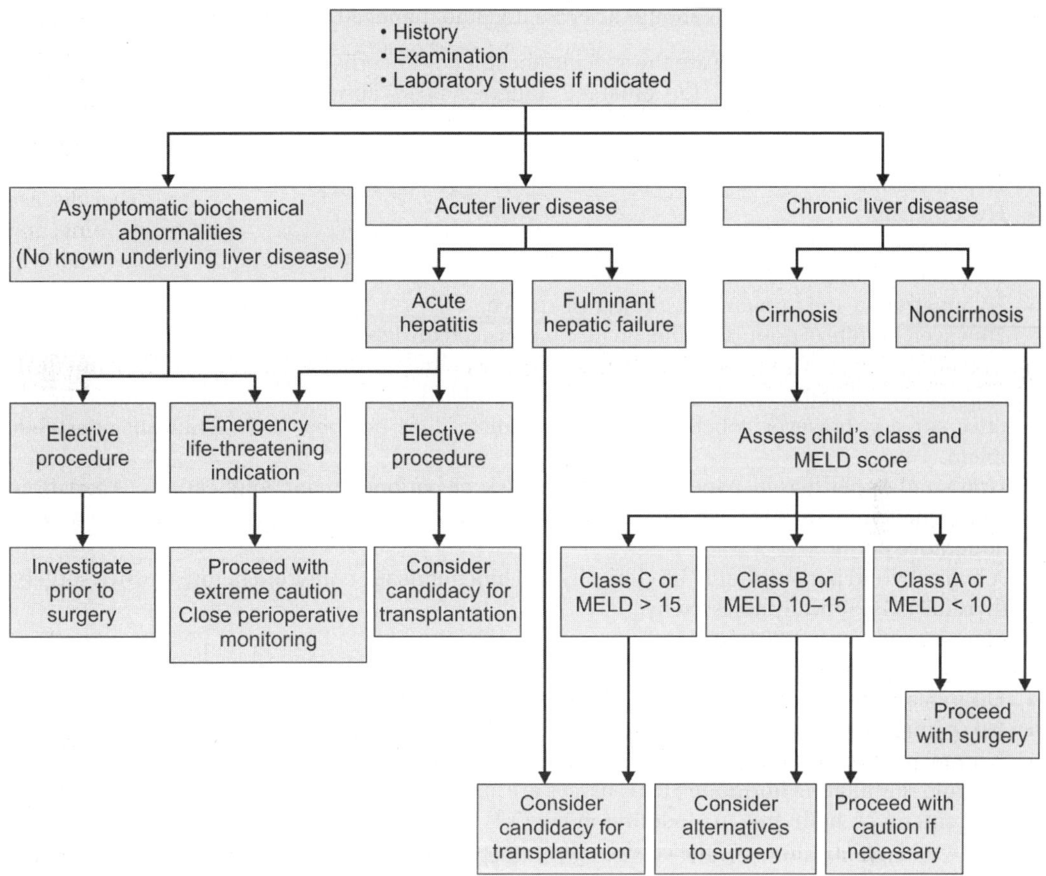

Evaluation of Endocrine System

Diabetes mellitus and thyroid function disorders are the most common endocrine diseases encountered in clinical anesthesia practice.

Screening for diabetes/risk of hyperglycemia can be based on patient history and examinations or investigations of glycemic control. Association has been identified between impaired glucose metabolism and poor perioperative outcome and it has been suggested that 'some effort' should be made to identify these patients in the preoperative period.

As diabetes mellitus increases the possibility of coexisting renal and/or cardiac disease; they should be assessed according to the guidelines for assessment of patients at high-risk of cardiovascular or renal disease. Diabetic patients are also at higher risk of difficult airway, so careful airway assessment in these patients would seem logical. In a diabetic patient it is prudent to find out long-term complications such as atherosclerotic cardiac disease, chronic renal disease, diabetic autonomic neuropathy, etc.

A plan of perioperative glucose control should be formulated from the current medication status of the patients and invasiveness of the surgery. In poorly controlled diabetic patient, careful attention should be paid to prevent short-term complications of diabetes such as diabetic keto-acidosis and hyperosmolar nonketotic coma (HONC).

Thyroid function disorders also affect perioperative management to a significant extent. Both hyper and hypothyroid patients should be evaluated and managed before elective surgery.

Hypothyroidism: The following are the specific anesthetic concerns in a hypothyroid patient:

- Airway compromise—look for enlarged tongue, sleep apnea, large goiter and tracheal compression
- Hypodynamic cardiovascular system
- Hypoglycemia
- Hypothermia
- Hematological—anemia
- Respiratory—impaired CO_2 responsiveness
- Hyponatremia and impaired free water clearance.

However, in spite of popular belief, no RCT has proved till date that a hypothyroid patient require less anesthetic drug. However, they may be more sensitive to the respiratory depressant effects of opioids and inhalation anesthetic. Clinically hypothyroid patients should be optimized before elective surgery; however subclinical hypothyroidism does not pose any significant anesthetic problem.

Untreated hyperthyroid patients are also at risk of perioperative complications. Apart from airway related problem due to an enlarged thyroid gland, following issues should be assessed in the perioperative period:

A hyperthyroid patient should be clinically and biochemically euthyroid before elective surgery. Euthyroidism is clinically assessed by:

- Sleeping pulse rate < 90/min
- Progressive weight gain
- Disappearance of toxic symptoms like tremors, nervousness, anxiety, etc.
- No requirement of sedation for sleep.
- Normal pulse pressure, sinus rhythm, disappearance of cardiac murmurs.

Thyroid-stimulating hormone (TSH) assays are single best test to evaluate for hypothyroidism. Measurement of both free tri-iodothyronine (T3) and thyroxine (T4) and TSH is useful in hyperthyroid patients to avoid the confounding effects protein-binding on total hormone levels. If clinical symptoms of the patients and therapy have not changed, tests within the 6 month before surgery are usually acceptable.

COAGULATION DISORDERS

Routine use of coagulation tests is not recommended unless there are specific risk factors in the history. If coagulation disorders are suspected, the patient should be referred to a hematologist and proper correction of coagulopathy to be initiated to decrease intraoperative bleeding and transfusion requirements.

PREOPERATIVE INVESTIGATIONS

Preoperative testing is performed to evaluate existing medical conditions and to diagnose asymptomatic conditions based on known risk factors for particular diseases. The choices of laboratory tests should depend on the probable impact of the test results on the differential diagnosis and on patient management. A test should be ordered only if the results will impact the decision to proceed with the planned procedure or alter the anesthesia care plans (Table 4).

Table 4 | Preoperative testing guidelines for American Society of Anesthesiologists physical status I patients

Procedure type	*Invasive status*	*Tests*
Low risk, e.g. breast biopsy, knee arthroscopy, cataracts	Minimal	Baseline creatinine if procedure involves injection of contrast dye
Intermediate risk, e.g. inguinal hernia or lumbar laminectomy	Moderate	Baseline creatinine if procedure involves injection of contrast dye
High risk, e.g. thoracotomy, colectomy, or other procedures with expected fluid shifts or significant blood loss	High	Complete blood count with platelets, electrolytes, blood urea nitrogen, and creatinine

ASSESSMENT OF A CHILD BEFORE ELECTIVE SURGERY

Principles of preoperative evaluation of a child are essentially similar to an adult. However, alleviation of anxiety of both the parents and the child in the preoperative visit is of utmost importance. The aims of preoperative evaluation of a child are:

- Identify and optimize coexisting diseases that may alter perioperative care
- Alleviate anxiety of both the child and the parents
- Ensure that proper preoperative guidelines are followed.

A few controversial issues have been discussed below:

Upper Respiratory Tract Infection

Upper respiratory tract infection (URI) in children is associated with increased adverse airway events such as laryngospasm, bronchospasm, breath holding, desaturation and increased postoperative oxygen requirements. Patients undergoing airway surgery and who are less than one year old are at higher risk. However, children with mild isolated URI in the form of rhinorrhea and/or common cold can usually undergo surgery and anesthesia safely. Following clinical signs may predict adverse outcome in these children:

- Green/yellow productive sputum
- Lower respiratory tract signs—rhonchi, wheeze and creps
- Temperature >38.5
- Lethargy, changed behavior.

Prematurity

These infants may present with a wide variety of cardiorespiratory and neurological disorders including the risk of a perioperative apnea. The risk of apnea in infants less than 60 weeks postconceptional age is significant and preoperative plan should be formulated to monitor these children for at least 24 hours in the postoperative period. Even infants without a history of apnea may develop apnea after general anesthesia if they are less than 60 weeks postconceptional age. Risk factors for postoperative apnea include younger gestational age and hemoglobin less than 10 gm/dL. The risk of apnea does not decrease to below 1% until 56 weeks postconceptional age for infants born at 32 weeks gestation.

RISK STRATIFICATION

Studies have corroborated an association of mortality and morbidity with ASA physical status (ASA PS) scores (Fig. 1).

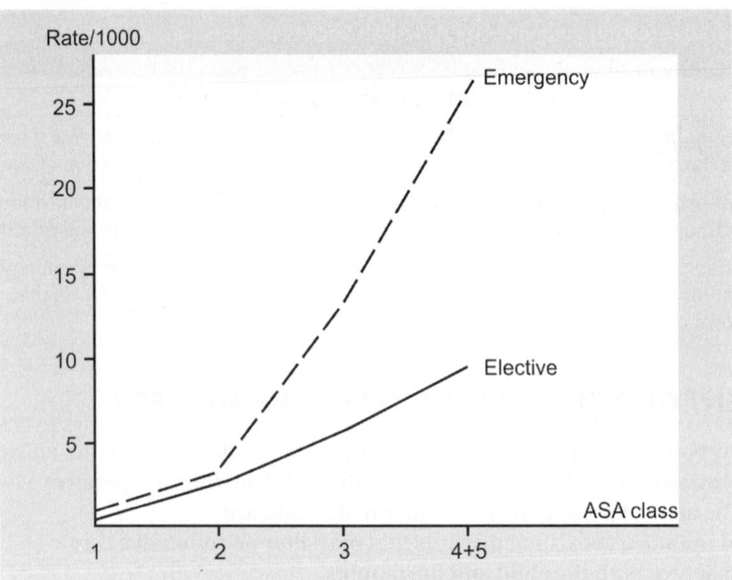

Fig. 1 Relationship of mortality with ASA physical status

American Society of Anesthesiologists Physical Status Classification (Table 5)

PS1: Healthy patient without organic, biochemical, or psychiatric disease.
PS2: A patient with mild systemic disease, e.g. mild asthma or well-controlled hypertension. No significant impact on daily activity. Unlikely impact on anesthesia and surgery
PS3: Significant or severe systemic disease that limits normal activity, e.g. renal failure or dialysis or class 2 congestive heart failure. Significant impact on daily activity. Likely impact on anesthesia and surgery.
PS4: Severe disease that is constant threat to life or requires intensive therapy, e.g. acute myocardial infarction, respiratory failure requiring mechanical ventilation. Serious limitation of daily activity. Major impact on anesthesia and surgery.
PS5: Moribund patient who is equally likely to die in the next 24 hours with or without surgery.
PS6: Brain-dead organ donor.
'E' added to the above (P1–P5) indicates emergency surgery.

Table 5 | ASA classification of physical status and the associated mortality rates (for elective and emergency cases)

ASA rating	*Mortality rate (%)*
ASA PS I	0.1
ASA PS II	0.2
ASA PS III	1.8
ASA PS IV	7.8
ASA PS V	9.4

BIBLIOGRAPHY

1. ACC/AHA 2007 guidelines on perioperative cardiovascular evaluation and care for noncardiac surgery: executive summary: a report of the American College of Cardiology/American Heart Association Task Force on Practice Guidelines (Writing Committee to Revise the 2002 Guidelines on Perioperative Cardiovascular Evaluation for Noncardiac Surgery). Anesth Analg. 2008;106:685-712.
2. Kheterpal S, O'Reilly M, Englesbe MJ, et al. Preoperative and intraoperative predictors of cardiac adverse events after general, vascular and urological surgery. Anesthesiology. 2009;110:58-66.
3. Lee TH, Marcantonio ER, Mangione CM, et al. Derivation and prospective validation of a simple index for prediction of cardiac risk of major noncardiac surgery. Circulation. 1999;100:1043-49.
4. Lerman J. Preoperative assessment and premedication in paediatrics. Eur J Anaesthesiol. 2013;30:645-50.
5. Practice advisory for preanesthesia evaluation: an updated report by the American Society of Anesthesiologists Task Force on Preanesthesia Evaluation. Anesthesiology. 2012;116:522-38.
6. Preoperative evaluation of the adult patient undergoing noncardiac surgery: guidelines from the European Society of Anaesthesiology. Eur J Anaesthesiol. 2011;28:684-722.
7. Ziser A, Plevak DJ, Wiesner RH, et al. Morbidity and mortality in cirrhotic patients undergoing anesthesia and surgery. Anesthesiology. 1999;90:42-53.

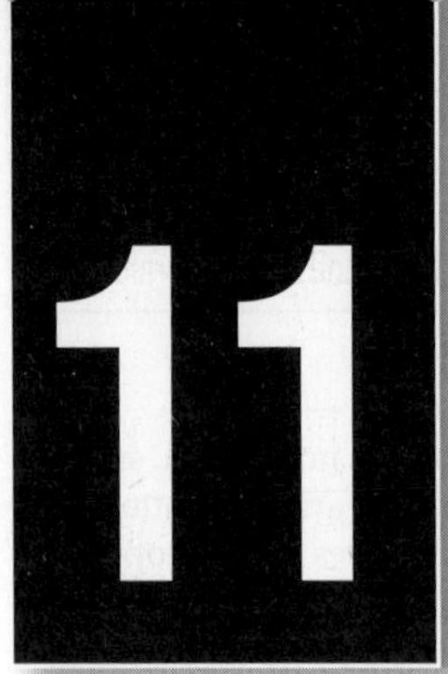

Legal Aspects of Anesthesia: Knowledge of Postgraduates in Anesthesiology

Sukdev Nayak

The courts expect a very high level of responsibilities from the anesthesiologists while discharging their duty. Any practicing anesthesiologists can be summoned to the court for any dereliction of duties and take to task. It is for the anesthesiologists to prevent the initiation of law suits occur against their name. At the present times, any patient or his relatives can knock the doors of justice for malpractice.

The law expects from all the anesthesiologists three things:

1. Essential obligations to assess and use that 'reasonable' degree of learning and skill which is 'ordinarily' possessed by other anesthesiologists in the same locality. The degree of learning and knowledge is the degree that might reasonably be expected from the average doctor in that area.
2. The doctor must use his best judgment. Judgment is the faculty of deciding wisely. It is not the best possible judgment, but his best judgment must bring to bear.
3. He must keep abreast of the times and follow the approved methods in general use.

LEGAL MASTER-SERVANT RELATIONSHIP

Prior to 1942 the relationship between the surgeon and the anesthetists was that of a master-servant, i.e. the anesthesiologist had no indemnity for any mishap during surgical period. The surgeon was taking full charge of the operating period, including anesthesia. If a patient suffered or died from the anamnesis, the surgeon was held responsible though the anesthetists would be joined in the action. But now the anesthetist alone may be held responsible for trouble arising during anesthesia and amnesia but not the surgical interventions. This has put the anesthesiologists to own up their fair responsibility in providing health care.

Hence, the anesthesiologist should now be fully aware of the legal angle. Proper assessment of the risks of anesthesia by taking patient's history and physical state prior to administering the anesthetic is very important. It has to be done by the person himself or by another person on vicarious responsibility. Detailed physical examination is to be done by the anesthesiologist himself/herself to ascertain the patient's condition. Anesthesiologist's notes written in own handwriting are recorded prior to operation to establish this fact. These notes are the safeguards. The risks must be explained to the patients and relatives in a language, they understand and comprehend.

Types of legal cases: An anesthesiologist can be dragged to court either in a criminal or a civil case. In a criminal case, the aggrieved party files a complaint against the anesthesiologist in a police station which then investigates the case and the government prosecutes the concerned anesthesiologist. This happens only when the offense is of a serious nature. The idea of judicial proceedings in criminal cases is to punish the anesthesiologist concerned for the lapse on his part. Complainant does not get any compensation incriminal cases. In a civil case, the aggrieved party itself approaches the court to seek compensation for the harm caused by the action of the anesthesiologist. These cases can go to the common courts or to one of the consumer courts. After introduction of Consumer Protection Act (CPA), most of the cases relating to Medical Negligence go to the consumer courts. The reasons for this are the inexpensive and simple procedure and speedy disposal of the cases in these courts.

Grounds for action: Almost always the patient or their relatives blames the anesthesiologist on grounds of negligence. In a criminal case, it is criminal negligence and in a civil suit, it is negligence in torts.

STANDARDS OF CARE

The standard of care is a general formula describing how a doctor should act in a particular case. It is usually employed by a court or jury to determine whether the anesthesiologist performed his duty and if there was any omission or commission. It is subjective to the locality of the case, and at times could be specific to one particular case. It is based on standard textbooks, references, journals. It is also derived from different guidelines drawn by professional societies from time-to-time in the discipline of anesthesia. The court usually compares the case in question with any similar case which appears to be "prudent and reasonable" and performed by another anesthesiologist from the locality or anywhere around the country. The main standards are:

- The anesthesiologist or an equally qualified person should be present throughout the conduct of general and regional anesthetics and monitor anesthesia care.
- Evaluate continually oxygenation, ventilation, circulation, and temperature.
- Monitor blood oxygen level.

He should provide adequate and continuous ventilation to the anesthetized patient. This is accomplished through four methods:

1. Continually measuring clinical signs as "chest excursion, observation of the reservoir breathing bag, and the auscultation of the breathing sounds." Also, it is encouraged to monitor the level of expired carbon dioxide unless it was restricted by the patient, procedure, or equipment.
2. Ensuring the correct positioning of the endotracheal tube or laryngeal mask and identifying carbon dioxide in the expired gas, as well as performing postoperative capnography, capnometry or mass spectroscopy.
3. Attaching a device that detects whether a disconnection occurred in the breathing system when the patient's ventilation is controlled by a mechanical ventilator.
4. Observing the ventilation adequacy through continual observation of clinical signs and/or monitoring the level of expired carbon dioxide.

These standards came into practice in the early 90s because of sharp rise of premium of professional indemnity and simultaneous public outcry due to increased cases of compensation for anesthesia hazards. Broadcasting of the program on Australian Broadcasting Corporation in 1992 called, "The Deep Sleep, 6000 Will Die or Suffer Brain Damage". This program was iconic in the development of legal issues in anesthesia practice and portrayed a number of problems in anesthesia which could be preventable by appropriate means.

The subsequent increased public awareness pushed anesthesia patients to ask about safety procedures before entering the operating room.

EXPERT WITNESS

Because the judge and jury cannot comprehend the technical issues related to anesthesia malpractice the court assigns 'expert witnesses' to establish whether the minimum standards of care were maintained or not by the defendant-anesthesiologist. Expert witnesses may be any one and are not necessarily medical doctors. Persons with appropriate training may also be summoned to help the court of law. Witnesses should not be a personal friend of the defendant. They must be nationally reputed and acknowledged for their expertise in their field, and are expected to assist in the case, through their skills and training to explain the occurred events.

HOW TO AVOID A LAWSUIT?

To avoid a lawsuit, the anesthesiologist should receive a signed 'informed consent' of the patient or of his/her legal guardian was he/she underage or incapacitated to make his/her own decision. The consent should be preferably written rather than a verbal one since it would hold much better in court. The consent form should include a reasonable and clear explanation of the procedure, describing the risks that might occur with specific patients due to their particular conditions. In the rare case, the patient does not wish to be informed of the procedure and risks, then that should be mentioned in the consent form and preferably countersigned by the patient.

Ingredients of negligence: The opposite party (patient or plaintiff in legal parlance) has to prove four things to be successful in a suit for medical negligence, they are:

1. *Duty:* That the anesthesiologist owed the person a duty.
2. *Breach of duty:* That the anesthesiologist failed to fulfill his or her duty.
3. *Damages:* That actual damage resulted because of the acts of the anesthesiologist.
4. *Causation:* That a reasonably close causal relationship exists between the anesthesiologist's acts and the resultant injury.

Punitive damages or 'exemplary' damages are intended to punish the physician for his/her negligence. The patient's current status is compared to how it used to be had it not been for the anesthesiologist's actions. Exemplary damages are awarded as a deterrent to other physicians as not to repeat the same mistake.

IF A TRIAL IS TO OCCUR?

If the case might be and the four elements are all proved, then the anesthesiologist would probably be sued. If the case does make it to trial, the anesthesiologist would go through several phases and his conduct through them would determine the final outcome of his/her trial.

Phase 1

Primarily, the anesthesiologist must not discuss the details of the case with anyone, be them family members, friends or colleagues. There should never, repeat never any attempt to alter any records; instead all materials and records related to the case should be gathered and preserved. The physician should make notes of the case and cooperate fully with the attorney and investigating agency.

Phase 2

The phase 2 is also known as the 'Discovery' phase. At this stage, the physician and the attorney should work on gathering all facts connected to the case and on clarifying any issues in advance of the trial. Through this phase, the defendant is both assessed and harassed to determine whether he/she will make a good witness in court. The anesthesiologist should answer written interrogatives including information about his/her training, experience and qualifications. This process should be supervised by the attorney since careless or wrong facts or facts placed in a wrong manner can become troublesome later on and can be misinterpreted.

The defendant will also be deposed as a fact witness, while other anesthesiologists would be deposed as expert witnesses. The defendant is thus not allowed to give any opinion on the case, merely recount what happened. During these depositions, the anesthesiologist should refrain from doing the following things:

Do's and don'ts at the Deposition

Do's

- The anesthesiologist/defendant should be aware that a deposition is just as important as testifying in court.
- He/she should be factually prepared with all the details of the case, as well as carrying his/her current curriculum vitae.
- He/she should dress conservatively and appropriately to the situation.
- The defendant should be confident, concise and clear in his/her answers, speaking a bit slower than usual and ready with the correct spelling of a medical term if the clerk asks.
- He/she should be prepared before hand for the deposition by working on questions and rebuttals with the defense attorney.

Don'ts

- The deposition should not be taken in a familiar place to the defendant such as his/her office since it would give him/her a false sense of security and he/she would let his/her guard down.
- He/she should not be arrogant when giving his/her deposition nor should he/she be humorous and make jokes.
- He/she should not use technical medical jargon or volunteer extra information when not asked about it.
- He/she should not be evasive or hostile or admit that there are "definite authoritative textbooks" on which he/she relies on because such a statement would hold him/her reliable to the complete content of the textbook, whether he/she agrees with it or not.
- The defendant should not smoke and should avoid becoming angry or emotional.

Phase 3: The Trial

During the third phase, i.e. trial, the anesthesiologist should aim at convincing the court that he/she behaved in the manner of a prudent and competent physician; that his/her behavior would have been done by any other doctor placed in the same situation. He/she should specify the reasons behind his/her choosing a specific technique or procedure and not another, assuming his/her reasons are valid. If he/she created the impression that a number of procedures were possible and he/she adopted the optimum one, then that would greatly enhance his/her defense. Finally, he/she should not claim that he/she acted out of 100% certainty meaning the opposing witness is 100% wrong. This would decrease his/her credibility.

How to Decrease the Likelihood of a Lawsuit?

The preceding points refer to if the physician encountered a lawsuit.
However, how should one decrease the likelihood of encountering one?
There are five points to be adhered to:

1. The physician must improve his 'doctor-patient' relationship.
2. This is accomplished by spending as much time as possible with the patient and his/her family preoperatively describing the procedure, calming nerves and building a relationship of trust. The anesthesiologist should be aware of the patient's condition, be ready to follow-up actively, if any complications occur and explain it in full if it does. He/she should project a professional image and appear as a person to be trusted.
3. The anesthesiologist should adhere to the 'standards of care' through keeping his/her knowledge bank updated, being prudent in his/her choice of agents, and maintaining the patient's vital signs within a reasonable range.
4. The physician should maintain good records, adhering to the "If it is not written, it was not done" rule. He/she should always have a preoperative note which distinguishes the difference between a bad result and actual negligence. The physician should include a differential diagnosis. He/she should not write notes admitting any wrong doings nor accusing others.
5. The anesthesiologist should respond appropriately when an incident does occur through obtaining consultations and following up on the patient until his/her services are no longer needed and document that in the medical record. The physician should avoid 'Vicarious Liabilities'. He/she should supervise competent people since supervising assistants makes him/her liable for their actions. He/she should specify what equipment and techniques are to be used and not agree to supervise more simultaneous cases than he/she can safely handle. However, in the case of an anesthesiologist supervising a nurse anesthetist, he/she is not liable for the nurse's decision as long as he/she was not involved in the anesthetic management and the making of the decision.

Phase 4: Settling or Losing the Lawsuit

This is the fourth and last stage. In case the care was substandard, the lawsuit would be settled or lost and payment is to be given. The payments are largest in lawsuits for permanent and disabling injuries, lower for death, and lowest for temporary injuries. Finally, in the cases where the anesthesiologist did abandon the patient, inadequately supervised others, or billed a patient for services which was not rendered, then that would make it very hard to defend.

GOVERNMENT HOSPITALS

Right to life guaranteed under the fundamental rights in the Constitution of India is infringed by negligence of the Government doctors. Government or Private Hospitals: Prior to 1995, consumer courts in some cases held that the Government Hospitals are not covered by the Consumer Protections Act. However, the Supreme Court in its judgment in IMA versus V Shantha has clarified this point. In fact, CPA never differentiated between government or private hospitals. It only said that CPA does not cover services provided free of charge. Since most of the government hospitals provide services free of charge, they are not covered by the CPA. However, any hospital whether Government or private who collects charges from all or some of its patient is covered by the CPA after the Supreme Court Judgment. In these hospitals, even the patients treated free of charge are entitled to move the Consumer Courts for compensation for any deficiency in service.

VEXATIOUS COMPLAINTS

Since the approach to the Consumer Courts does not cost anything to the complainant, there is a possibility of this being misused or used as a tool for harassment. Even the courts have accepted this possibility. Though courts have awarded compensation to the respondents in cases of vexatious complaints, the amount is not sufficient to act as deterrent against lodging of frivolous or vexatious complaints and harassment of suppliers of goods and providers of services. Possibility of filing false and vexatious complaints with an intention to harass or speculate has been accepted by the courts also.

PREVENTION

Codes of practice improve standards and it is for the benefit of the medical profession and the patients who place themselves in its hands that further steps are taken expeditiously to achieve this objective. If the rising tide of medical litigation and professional indemnity premiums are to be checked it is necessary for individual anesthesiologist to know and to follow the minimum standards expected of them by the public, their profession and the law. The introduction of the AS A "Standards for Basic Intraoperative Monitoring" was accompanied by a decrease in the number of anesthesia-related liability claims. Improved monitoring, especially the greater use of pulse oxymetry and capnography, has undoubtedly contributed to the decrease in severe complications and the associated large awards. The key factors in the prevention of patient injury are vigilance, up-to-date knowledge, and adequate monitoring.

CONCLUSION

The anesthesiologist has a duty to own body and mind. Full competency and skill is absolute necessary for professional anesthesia practice. A perfect physical, psychosocial and spiritual health is paramount for a successful anesthesia career. Any doubts in the capacities calls for a decrease or cease in professional practice. A competent and prudent anesthesiologist while following appropriate guidelines and providing the proper standards of care, will always be safe from the jaws of malpractice lawyers, and lead a happy life.

BIBLIOGRAPHY

1. AB Kohn, Linda T, Corrigan, Janet M, Donaldson, Molla S (Eds). To Err is Human: building a Safer Health System 2000. Washington, DC. National Academies Press. p. 312. ISBN 978-0-309-06837-6.
2. Anesthesia Patient Safety Foundation. Comments From the Anesthesia Patient Safety Foundation.
3. Anesthesia Patient Safety Foundation. The establishment of the APSF by Ellison C. Pierce Jr.
4. Australian Broadcasting Corporation, The World Today: Concerns over medication errors in Australian hospitals.
5. Charatan Fred. Clinton acts to reduce medical mistakes. BMJ Publishing Group, 2000 Retrieved 2006-06-23.
6. Commonwealth Fund International Survey. Taking the Pulse of Health Care Systems: Experiences of Patients with Health Problems in Six Countries, 2005.
7. David M Gaba. Anesthesiology as a model for patient safety in health care. Medical Care 320 (7237):785–788. doi:10.1136/bmj.320.7237.785. PMC 1117775. PMID 10720368. Retrieved 2006-06-24.
8. Department of Health Expert Group. An organisation with a memory, 2000. Department of Health, United Kingdom. Retrieved 2006-07-01.
9. Dr. P Narsimha Rao versus V G Jaiprakash A.P. Law Journal Vol. XLIII, p. 491.
10. Elizabeth A. Henneman, RN, Unreported Errors in the Intensive Care Unit: a case study of the way we work. Critical Care Nurse 27(5):27-34. PMID 17901458. Retrieved 2008-03-23.

11. Fahrenkopf AM, Sectish TC, Barger LK, et al. 2007; Rates of medication errors among depressed and burnt out residents: prospective cohort study. BMJ 336 (7642): 488–91. doi:10.1136/bmj.39469.763218.BE. PMC 2258399. PMID 18258931.
12. G Ross Baker, Peter G Norton, et al. 2008. The Canadian Adverse Events Study: the incidence of adverse events among hospital patients in Canada. Canadian Medical Association Journal. 2004;170(11):1678-1685. doi:10.1503/cmaj.1040498. PMC 408508. PMID 15159366. Retrieved 2006-07-04.
13. Harold C, Sox Jr, Steven Woloshin. How Many Deaths Are Due to Medical Error? Getting the Number Right. Effective Clinical Practice, 2000. Retrieved 2006-06-22.
14. Institute of Medicine. To Err Is Human: Building a Safer Health System (page 4). The National Academies Press, 2000. Retrieved 2006-07-01.
15. Jacob Mathew versus State of Punjab and Another, AIR 2005 Supreme Court 3183.
16. Janice Tomlin (producer): The Deep Sleep: 6,000 will die or suffer brain damage, WLS-TV Chicago, 20/20. April 22, 1982.
17. J Bryan Sexton, Eric J Thomas, Robert L Helmreich. Error, stress, and teamwork in medicine and aviation. British Medical Journal. 2000;320(7237):745-749. doi:10.1136/bmj.320.7237.745. PMC 27316. PMID 10720356. Retrieved 2006-06-24.
18. Landrigan CP, Rothschild JM, Cronin JW, et al. Effect of reducing interns' work hours on serious medical errors in intensive care units. N Engl J Med. 2004;351(18):1838-48. doi:10.1056/NEJMoa041406. PMID 15509817.
19. Nocera A, Khursandi DS. Doctors' working hours: can the medical profession afford to let the courts decide what is reasonable? Med J Aust. 1998;168(12):616–8. PMID 9673625.
20. Patrick A Palmieri, et al. The anatomy and physiology of error in averse health care events. Advances in Health Care Management. 2008;7:33-68. doi:10.1016/S1474-8231(08)07003-1.
21. State CDR Commission, Chandigarh. Nihal Kaur and Ors. Versus. Director Postgraduate Institute of Medical Science and Research and Ors. III (1996) CPJ 112.
22. The Anesthesia Patient Safety Foundation: a Brief History.
23. The Joint Commission's Annual Report on Quality and Safety 2007: Improving America's Hospitals (Accessed 2008-04-09).
24. Wilson RM, Runciman WB, Gibberd RW, Harrison BT, Newby L, Hamilton JD. The Quality in Australian Health Care Study. Med J Aust. 1995;163(9):458-71. PMID 7476634.
25. Wu AW, Folkman S, McPhee SJ, et al. Do house officers learn from their mistakes? JAMA. 1991; 265(16):2089-94. doi:10.1001/jama.265.16.2089. PMID 2013929.
26. Adverse Events in New Zealand Public Hospitals: Principal Findings from a National Survey. New Zealand Ministry of Health. December 2001. Retrieved 2006-07-15.
27. World Alliance for Patient Safety. Organization Website. World Health Organization. Retrieved 2008-09-27.
28. abc Weingart SN, Wilson RM, Gibberd RW, Harrison B (March 2000). Epidemiology of medical error. BMJ 320(7237):774-7. doi:10.1136/bmj.320.7237.774. PMC 1117772. PMID 10720365.
29. ab Gardner, Amanda (6 March 2007). "Medication Errors During Surgeries Particularly Dangerous". The Washington Post. Retrieved 2007-03-13.

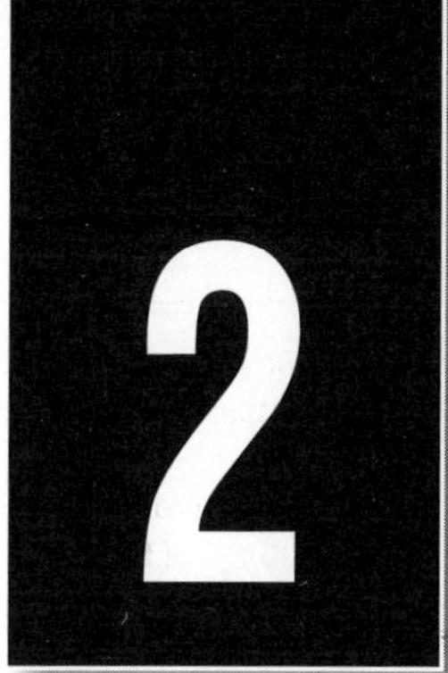

LONG CASES

CHAPTERS

12

Mitral Stenosis during MD (Anesthesiology) Examination

Deepak K Tempe, Indira Malik

1. What is your case? (Must know)

Ans. The patient, Satveer Singh, male, aged 46 years, resident of Bulandshahr, Uttar Pradesh, India working as a shopkeeper, was admitted to the hospital on 14.8.2013 with the chief complaints of shortness of breath since 6 months and palpitation for the past 2 months. The shortness of breath was mild, gradually progressive and nonseasonal. Past history is unremarkable with no history of hoarseness of voice, dysphagia, chest pain, coughing up of blood, fever with joint pain or sudden breathlessness in the middle of the night. There is no history of loss of consciousness, neurological deficit, abdominal or leg swelling. Patient is married. Family history and psychological history is unremarkable. Patient is currently on digoxin, frusemide and spironolactone.

On examination, the patient is alert, conscious and cooperative. His facies and decubitus are normal and build and nutrition is average. There is no pallor, cyanosis, clubbing or ankle edema. Patient is breathing comfortably and temperature is normal. Pulse is 110/min, low volume and irregularly irregular. All peripheral pulses are palpable equally. Blood pressure (BP) is 110/70 mm Hg in supine position and the neck veins are engorged with a vertical height of 8 cm above the sternal angle. There is no deformity of the precordium. On palpation, the apex beat is tapping in nature, and not displaced. A diastolic thrill is palpable in the mitral area which is best felt in the left lateral position and in full expiration. There is absence of left parasternal heave. On auscultation, the first heart sound (S1) is loud with varying intensity, and the second heart sound (S2) is audible. There is a low pitched mid-diastolic rumbling murmur of grade IV intensity at the apex without any radiation. The murmur is best audible with the bell of the stethoscope in the left lateral position at the height of expiration. Auscultation of lower left sternal border reveals a low pitched pansystolic murmur of grade II intensity with inspiratory accentuation and diminishing nature during forced expiration. Auscultation of other chest areas is unremarkable.

Examination of the respiratory system reveals bilateral vesicular breath sounds with no adventitious sounds. There is no hepatosplenomegaly or ascites. Airway examination is unremarkable with Malampatti grade II, adequate mouth opening and neck extension with thyromental distance and mandibular occlusion within acceptable limits. No spinal abnormalities are detected.

The laboratory and other investigations revealed a hemoglobin of 12.8 gm/dL with normal white cell and platelet counts. Patient is nondiabetic with normal renal function. His coagulation profile is normal. Liver function test reveals mildly elevated transaminase values, other parameters remaining acceptable. Serum sodium and potassium levels are 132 and 3.7 mEq/L respectively. His blood group is O positive and serology is nonreactive. Erythrocyte sedimentation rate, C reactive protein and antistreptolysin O titer are within normal range.

ECG shows atrial fibrillation (AF): X-ray of the chest shows straightening of the upper left border of the cardiac silhouette and prominence of the main pulmonary artery. A double contour of the right border of the heart is visible. Dilatation of the upper lobe pulmonary veins is seen.

Echocardiography reveals severe mitral stenosis (MS) with a mitral valve orifice area of 0.8 cm^2 due to rheumatic heart disease, moderate tricuspid regurgitation (TR) and severe pulmonary hypertension with good left ventricular function. Left atrium (LA) size is 4.0 cm. There is presence of spontaneous echo contrast and thrombus in the LA.

Coronary angiography performed to rule out coronary artery disease (CAD) revealed normal vessels.

Provisional diagnosis: It is a case of severe MS most likely due to rheumatic valvular heart disease with functional TR due to pulmonary hypertension with atrial fibrillation without presence of heart failure.

2. What is the etiology of MS? (Must know)

Ans. Clinically significant MS in adult patients in developing countries is usually a result of rheumatic heart disease.[1] Congenital abnormalities of the mitral valve represent a rare cause of MS in younger patients. Other uncommon conditions that do not directly involve the mitral valve apparatus but may limit left ventricular inflow and simulate the clinical findings of MS include cor triatriatum, large LA neoplasms and pulmonary venous obstruction.[2]

3. What is the pathophysiology of MS? (Must know)

Ans. Rheumatic MS causes thickening of the valve leaflets and commissural fusion, later progressing to leaflet calcification and subvalvular fusion. These changes reduce the effective mitral valve area and restrict diastolic inflow into the left ventricle (LV). Obstruction of the blood flow across the mitral valve generates a pressure gradient between the LA and LV. The effects are seen both proximal and distal to the obstructed valve.

As a result of restriction of the diastolic inflow to the LV, it remains chronically underloaded with a limited preload reserve. This causes a reduction of the LV end-diastolic pressure and volume, consequently reducing the stroke volume and therefore the cardiac output.

The LV also suffers from systolic as well as diastolic dysfunction in patients with MS. LV contractility may be depressed and may manifest as ejection fraction (EF) <50%. The LV dysfunction may persist after surgery, thus indicating that the limitation of diastolic flow is not the only reason for a decreased EF. This has been attributed to a sudden increase in the diastolic filling of a chronically underloaded ventricle. Intrinsic myocardial depression may occur due to rheumatic myocarditis[3] and angiographically demonstrable contraction abnormalities have been reported in 20% of patients.[4] Thickening and calcification of the mitral valve apparatus may alter the LV geometry and lead to systolic dysfunction. Vasoconstriction may occur in response to a chronically reduced cardiac output while inadequate myocardial wall thickness may also cause increase in the afterload.

Mitral stenosis (MS) creates an obvious impairment of diastolic filling due to reduced compliance which may occur as a result of the rheumatic disease process. The internal constraint may be created due to tethering of the papillary muscles to a rigid valve apparatus.

The changes occurring proximal to the obstructed valve reflect upon the LA and the pulmonary vasculature. According to the Gorlin formula:

$$\text{Valve area} = \text{Transvalvular flow} \div \text{constant} \times \sqrt{\text{Pressure gradient}}$$

Reduction in valve area causes increase in the pressure gradient to maintain the transvalvular flow rate if the heart rate remains normal. However, when tachycardia occurs, diastolic period is shortened. Thus, to maintain cardiac output and to increase the flow rate, the pressure gradient increases by the square of the increase in flow rate. This leads to the occurrence of symptoms in the patient due to increase in LA pressure and pulmonary congestion. This is the mechanism by which pregnancy, thyrotoxicosis or fever may precipitate symptoms of dyspnea in an otherwise asymptomatic patient with MS. Over a long period of time, elevated transmitral pressure gradient leads to dilatation of the LA. In developing countries, patients often present at a very late stage with massive LA dimensions of up to 10–12 cm (normal up to 3.5 cm). Increase in the LA pressure reflects upon the pulmonary vasculature causing pulmonary venous hypertension followed by pulmonary arterial hypertension (PAH). With the progression of the disease, permanent changes in the vasculature result in increased pulmonary vascular resistance (PVR) and PAH. This further culminates in right ventricular (RV) dilatation, hypertrophy and eventually failure. The full blown picture of congestive heart failure comprises of TR, distended neck veins, hepatomegaly, peripheral edema and ascites. Poor lung compliance due to increased pulmonary blood volume and extravascular lung water exacerbates ventilation-perfusion mismatch, which may cause hypoxemia further worsening the PAH. Distension of the LA also distorts the depolarization pathways leading to arrhythmias, most commonly AF with fast ventricular response, which may become the precipitating factor for appearance of symptoms.

Left ventricular pressure-volume loop in MS: This can be generated by real time measurement of pressure and volume within the LV (Figs 1 and 2). Several physiologically relevant hemodynamic

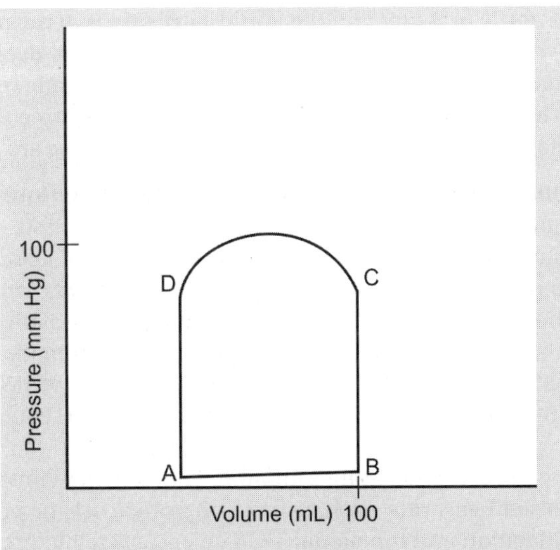

Fig. 1 A normal left ventricular pressure-volume loop. Refer to the text for details (This is a diagrammatic and not an accurate representation)

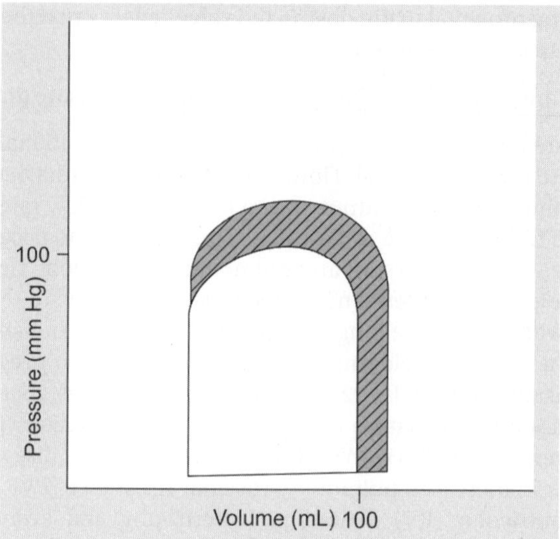

Fig. 2 Pressure-volume loop in a patient with mitral stenosis (clear area) against normal (shaded area). Note the "underloaded" left ventricle, both in terms of pressure and volume. (This is a diagrammatic and not an accurate representation)
Source: Tempe DK. Clinical Practice of Cardiac Anaesthesia, 3rd edn. Delhi: CBS Publishers, 2012)

parameters such as LV compliance, stroke volume, cardiac output, EF, myocardial contractility can be determined from these loops.

Alterations in LV pressure with respect to volume occur in a counterclockwise fashion over time (Fig. 1). The mitral valve opens at point A and ventricular filling begins. Mitral valve closes at point B and ventricular systole begins. Segment BC depicts isovolumic contraction which ends when the LV pressure exceeds the aortic pressure and the aortic valve opens at the point C. This is followed by the ejection phase which ends at point D, when the LV pressure decreases below the aortic pressure and the aortic valve closes. Segment DA represents isovolumic relaxation. In MS, the LV is underloaded both in terms of pressure and volume. LV filling during diastole, the isovolumic contraction phase, cardiac output and the isovolumic relaxation phase are all reduced (Fig. 2).[1]

4. What are the presenting symptoms in a patient with MS? (Must know)

Ans. In developing countries, patients suffer from inadequate nutrition, sanitation and medical care. Consequently, many of them suffer from recurrent episodes of endocarditis and severe MS develops within 5 years of the initial episode. Therefore, the patients are very young, usually in the second decade of life. In contrast, in developed countries, rheumatic fever is rare and there is a latency period of 3–4 decades between the initial bout of rheumatic fever and the onset of symptoms. Therefore, patients usually present in the 4th–6th decade of life. This also explains why associated CAD in patients with MS is more common in the developed countries but is not so in the developing countries.

Dyspnea is the most common presenting symptom, generally precipitated by some unrelated condition causing increased heart rate such as fever, thyrotoxicosis or pregnancy. PAH leads to RV pressure overload, dilatation and functional TR. The end-stage picture of biventricular failure with pulmonary and hepatic congestion, peripheral edema and ascites follows, if the patient is left untreated.

5. Explain the following unusual clinical findings in MS. (Useful to know)

Ans.

1. *Causes of muffled S1 in MS in place of loud S1:*
   a. Mitral regurgitation (MR)/severe aortic regurgitation
   b. Mitral valve calcification
   c. Active rheumatic carditis/digitalis overdose (prolonged PR interval)
   d. Acute myocardial infarction
   e. Emphysema/obesity/thick chest Wall
2. *Displaced apex beat in MS:*
   a. *Outward displacement:* RV hypertrophy due to PAH
   b. *Outward and downward displacement:* LV hypertrophy due to accompanying regurgitant lesions.
3. *Undetectable mid-diastolic murmur in MS:* Markedly reduced cardiac output (silent MS)[5]

6. How do you assess the severity of MS? (Must know)

Ans.

Clinical:

a. *Symptoms:* Severity of the symptoms depend upon the severity of the stenosis. Symptoms are usually present at rest if the valve area is < 1 cm^2. However, initiation of medical therapy may reduce the severity of the symptoms, therefore it is necessary to elicit an accurate drug history at the time of presentation.
b. Proximity of A2 — opening snap gap (A2 = Aortic valve closure).
c. Longer duration of mid-diastolic murmur in patients with preserved CO.

Echocardiographic (Table 1):1

a. Mitral valve area
b. Gradient across the mitral valve
c. Severity of PAH
d. LA size

Table 1 | Echocardiographic grading of mitral stenosis

Parameter/severity	Normal	Mild	Moderate	Severe
Valve area (cm^2)	4–6	1.6–2.5	1.1–1.5	<1.0
Mean gradient (mm Hg)	< 2	< 5	5–10	> 10

The other useful information provided by echocardiography is size and function of the ventricles and an estimation of pulmonary artery pressures.

Cardiac catheterization: The utility of left and right heart catheterization is realized when there is a discrepancy between the clinical severity and the findings on 2D transthoracic echocardiography that cannot be resolved with either transesophageal echocardiography (TOE) or cardiac magnetic resonance imaging. In patients who are at high-risk for CAD, especially those with positive noninvasive stress tests for myocardial ischemia, coronary angiography is advisable preoperatively to identify patients with critical coronary obstruction that should be bypassed at the time of valve surgery. Computerized tomographic coronary angiography is commonly used to screen patients preoperatively for the presence of CAD. Since, there is a good correlation between continuous wave Doppler derived pressure gradients and that determined by the catheterization, assessment of MS does not necessarily require catheterization.

7. What is the differential diagnosis of mid-diastolic murmur? (Useful to know)

Ans.

a. *Carey-Coombs murmur:* Found in active rheumatic valvulitis. The murmur varies in intensity from day-to-day and disappears after the acute attack. There is absence of diastolic thrill, opening snap and Loud S1.
b. *Austin-Flint murmur:* Functional murmur in severe aortic regurgitation. It is not intensified in presystole, is not associated with loud S1 or opening snap and becomes softer with administration of amyl nitrite. Most importantly aortic regurgitation murmur is present in aortic area.
c. *Functional murmur:* Due to severe MR, ventricular septal defect or patent ductus arteriosus. This diastolic murmur commences slightly later than in patients with MS, and there is often clear-cut evidence of LV enlargement. An opening snap and increased P_2 are absent, and S_1 is soft or absent.
d. *LA myxoma:* The auscultatory findings may change markedly with body position.[5]

8. What is the Graham-Steell murmur? (Nice to know)

Ans. A high-pitched, early diastolic, decrescendo blowing murmur heard in the second intercostal space to the left of the sternum due to pulmonary insufficiency, resulting from dilatation of the pulmonary valve ring and occurs in patients with mitral valve disease and severe PAH. This murmur may increase in intensity with inspiration and is accompanied by a loud and often palpable P2.[5]

9. Describe the treatment strategy for MS. (Useful to know)

Ans.

I. Medical therapy for MS aims to:
  a. Reduce recurrence of rheumatic fever
  b. Prophylaxis for endocarditis
  c. Reduce symptoms of pulmonary congestion
  d. Control the ventricular rate if AF is present
  e. Prevention of thromboembolic complications
    - Penicillin prophylaxis of group A hemolytic streptococci (GAS) infections for secondary prevention of rheumatic fever is important for at risk patients with rheumatic MS. Factors that determine the duration of prophylaxis are:
      i. Number of previous attacks
      ii. Time elapsed since the last attack
      iii. Risk of exposure to GAS infections
      iv. Age of the patient
      v. Presence or absence of cardiac involvement

      Sulfonamides (e.g. sulfadiazine, neotrizine) or macrolides (e.g. erythromycin, clarithromycin) are acceptable choices in patients allergic to penicillin.
    - The 2008 focussed update on infective endocarditis by the American College of Cardiology/American Heart Association recommend antibiotic prophylaxis against infective endocarditis for dental procedures, in the following situations:[6]
      i. Patients with prosthetic heart valves or prosthetic material used for valve repair.
      ii. Previous history of infective endocarditis.
      iii. Patients with congenital heart diseases.
      iv. Cardiac transplant recipients with valve regurgitation.
    - Symptoms of pulmonary congestion are reduced by restriction of sodium intake and oral diuretics.
    - Beta blockers, nondihydropyridine calcium channel blockers and digoxin are useful in controlling the ventricular rate in patients with AF.

- Warfarin dose titrated to an international normalized ratio of 2–3 should be administered to patients with MS with history of thromboembolism. Patients with mild to moderate MS with recent onset of AF can undergo pharmacological or electrical cardioversion. They must receive anticoagulation therapy prior to cardioversion for at least 3 weeks. Alternatively, a TOE can be performed to exclude the presence of LA thrombus prior to cardioversion. Patients who are successfully cardioverted should receive long-term anticoagulation and antiarrhythmic drugs.[7]

II. Surgical therapy for MS includes mitral valvotomy (surgical or percutaneous) or mitral valve replacement (MVR). Surgical mitral valvotomy can be performed by closed or open technique.

Balloon mitral valvotomy (BMV) is widely preferred over surgical management of MS. However, if the valve is unsuitable, coexisting MR or LA thrombus is present, it is not feasible. Echocardiographic grading scale (Wilkins score) has been developed to evaluate mitral leaflet mobility, thickness, calcification and subvalvular fusion. Each of these parameters is graded on a scale of 1–4, and patients who have a score < 9 are suitable for BMV.[8] BMV shortens the hospital stay and eliminates the risk imposed by thoracotomy and anesthesia. However it is necessary that a skilled cardiologist along with a back up team of cardiac surgeon and anesthesiologist is available. This is important as the patient may develop acute MR and require urgent valve replacement.

Due to economic reasons and sheer number of patients, closed mitral valvotomy (CMV) is still the preferred operation in developing countries. The long-term results of this operation are reported to be satisfactory. A significant decrease in the mean left atrial diameter and pulmonary artery systolic pressure (PASP), along with reduction of transmitral gradient and improvement in valve area has been observed.

Open mitral valvotomy (OMV) is considered a better operation and is preferentially performed in developing countries. Relief of valvular and subvalvular obstructive elements can be dealt with much better under direct vision.

The above discussion indicates that in developing countries, the choice of treatment for MS should be as follows:

i. *BMV:* If the facility is available, it should be preferred in patients with New York Heart Association (NYHA) class II, III, or IV symptoms when valve morphology is favorable and there is no MR or LA thrombus. It is also advised for asymptomatic patients with moderate to severe MS and PAH (PASP > 50 mm Hg, at rest, PASP > 60 mm Hg with exercise)
ii. *CMV:* If BMV is unavailable or contraindicated
iii. *OMV/MVR:* It is recommended in patients with moderate to severe MS with NYHA III or IV symptoms if BMV is: (i) unavailable, (ii) contraindicated, (iii) valve morphology is unfavorable. It is also recommended for symptomatic patients with moderate to severe MS who also have moderate to severe MR.[9]

10. How would you optimize this patient on anticoagulant medication in the preoperative period?

Ans. Warfarin, if being given for thromboprophylaxis in a patient with MS with AF should be stopped 5 days before surgery and low molecular weight heparin should be initiated. It has to be discontinued 12 hours preoperatively. If intravenous heparin is being given as bridging therapy, it must be stopped 4–6 hours prior to surgery. Postoperatively, warfarin may be started 12–24 hours later, if adequate hemostasis has been achieved and there is no evidence of ongoing bleeding.

11. How would you premedicate this patient?

Ans. Adequate premedication is essential to prevent anxiety and tachycardia. However, oversedation must be avoided as these patients are sensitive to even small doses of narcotics and hypnotics. Appropriate monitoring and supplemental oxygen therapy should be available. Morphine

(0.1 - 0.2 mg/kg) along with promethazine (12.5 - 25 mg/kg) given intramuscular 1-2 hours before surgery is an adequate premedication for these patients. A small dose of benzodiazepine may also be used. Scopolamine is another alternative as it directly avoids tachycardia.[1]

12. What are the intraoperative goals of hemodynamic management? (Must know)

Ans. *Preload:* Maintain adequate intravascular volume, but overly aggressive use of fluids can precipitate pulmonary edema. Also remember that a small amount of blood loss or vasodilatation may produce significant hypotension as the preload reserve is limited in these patients.

Heart rate: Tachycardia causes the gradient across the stenotic valve to increase, therefore it is essential to maintain heart rate between 80-90/minute. Since the LV filling is substantially dependent on atrial contraction, normal sinus rhythm should be preserved as far as possible.

Contractility: Maintain

Systemic vascular resistance: Maintain

Pulmonary vascular resistance: Should be reduced to keep RV afterload low. Hypoxia, hypercapnia and acidosis must be avoided to achieve this goal. In addition, pulmonary vasodilator (Nitroglycerin, Sodium nitroprusside) may be used.[2]

13. How would you monitor this patient in the intraoperative period? (Must know)

Ans. In addition to all the standard monitoring for any case as recommended by American Society of Anesthesiologists, the patient must have an invasive arterial line (preferably radial), central venous catheter and in patients with severe PAH with RV dysfunction, a PA catheter may also be considered. It should be remembered that the utility of PA catheter in these patients is limited to monitoring the PA pressure and not the left sided filling pressure as the pulmonary vasculature is abnormal. After induction of general anesthesia (GA), insertion of a TOE probe (if available) would be desirable to confirm the valvular pathology, assess other valves and LV function. After valvotomy or valve replacement, it enables the assessment of proper working of the prosthesis, any paravalvular leaks and assess post bypass LV function.[1]

14. What anesthetic technique would you adopt for the patient? (Must know)

Ans. General anesthesia (GA) with endotracheal intubation is preferred. In patients undergoing open heart procedures, a high-dose narcotic technique with pancuronium or vecuronium should be preferred. The maintenance of hemodynamic stability is most important and is more challenging if the disease is severe. It is a good practice to administer increments of small doses of anesthetic agents to avoid precipitous changes in hemodynamics. A wide bore venous cannula should also be in place to administer fluids quickly, if required. Fentanyl (5–7 μg/kg), thiopentone (1–2 mg/kg) and pancuronium or vecuronium (0.08–0.12 mg/kg) would be ideal for induction. The choice of muscle relaxant should be based on the basal heart rate. If the basal heart rate is less (60–70/min), pancuronium or rocuronium should be preferred as they increase the heart rate. If the basal heart rate is fast (≥ 100/min), vecuronium should be preferred. While choosing the muscle relaxant, it should also be remembered that high-dose opioids also decrease the heart rate. Maintenance of anesthesia with vecuronium or rocuronium infusion with volatile agents may be continued during the conduct of cardiopulmonary bypass (CPB). In the modern era of fast tracking, anesthetic combinations using smaller doses of narcotics or short acting narcotics (remifentanil), propofol, inhalational agents and intermediate acting muscle relaxants may be used to ensure early recovery and extubation. Monitoring of mean arterial pressure, blood gases, electrolytes, glucose, urine output and temperature is carried out during CPB. After the valve is replaced successfully, the patient is gradually weaned off bypass with the help of inotropes to improve the LV function and reduce RV afterload. Vasodilators like nitroglycerin or nitroprusside 0.5–1 μg/kg/min are useful in patients having severe PAH. Adrenaline, dopamine or dobutamine may be used to treat episodes of hypotension but with a cautious watch on filling conditions in order to avoid increase in RV afterload. Milrinone, a phosphodiesterase inhibitor, is a selective pulmonary vasodilator, thus effectively reduces RV afterload and also has positive inotropic effect.[1]

15. What is the postoperative management? (Useful to know)

Ans. It is important to avoid even mild hypercarbia (up to 48 mm Hg) which causes significant increase in PVR and RVEDP. Therefore, it is desirable to electively ventilate the patients for sometime postoperatively and maintain normocarbia at all times. Increased pulmonary blood volume and extracellular lung water lead to decrease in lung compliance and exacerbate ventilation-perfusion mismatch. Therefore, these are additional reasons to electively ventilate the patient postoperatively. Inotropic and vasodilator therapy should be continued for 24–48 hours in patients having severe PAH.[1]

16. Management of a pregnant patient with MS. (Must know)

Ans. The MS is the most common cardiac lesion seen in women of child-bearing age group. Due to the hyperdynamic circulation during pregnancy, symptoms may be manifested for the first time during pregnancy. The CMV can be performed safely at any stage of the pregnancy giving significant functional and clinical improvement without adversely affecting the fetus. The BMV can also be successfully performed anytime before term. However, no intervention is required in patients with mild MS and the pregnancy may be allowed to continue.

An elective cesarean section should be preceeded by either of the procedures mentioned above. If this is not possible, epidural or general anesthesia is preferred for patients with mild-to-moderate stenosis. Continuous lumbar epidural analgesia is useful but hypotension must be anticipated and prevented or treated promptly. A careful extension of the epidural block (if the catheter is in place for labor analgesia) may be carried out in patients with mild-to-moderate MS requiring cesarean section. Intravascular volume must be maintained with intravenous fluids. Inotropic support with dopamine or dobutamine (5–10 μg/kg/min) may be needed if PAH or RV dysfunction is present. Administration of ergometrine is avoided after delivery of the fetus as it may cause transient increase in BP and also uterine retraction leading to autotransfusion effect. Therefore, oxytocin infusion is preferred for control of hemorrhage

Patients having severe MS are not ideal candidates for regional anesthesia as the consequences of decreased venous return or systemic vascular resistance may be disastrous. Opioid based general anesthesia is good for maintaining hemodynamic stability but may cause severe respiratory depression in the newborn baby. However, hemodynamic stability should always be given priority as compromise of hemodynamics will also threaten the fetus. Therefore, fentanyl 10–20 μg/kg (total) or morphine 0.5–1 mg/kg (total) may be used. The fetus may be resuscitated for respiratory depression. All precautions to prevent aspiration must be taken before induction of GA. Rapid sequence induction may not be tolerated by these patients as it can result in dramatic cardiovascular changes. Elective postoperative ventilation is usually required.

Invasive hemodynamic monitoring is indicated for all patients irrespective of the technique being used for anesthesia. An intra-arterial line and a CVP line are essential. A PA catheter may provide additional help in cases with some degree of PAH.[1]

17. What are the other concomitant valve lesions?

Ans. In about 25% patients with rheumatic heart disease, pure MS is manifested and an additional 40% have combined MS and MR. Other concomitant valve lesions may be aortic stenosis, aortic regurgitation and TR.[1]

REFERENCES

1. Tempe DK. Clinical Practice of Cardiac Anaesthesia, 3rd edn. Delhi: CBS Publishers, 2012
2. Kaplan JA. Kaplan's Cardiac Anesthesia: The echo era, 6th edn. Missouri: Elsevier Saunders, 2011
3. Gash AK, Carabello BA, Cepin D, et al. Left ventricular ejection performance and systolic muscle function in patients with mitral stenosis. Circulation. 1983;67:148-54.
4. Heller SJ, Carleton RA. Abnormal left ventricular contraction in patients with mitral stenosis. Circulation. 1970;42:1099-110.
5. Longo DL. Harrison's Principles of Internal Medicine, 18th edn. Boston MA: McGraw-Hill Professional, 2011.
6. Nishimura RA, Carabello BA, Faxon DP, et al. American College of Cardiology/American Heart Association 2008 Guideline update on valvular heart disease: focussed update on infective endocarditis: a report of the ACC/AHA taskforce on practice guidelines. Circulation. 2008;118:887-9.
7. Fuster V, Ryden LE, Cannom DS, et al. American College of Cardiology Foundation/American Heart Association/Heart Rhythm Society Focussed updates incorporated into the American College of Cardiology Foundation/American Heart Association/European Society of Cardiology 2006 guidelines for the management of patients with atrial fibrillation: A report of the ACCF/AHA task force on practice guidelines. Circulation. 2011;123:e269-e367.
8. Wilkins G, Weyman A, Abascal V, et al. Percutaneous balloon dilatation of the mitral valve: an analysis of echocardiographic variables related to outcome and the mechanism of dilatation. Br Heart J. 1988;60:299-308.
9. Nishimura RA, Carabello BA, Faxon DP, et al. Focussed update incorporated into the American College of Cardiology/American Heart Association 2006 guidelines for the management of patients with valvular heart disease. J Am Coll Cardiol. 2008;52:e1-e142.

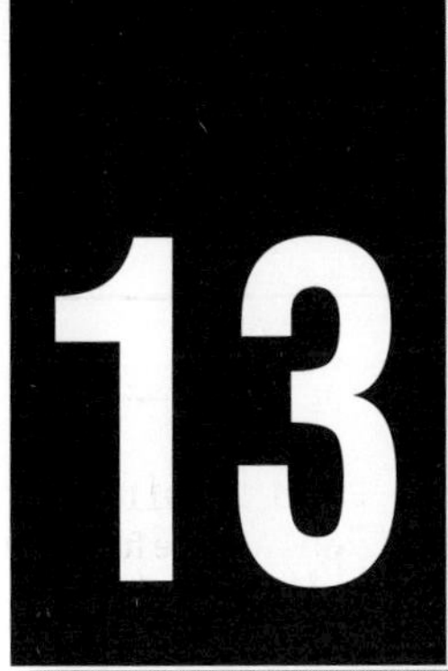

Anemia in Pregnancy

Sagarmoy Basu

CASE SUMMARY

A 30-year-old lady, in 37 weeks of gestation, G2P1, has been posted for cesarean section (c/s). There is no significant medical or surgical history except that she had a cesarean section 4 years back. Her vitals are PR—104/min, regular, average volume, BP—118/64 mm Hg. Clinically, she has moderate pallor. Systemic examination is within normal limits. Airway examination is unremarkable, with MG I. Investigations reveals her Hb to be 9.0 gm/dL.

1. What is your case? (Must know)

Ans. Case summary (pregnant lady posted for c/s with anemia).

2. How do you define anemia? (Must know)

Ans. It is defined as the deficiency in the oxygen carrying capacity of the blood due to a diminished qualitative or quantitative erythrocyte mass or hemoglobin or both in a normovolemic or near normovolemic person.

The World Health Organization defines anemia as a hemoglobin level <13 gm/dL in men and <12 gm/dL in women.

Anemia in pregnancy is defined by WHO as hemoglobin concentration of less than 11 gm/dL or hematocrit <0.33 in the first and third trimesters, while in the second trimester a fall of 0.5 gm/dL due to increased plasma volume and the value is accepted at 10.5 gm/dL or hematocrit <0.32 and have an increased risk of perinatal morbidity.

3. What is the incidence of anemia in women of childbearing age?

Ans. It has been estimated by World Health Organization that a large proportion of women both in industrialized (18%) and developing (35–75%) countries become anemic during pregnancy.

4. What are the principal causes of anemia in pregnancy? (Must know)

Ans. a. Physiological

b. Pathological or acquired

Physiological or dilutional: It is the relative rise in plasma volume (from 40 mL/kg–70 mL/kg.) compared to relatively less rise in volume of (25–30 mL/kg) in RBC volume. The changes start from around 6 weeks of gestation and continues till 3rd trimester.

Pathological or Acquired Causes

The most common causes in India:
- Nutritional deficiency is the most common in our country
- Nutritional deficiency occurs due to deficiency of iron, folic acid and vitamin B_{12}
- Inadequate intake of food or food deficient in iron, folic acid, vitamin B_{12} and repeated pregnancies within short interval.

Iron Deficiency Anemia (60%)

It is said that it takes about two years to replenish the iron stores in mother unless mother is supplemented with hematinic factors.

The prepregnant iron stores is not adequate to meet the increased demand of pregnancy due to expansion of blood volume in the latter half of pregnancy. Normal supplementation of iron in diet of pregnant woman is 60 mg per day (approx.).

Macrocytic Anemia (10%)

It occurs due to deficiency of folic acid and/or vitamin B_{12}.

Folic acid requirement usually doubles during pregnancy especially in last trimester. The body stores of folic acid is limited and further renal clearance of it increases to substantial amount during normal pregnancy leading to fall in concentration of plasma folate. Unless there is dietary supplementation anemia is likely to occur. Folate deficiency is suspected when there is poor response to iron supplementation as well as the increase in MCV. Folate supplements, up to 4 mg/day orally for 3 weeks will treat acute deficiency which should be followed by 5 mg once weekly as maintenance therapy. It is said women planning for pregnancy should have folic acid 4 mg daily as a prophylactic from preconception state to throughout the 1st trimester to prevent the risk of neural tube defects (spina bifida, anencephaly and encephalocele) due to imperfect closure of the neural tube taking place 3–4 weeks after conception. Others may take 400 μg daily.

Vitamin B_{12} deficiency: Women principally on vegetarian diet lead to deficiency causing pernicious anemia.

Blood loss (acute or chronic): It is are quite common from any part of gastrointestinal tract or per vaginum.

Hookworm infestation is common in rural India while schistosomiasis is common in Western countries. Antepartum hemorrhage is another important cause.

Infections

Malaria can cause hemolysis, HIV infection, presence of anemia with leukopenia, thrombocytopenia, lymphadenopathy and oral candidiasis is a cause of suspicion.

Hemoglobinopathies: Sickle cell disease and thalassemia, enzyme deficiencies: G6PD (Glucose-6-phosphate dehydrogenase) deficiency reduces the life span of RBC with a number of drugs having the capacity to precipitate hemolytic crisis. Precipitating drugs of anesthetic importance are aspirin, phenacetin and sulfonamides. Procaine is contraindicated as reduction of methemoglobin is impaired.

5. What are the body's compensatory factors to combat this dilutional anemia? (Must know)

Ans. a. Increased cardiac output

b. Lowered blood viscosity

c. Increased 2–3 diphosphoglycerate (2,3-DPG) concentration in the RBC shifts of oxy-hemoglobin dissociation curve to the right promoting release of oxygen to the tissues.

6. Discuss in brief morphological classification of anemia. (Must know)

Ans. Based on average size of RBC and hemoglobin content:

- *Microcytic hypochromic (MCHC<32%):* MCV, MCH and MCHC all are reduced. It is commonly found in iron deficiency anemia and in a few noniron deficiency anemia (e.g. thalassemia)
- *Normocytic normochromic:* MCV, MCH, MCHC all are normal. Commonly observed in acute blood loss, hemolytic anemia, bone marrow failure.
- *Macrocytic anemia:* MCV is above normal and is commonly seen in megaloblastic anemia due to deficiency of vitamin B_{12} or folic acid.

7. How do you classify anemia in pregnancy? (Must know)

Ans. Classification of anemia in pregnancy:

Iron deficiency anemia: Blood loss: Gastrointestinal loss (peptic ulcer, gastritis, polyposis, malignancy in the gastrointestinal tract, hookworm and schistosomiasis infestation, exacerbation due to chronic use of aspirin and NSAIDs causing erosion of intestinal mucosa and impair platelet function. Women at childbearing age cyclical blood loss, pregnancy and breastfeeding may cause iron deficiency anemia by depleting iron stores. Chronic hemoptysis (due to pulmonary tuberculosis or lung malignancy), hematemesis due to any cause or hematuria (due to lesion anywhere in the urinary tract), bleeding per anum (commonly due to hemorrhoids).

Malabsorption: Release of iron from food and maintaining it in soluble form requires the help of acid gastric juice. Hypochlorhydria in the elderly or due to proton pump inhibitors, previous gastric surgery may contribute to lack of availability of iron from the diet. Iron is actively absorbed from the upper small intestine and likely to be affected by celiac disease (immunologically mediated inflammatory disease of small bowel resulting mal absorption of gluten free diet).

Physiological demands: Rapid growth in infancy and puberty, cyclical loss in women, pregnancy and parturition,

Megaloblastic anemia:
It occurs due to vitamin B_{12} deficiency.
Average daily requirement: 5–30 μg
Source: Meat, fish, eggs.
Dietary deficiency: Gastric factors, pernicious anemia (autoimmune disorder of gastric mucosa, loss of parietal cells causing deficiency of intrinsic factor).

Folate deficiency: Anemia of chronic disease: It may be due to chronic infections, inflammation or neoplasia.

Miscellaneous causes: Hemolysis, congenital (inherited red cell defects of structure or metabolism. The principal defects are in red cell membrane (hereditary spherocytosis), glucose 6 phosphate dehydrogenase (G6PD) deficiency, hemoglobinopathies, bone marrow suppression.

8. Describe the management of anemia in pregnancy. (Must know)

Ans.

A. *Prophylaxis of nutritional anemia:*
   i. Proper balanced diet
   ii. Supplementary iron (60 mg elemental iron) and folate (1 mg/day) therapy
   iii. Providing protein-rich diet with vitamin C (100 mg/day)

iv. Adequate treatment of infections or infestations
v. Proper antenatal care.

B. *Correction of pre-existing anemia:*

i. *Oral iron therapy:* Ferrous sulfate tablets 200 mg, 3 times a day along with folate supplement may raise the Hb @1–1.5 gm/dL/week.

ii. *Parenteral iron therapy:*

a. *Repeated deep intramuscular injections (advantage is less gastrointestinal tract discomfort):* Administered in the upper outer quadrant of gluteal region using Z track technique. Dose calculated vide infrapreviously.

Iron-sorbitol-citric acid complex (50 mg/mL of elemental iron) is preferably used for intramuscular route.

Iron-dextran (50 mg/mL of elemental iron) may be used in both intramuscular or intravenous route being available in 2 mL and 1 mL vials

b. *Intravenous route:* Total dose infusion (TDI)

Iron-dextran (50 mg/mL of elemental iron) is used.

Total deficit infused in a single sitting with an infusion.

Mode of administration:

To be preceded by test dose: Total dose of iron required (mg) (formula varies by manufacturer)

0.3 × (100-Hb%) × weight (in lbs), or (15-Hb% of patient) × body weight in kg × 3. Additional 50% added for replenishment of stores.

Caution: Renal disorder, cardiorespiratory disease, allergy are contraindication to parenteral therapy.

iii. *Blood transfusion:* Decision lies with level of hemoglobin and clinical condition of the patient (significant acute bleeding leading to risk of hypoxia, anemia discovered at term, possibility of coronary insufficiency).

General guidelines for transfusion:

I. *During antenatal period:*

a. *Less than 36 weeks*
- Hemoglobin 5.0 gm/dL or less even in absence of clinical signs or hypoxia
- Hemoglobin between 5.0 gm/dL and 7.0 gm/dL in presence of established or incipient cardiac failure or clinical evidence of hypoxia, pneumonia, or bacterial/parasitic infection, malaria, pre-existing cardiac disease not due to anemia.

b. *36 weeks or more*
- Hb 6.0 gm/dL or below
- Hb between 6 gm and 8 gm/dL in presence of established or incipient cardiac failure or clinical evidence of hypoxia, pneumonia or any other serious bacterial/parasitic infection malaria or pre-existing heart disease not due to anemia.

II. *Elective cesarean section:*
- Having history of antepartum hemorrhage (APH), postpartum hemorrhage (PPH), previous cesarean section
- When Hb is between 8.0 gm and 10 gm/dL with confirmed blood group, freshly taken serum for cross matching should be saved. If Hb is 8.0 gm/dL two units of blood should be cross matched and kept ready in the theater.

Cautions during transfusion: Added circulating volume may lead to congestive cardiac failure in already stressed myocardium. Packed cell transfusion has the advantage of minimal expansion of circulating volume. Diuretics may be of help.

If it is a planned case without any life-threatening urgency then blood should be transfused at least 48 hrs prior to surgery to enable: (a) restoration of intravascular volume and blood viscosity (b) reducing Valtis-Kennedy effect of old banked blood so that ideal oxygen carrying capacity is restored.

9. What are the problems of anesthesia in anemia in pregnancy? (Must know)

Ans. Tissue oxygenation is hampered by low oxygen carrying capacity of the blood. However body's compensatory mechanisms (as stated earlier) may help to a large extent.

10. Outline the anesthetic management of this patient. (Must know)

Ans.

A. *Principles of anesthesia:*
   - Prevention of hypoxia (proper preoxygenation) and maintenance proper oxygenation throughout the procedure.
   - *Prevention of hypotension:* Prevention of aortocaval compression, care during regional analgesia
   - Prevention of circulatory overload
   - Prevention of hypercarbia

   At the outset the Hb level should be judged and necessary preoperative preparation is needed.

B. *Anesthetic considerations:*
   - *History and general survey:* Hb level and clinical features of bleeding, drug intake (aspirin), mental disturbances and subacute combined degeneration of the cord (symmetrical paresthesia with loss of proprioceptive and vibratory senses especially in lower limbs, unsteady gait, diminished tendon reflexes) may be the feature of vitamin B_{12} deficiency. If present these findings should be carefully mentioned in the history sheet to avoid unwanted medico-legal problems in the postoperative period. History of chronic renal failure (inadequate production of erythropoietin), endocrine dysfunction (hypothyroidism) should be looked for.
   - Routine investigation and necessary investigations

C. *Administration of anesthesia:*

   Principles as mentioned earlier.
   - *Regional anesthesia:* Crystalloid infusion is needed to fill up the increased vascular bed due to sympathetic block.

   Fall in Hb by 20% occurs if 2 liters of Ringer Lactate/Normal saline is infused in a standard 60–65 kg woman. This can exacerbate anemia precipitating heart failure. A cautious approach is necessary to switch over to vasoconstrictor/blood transfusion of after an interval. A CVP line is helpful in such a situation.

   Regional anesthesia should preferably be avoided in megaloblastic anemia due to possibility of medicolegal problems.
   - *General anesthesia:*
     i. Awareness may occur due to raised FiO_2
     ii. Hypothermia and alkalosis are to be avoided to prevent undue shift of the dissociation curve.
     iii. Normocarbia is to be maintained during ventilation.
     iv. Theoretically nitrous oxide (however for longer duration) is not appropriate for macrocytic anemia as it may suppress bone marrow.
     v. Spontaneous ventilation with high concentration of inhalational agent likely to depress respiration and myocardial performance both of which are essential for maintenance of adequate Oxygen flux.

vi. Adequate tissue perfusion is judged clinically by blanching ear lobes, nose and forehead and time taken for pallor to disappear.
vii. Posture need be changed cautiously as it may lower the blood pressure and cardiac output.

D. *Postoperative care:*
   i. Extubation should be done when the relaxant effect has worn off, help of a nerve stimulator is ideal.
   ii. Hypoxia should be prevented
   iii. Shivering must be avoided
   iv. First 24 hrs should be cared in a high dependency ward
   v. Regular monitoring of pulse, BP, oxygen saturation, CVP, fluid intake and output are to be recorded.

11. What are the less common anemias and the management? (Must know)

Ans.

A. *Sickle cell disorders:*
   Points to remember:
   i. Patients are to be well hydrated as these patients cannot concentrate urine. Early fluid replacement will prevent impending crisis.
   ii. A Hb level of 6–9 gm/dL is accepted as steady state. This level of Hb is well tolerated by patients with HbS having lowered oxygen affinity than HbA. Attempt to raise the Hb will increase the blood viscosity leading to possibility of crisis.
   iii. RBC enriched with 2–3 DPG displaces the dissociation curve to right. Infusion of isotonic bicarbonate at a rate 3 mmol/kg/hr during surgery is a compromise.
   iv. Hypoxia is to be avoided at all cost to prevent crisis. Up to 50% oxygen has been advocated by some authorities to avoid hypoxia.

B. *Thalassemias:*
   Points to consider:
   i. Apart from Hb estimation platelet count, prothrombin time should be checked
   ii. Iron overload (due to increased absorption from gastrointestinal tract) and repeated transfusion may lead to functional abnormalities in the liver heart and endocrine system.

BIBLIOGRAPHY

1. Cambell M. Obstetrics by Ten Teachers, 17th edn. London, Arnold; 2000.
2. Gary F Cunningham et al. William's Text Book of Obstetrics, 21st edn, 2001.
3. Kumar. Robbins & Cotran Pathologic Basis of Disease, 8th edn.
4. Oxford Handbook of Anesthesia, 2nd edn.
5. Problem Oriented Patient Management. In: Yao & Artusio's Anesthesiology, 6th edn, 2010.

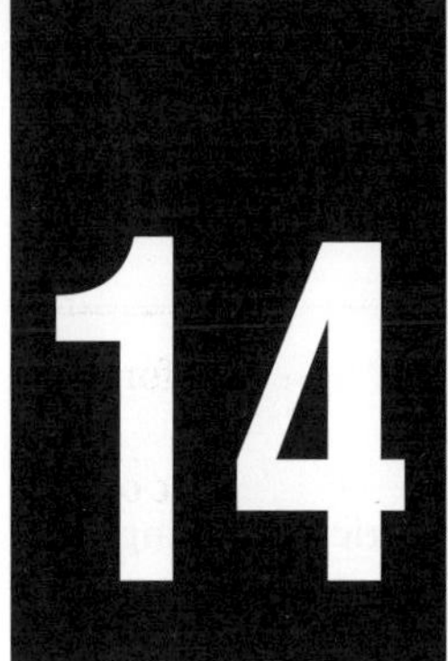

Anesthetic Management of a Patient with Permanent Pacemaker/Cardiac Implantable Electronic Device

Sumitra Bakshi, JV Divatia

Interventional cardiology has grown and is extensively practiced all over our country. Cardiac pacing and implantable defibrillators are being extensively used in the treatment of patients with cardiac arrhythmias. It is not unusual for the anesthesiologist to encounter a patient with these devices for an elective/emergency surgery. Perioperative management of these patients should include the following:

- Establishing whether patient has a cardiac implantable electronic device (CIED)
- Basics of pacemaker and CIED
- Preoperative and intraoperative device functioning
- Postoperative care and instructions
- Specific clinical scenarios.

ESTABLISHING WHETHER PATIENT HAS A CIED (MUST KNOW)

History: In majority of cases the patient would give a history of placement of implantable device.

It is essential to elicit vital information with respect to indication of CIED placement, device functioning, patients underlying cardiac function and associated co-morbidities.

Indication of CIED placement

- After myocardial infarction there can be damage to impulse formation and conduction system of the heart following MI. Indication for pacemaker include:
  - Persistent complete heart block
  - Newly acquired bundle branch block with first degree heart block
  - Newly acquired bifascicular bundle branch block
- Symptomatic bradycardia (history of loss of consciousness)
  - AV block (second-third degree) with symptoms
  - Bifascicular or trifascicular block with symptoms

- Sinus node dysfunction
  - As a result of long-term drug therapy
  - Symptomatic chronotropic incompetence
- Heart failure needing a cardiac resynchronization therapy by using a biventricular pacing
- Hypertensive carotid sinus and neurocardiac syndromes
  - Recurrent syncope associated with carotid sinus stimulation
  - Asystole of > 3 sec duration in absence of any medication.

History with respect to device functioning: Presence of preimplantation symptoms like lightheadedness, dizziness or fainting which occurs after pacemaker insertion implies device failure and will need cardiac consultation.

Evaluation of the pacemaker: Every device would have a card by the manufacture it would be as Figure 1:

Pacemaker Interrogation

It is a routine 'check-up' of pacemaker (Fig. 2) which is done at regular intervals or prior any planned surgical procedure. The cardiologist extracts information about the pacemakers through a device connected to the computer which is held over the patient's chest. Information regarding pacemaker/CIED battery status and lead status is obtained. The pacemaker can also be reprogrammed in this interrogation. Occasional, patient's experience a feeling of lightheadedness during the interrogation.

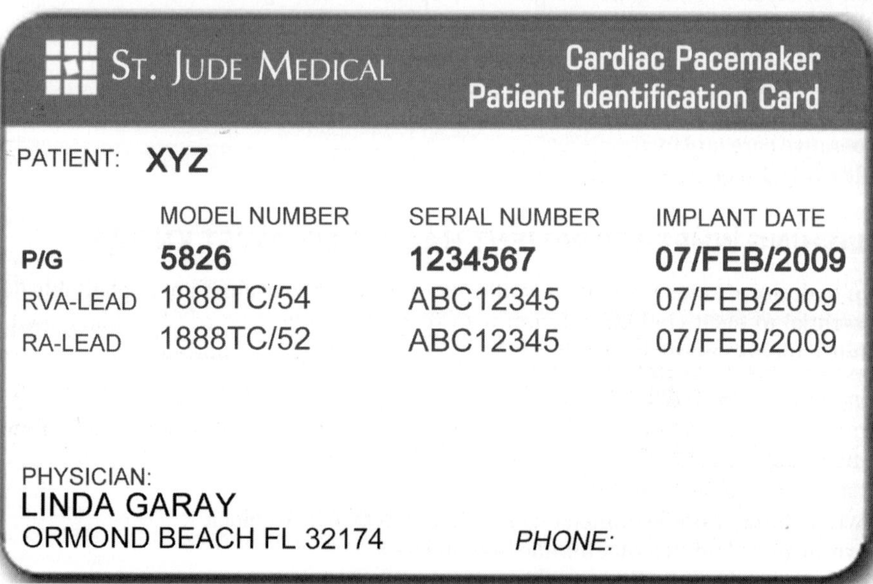
ST. JUDE MEDICAL

Cardiac Pacemaker Patient Identification Card

PATIENT: XYZ

	MODEL NUMBER	SERIAL NUMBER	IMPLANT DATE
P/G	5826	1234567	07/FEB/2009
RVA-LEAD	1888TC/54	ABC12345	07/FEB/2009
RA-LEAD	1888TC/52	ABC12345	07/FEB/2009

PHYSICIAN:
LINDA GARAY
ORMOND BEACH FL 32174 PHONE:

Fig. 1 Sample of a pacemaker card

Device: **EnRhythm P1501DR**
Serial Number: **PNP453333H**

Date of Visit: **15-Sep-2010 08:43:40**
9987 Software Version 7.0

Parameters **Page 1**

Pacing Summary

Mode		Rates		AV Intervals	
Mode	AAIR<=>DDDR	Lower	50 bpm	Paced AV	180 ms
Mode Switch	On	Upper Track	130 bpm	Sensed AV	150 ms
		Upper Sensor	120 bpm		

Pacing Details

Rate Response	
Rate Response	7
Activity Threshold	Medium Low
Activity Acceleration	30 sec
Activity Deceleration	5 min

AV Therapies	
Rate Adaptive AV	Off

	Atrial	RV
Amplitude	2 V	2 V
Pulse Width	0.5 ms	0.5 ms
Sensitivity	0.3 mV	0.9 mV
Pace Polarity	Bipolar	Bipolar
Sense Polarity	Bipolar	Bipolar

Arrhythmia Interventions	
A. Rate Stabilization	Off
A. Preference Pacing	Off
Post Mode Switch	Off
V. Rate Stabilization	Off

Device: **EnRhythm P1501DR**
Serial Number: **PNP453333H**

Date of Visit: **15-Sep-2010 08:43:40**
9987 Software Version 7.0

Parameters **Page 2**

Refractory/Blanking	
PVARP	310 ms
PVAB Interval	150 ms
PVAB Method	Partial
A. Blank Post AP	200 ms
A. Blank Post AS	100 ms
V. Blank Post VP	200 ms
V. Blank Post VS	120 ms

Additional Features	
Non-Comp Atrial Pacing	On
NCAP Interval	300 ms
PMT Intervention	Off
PVC Response	On
V. Safety Pacing	On

Device Information

Device	Medtronic	EnRhythm P1501DR	PNP453333H	Implanted: 26-Jan
Atrial	Medtronic	5076 CapSureFix® N...	PJN1138506	Implanted: 26-Jan
RV	Medtronic	5076 CapSureFix® N...	PJN1163355	Implanted: 26-Jan

Fig. 2 Pacemaker interrogation

Other relevant patient history: Since substantial number of these patients suffers from coronary artery disease (50%), hypertension (20%) and diabetes (10%), one should know:

- The severity of the cardiac disease
- The current functional status
- Medication the patient is on.

Clinical Examination

Other than routine clinical examination especially look for:

- Signs of CCF, Bruits
- Physical examination for scars, palpating the device (Generally, generator for the epicardial electrodes is kept in the abdomen and over one of the pectoris muscles for the endocardial electrodes).

Investigations

- Routine biochemical and hematological investigations should be performed as indicated on an individual basis. Measurement of serum electrolytes (especially K^+) should be performed.
- A 12 lead electrocardiogram.

Information from 12 Lead ECG (Fig. 3)

Nature of pacing: In atrial pacing, an electrical spike appears before the P wave and the QRS complex is usually normal. In ventricular pacing, there are two spikes, one before the P wave and another preceding the QRS complex.

Patient's intrinsic activity will be reflected by normal QRS complex with or without preceding P wave.

In emergency cases—when history/interaction of patient is not possible—an X-ray chest helps in picking up presence of pacemaker/CIED *in situ* (Fig. 4).

In all patients with CIED, a X-ray should be ordered for visualization and confirmation of continuity of pacing wires.

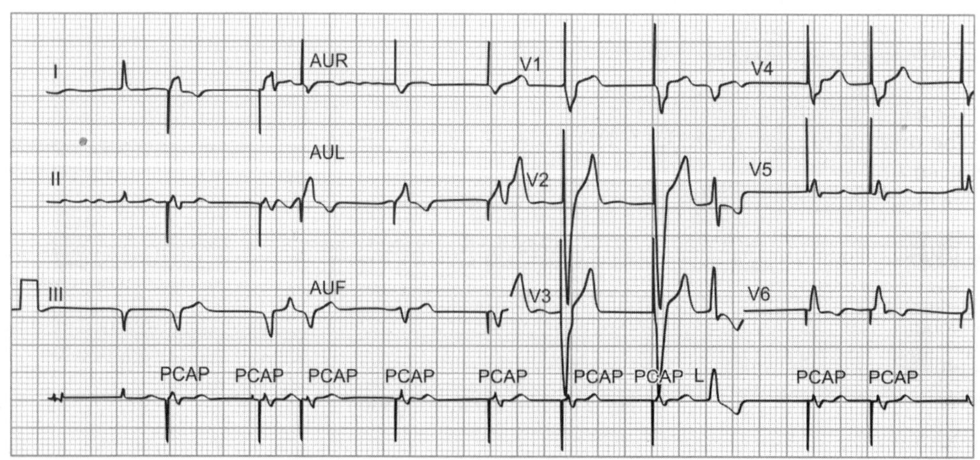

Fig. 3 Lead ECG of a patient with pacemaker

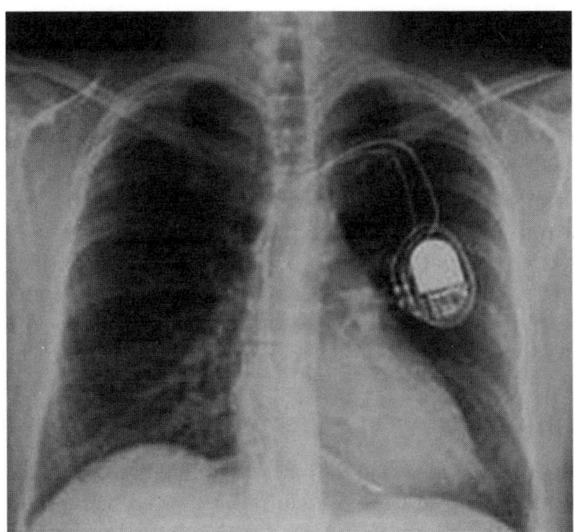

Fig. 4 X-ray with CIED *in situ*

Evaluation of Cardiac Status

Dobutamine stress test: Despite the presence of chronotropic incompetence among pacemaker-dependent patients, there is preservation of both a positive inotropic response to dobutamine with increased myocardial contractility and changes in left ventricular loading conditions leading to increased myocardial oxygen demand. The demonstration of inducible ischemia during these conditions suggests that HR increase may not be necessary to provoke ischemia. Because dobutamine can provoke ischemia on the basis of factors independent of HR, this tests may still be diagnostic despite a blunted HR response and failure to achieve a specific target HR.

BASICS OF PACEMAKER AND CIED

Pacemakers can be classified as per the method of insertion, location of leads, etc.

- Transvenous
- Transcutaneous
- Epicardial
- Transesophageal

The original nomenclature by ICHD (Intersociety Commission for Heart Disease) Resources involved a three letter code. This code has been extended to five letters. Table 1 gives these generic codes for pacemaker.

Table 1 | Generic codes of pacemaker

Pacing	*Sensing*	*Response*	*Programmability*	*Tachycardia*
O–None	O–None	O–None	O–None	O–None
A–Atrium	A–Atrium	I–Inhibited	C–Communicating	P–Pacing
V–Ventricle	V–Ventricle	T–Triggered	P–Simple programmable	S–Shock
D–Dual (A+V)	D–Dual (A+V)	D–Dual (I+T)	M–Multiple programmable	D–Dual (P+S)
			R–Rate modulation	

Modern day pacemakers are programmable into one of three modes:

1. Asynchronous pacing or fixed rate (AOO, VOO, DOO)—pace at preset rate that is independent of the inherent heart rate. Most dangerous complication is ventricular fibrillation due to R on T phenomenon.
2. Single chamber demand pacing (AAI, VVI) paces at a preset rate when spontaneous heart rate falls below pre set rate.
3. Dual chamber AV sequential pacing requires two pacemaker leads, one in atrium and one in the ventricle. The atrium is stimulated to contract first, and after an adjustable PR interval the ventricle is stimulated to contract.

Dual chamber pacing is indicated when ventricular pacing alone cannot maintain adequate cardiac output and atrial pacing alone cannot be done as in third degree AV block. Major advantage is ability to increase cardiac output and reduce incidence of atrial fibrillation.

Common Terminology used with Pacemaker (Good to know)

Pulse generator: It includes the energy source (battery) and electric circuits for pacing and sensory function. Mercury–Zinc batteries that were used in the early days had a short useful life (2–3 years). Currently Lithium-iodide batteries are being used which have longer life (5–10 years) and high energy density.

Leads: These are insulated wires connecting pulse generator and electrodes.

Electrode: It is an exposed metal end of the lead in contact with the endocardium or epicardium.

Unipolar pacing: There is one electrode, the cathode (negative pole) or active lead. Current flows from the cathode, stimulates the heart and returns to anode (positive pole) on the casing of pulse generator via the myocardium and adjacent tissue to complete the circuit. Unipolar pacemaker is more likely to pick up extracardiac signals and myopotentials. Pacemaker spikes are large in this pacing.

Bipolar leads: Consist of two separate electrodes, anode (positive pole) and cathode (negative pole), both located close to each other within the chamber that is being paced. As the electrodes are very close, circuit is small and the possibility of extraneous noise disturbance is less also the signals are sharp. Pacemaker spikes are very small in this type of pacing.

Endocardial pacing: It is also called as transvenous pacing which implies that the leads/electrodes system has been passed through a vein to the right atrium or right ventricle. It can be unipolar or bipolar.

Epicardial pacing: This type of pacing is accomplished by inserting the electrode through the epicardium into the myocardium and is generally done following cardiac surgery. This can also be unipolar or bipolar.

Pacing threshold: This is the minimum amount of energy required to consistently cause depolarization and contraction of the heart. Pacing threshold is measured in terms of both amplitude and duration for which it is applied to the myocardium. The amplitude is programmed in volts (V) or in milliamperes in some devices, and the duration is measured in milliseconds.

Sensitivity: It is the minimal voltage level of intrinsic R wave or P wave that must be exceeded to detect R or P wave to activate the sensing circuit of the pulse generator and thus inhibit or trigger the pacing circuit.

Resistance: It can be defined as impedance to the flow of current. In the pacemaker system it amounts to a combination of resistance in lead, resistance through the patient's tissue and polarization that takes place when voltage and current are delivered into the tissues. Abrupt changes in the impedance may indicate problem with the lead system. Very high resistance can indicate a conductor fracture or poor connection to the pacemaker. A very low resistance indicates an insulation failure.

Hysteresis: It is particularly useful in patients with sick sinus syndrome. This feature allows a longer escape interval after a sensed event, giving the heart a greater opportunity to beat on its own. Here pacemaker is programmed to upper and lower rate and a programmable lower hysteresis rate.

Runaway pacemaker: This is pacemaker dysfunction characterized by fast and erratic spikes. This occurs with generator dysfunction due to battery failure or damage produced by leakage of the tissue fluids into the pulse generator. Treatment with antiarrhythmic drugs or cardioversion may be ineffective in such cases. It is necessary to change the pacemaker to an asynchronous mode, or reprogram it to lower outputs. If the patient is hemodynamically unstable temporary pacing should be done followed by changing of pulse generator.

Programmable pacemakers: Our physiologic pacemaker, SA node responds to body's changing demands by increasing or decreasing heart rate. Patients on modes like DDD, VVI, and AAI modes cannot increase or decrease heart rate according to the metabolic demands. To overcome this problem recent generation pacemakers provide flexibility to adapt the device to patient's changing metabolic needs. The various factors, which can be programmed are pacing rate, pulse duration, voltage output, R wave sensitivity, refractory periods, PR interval, mode of pacing, hysteresis (difference between intrinsic heart rate at which pacing begins and pacing rate), and atrial tracking rate. Various types of sensors have been designed which respond to the parameters such as vibration, acceleration, minute ventilation, respiratory rate, central venous pressure, central venous pH, QT interval, pre-ejection period, right ventricular contractility, mixed venous oxygen saturation, and right atrial pressure. Out of these, sensors capable of detecting body movements (vibrations), changes in ventricular repolarization, central venous temperature, central venous oxygen saturation, respiratory rate and depth, and right ventricular contractility are commonly used in clinical practice.

Biventricular pacemakers: Electrical depolarization is normally initiated throughout both ventricles by the His-Purkinje system. In patients with systolic dysfunction with conduction disturbances as manifested by prolonged QRS complex, conduction of the wave of depolarization in the left ventricle is markedly altered. As a result left ventricular contraction becomes dyssynchronous, with resultant decrease in stroke volume, increased wall stress, and delayed relaxation. A biventricular pacemaker, also known as CRT (cardiac resynchronization therapy) is a type of pacemaker that paces both the septal and lateral walls of the left ventricle. By pacing both sides of the left ventricle, the pacemaker can resynchronize a heart to contract in synchrony. CRT devices have at least two leads, one in the right ventricle to stimulate the septum, and another inserted through the coronary sinus to pace the lateral wall of the left ventricle. For patients in normal sinus rhythm, there is also a lead in the right atrium to facilitate synchrony with the atrial contraction. Thus, timing between the atrial and ventricular contractions, as well as between the septal and lateral walls of the left ventricle can be adjusted to achieve optimal cardiac function.

Pacemaker syndrome: It is also known as AV dyssynchrony syndrome represents the clinical consequences of AV dyssynchrony or suboptimal AV synchrony, regardless of the pacing mode. (Ellenbogen KA, Gilligan DM, Wood MA, et al. The pacemaker syndrome—a matter of definition. Am J Cardiol. 1997;79(9):1226-9). This leads to a variety of clinical signs and symptoms resulting from deleterious hemodynamics. These include hypotension, syncope, vertigo, light-headedness, fatigue, exercise intolerance, malaise, weakness, lethargy, dyspnea, and induction of congestive heart failure. Cough, awareness of beat-to-beat variation of cardiac response from spontaneous to paced beats, neck pulsation or pressure sensation in the chest, neck, or head, headache, and chest pain are the other symptoms. Symptoms may vary from mild to severe, and onset may be acute to chronic. The main mechanisms behind these symptoms are—loss of atrial kick with resultant drop in cardiac output, increased atrial pressure leading to symptomatic pulmonary and hepatic congestion, retrograde ventriculoatrial conduction leading to delayed, nonphysiologic timing of atrial contraction in relation to ventricular contraction and nonphysiologic ventricular depolarization pattern.

Pacing Threshold and Factors Affecting

Pacing threshold is the minimum amount of energy required to consistently cause depolarization and therefore contraction of the heart. Pacing threshold is measured in terms of both amplitude and duration for which it is applied to the myocardium. The amplitude is programmed in volts (V) or in milliamp in some devices, and the duration is measured in milliseconds. Table 2 lists the factors affecting pacing threshold.

Table 2 | Factors affecting pacing threshold

Factors which increase pacing threshold	*Factors which decrease pacing threshold*
• 1–4 weeks after implantation	• Increased catecholamines
• Myocardial ischemia/infarction	• Stress, anxiety
• Hypothermia, hypothyroidism	• Sympathomimetic drugs
• Hyperkalemia, acidosis/alkalosis	• Anticholinergics
• Antiarrhythmics (class IA, IB, IC)	• Glucocorticoides
• Severe hypoxia/hyperglycemia	• Hyperthyroidism
• Inhalation-local anesthetics	• Hypermetabolic status

If pacing threshold of myocardium increases more than that of pacemaker due to any of the above-mentioned reasons, pacemaker will fail to pace (failure to capture).

Factors Important from Anesthesia Point of View

Physiological effects: During the first two weeks, there is an initial sharp increase in the pacing threshold, i.e. up to ten times the acute level because of the tissue reaction around the electrode tip. Then it decreases to two to three times the acute level because of the scar formation. In chronic state, it reaches the initial level in 80% of patients. But this has become far less of a problem with the introduction of steroid-eluting leads and other refinements in the lead technology.

Potassium: This is an important electrolyte that determines the resting membrane potential (RMP). A mild to moderate increase in serum potassium causes an increase in myocardial excitability, but further increase leads to impaired myocardial responsiveness, including that to pacing stimulation.

Myocardial infarction: Its scar tissue is unresponsive to electrical stimulation and may cause loss of pacemaker capture.

Antiarrhythmic drug therapy: Class Ia (quinidine, procainamide), Ib (lidocaine, diphenylhydantoin), and Ic (flecainide, encainide, propafenone) drugs have been found to increase the pacing threshold.

Acid-base status: Alkalosis and acidosis both cause increase in pacing threshold.

Hypoxia: It increases pacing threshold.

Anesthetic drugs: These drugs are not likely to change the pacing threshold. It is notable that addition of equipotent halothane, enflurane, or isoflurane to opiate based anesthesia after cardiopulmonary bypass did not increase pacing threshold.

Implantable Cardioverter-defibrillator (ICD)

A ICD system consists of a pulse generator and leads for tachyarrhythmia detection and therapy. It provides antitachycardia and antibradycardia pacing, synchronized or nonsynchronized shocks, telemetry and diagnostics including storing even electrograms and history logs. Modern ICD use transvenous lead systems for sensing, pacing and shocks. Epicardial leads are still in use for infants and children. Current ICD have any programmable features, essentially measure each cardiac R-R interval and categorize the rate as normal, too fast or two slow. When the device detects a sufficient number of short R-R intervals within a period of time it will declare a tachycardia episode. The internal computer will decide between antitachycardia pacing and shock based on its programmed algorithm typically ICD delivers no more than six shocks per episode. Once a shock is delivered, the ICD will redetect to determine whether the shock successfully terminated the arrhythmia. Table 3 shows types of ICD-NASPE/BPEG generic defibrillator (NBD) code.

Table 3 | Types of ICD-NASPE/BPEG generic defibrillator (NBD) code

Letter I	*Letter II*	*Letter III*	*Letter IV*
Shock chamber(s)	Antitachycardia pacing chamber	Tachycardia detection	Antibradycardia pacing chamber(s)
O–None	O–None	E–Electrogram	O–None
A–Atrium	A–Atrium	H–Hemodynamic	A–Atrium
V–Ventricle	V–Ventricle		V–Ventricle
D–Dual (A+V)	D–Dual (A+V)		D–Dual (A+V)

Indications

- Hemodynamically significant ventricular tachycardia or ventricular fibrillation
- Spontaneous sustained VT with structural heart disease
- Syncope of undermined origin with clinically relevant, hemodynamically significant sustained VT or VF induced at EPS.

PREOPERATIVE AND INTRAOPERATIVE DEVICE FUNCTIONING (MUST KNOW)

Preoperative preparation includes the following:
- Determine whether electromagnetic interference (EMI) is likely to occur during the planned procedure
- Determining whether reprogramming the cardiac rhythm management device (CRMD), i.e. changing to an asynchronous pacing mode or disabling any special algorithms, including rate-adaptive functions is needed

- Suspending antitachyarrhythmia function, if present
- Advising the surgeon performing the procedure to consider use of a bipolar electrocautery system or ultrasonic scalpel to minimize potential adverse effects of EMI on the pulse generator or leads
- Assuring the availability of temporary pacing and defibrillation equipment
- Evaluating the possible effects of anesthetic technique on CIED function and patient CIED interactions.

Effect of the Magnet Application on Pacemaker Function

Magnet application is an extremely important function. Most pacemakers and ICDs have built-in magnetic reed switches that are designed to switch 'on' or 'off' circuitry in response to magnets. The magnet is placed over the pulse generator to trigger the reed switch present in the pulse generator resulting in a nonsensing asynchronous mode with a fixed pacing rate (magnet rate). In an ICD system magnet cannot convert the pacemaker to asynchronous mode, it only disables tachycardia detection and therapy of the ICD.

Clinical magnets, made of ferrous alloy, come in various shapes (ring or doughnut, horseshoe, and rectangle or bar). The site of magnet placement is important since a poorly positioned magnet may not produce the desired effect. Magnets are best placed directly on top of the device.

It is advisable to consult the manufacturer to know the magnet response before use. The patient must be connected to an electrocardiograph recorder before the magnet is applied and, remain connected, until after the magnet is removed. The first few paced complexes after magnet application provide information regarding the integrity of the pulse generator and its lead system. A 10% decrease in magnet rate from the time of implantation indicates power source depletion and is an indicator of end of life requiring elective replacement of battery.

If magnet application on a pacemaker site does not produce any response on the surface ECG pacing rate or mode, the magnet may be repositioned. If no change is still observed, reasons may be:

- A depleted pacemaker battery
- The pacemaker is programmed to ignore the magnet (St. Jude, Boston Scientific, and Biotronik synchronous mode)
- The magnetic field does not reach the device, as in the case of those with deeper (abdominal or submuscular) implants or in very obese patients
- End of life or lower battery life. The most current devices should be considered programmable unless known otherwise.

Reprogramming of the Implantable Cardioverter-defibrillator Preoperatively

Implantable cardioverter-defibrillator (ICD) can be reprogrammed to disable the antitachycardia function before surgery in operating room where a defibrillator is readily available. A magnet can be placed over the ICD to disable the antitachycardia function in the operating room. The advantage of placing a magnet on an ICD is that the magnet can be easily removed and antitachycardia function is quickly enabled in case of VT/VF during surgery.

Equipment to be Kept Ready in the Operating Room

- Continuous ECG monitoring
- External transcutaneous and intravenous pacing

- Defibrillator
- Drugs for resuscitation.

Routes of establishing temporary pacing includes

Transcutaneous: Defibrillating electrodes such as Zoll Pads preferred. They can be connected to a defibrillator/pacemaker. The electrodes should be placed as far (more than 6 inch or 15 cm) from a CRMD. Three recommended electrode placements are as follows:

1. *Anteroposterior placement:* The right arm (RA) electrode placed under the left scapula and the left leg electrode at apex of the heart.
2. *Posteroanterior placement:* The RA electrode placed under the right clavicle and the LL electrode at the apex of the heart.
3. *Apex posterior placement:* The RA electrode placed over the right scapula and the LL electrode at the apex of the heart.

Transesophageal

Transesophageal atrial pacing is feasible in almost all patients because of the proximity between the esophagus and the posterior aspect of the atria. Transesophageal pacing and recording is done using specialized or nonspecialized catheters. There are two different lead types:

1. The pill electrode, connected to a flexible wire that the patient swallows with water.
2. A flexible catheter that can even be used in comatose or intubated patients and passed nasally. It is positioned into the esophagus in order to record the posterior paraseptal atrial electrogram.

There is a relationship between the site of maximal atrial amplitude and the lowest atrial pacing threshold. The optimal atrial pacing site is usually found around 40 cm from the nares.

There are a few limitations to the technique:

- There is only one site of atrial pacing and recording
- There is no ventricular pacing
- Sometimes atrial capture can be difficult to assess on the surface ECG
- Leads to patient discomfort most frequently described as mild burning or chest discomfort like indigestion.

Intraoperative Monitoring for Patients with Pacemakers

Intraoperative monitoring should be based on the patient's underlying disease and the type of surgery.

Continuous ECG monitoring is essential to monitor pacemaker functioning. The artifact filter on the ECG monitor should be disabled in order to detect the pacing spikes.

In addition, mechanical evidence of the cardiac contraction should be monitored by palpation of the pulse, pulse oximetry, precordial stethoscope and arterial line, if indicated.

Presence of pacemaker is not an indication for insertion of pulmonary artery (PA) or central venous catheter. If these are indicated, care should be taken during insertion of the guidewire or central venous catheter as they are potentially arrhythmogenic and can also dislodge pacemaker leads, especially in recently implanted CRMDs. It is best to avoid the insertion of PA catheter.

Since these patients frequently have underlying cardiac dysfunction other parameters of perfusion should also be monitored. These include capillary refill, urine output, peripheral temperature, etc.

Choice of Anesthesia Technique

The anesthetic technique should be used according to the need of the patient.

Though there are no guidelines favoring or contradicting use of regional anesthesia in patients with pacemaker, few case reports of use of regional techniques in obstetric are available. One must remember that a paced heart cannot compensate for hypotension by tachycardia and hence spinal anesthesia should be used cautiously and preferably avoided in cases of anticipated blood loss or fluid shift.

Intraoperative management in case of GA: Both narcotics and inhalational techniques can be used safely. These anesthetic agents do not alter current and voltage thresholds of the pacemaker. Skeletal myopotentials commonly encountered with succinylcholine, myoclonic movements, or direct muscle stimulation can inhibit or trigger pacemaker and should be avoided.

Perioperative hypothermia should be avoided as muscle activity caused by shivering may affect pacemaker functioning. Use of nondepolarizing muscle relaxants is safe. In induction agents etomidate and ketamine should be avoided as these can sometimes cause myoclonic movements.

1. **Is there a need to reprogram the pacemaker and convert it to asynchronous mode for every surgery?**

Ans. Reprogramming the pacemaker to asynchronous fixed mode puts patient at risk of developing R on T phenomenon and ventricular tachycardia especially for patients with good underlying rate. When the risk of electromagnetic interference (EMI) is unlikely to interfere with pacemaker as in surgeries below umbilicus, contralateral arm, eyes or on face or surgeries not requiring use of cautery, pacemaker need not be reprogrammed. Also for patients who are not dependent on pacemaker as elicited from history and preoperative assessment, it is better to leave pacemaker on demand mode. But in all situations rate responsive function should be suspended.

Effect of Electrocautery on Pacemaker

The responses of pacemakers to electrocautery includes:
- Inhibition of pacing
- Asynchronous pacing
- Reset to backup mode
- Myocardial burns (rare)
- VF (rare).

Responses of ICD include:
- Inhibition of pacing
- Asynchronous pacing
- Inappropriate tachytherapy
- Inhibition of tachytherapy.

One should apply the following measures to decrease the possibility of adverse effects due to electrocautery.
- Bipolar cautery should be used as much as possible as it has less EMI.
- If unipolar cautery is to be used during operation, the grounding plate should be placed close to the operative site (active cautery tip) and as far away as possible from the site of pacemaker, usually on the thigh and should have good skin contact.
- Electrocautery should not be used within 15 cm of pacemaker.
- Frequency of electrocautery should be limited to 1 second bursts in every 10 seconds to prevent repeated asystolic periods. Short bursts with long pauses of cautery are preferred.

- Pacemaker may be programmed to asynchronous mode by a magnet or by a programmer. Before using cautery, the programmer must be available in the operation theater (OT). During the use of cautery, magnet should not be placed on pulse generator as it may cause pacemaker malfunction.
- Provision of alternative temporary pacing (transvenous, noninvasive transcutaneous) should be ready in the OT.
- Positive chronotropic drugs such as isoproterenol and atropine should be available.
- If defibrillation is required in a patient with pacemaker, paddles should be positioned as far away as possible from the pacemaker generator. If possible, anterior to posterior positioning of paddles should be used. Although permanent pacemakers have protective circuits to guard against externally applied high voltage, pulse generator malfunction has been reported.
- In elective cardioversion, the lowest voltage necessary should be utilized. However, even with these precautions, defibrillation may result in acute increase in the stimulation threshold, with resultant loss of capture. If this occurs, immediate reprogramming or temporary pacing should be done with increased generator output.
- Careful monitoring of pulse, pulse oximetry and arterial pressure is necessary during electrocautery, as ECG monitoring can also be affected by interference.
  The device should always be rechecked after operation.

POSTOPERATIVE CARE AND INSTRUCTIONS

In patients with rate responsive pacemakers, rate responsive mode should be deactivated before surgery. If this is not possible for some reason, the mode of rate response must be known so that conditions causing changes in paced heart rate can be avoided. For example, shivering and fasciculations should be avoided, in the postoperative period. If the pacemaker is 'activity' rate responsive-ventilation should be kept controlled and constant and temperature must be kept constant in 'temperature' rate responsive pacemakers.

Specific Clinical Scenarios

2. In the middle of surgery, the patient develops ventricular tachycardia. What would you do?
Ans. For a patient with an ICD and magnet disabled therapies/programming disabled therapies:
- Avoid all sources of EMI (electro-magnetic interference)
- Remove the magnet/re-enable therapies through programming if programmer available
- Observe patient for appropriate CIED therapy
- If above activities does not start the ICD function proceed with external defibrillation/cardioversion. For external cardio version place pads or paddles as far a possible from CRMD. Place defibrillator pads perpendicular to the major axis of CIED to the extent possible by placing them in an anteroposterior location. If technically impossible to place the pads or paddles in location that help to protect the CIED, Defibrillate/cardiovert the patient in the quickest possible way and be prepared to provide pacing through other routes.

3. In a patient with pacemaker for ECT, what care would you take?
Ans. ECT appears safe for patients with pacemakers, since little current flows within the heart because of the high impedance of body tissue, but the seizure may generate myopotentials which may inhibit the pacemaker. Thus ECG monitoring is essential and pacemakers should be changed to nonsensing asynchronous mode (fixed mode).

4. Any others areas where one needs to excise caution with patient with pacemaker?

Ans. *Transurethral resection of prostate (TURP) and uterine hysteroscopy:* Coagulation current used during TURP procedure has no effect, but the cutting current at high frequencies (up to 2500 kc/sec) can suppress the output of a bipolar demand ventricular pacemaker. When electrosurgical unit (ESU) use is anticipated reprogramming of pacemaker preoperatively to the asynchronous (fixed rate) mode should be performed.

Radiation: Cases where radiation therapy is planned for deep seated tumors, therapeutic radiation can damage the complementary metal oxide semiconductors (CMOS) that are the parts of most modern pacemakers. Generally, doses in excess of 5000 rads are required to cause pacemaker malfunction but as little as 1000 rads may induce pacemaker failure or cause runaway pacemaker. If pacemaker cannot be shielded from the field of radiation, consideration should be given to reimplanting the pacemaker generator at distant site. Temporary damage to pacemaker may recover after reprogramming but there may be permanent damage to the pacemaker as well.

Nerve stimulator testing or transcutaneous electronic nerve stimulator unit (TENS): TENS is now a widely used method for pain relief. TENS unit consists of several electrodes placed on the skin and connected to a pulse generator that applies 20 μsec rectangular pulses of 1–200 V and 0–60 mA at a frequency of 20–110 Hz. This repeated frequency is similar to the normal range of heart rates, so it can create a far field potential that may inhibit a cardiac pacemaker. Adverse interaction between these devices has been frequently reported, so these patients should be monitored during initial application of TENS. Pacemaker mediated tachycardia has been induced by intraoperative somatosensory evoked potential stimulation.

Studies and case reports suggest that unipolar electrode seems to be most susceptible to interferences. One case of pacemaker interference caused by activation of a nerve stimulator has been reported. However, with the advancements of modern pacemakers technology, a prospective study from Mayo clinic shows that interscalene nerve blocks and other peripheral nerve blocks using the nerve stimulator can be performed in patients with pacemakers without notable interferences with pacemaker functions.

Lithotripsy: Anesthesia may be required in patients undergoing extracorporeal shockwave lithotripsy (ESWL) for immobilization and to avoid pain in flank at entry site of waves. There may be electrical interference from hydraulic shock waves and can cause mechanical damage. High-energy vibrations produced by lithotripsy machine can cause closure of reed switch causing asynchronous pacing. 'Activity' rate responsive pacemaker can be affected due to the damage caused to the piezoelectric crystals by ESWL. The shock waves can produce ventricular extrasystoles, if not synchronized with R wave. Pacemaker malfunction can occur in patients undergoing ESWL, requiring adequate preparation prior to procedure. Focal point of the lithotripter should be kept at least six inches (15 cm) away from the pacemaker. Dual chamber demand pacemaker is especially sensitive to shock waves and should be reprogrammed to a simpler mode (VOO, VVI) preoperatively.

MRI: Three types of powerful forces exist in the MRI suite.

1. *Static magnetic field:* An intense static field is always present even if the scanner is not imaging. Most of the pacemakers contain ferromagnetic material, which gets attracted to the static magnetic field in the MRI and may exert a torque effect leading to discomfort at the pacemaker pocket. The reed switch activation by high static field of 0.5–1.5 T can result in switching of pacemaker to a nonsensing asynchronous pacing.
2. *Radiofrequency field (RF):* This field is switched on and off during magnetic resonance imaging and has a frequency of 21–64 MHz depending on the strength of magnetic field. The radiofrequency signals can cause interference with pacemaker output circuits resulting in rapid

pacing at multiple of frequency between 60 and 300 bpm causing rapid pacing rate. It may cause pacemaker reprogramming and destruction of electronic components. It may also cause heating at the electrode-tissue boundary, which may cause thermal injury to endocardium and myocardium.

3. *Gradient magnetic field:* It is used for spatial localization, changes its strength along different orientations and operates at frequencies in order of 1 kHz. Gradient magnetic field may also interact with reed—switch in pacemaker. Inappropriate sensing and triggering because of the induced voltages can occur.

   Patients with pacemakers should not routinely undergo MRI scanning. Further studies are necessary to refine the appropriate strategies for performing MRI safely in a patient with implanted pacemaker. The risk benefit ratio must be individually evaluated in every patient with a pacemaker. Patients, who require head MRI scanning without alternative diagnostic possibilities, may be best served in a carefully monitored setting. Appropriate patient selection should be done and equipment for resuscitation and temporary pacing should be available. A cardiologist should be present. Also patients should be closely monitored with ECG and oxygen saturation.

Radiofrequency (RF) ablation: Care should be taken to keep the RF current path as far away from pulse generator and lead system.

BIBLIOGRAPHY

1. Anesthesiology Problem-Oriented Patient Management Yao & Artusio's, 6th edn, 2010.
2. G Adward Morgan. Clinical anesthesiology, fourth edition, 2006.
3. Practice Advisory for the Perioperative Management of Patients with Cardiac Implantable Electronic Devices: Pacemakers and Implantable Cardioverter-Defibrillators an Updated Report by the American Society of Anesthesiologists Task Force on Perioperative Management of Patients with Cardiac Implantable Electronic Devices. Anesthesiology. 2011;114:247-61.
4. Rastogi S, Goel S, Tempe D, et al. Anesthetic management of patients with cardiac pacemakers and defibrillators for noncardiac surgery. Annals of Cardiac Anaesthesia. 2005;8:21-32.

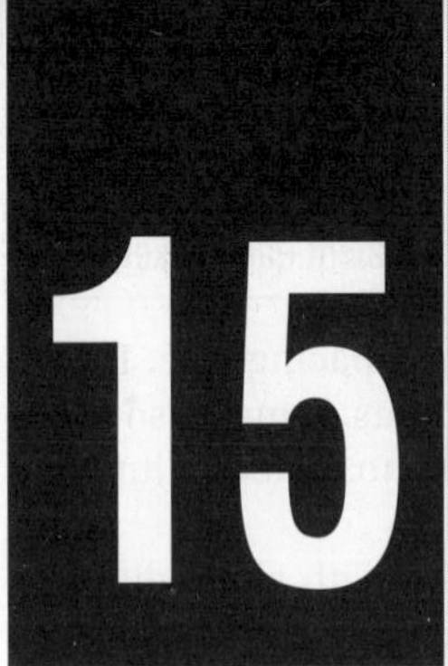

Anesthetic Management of a Patient with Chronic Renal Failure Posted for Elective Surgery

Nibedita Pani, Dhanee Majhi

Definition: Chronic kidney disease (CKD) is defined as either a glomerular filtration rate (GFR) of < 60 mL/min/1.73 m^2 for 3 months or more, irrespective of cause, or kidney damage leading to a decrease in GFR, present for 3 months or more. The damage may manifest as abnormalities in the composition of blood or urine, on radiological imaging, or in histology. It is classified into five stages depending on GFR.[1]

1. Describe the classification of CKD. (Must know)

Ans. *Stage 1:* Normal GFR; GFR ≥ 90 mL/min/1.73 m^2 with other evidence of chronic kidney damage*

Stage 2: Mild impairment; GFR 60–89 mL/min/1.73 m^2 with other evidence chronic kidney damage*

Stage 3: Moderate impairment; GFR 30–59 mL/min/1.73 m^2

Stage 4: Severe impairment; GFR 15–29 mL/min/1.73 m^2

Stage 5: Established renal failure; GFR, <15 mL/min/1.73 m^2 or on dialysis.

Ref: **Adapted from:** Joint Specialty Committee on Renal Medicine of the Royal College of Physicians and the Renal Association, and the Royal College of General Practitioners.[2]

2. What is the etiology of renal failure?[1] (Nice to know)

Ans.

- Diabetes mellitus
- Chronic glomerulonephritis
- Pyelonephritis

---

*The 'other evidence of chronic kidney damage' may include: persistent microalbuminuria; persistent proteinuria; persistent hematuria, after exclusion of other causes, e.g. urological disease; structural abnormalities of the kidneys demonstrated on ultrasound scanning or other radiological tests, e.g. polycystic kidney disease, reflux nephropathy; biopsy-proven chronic glomerulonephritis.[1]

- Renovascular disease
- Polycystic kidneys
- Hypertension
- Uncertain etiology/glomerulonephritis unproven
- Systemic lupus erythematosus
- Interstitial nephritis
- Other.

3. What is the prevalence of chronic renal failure? (Nice to know)

Ans. In the United States, the National Institute of Diabetes and Digestive and Kidney Diseases (NIDDK) reports that 1 in 10 American adults has some level of chronic kidney disease (CKD). Kidney disease is the ninth leading cause of death in the United States. There is a rising incidence of chronic kidney disease that is likely to pose major epidemiology and risk factors of chronic kidney disease in India—results from the SEEK (Screening and Early Evaluation of Kidney Disease) study. In India, it has been recently estimated that the age-adjusted incidence rate of ESRD to be 229 per million population (pmp), and >100,000 new patients enter renal replacement programs annually.[3]

4. Describe the pathophysiology of CKD.[4] (Good to know)

Ans. A normal kidney contains approximately 1 million nephrons, each of which contributes to the total glomerular filtration rate (GFR). In the face of renal injury (regardless of the etiology), the kidney has an innate ability to maintain GFR, despite progressive destruction of nephrons, as the remaining healthy nephrons manifest hyperfiltration and compensatory hypertrophy. This nephron adaptability allows for continued normal clearance of plasma solutes. Plasma levels of substances such as urea and creatinine start to show measurable increases only after total GFR has decreased to 50%.

The plasma creatinine value will approximately double with a 50% reduction in GFR. For example, a rise in plasma creatinine from a baseline value of 0.6 mg/dL to 1.2 mg/dL in a patient, although still within the adult reference range, actually represents a loss of 50% of functioning nephron mass.

The hyperfiltration and hypertrophy of residual nephrons, although beneficial for the reasons noted, has been hypothesized to represent a major cause of progressive renal dysfunction. The increased glomerular capillary pressure may damage the capillaries, leading initially to secondary focal and segmental glomerulosclerosis (FSGS) and eventually to global glomerulosclerosis.

Factors other than the underlying disease process and glomerular hypertension that may cause progressive renal injury include the following:

- Systemic hypertension
- Nephrotoxins [e.g. nonsteroidal anti-inflammatory drugs (NSAIDs), intravenous contrast media]
- Decreased perfusion (e.g. from severe dehydration or episodes of shock)
- Proteinuria (in addition to being a marker of CKD)
- Hyperlipidemia
- Hyperphosphatemia with calcium phosphate deposition
- Smoking
- Uncontrolled diabetes.

Knowledge of the pathophysiologic derangements as well as external (sometimes iatrogenic) insults that can arise in the perioperative period in patients with CKD is vital in the evaluation and management of these patients. Impairment of the excretory function of the kidney results in an elevation in blood urea nitrogen (BUN), creatinine, and various protein metabolic products. Impairment in the synthetic function results in a decrease in the production of erythropoietin (causing anemia) and active vitamin D-3 (causing hypocalcemia, secondary hyperparathyroidism, hyperphosphatemia, and renal osteodystrophy). Impairment in synthetic function also results in a reduction in acid, potassium, salt, and water excretion (causing acidosis, hyperkalemia, hypertension, and edema) and in platelet dysfunction, leading to an increase in bleeding tendencies.[5]

5. What are the pathophysiological changes in CKD?[1] (Must know)

Ans. Chronic kidney disease (CKD) is associated with pathophysiological changes in many systems, which have implications for the safe conduct of anesthesia.

Cardiovascular system

- Salt and water retention, hypertension, and LVH
- Cardiomyopathy, congestive cardiac failure, and subclinical pulmonary
- Edema
- Accelerated atherosclerosis and stiffening of large capacitative arteries
- Altered lipoprotein metabolism
- Complications of AVF/shunts, e.g. heart failure, limb ischemia, steal syndrome, pulmonary atheroembolism
- Uremic pericarditis
- Cardiovascular autonomic neuropathy with reduced baroreceptor sensitivity, sympathetic hyperactivity, and parasympathetic dysfunction
- Calciphylaxis and vascular calcification resulting in valvular heart disease and calcified atherosclerotic lesions
- Anemia.

Hemostasis and coagulation

- Uremic thrombocytopathy
- Prothrombotic tendency/hypercoagulation and reduced fibrinolysis
- Vascular access thrombosis.

Metabolic acidosis

- Bone resorption
- Negative nitrogen balance, muscle wasting, growth retardation.

Musculoskeletal system

- Renal osteodystrophy
- Rhabdomyolysis after major surgery.

Endocrine system

- Secondary and tertiary hyperparathyroidism, vitamin D deficiency
- Diabetes mellitus.

Gastrointestinal system

- Delayed gastric emptying
- Anorexia, vomiting, reduced protein intake, malnutrition
- Reduced calcium absorption.

Immune system: Immunosuppression due to uremia or drugs

Fluid and electrolyte homeostasis

- Hyperkalemia
- Volume overload
- Dehydration.

Neurological abnormalities
- Abnormal in central nervous system (CNS) and peripheral nervous system
- CNS changes—mild personality alterations to asterixis, myoclonus, encephalopathy and convulsions
- Peripheral neuropathy, glove and stocking sensory loss progressing to motor changes.

6. What are the common clinical manifestations of CRF?[6] (Must know)

Ans.
- *Electrolytes imbalance:* Volume expansion, hyponatremia, hyperkalemia, metabolic acidosis, hyperuricemia, hyperphosphatemia, hypocalcemia, hypermagnesemia
- Unpredictable intravascular fluid volume status
- *Gastrointestinal:* Gastroparesis nausea vomiting, pancreatitis, peptic ulcer disease, gastro-intestinal bleeding
- *Cardiovascular:* Accelerated atherosclerosis, systemic hypertension, left ventricular hypertrophy, congestive cardiac failure, pulmonary edema, cardiomyopathy, pericarditis, hyperdynamic circulation
- *Hematologic:* Anemia, B- and T-cell dysfunction, qualitative platelet dysfunction, bleeding diathesis
- *Musculoskeletal:* Muscle weakness, uremic osteodystrophy (osteomalasia, osteosclerosis, osteitis fibrosa cystica)
- *Neurologic:* Encephalopathy, loss of memory, seizures, peripheral neuropathy, autonomic dysfunction (postural hypotension), myoclonus, asterixis, dialysis disequilibrium (dehydration,weakness, nausea and vomiting, hypotension and occasionally seizure and coma)
- *Endocrine:* Vitamin D deficiency, secondary hyperparathyroidism carbohydrate intolerance, hypertriglyceridemia.

7. What is azotemia? (Good to know)

Ans. Due to progressive renal insufficiency, retention of nitrogenous waste product occur causing rise in blood urea and serum creatinine.

8. What is uremic syndrome? (Good to know)

Ans.
- Constellation of signs and symptoms (anorexia, nausea, vomiting, pruritus, anemia, fatigue, coagulopathy) that reflect the kidney's progressive inability to perform its excretory, secretory, and regulatory functions. BUN concentration is a useful clinical indicator of the severity of the uremic syndrome and patient response to therapy
- Treatment dietary protein restriction results in decreased protein catabolism and urea production.

9. What is the cause of uremic bleeding? What is the treatment?[7] (Good to know)

Ans. Patients with chronic renal failure have an increased tendency to bleed despite the presence of normal laboratory coagulation studies (platelet count, prothrombin time, plasma thromboplastin time). The bleeding time is the screening test that best correlates with the tendency to bleed (Table 1). Hemorrhagic episodes (gastrointestinal bleeding, epistaxis, hemorrhagic pericarditis, subdural hematoma) remain major factors contributing to the morbidity and mortality associated with anemia.

Table 1 | Treatment of uremic bleeding

Drug	*Dose*	*Onset of effect*	*Peak effect*	*Duration of effect*
Cryoprecipitate	10 units IV over 30 min	<1 hr	4–12 hrs	12–18 hrs
DDAVP (Desmopressin)	0.3 µg/kg IV or SC	<1 hr	2–4 hrs	6–8 hrs
Conjugated estrogen	0.6 mg/kg/day IV for 5 days	6 hrs	5–7 days	14 days

10. What are the causes of anemia? (Nice to know)

Ans.

- Decreased production of renal erythropoietin
- Suppression of bone marrow with uremic toxins
- Hemolysis
- Associated bleeding tendency with increased red blood cell (RBC) fragility
- Nutritional deficiency
- *Other causes:* BM fibrosis, chronic infection, hemoglobinopathies.

Compensated by: Increase in cardiac output, right side shift of oxyhemoglobin dissociation curve.

11. How should anemia be managed in patient with ESRD?[8] (Nice to know)

Ans. Patients can be treated with erythropoiesis-stimulating agents (ESAs) to increase hemoglobin levels. The preponderance of the evidence suggests that although ESAs raise hemoglobinA_{1c} and improve quality of life, targeting the complete correction of anemia with ESA is inadvisable. If patients with renal failure returned to normal hematocrit, they run a higher risk for composite death resulting from stroke, myocardial infarction, congestive heart failure, poorly controlled blood pressure, and thrombotic events. The practice at this time is to maintain a conservative target hemoglobin of 11–12 g/dL, but not greater than 13 g/dL with ESA treatment.

Intravenous or oral iron supplements are also used to treat anemia. Other novel agents are under investigation. For example, a continuous erythropoietin receptor activator allows less frequent dosing of an ESA. An intravenous iron nanoparticle (ferumoxtol) can raise hemoglobin more than oral iron.

12. What are the hazards of blood transfusion to raise hemoglobin? (Nice to know)

Ans.

- Risk of infection
- Risk of transmission of antibodies
- Risk of overload
- Risk of hyperkalemia
- Risk of hemosiderosis.

13. Cause of exacerbation of hyperkalemia in ESRD. (Nice to know)

Ans.

- Excessive dietary intake
- Hemolysis
- Hemorrhage
- Massive blood transfusion
- Metabolic acidosis

- Beta-adrenergic blockade
- Angiotensin-converting enzyme inhibitors
- Angiotensin receptor blockers
- Insulin deficiency or resistance
- Hyperosmolality
- Hyperglycemia
- Rhabdomyolysis
- Succinylcholine
- Digoxin overdose or potassium sparing diuretics.

14. What are the ECG manifestations of hyperkalemia? (Must know)

Ans.

- Peaked T waves
- Flattened P waves
- Lengthened PR interval
- Disappearance of P wave
- Widened quality rating system (QRS) "complex that can progress to a sine wave", "ventricular asystole or ventricular fibrillation".

15. What are the drugs associated with hyperkalemia? (Must know)

Ans. Succinylcholine, nonsteroidal anti-inflammatory drugs, Beta-adrenergic receptor blockers, heparin, ACE inhibitors and ARBs, digoxin, spironolactone, amiloride and triamterene, ciclosporin and tacrolimus.

16. What is the drug treatment for hyperkalemia?[9] (Must know)

Ans. Table 2 shows drug treatment of hyperkalemia.

Table 2 | Drug treatment of hyperkalemia

Drug	*Dose*
Calcium chloride	5 mL of 10% solution over 2 min (monitor for bradycardia)
Calcium gluconate	10 mL of 10% solution over 2 min
Insulin	5–10 units of regular insulin with 1–2 amps D50 W IV bolus
Sodium bicarbonate	1 mEq/kg slow IV push or continuous drip; not to exceed 50–100 mEq
β-agonist (albuterol)	2.5 mg mixed with 3 mL isotonic saline through nebuliser every 20 min as tolerated
Diuretics (furosemide)	20–40 mg IV push
Magnesium	1–2 g IV over 30–60 sec; repeat every 5–15 min as required or 3–10 mg/min IV infusion

17. How would you evaluate the patient preoperatively? (Must know)

Ans. *History and Physical Examination*[5]

Conduct a thorough history and physical examination because they are essential in the evaluation of patients with CKD prior to surgery. Obtain information on the following during the history and physical examination:

- Blood pressure and sugar trends
- Presence of anemia
- Radiocontrast exposure
- Prior surgical experiences

- Bleeding tendencies
- Allergies
- Use of potentially nephrotoxic drugs
- Nutritional and volume status
- Significant history of cardiac disease or peripheral arterial disease (PAD)
- Presence of comorbid disease
- Functional capacity.

Other Important History[5]

- Stable or unstable angina, history of myocardial infarction
- Arrhythmias (atrial fibrillation)
- Comorbid disease (e.g. pulmonary disease, history of stroke, transient ischemic attacks). Obtain the patient's functional capacity by using simplified questions of usual daily activities (e.g. climbing flights of stairs, playing tennis, shoveling snow in the winter). Strenuous activities, such as swimming, tennis, or basketball, have estimated energy requirements of at least 10 metabolic equivalents (METs)
- Perform a thorough physical examination, particularly to obtain evidence of volume overload and cardiovascular abnormalities (e.g. murmurs, carotid bruits, pericardial effusion, abnormal peripheral pulses)
- Note the presence or absence of hair on the lower extremities because this information may herald undiagnosed PAD. Record all extremity pressures, and calculate the ankle-brachial index (ABI).

Investigations

- *Blood:* Hb%, complete blood count, PCV
- RBS
- *LFT:* Plasma proteins, total albumin, globulin
- Serum electrolytes-k, Ca, Raised phosphates, Mg
- *RFT:* Blood urea, serum creatinine, uric acid
- GFR
- *Coagulation profile:* Platelet count
- *Lipid profile:* Hyperlipidemia
- *ABG analysis:* To evaluate oxygen delivery and tissue perfusion or metabolic failure
- *X-ray chest:* To rule out pleural effusion and signs of congestive heart failure
- *ECG:* To rule out LVH, IHD, Changes of hyperkalemia, ventricular ectopics
- *2D ECHO:* To know EF, cardiomyopathy, pericardial effusion
- *Urine analysis:* Specific gravity, osmolality, urine sodium
- HBs Ag and HIV status
- Renal scan/USG/CT/MRI scan for kidney status
- *Specific tests:* ABO tissue compatibility, HLA/Tissue typing, lymphocyte typing, microcytotoxicity typing (in renal transplant).

18. What are the risk factors for patient of CRF undergoing surgery? (Must know)

Ans.

- Low oxygen carrying capacity
- Altered intravascular volume status
- Multisystem involvement
- Immunosuppression
- Delayed gastric emptying time
- Delayed drug excretion

- Bleeding tendency
- Care of shunt, difficult venous assess
- Hepatitis carrier.

19. Described major clinical predictors to be used for the perioperative management of a patient with chronic renal failure.[5] (Good to know)

Ans. See Flow chart 1.

Flow chart 1 Major clinical predictors to be used for the perioperative management of a patient with chronic renal failure

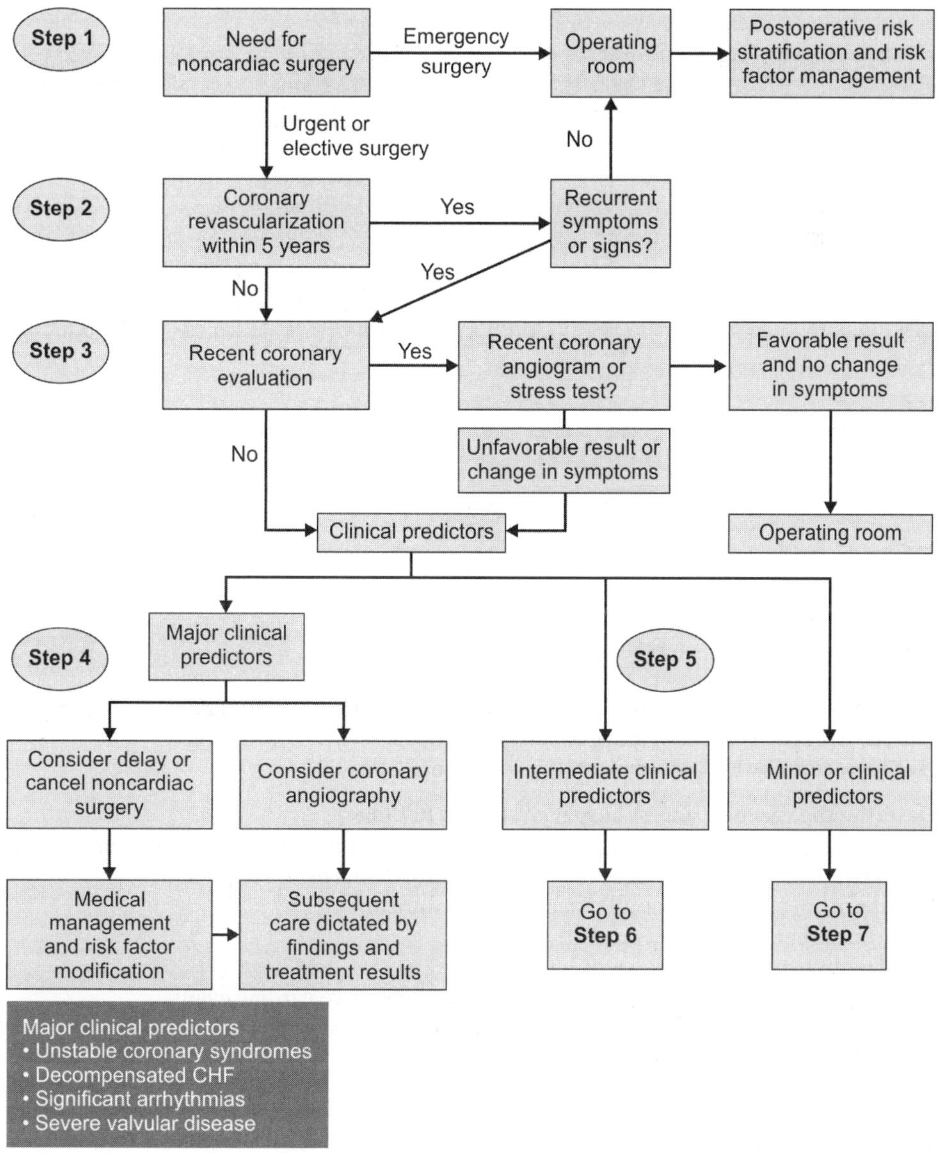

20. Describe intermediate clinical predictors to be used for the perioperative management of a patient with chronic renal failure.[5] (Good to know)

Ans. See Flow chart 2.

Flow chart 2 Intermediate clinical predictors to be used for the perioperative management of a patient with chronic renal failure

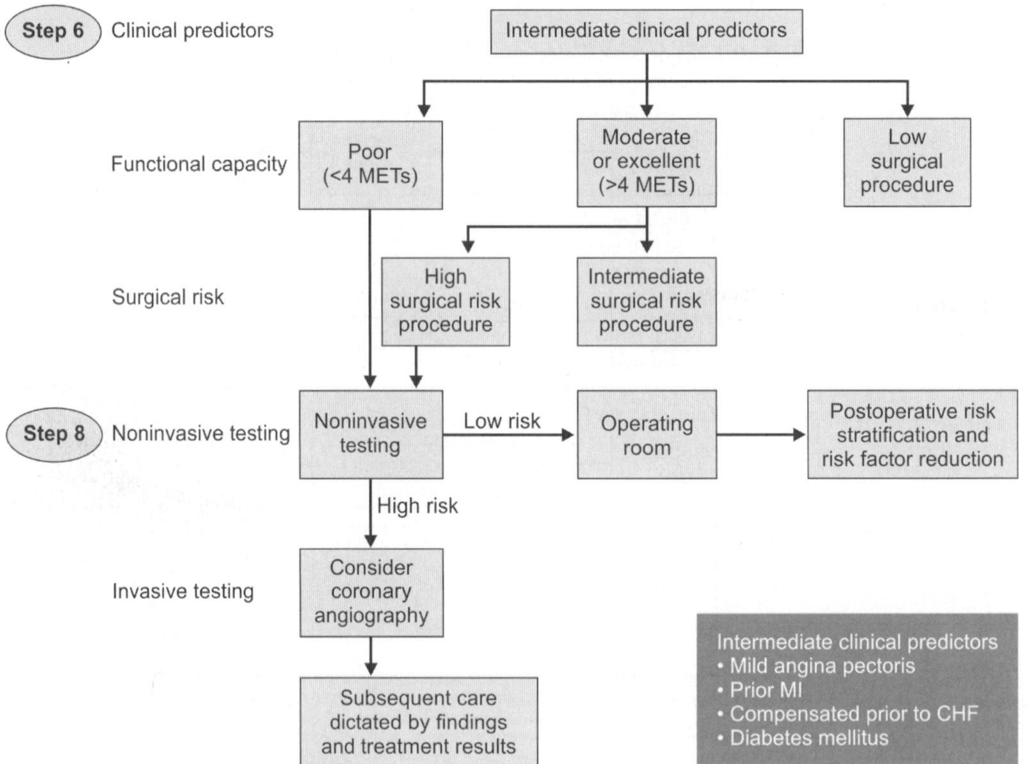

21. Describe minor clinical predictors to be used for the perioperative management of a patient with chronic renal failure.[5] (Good to Know)

Ans. See Flow chart 3.

22. Describe the vascular access surgery.[10] (Good to know)

Ans. Patients with ESRD undergoing renal replacement therapy with intermittent hemodialysis will often require anesthesia and surgery to form an arteriovenous fistula or graft.

The aims of anesthesia for vascular access surgery are to:

- Ensure intraoperative patient comfort
- Optimize surgical conditions
- Minimize risk of anesthetic complications, e.g. perioperative cardiac events
- Optimize postoperative state—avoidance of prolonged sedation, minimal requirement for strong postoperative analgesia.

Anesthetic techniques include

- Local anesthetic (LA) infiltration (with or without sedation)
- Regional anesthesia (RA) using brachial plexus local anesthetic block (with or without sedation)
- General anesthesia (GA).

Flow chart 3 Minor clinical predictors to be used for the perioperative management of a patient with chronic renal failure

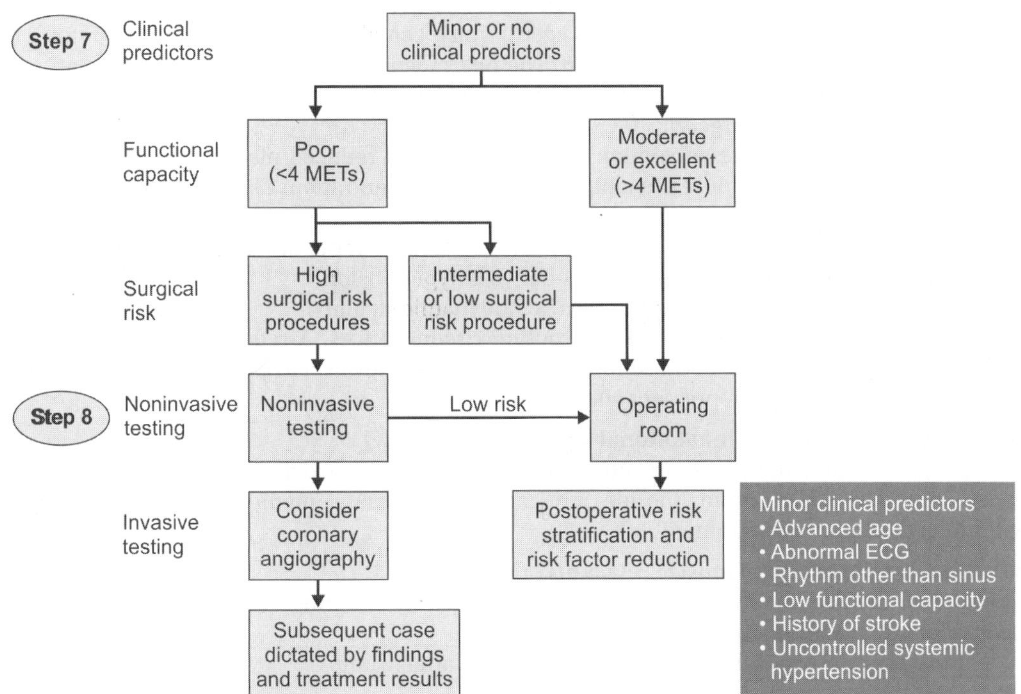

Vascular Access[1] (Good to Know): Maintenance of vascular access patency is of vital importance in patients with Stage 5 CKD on HD. Vascular access may be either permanent or temporary. Options for permanent access include native arteriovenous fistulae (AVF), arteriovenous grafts (AVG), and long-term catheters. Temporary vascular access includes: acute short-term noncuffed catheters which may or may not be tunneled; long-term tunneled cuffed catheters; and subcutaneous port catheter systems.

Insertion Site (Good to Know): The right internal jugular vein is the preferred site as the risk of complications is lower. In particular, it is the risk of stenosis of the vein that is reduced when using this route. The left internal jugular site is associated with a poorer blood flow rate and a greater rate of stenosis and thrombosis. The subclavian route should be avoided as the risk of stenosis after catheterization is unacceptably high, with 40–50% of patients demonstrating some degree of stricture on venography. Subclavian vein stenosis can result in fistula dysfunction with elevated venous dialysis pressures and painful arm edema. In patients who are candidates for renal transplantation, the femoral route should be avoided to prevent stenosis of the external iliac vein, as the transplanted kidney is anastomosed to it. The femoral route is also associated with the greatest risk of infection.

Complications (Good to Know): Problems relating to vascular access are a leading cause of hospitalization, morbidity and the need for anesthesia in patients with stage 5 CKD. These include infection, stenosis, thrombosis, aneurysm, limb ischemia, limb edema, heart failure, pulmonary atheroembolism, steal syndrome, and recirculation.

PHARMACOLOGY[1]

23. What are the effects of induction agents? (Must know)

Ans. Propofol is an intravenous induction agent, which can also be administered by continuous infusion to maintain anesthesia or sedation. The pharmacokinetics of bolus administration, and of maintenance infusion, do not seem to be markedly altered in ESRD patients (including those dialysed 12 hours prior to surgery).

Thiopental has an increased volume of distribution and reduced plasma protein binding in renal failure. The brain is exposed to a higher free drug concentration. The rate of administration should be reduced.

Ketamine pharmacokinetics is not significantly altered by renal disease, but its hypertensive effects make it undesirable in patient with underlying hypertension.

Etomidate is well tolerated and preserves hemodynamic stability.

Propofol or etomidate can be used in routine circumstances. A reduced induction dose of propofol may be considered because lower plasma protein levels and postdialysis hypovolemia can exaggerate their cardiodepressant effects.

24. What are the effects of inhalational agents? (Must know)

Ans. Desflurane and isoflurane are not associated with renal toxicity and appear safe to use in patients with CKD. Serum fluoride induced nephrotoxicity: methoxyflurane>sevoflurane> enflurane>desflurane>isoflurane.

25. What are the choice of muscle relaxants? (Must know)

Ans. Choice of MR for maintenance of skeletal muscle paralysis during surgery is influenced by the clearance mechanisms of the drugs.

Suitable neuromuscular blocker: Cisatracurium and atracurium.

26. What are the effects of various anesthetics on renal function?[11] (Must know)

Ans. See Table 3.

Table 3 | Effects of anesthetics on renal function

	RBF	*GFR*	*Urine output*	*Urine solutes*
General anesthesia	↓	↓	↓	↓
Intravenous anesthetics				
Thiopental	↔	↓	↓	↓
Midazolam	↔	↔	↓	↔
Fentanyl/droperidol	↔	↔	↓	↓
Fentanyl (high dose)	↔	↔	↔	↔
Inhaled anesthetics				
Halothane	↔	↓	↓	↓
Enflurane	↓	↓	↓	↓
Isoflurane	↔	↓	↓	↓
PEEP	↓	↓	↓	O
Regional anesthesia				
Epidural (with epinephrine)	↓	↓	↓	O
Epidural (without epinephrine)	↔	↔	↔	O
Spinal	↔	↔	↔	O

Key: ↔, no significant change; O, significant data; ↓, decrease

27. What are the effect of reversal agent? (Must know)

Ans. Neostigmine clearance is reduced and its half-life is prolonged in CKD, result in parasympathomimetic response bradycardia, AV block, when combined with atropine than glycopyrronium.

Sugammadex—helpful in preventing postoperative residual curarization (PORC) when patient have received an aminosteroid NMBA. It has got relative few side effects.

28. What are the preferred analgesia? (Must know)

Ans. Fentanyl, alfentanil, sufentanil and remifentanil.

29. Describe characteristics of opioids in renal failure and dialysis.[12] (Must know)

Ans. See Table 4.

Table 4 | Characteristics of opioids in renal failure and dialysis

Opioids	*Accumulation in renal failure*	*Safety profile in HD patient*
Morphine	Yes	Reduce dose and increase interval extreme caution required
Fentanyl	Parent compound may accumulate	Safe—reduce dose
Alfentanil	No	Safe—reduce dose due to increased free fraction
Remifentanil	No	Safe
Codeine	Yes	Avoid serious adverse effects have been reported
Oxycodeine	Yes	Ideally avoid if used, reduce dose and increase interval. Extreme caution required
Tramadol	Yes	Avoid—lowered seizure threshold and altered mental status
Meperidine	Normeperidine accumulates	Avoid—metabolite accumulation causes seizures
Methadone		Appears safe
Hydromorphone	Yes	Neuroexcitation possible use lower dose or longer interval. If used, additional dose may be needed after HD

- Acetaminophen prolonged use of acetaminophen is associated with analgesic nephropathy, but occasional or moderate use is safe. The use of acetaminophen in the perioperative period is safe and does not require dose adjustment.[13]
- Nonsteroidal anti-inflammatory agents the adverse effects of the nonsteroidal anti-inflammatory drugs (NSAIDs) are likely to outweigh any potential benefit in the perioperative period. They exacerbate hypertension and precipitate edema, hyponatremia, and hyperkalemia. There is an increased risk of gastrointestinal bleeding, which may be aggravated by the combined effects of uremic thrombasthenia and drug-induced platelet inhibition. Their use is associated with an increased risk of cardiovascular complications in this at risk population.[14] They are nephrotoxic agents that precipitate an acute decrease in GFR and may also cause acute interstitial nephritis as part of an idiosyncratic reaction. The renal effects of the COX-2 inhibitors are similar to those of the nonselective NSAIDs.[15]

30. What unusual situations can prolong neuromuscular blockade?[16] (Must know)

Ans. *Drugs:*

- *Antibiotics:* Aminoglycosides and tetracycline
- *Local anesthetics:* Small doses of local anesthetic enhances neuromuscular blockade, and large doses block neuromuscular transmission. Depending on the dose, local anesthetics interfere with the prejunctional release of acetylcholine, stabilize postjunctional membranes, and directly depress skeletal muscle.
- *Cardiac antidysrhythmic drugs:* lidocaine can augment pre-existing neuromuscular blockade. Quinidine interferes with the prejunctional release of acetylcholine and potentiates depolarizing and nondepolarizing drugs.
- *Diuretics:* Enhances nondepolarizing agents by inhibiting cAMP, leading to decreased prejunctional release of acetylcholine
- *Phenytoin:* Causes resistance to nondepolarizing drugs
- Lithium
- Calcium channel blockers.

Electrolytes

- *Potassium:* Hypokalemia increases the transmembrane potential, causing hyperpolarization of cell membrane. This leads to resistance to depolarizing drugs and increase sensitivity to nondepolarizing drugs. Hyperkalemia lowers the resting transmembrane potential and partially depolarizing the cell membrane. This increases the effect of depolarizing drugs and opposes the action of nondepolarizing drugs.
- *Magnesium:* Hypermagnesemia enhances nondepolarizing agents.

Acid-base imbalance

- Respiratory acidosis enhances neuromuscular blockade and opposes reversal with neostigmine
- The effects of metabolic acidosis and respiratory and metabolic alkalosis are inconsistent.

Temperature

- *Hypothermia:* Reduces hepatic enzyme activity, slowing of muscle contraction and relaxation and thereby enhancing the block.

31. What is the effect of anesthesia in persons with CKD?[5] (Good to know)

Ans. The administration of general anesthesia may induce a reduction in renal blood flow in up to 50% of patients, resulting in the impaired excretion of nephrotoxic drugs. In addition, the function of cholinesterase, an enzyme responsible for breaking down certain anesthetic agents, may be impaired, resulting in prolonged respiratory muscle paralysis if neuromuscular blocking agents are used. *N*-acetyl-procainamide, a metabolite of procainamide, accumulates in persons with CKD and, when used in combination with H_2-blockers, causes prolongation of the QTc. The dose should be adjusted, or a substitute should be used.

Fluorinated compounds, such as methoxyflurane and enflurane, are nephrotoxic and should be avoided in patients with CKD. Succinylcholine, a depolarizing blocker, causes hyperkalemia.

32. What is the effect of surgery in persons with CKD?[5] (Good to know)

Ans. Hyperkalemia may be precipitated by tissue breakdown, transfusions, acidosis, ACE inhibitors, beta-blockers, heparin, rhabdomyolysis, and the use of ringer lactate solution as a replacement fluid. Ringer lactate solution contains potassium, which is often disregarded but can cause hyperkalemia. Third-space fluid loss, diarrhea, vomiting, and nasoenteric suction result in both volume contraction and hypokalemia. Hypokalemia is sometimes followed concomitantly with hypomagnesemia.

Most patients with CKD have chronic acidosis; surgical disease can further complicate the acidemia. Such patients are at a higher risk for hyperkalemia, myocardial depression, and cardiac arrhythmia.

Hypocalcemia and hyperphosphatemia may be caused by rhabdomyolysis. Hyponatremia may occur from hypotonic fluids or inappropriate secretion of antidiuretic hormone.

33. What are the effects of fluid and electrolytes?[5] (Must know)

Ans. However, there is evidence that patients with CKD develop fluid overload early and this may be a stimulus for inflammation and accelerated progression of renal disease. It is possible that edema is associated with altered gut permeability and an associated inflammatory response. Patients with CKD are unable to adapt to large variations in salt intake and have an impaired ability to concentrate and dilute urine. Maximum sodium excretion is a function of GFR. The impaired ability to excrete a sodium load predisposes these patients to volume overload, especially when large volumes of saline solutions are administered. Infusion of large volumes of saline will also result in hyperchloremic metabolic acidosis. The deleterious effects of metabolic acidosis include depression of myocardial contractility, reduced cardiac output, and reduced renal blood flow. Furthermore, hyperchloremia can reduce renal blood flow and GFR. If access to free water is restricted in the perioperative period, the inability to concentrate urine will result in hypernatremia and hypertonicity. In managing patients on dialysis, the anesthetist should establish the patient's dry weight and compare it with their weight immediately before coming to theater. Failure to achieve dry weight with dialysis is a common problem, particularly with short duration dialysis prescriptions. Nevertheless, patients with CKD are at risk of developing hyperklemia if challenged with excessive exogenous potassium or transcellular potassium shifts. In this respect, acidemia, insulin deficiency, hypertonicity, and acute beta-adrenergic receptor block should be avoided. Intravenous fluids containing hydroxyethyl starch have adverse effects on renal function in renal transplant recipients and in critically ill patients with severe sepsis or septic shock.

34. What should be the intravenous fluid? (Must know)

Ans. Patients dependent on hemodialysis require special attention with respect to perioperative fluid management. An absence of renal function narrows the margin of safety between insufficient and excessive fluid administration to these patients. Noninvasive operations require replacement of only insensible water losses with 5% glucose in water (5–10 mL/kg IV). The small amount of urine output can be replaced with 0.45% sodium chloride. Thoracic or abdominal surgery can be associated with loss of significant intravascular fluid volume to the interstitial spaces. This loss is often replaced with balanced salt solutions or 5% albumin solutions. Blood transfusions may be considered if the oxygen-carrying capacity must be increased or if blood loss is excessive. Measuring the central venous pressure may be useful for guiding fluid replacement.

35. Describe the general aspects of anesthetic associated concerns. (Must know)

Ans.

- Intramuscular injection should be avoided in consideration of low muscle mass and uremic platelet dysfunction.
- Attention to patient positioning on the operating table as poor nutritional status render the skin particularly prone to bruising and sloughing, and extra padding is required to protect vulnerable nerves.
- Intravenous access and blood pressure monitoring should be avoided the AV fistula arm.
- Patient identification armbands must not encroach on the fistula and compression of the fistula during surgery must not occur
- Subclavian venous access should be avoided (increase rate of stenosis)

- Immune suppression increases risk of postoperative sepsis.
- Many patients with chronic renal failure receive prophylactic antibiotic for surgical procedures, particularly dialysis for surgical procedures, and for dialysis graft procedures.

36. What are the intraoperative management? (Must know)

Ans. The aim is to maintain adequate renal perfusion pressure. The following may allow optimal intraoperative care:

- Appropriate intravascular volume replacement.
- Avoidance of nephrotoxic drugs.
- Urinary catheter aiming for a urine output > 0.5 mL/kg/hr
- Maintenance of a suitable mean arterial pressure (MAP) for the patient and operation (avoid hyper- or hypovolemia)
- Monitoring of central venous pressure (CVP)
- Monitoring of cardiac output
- Vasopressors
- Anticipation of anesthetic and surgically induced hemodynamic pertubations both intra- and postoperatively.

Intraoperatively the neurohumoral response to surgery causes a sympathetic response, releasing vasopressin, aldosterone and cortical in the 'fight or fight' response. One of the aims of this is to aid salt and water retention protecting the renal vasculature. Anesthetic agents, ACE inhibitors and NSAIDs will alter this protective response.

37. Is invasive monitoring required during surgery?[17] (Must know)

Ans.

- *CVP:* Adequate hydration is an important part of the anesthetic management. Measuring CVP is not an absolute requirement. External jugular venous pressure has been used as an alternative to CVP monitoring. The CVP or pulmonary artery pressure can be used to guide fluid therapy. As postdialysis patients have intravascular volume depletion. To decrease the incidence of postoperative acute tubular necrosis, a liberal hydration policy is employed intraoperatively.
- *IABP:* An arterial line is not absolutely required. It should be placed if a patient has an advanced comorbid condition(s) that requires close monitoring of blood pressure and acid base status. Often, placement of an intra-arterial line is difficult, because many recipients have poor arterial access secondary to diabetes, peripheral vascular disease, arteriovenous fistula and shunts. Major swings in blood pressure may occur, with hypotension (49.6%) being more likely than hypertension (26.8%).
- *Pulmonary artery catheter:* Not routinely placed but patient with severe comorbid conditions, such as symptomatic coronary artery disease, LV dysfunction, congestive heart failure, valvular heart disease, or severe chronic obstructive pulmonary disease, can be monitored precisely.
- Transesophageal echocardiography (TEE) can help determine if hypotension is caused by hypovolemia or myocardial infarction.

38. Describe renal risk assessment and interventions.[5] (Good to know)

Ans. *Patients with CKD treated conservatively:* Patients who are euvolemic, responsive to diuretic therapy, and/or have no significant electrolyte abnormalities or bleeding tendencies are uncomplicated and do not require dialysis before surgery. Patients with edema, CHF, or pulmonary congestion or those who are responsive to diuretic therapy require further cardiovascular evaluation. If the results of the cardiovascular evaluation are optimal, then fluid overload can be attributed to CKD. Combination diuretic therapy can help treat these patients to achieve euvolemia prior to surgery. Patients with diabetes have a greater tendency of having volume overload or cardiovascular disease. CKD may be so advanced that the patient develops diuretic resistance, with progressive edema. Preoperative dialysis may be considered in these patients. If postoperative dialysis is imminent, the surgeons should be advised to place a temporary catheter intraoperatively. This avoids the use of femoral cannulation, which carries a higher risk of infection. Permanent vascular access placement can then be arranged when the patient is more stable.

Further deterioration in renal function can be avoided by identifying and eliminating potential nephrotoxic agents. These include substitution or dosage adjustment for antibiotics (e.g. aminoglycosides, acyclovir, amphotericin), sedatives, and muscle relaxants. NSAIDs and COX-2 inhibitors should be avoided, as should radiocontrast material. Demerol (meperidine) used for postoperative pain should be avoided because accumulation of its metabolite normeperidine can cause seizures in patients with CKD, especially those on dialysis. All drug interactions and potential nephrotoxicity must be identified and either stopped or the dose of the drug adjusted for the level of renal function. Electrolyte abnormalities must be identified and corrected perioperatively.

39. Patients already on dialysis or those who have a renal transplant, how will you manage?[5] (Good to know)

Ans. For patients already on dialysis, dialysis adequacy, preoperative dialysis needs, postoperative dialysis timing, and dosage requirements for all medications should be determined. Patients on hemodialysis usually require preoperative dialysis within 24 hours before surgery to reduce the risk of volume overload, hyperkalemia, and excessive bleeding. Patients with peritoneal dialysis who are undergoing abdominal surgery should be switched to hemodialysis until wound healing is complete. Peritoneal dialysis should be continued for those undergoing nonabdominal surgery.

Because of complicated interactions and immunosuppressive dosing, monitoring, and adjustment, a nephrologist with specialized knowledge of renal transplantation should be involved in the preoperative evaluation of patients with CKD who have received kidney transplantation.

40. What preoperative work-up would you order for dialysis patient? (Must know)

Ans. *Medical optimization include:*

- Dialytic correction of metabolic status
- Management of anemia erythropoietin, darbepoetin alfa[18]
- *Tailoring of blood pressure and heart failure treatment*: Hypertension is common in hemodialysis patients and good control should be achieved to minimize perioperative instability. Angiotensin converting enzyme inhibitors and angiotensin receptor blockers are omitted on the day of surgery because of the risk of significant hypotension at induction of anesthesia.
- *Blood glucose control:* Dialysis patients are also at increased risk of hypoglycemia with fasting. Safe glucose levels, generally considered to be target levels < 180 mg/dL or 10 mmol/L.[19]
- *Calcium, phosphate and parathyroid hormone management:* Medical management includes the use of phosphate binders and vitamin D analogs.
- *Fluid and electrolyte status:* Close attention should be paid to establishing the correct 'dry weight' for the patient, i.e. the weight at which they are euvolemic.
- *Nutritional status:* Malnutrition is common in ESRD patients receiving hemodialysis and the pathogenesis is complex. Under-dialysis leads to anorexia and abnormalities in taste which impact dietary nutrition intake. In the case of elective surgery, there should be adequate time to involve a dietician, increase dialysis adequacy, and improve nutritional intake prior to surgery. In cases where this is not possible via the enteral route, total parenteral nutrition (TPN) can be used to supplement or replace oral intake, and can be administered during dialysis sessions.
- *Hemodialysis vascular access:* This is often described as the patient's 'lifeline'. If the patient as a known central venous stenosis, this anesthetist and surgeon should be informed as it may have implications for their practice or the planned procedure. As general rule, hemodialysis catheters should not be used for purposes other than dialysis (e.g. blood sample, CVP monitoring, drug administration) except in an emergency.

- *Infection control issue:* ESRD patients are at increased risk of bacterial colonization and infection by virtue of altered neutrophil and monocyte function, impaired lymphocyte activation or number, cytokinemia and abnormal pathogen recognition.[20]
- *Reduction in bleeding risk:* Low molecular weight heparin, popular for DVT prophylaxis, undergoes predominantly renal excretion and accumulates in ESRD, increasing bleeding risk. If used, doses should be significantly reduced. Although low-dose aspirin has been safely continued through the perioperative period, clopidogrel should be discontinued 7 days prior to surgery unless there are specific indications for its use. Adequate dialysis and uremia reduction in the perioperative period will help improve platelet function. In circumstances where other techniques have failed, tranexamic acid may be effective, although it accumulates in renal failure.[21]

41. What are the postoperative management? (Must know)

Ans.

- Admission to high dependency or intensive care facilities may be suitable for patients with significant comorbidity and after major surgical procedures.
- Postoperative cardiac assessment must be performed and continued for 3–5 days with daily ECGs and screening of cardiac enzyme levels to detect and treat possible perioperative MI. Perioperative MI occurs mostly within the first 72 hours; however, most occurrences are silent. The incidence rate of perioperative MI is approximately 1% but carries a high mortality rate of almost 50%. Therefore, any enzyme elevations are not diagnostic in and of themselves. The diagnosis of postoperative MI should be made based on a combination of clinical, laboratory, and ECG evidence.
- Hemodialysis should ideally be delayed until the risk of fluid shifts and hemorrhage has fallen (some suggest at least 24 hours postoperatively) and, depending on the nature of surgery, anticoagulation may need to be reduced or omitted.
- Require close attention to fluid and electrolyte balance. Keep CVP in between 10 and 12 cm H_2O. Electrolyte, urea and creatinine levels should be checked in the early postoperative period and as indicated thereafter.
- A multimodal approach to postoperative analgesia should be employed. Paracetamol are effective and beneficial and markedly diminish opioid requirements.
- *Intraoperative local anesthesia (LA) infiltration. Advantages:* This is the simplest form of postoperative analgesia, often used in conjunction with other techniques. LA infiltration is often inadequate with a finite duration of action.[10]
- *Regional analgesia (e.g. epidural analgesia, brachial plexus block). Advantages:* RA provides both intra- and postoperative analgesia with reduced requirement for systemic analgesic drugs. Potential complications such as analgesic failure or hypotension.[10]
- With regard to management of hypertension, ischemic heart disease, and heart failure, the aim should be to re-establish the patient on his/her normal medications as soon as is feasible in the postoperative period.
- For abdominal surgery patients, placing feeding tube distal to the pylorus at the time of surgery will facilitate enteral drug administration even in the presence of reduced gastric emptying.

42. What are the choice of anesthesia: depend upon the duration and type of surgery? (Must to know)

Ans.

- *Spinal anesthesia:* Relative contraindication mainly due to coagulation defect.
- *Epidural anesthesia:* Uremic bleeding tendency combined with the effects of residual heparin given during dialysis increases risk of hemorrhage into the epidural space. Underlying hepatic disease can also alter platelet function and decrease coagulation factor level.

- The use of hypotensive epidural anesthesia in 50 patients, with CKD stage 3 or more undergoing total hip replacement, did not result in any acute deterioration of renal function or other complications from epidural anesthesia.[22]
- There may be an association between HD (hemodialysis) and spontaneous epidural hematoma formation. HD is associated with a rise in intracranial pressure that may play a role in its pathogenesis. Epidural anesthesia in poorly controlled hypertensive patients may result in hemodynamic instability that could potentially compromise renal perfusion and increase the likelihood of acute kidney injury. Although there may be patients with CKD for whom the benefits of epidural anesthesia outweigh the risks, a careful analysis of the individual case is enquired.[23]

43. Renal replacement therapy (RRT). (Good to know)

Ans. *There are five indications for renal replacement therapy (RRT):* Volume overload, hyperkalemia, severe metabolic acidosis, symptomatic uremia, and intoxication of dialyzable substances. Patients with end stage kidney disease require RRT or a renal transplant. There are two basic modes of RRT in patients with end-stage kidney disease: intermittent hemodialysis and peritoneal dialysis. The patient with chronic renal failure on hemodialysis should undergo hemodialysis the day before elective surgery. If a patient with renal failure presents emergently for surgery and has an acute indication for dialysis but is hemodynamically unstable intraoperative continuous venovenous hemodialysis should be used if available.[24]

CONCLUSIONS

In managing patients with CKD, the anesthetist aims to minimize the risk of perioperative complications. This requires careful patient assessment and efforts to modify identified risk factors, for example, hyperkalemia, to improve patient outcome. Recent developments in this regard include: a refined appreciation of the association between CKD and cardiovascular disease, knowledge of the importance of blocking the renin-angiotensin system (RAS) to delay regression of the condition, and new insights into the complex prothrombotic and hemostatic abnormalities involved. It is clear that temporary vascular access for HD is to be avoided and subclavian HD catheters are associated with an unacceptably high-risk of subclavian vein stenosis. The pharmacokinetic and pharmacodynamic changes must be taken into consideration: many drugs having reduced renal and nonrenal clearance in CKD. PORC remains a risk.[1]

REFERENCES

1. Craig RG, Hunter JM. Recent developments in the perioperative management of adult patients with chronic kidney disease. BJA. 2008;101(3): 296-310.
2. Joint Specialty Committee on Renal Medicine of the Royal College of Physicians of London and the Renal Association, and the Royal College of General Practitioners. Chronic Kidney Disease in Adults: UK Guidelines for Identification, Management and Referral. London: Royal College of Physicians, 2006.
3. Singh AK, Youssef MK Farag, Mittal BV, et al. Epidemiology and risk factors of chronic kidney disease in India - results from the SEEK (Screening and Early Evaluation of Kidney Disease) study. BMC Nephrology. 2013; 14:114.
4. Richard SK, Schraga ED. Dialysis Complications of Chronic Renal Failure MEDSCAPE online text book of Medicine www.emedicine.com.
5. Moro OS, Kenneth EO. Perioperative Management of the Patient With Chronic Renal Failure emedicine Updated: Jun 3, 2010.
6. Thomas R, Kanso A, Sedar JR. Chronic kidney diseases and its complication. Primary Care. 2008;35:329-44.
7. Adapted from Tolkoff-Rubin NE, Pascual M. Chronic renal failure. Sci Am Med. 1998;1-12.

8. Novak JE, Szczech LA. Triumph and tragedy: anaemia management in chronic kidney disease. CurrOpin Nephrol Hypertension. 2008;17:580-8.
9. Hamish T, Ross M. Fluid and electrolyte problems in renal dysfunction. Anaesthesia Intensive Care Med. 2009;10:289-92.
10. Simon T Rang, Nigel L West, Jeremy Howard, et al. Anaesthesia for chronic renal disease and renal transplantation Eau-Ebu Update Series. 2006;4:246-56.
11. Miller RD (Ed). Miller's Anesthesia. 7th edn. Philadelphia: Churchill Livingstone; 2010. p.2114
12. Dean M. Opioids in renal failure and dialysis patients. J Pain Symptom Manae. 2004;28(5):497-504.
13. Kurth T, Glynn RJ, Walker AM, et al. Analgesic use and change in kidney function in apparently healthy men. Am J Kidney Dis. 2003;42:234-44.
14. Mukherjee D, Nissen SE, Topol EJ. Risk of cardiovascular events associated with selective COX-2 inhibitors. J Am Med Assoc. 2001;286:954-9.
15. Launay-Vacher V, Karie S, Fau JB, et al. Treatment of pain in patients with renal insufficiency: The World Health Organization three-step ladder adapted. J Pain. 2005;6:137-48.
16. Stoelting RK, Hillier SC. Pharmacology and Physiology in Anaesthetic Practice. 4th edn. Philadelphia: Lippincott Williams & Wilkins; 2006. pp. 224-7.
17. Miller RD (Ed). Miller's Anesthesia.7th edn. Philadelphia: Churchill Livingstone;2010. pp. 2164-65.
18. Singh AK, Szczech L, Tang KL, Barnhart H, Sapp S, Wolfson M, et al. CHOIR Investigators: Correction or anemia with epoetin alfa in chronic kidney disease. N Engl J Med. 2006;355(20):2085-98.
19. Sheehy AM, Gabbay RA. An overview of preoperative glucose evaluation, management, and perioperative impact. J Diabets Sci Technol. 2009;3(6):1261-9.
20. Kato S, Chmielewski M, Honda H, Pecoits-Filho R, Matsuo S, Yuzawa Y, Tranaeus A, Stenvinkel P, Lindholm B. Aspects of immune dysfunction in end-state renal disease. Clin J Am Soc Nephrol. 2008;3(5): 1526-33.
21. Gallieni M, Cozzolino M, Ronga C, et al. Low-molecular-weight heparins should be used with caution in patients with chronic kidney disease. Nat Clin Pract Nephrol. 2008;4(9):488-9.
22. Sharrock NE, Beksac B, Flynn E, et al. Hypotensive epidural anaesthesia in patients with preoperativerenal dysfunction undergoing total hip replacement. Br J Anaesth. 2006;96:207-12.
23. Shahlaie K, Fox A, Butani L, et al. Spontaneous epidural hemorrhage in chronic renal failure. A case report and review. Pediatr Nephrol. 2004;19:1168-72.
24. Gebhard Wagener, Tricia E Brentjens. Anesthetic concernsin patients presenting with renal failure. Anesthesiology Clin. 2010;28:39-54.

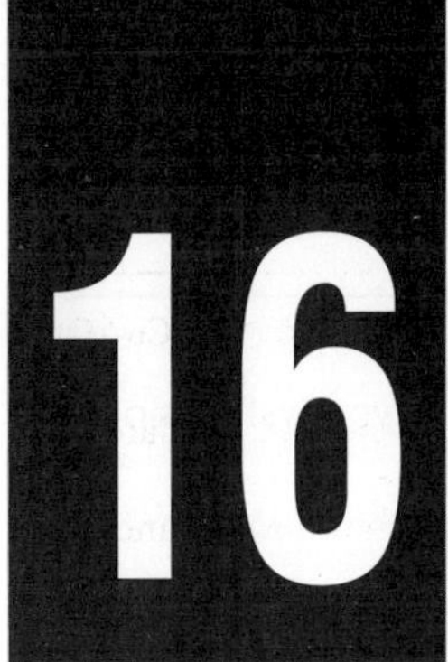

A Patient with Surgical Jaundice to Undergo Anesthesia for Laparotomy

Jayashree Sood

HISTORY

1. What are the relevant questions to be asked? (Must know)

Ans. Onset of jaundice—sudden, gradual, progressive?

- Duration—weeks, or months
- Prodromal symptoms before onset—viral hepatitis (release of endogenous interferon)
- Associated abdominal pain
  - Biliary colic—severe, intermittent, colicky pain
  - Pancreatic pain—continuous, dull pain, radiating to back, aggravated by food, relieved by sitting up or leaning forward
- Hepatomegaly—suggested by dull, continuous dragging pain in the right hypochondrium due to stretching of Glisson capsule.
- History of fever
  - Fever with arthralgias at onset of jaundice—viral hepatitis
  - Fever with rigors—cholangitis
  - Low grade fever—neoplasm
- History of high-colored urine, clay-colored stool, pruritus—obstructive jaundice
- History anorexia, weight loss and easy fatigability:
  - May be prodromal symptoms of alcohol or drug-induced hepatitis
  - Significant weight loss—malignancy
- History of gastrointestinal bleeding may indicate:
  - Ampullary malignancy
  - Development of portal hypertension
- History of medications
- History of injections, blood or blood product transfusion
- Contact with jaundiced patients
- Travel to hepatitis endemic areas—hepatitis A and E enterally transmitted
- History of upper abdominal surgery.

2. What are significant past history questions?

Ans.
- History of anesthesia exposure—halothane hepatitis, postoperative liver dysfunction
- History of gallstones.

Ref: Wylie and Churchill and Davidson's.

3. What should be asked in family history? (Must know)

Ans. *Family history of jaundice:*
- Wilson's disease
- Dubin-Johnson and Rotor syndrome—progressive familial intrahepatic cholestasis syndrome
- α_1-antitrypsin deficiency.

SOCIAL HISTORY

Alcohol consumption can cause alcoholic hepatitis leading to cholestasis.
Ref: Wylie and Churchill and Davidson's.

4. What will you do in general examination? (Must know) (Hutchison's Clinical Methods, 21st edn)

Ans.
- General condition
- Lying or sitting comfortably in bed or not
- Vital signs—pulse, blood pressure, respiration
- Pallor may indicate hemolysis, gastrointestinal bleeding
- Scratch marks—pruritus—obstructive jaundice
- Pedal edema—indicates hypoproteinemia or development of cirrhosis
- Bruises indicate coagulopathy
- Xanthoma—hypercholesterolemia
- Ecchymosis—vitamin K deficiency
- Lymphadenopathy—it supraclavicular, secondary involvement in gastrointestinal tract (GIT) malignancies.

Ref: Wylie and Churchill and Davidson's.

5. How will you present the clinical findings of the abdomen? (Must know) (Hutchison's Clinical Methods, 21st edn)

Ans. *Abdomen*

Inspection: Look for abdominal distension—ascites dilated abdominal vessels—cirrhosis operation scars umbilicus

Palpation: Right upper quadrant

Tenderness: Murphy's sign—cholecystitis cholangitis

Hepatomegaly: Tender—acute hepatitis, right heart failure nontender—malignancy, infiltrative process—amyloidosis

Distended, palpable gallbladder (Courvoisier's sign)—Malignant obstruction of common bile duct (CBD)

Splenomegaly: Hemolytic anemia, portal hypertension

Free fluid: Ascites—malignant or nonmalignant

Percussion: Shifting dullness—ascites

Auscultation: Bruits.

Ref: Wylie and Churchill and Davidson's.

6. Describe provisional diagnosis. (Must know)

Ans. If history of jaundice—slow onset, gradually progressive

- Occasional fever
- Dark colored urine
- Clay colored stools.

Pain abdomen: Intermittent, dull ache

On examination—Weight loss, anorexic, generalized icterus, vitals stable

Abdomen—no positive finding on inspection

Palpation on deep palpation lump felt, nontender.

7. What is the provisional diagnosis, you will tell?

Ans. A 60 years male with history of jaundice, progressive in nature.

Probably—obstructive jaundice due to growth in CBD, head pancreas or gallbladder.

8. What are the causes of intermittent jaundice and progressively worsening jaundice?

Ans. *Intermittent jaundice:*

- Choledocholithiasis
- Ampullary carcinoma
- Relapsing viral hepatitis.

Progressively worsening jaundice:

- Malignant obstruction
- Primary sclerosing cholangitis
- End stage liver disease.

9. Define jaundice.

Ans. Jaundice is yellowish discoloration of skin and mucous membranes due to increase in serum bilirubin.

10. Tell the sites to look for jaundice.

Ans. Sclera, under surface of tongue, palms, nails, skin.

11. Name differential diagnosis of family history of jaundice.

Ans.

- Wilson's disease
- α_1 antitrypsin deficiency
- Familial intrahepatic cholestasis syndrome (Dubin Johnson and Rotor syndrome).

12. Drugs which can produce cholestatic jaundice.

Ans.

- *Fatty liver*—tetracycline, valproate
- *Hepatitis*—INH, halothane, phenytoin, methyldopa, acetaminophen
- *Cholestatic*—oral contraceptives
- Chlorpromazine, erythromycin, rifampicin.

13. Explain the causes of hyperbilirubinemia. (Must know)

Ans. See Table 1.

Table 1 | Causes of hyperbilirubinemia

Unconjugated (Indirect) lipid soluble	Hemolysis (↑ production) Immaturity of enzyme system • Physiological jaundice of newborn • Jaundice of prematurity *Inherited* • Gilbert's • Crigler-Najjar syndrome Drugs
Conjugated (Direct) water soluble	Hepatocellular disease (hepatitis, cirrhosis) Intrahepatic cholestasis (pregnancy)
Intrahepatic primary biliary cirrhosis	Congenital conjugated hyperbilirubinemia Dubin-Johnson syndrome Rotor's syndrome
Extrahepatic calculus, stricture	Obstructive jaundice

Ref: Barash 6th Edition.

14. What are the causes of obstructive jaundice? (Must know)

Ans.

- **Intrahepatic**
  - Familial—Dubin-Johnson syndrome, cholestatic jaundice of pregnancy
    Recurrent intrahepatic cholestasis
  - Acquired—cholestatic drugs
    Viral and alcoholic hepatitis
    Biliary cirrhosis
    Sclerosing cholangitis
- **Extrahepatic**
  - Benign—gallstones, choledocholithiasis
    Chronic pancreatitis
    Strictures—iatrogenic, trauma
    Parasitic—ascariasis
    Biliary atresia
    Choledochal cysts
  - Malignant—gallbladder, ampulla
    Ca pancreas, bile duct.

15. What are the clinical features of a patient with cholelithiasis?

Ans. *History of dyspepsia:*

- Intermittent fever, pain, jaundice—Charcot's triad
- On examination—Murphy's sign.

16. What are the clinical features of a patient with malignant pancreas or gallbladder?

Ans. History of weight loss, anorexia painless, progressive deep jaundice

On examination—Courvoisier's sign—palpable gallbladder

Exception ampullary Ca—intermittent jaundice—due to sloughing of tumor cells

17. Describe the structural and functional units of the liver. (Must know)

Ans. *Structure (anatomy):*

- Largest gland 1.8 kg
- Covered by peritoneum—Glisson's capsule
- Divided into right, left, caudate and quadrate lobes
- Falciform ligament separates the right and left lobes.

Functional Units (Couinaud's Nomenclature)

Eight functionally independent segments—with their own vascular inflow, outflow and biliary drainage. This assists the surgeons to do limited segmental resection of the liver with relatively bloodless dissection.

Ref: Barash 6th Edition.

18. What are the normal values of serum bilirubin and LFTA?

Ans: *Serum bilirubin:*

Total	4–7 μmol/L
Unconjugated	<0.3 μmol/L
AST	10–40 μL^{-1}
ALT	10–37 μL^{-1}
ALK phosphatase	35–100 μL^{-1}

Ref: Wylie and Churchill and Davidson's.

19. Describe the blood supply of the liver and different factors affecting it. (Must know)

Ans. Increased by—Supine
Food
Hypercapnia
Acute hepatitis
Drugs: Barbiturates, P450 enzyme inducers, beta-agonists

Decreased by—Upright position
IPPV/PEEP
Hypocapnia, hypoxia
Cirrhosis
Anesthetic agents—Inhalation, intravenous beta-blockers
Surgical manipulation.

Intrinsic Regulation

It includes autoregulation and arteriovenous reciprocity.

Autoregulation occurs uptil a pressure of 80 mm Hg, below this the flow becomes pressure dependent. Arteriovenous reciprocity—is a phenomenon by which a fall in portal venous blood flow reduces hepatic arterial resistance and increases arterial flow and vice versa.

Extrinsic Regulation

Includes surgery, ventilation, hemorrhage and α- and β-receptors in the hepatic arterial bed.

Ref: Wylie and Churchill and Davidson's.

20. Describe the functions of liver. (Must know)

Ans. *Blood reservoir:* 10–15% of total blood volume, 25–30 ml of blood/100 gm of tissue.

- The autonomic innervation, allows rapid, control of reservoir volume.
- Sympathetic nervous system stimulation (pain, hypoxia, hypercarbia) decrease blood flow and volume.
- 80% of hepatic blood volume can be expelled within seconds.
- Anesthetics suppress sympathetic system and thus impair this reservoir function.
- Severe liver disease impairs the vasoconstrictive responses to catecholamines.

- *Regulator of blood coagulation:*
  - Responsible for synthesis of factors involved in coagulation, anticoagulation and fibrinolysis. All procoagulation factors are derived in the liver with the exception of factor VIII (vWF).
  - Vitamin K dependent factors are synthesized—II, VII, IX and X.
  - Vitamin K deficiency results in production of nonfunctional factors II, VII, IX and X.
- It synthesizes anticoagulant factors—antithrombin III, protein C and S and fibrinolytic factors
- *Endocrine organ:*
  - Synthesizes and secretes insulin like growth factor, angiotensinogen, thrombopoietin.
  - Liver converts T4 to T3 and synthesizes thyroid binding globulin.
- *Erythrocyte breakdown and bilirubin formation and excretion:*
  - Breakdown of Hb into heme and globin by the RE system. Heme is oxidized to biliverdin which is then converted to unconjugated bilirubin and released in bloodstream and along with albumin is transported to liver. Now bilirubin combines with cytoplasm protein and forms water soluble conjugated bilirubin which is then excreted into bile canalicula. In the large intestine the conjugated bilirubin is converted to urobilinogen, some of it is absorbed while remaining is excreted in stools.
- *Metabolic functions:*

  Carbohydrate metabolism
  - Maintains euglycemia, by glycogenesis and glycogenolysis
  - Also induces gluconeogenesis when required

  Lipid metabolism:
  - Liver is the major site for synthesis of fatty acids from excess sugar, protein and lipid.
  - Fatty acids are esterified to form triglycerides and cholesterol. Oxidation of FA to ketone bodies.

  Amino acid metabolism: Deamination of AA and urea formation.
  - Major site for protein and amino acid metabolism. After protein ingestion, the proteolytic enzymes hydrolyze the protein into amino acids which are absorbed and transported to liver. These are then converted to protein, as required.
  - Protein catabolism also takes place here. Proteins are degraded to aminoacids, which either undergo gluconeogenesis or are catabolized to ketoacids, NH_3 and glutamine. The urea cycle converts ammonia to urea which is then excreted via kidneys. Therefore in liver dysfunction, the urea cycle cannot convert NH_3 to urea and the NH_3 levels keep rising resulting in hepatic encephalopathy.
  - Since urea is synthesized in liver, a normal or low urea levels in liver disease are no indication that GFR is normal.

  Protein synthesis:
  - Albumin, α_1 glycoprotein, creative protein, haptaglobin and pseudocholinesterase. Hepatocytes synthesize albumin, all coagulation factors except factor VIII and globulins.
  - Half-life of serum albumin is 20 days and so it is not a reliable indicator of liver's residual synthetic capacity in acute liver disease.

- *Immunological function:*
  - Largest organ in the RE system.
  - 10% of liver mass constitutes the Kupffer cells which participate in immune surveillance, with phagocytosis of antigens from GIT.

Ref: Barash 6th Edition.

21. What is hepatic drug metabolism?

Ans. Phase I reactions—include oxidation by cytochrome P450 to make the molecule water soluble. Phase II reactions—include conjugation and glucuronidation making the molecule inactive water soluble.

Ref: Wylie and Churchill and Davidson's.

22. How will you investigate the patient to confirm your diagnosis? (Must know)

Ans. See Table 2.

Table 2 | Investigation of a patient with obstetric jaundice

	Prehepatic	*Hepatic*	*Post-hepatic*
S. bilirubin (Van den Berg test)	↑ unconjugated	↑ conjugated	↑ conjugated
Urine urobilinogen	++	+	–
Urine bile salts	Absent	±	+
Urine bilirubin	–	±	+
Fecal stercobilinogen	++	N or ↓	–
Fecal fat	N	N or ↑	↑↑
LFT Enzymes (AST, ALT)	N	↑↑ > 800 IU/L	↑↑ 50–100 IU/L
Alkaline PO_4	N	N	↑↑
S. albumin	N	↓	N or ↓
Prothrombin time (PT)	N	↑↑	↑↑ corrected by Vitamin K
Blood urea nitrogen (BUN)	N	N	N

23. What are surgeries done for obstructive jaundice?

Ans.

- Ca gallbladder—radical cholecystectomy with wedge resection and CBD excision
- Choledocholiathiasis—Endoscopic retrograde cholangiopancreatography (ERCP) removal or CBD exploration
- Cholangio Ca—Liver resection
- Biliary stricture—hepaticojejunostomy
- Periampullary Ca—Whipple's procedure
- Chronic pancreatitis—Whipple's procedure.

24. Explain the steps in Whipple's procedure.

Ans.

- Transection of jejunum from Dubin-Johnson flexure
- Transection of neck of pancreas
- Pancreaticojejunostomy
- Hepaticojejunostomy

- Gastrojejunostomy
- Feeding jejunostomy.

25. Describe the vascular supply of liver. (Must know)

Ans.

- Liver receives 25% of cardiac output (i.e. 100–130 mL/mt/100 kg)
- Hepatic A—delivers 25% of total hepatic blood flow, but 50% of hepatic oxygen delivery
- Portal V—delivers 75% of total hepatic blood flow, but only 50% of hepatic oxygen delivery
- Common hepatic A arises from the celiac trunk
- Portal vein is formed by confluence of splenic and superior mesenteric vein.
- The portal vein, hepatic artery and bile duct travel together.
- The vessels diminish in caliber and the terminal vessels directly drain into the hepatic sinusoids.
- Hepatic A pressure equals aortic pressure.
- Mean portal vein pressure is approximately 6–10 mm Hg.
- These two systems merge in the sinusoids where the pressure is about 2–4 mm Hg above that of the IVC.
- Blood from the sinusoids drains into the central vein which join to form the right, middle and left hepatic veins which enter the IVC.
- The PV, HA and the BD together form the portal triad; surrounded by the sinusoids.

Ref: Barash 6th Edition.

26. Describe microanatomy of liver.

Ans.

- Classic liver lobule is hexagonal on cross-section.
- Six vertically aligned portal canals at the corners. They contain the portal triad.
- In the center is the central vein.
- In between are the hepatocytes and sinusoids.

27. What is acinus lobule concept?

Ans. Small parenchymal mass around the portal triad.

Blood enters the center of the acinus and flows centrifugally to the hepaic venules (CV).

Therefore hepatic venule is at center of classic lobule but at periphery of acinus.

The acinus has zone 1, 2 and 3.

Zone 1 Maximum oxygen tension and nutrient supply

Zone 3 Minimum oxygen tension and nutrient supply

28. What are the pathophysiological consequences of obstructive jaundice?

Ans.

- Retention of bile solutes in liver decreases hepatocyte function. Reduced synthesis of albumin and clotting factors. Cytochrome 450 and Kuppfer cells ↓
- Jaundice, ↑ conjugated bilirubin, pruritus, CVS depression, nephrotoxicity hypercholesterolemia
- Absence of bile in intestines, leads to escape of endotoxins into portal blood. Malabsorption of Vitamins A, D, E and K.

29. Name other tests which are used to diagnose hepatic pathology? (Nice to know)

Ans. *Ultrasound:*

- Shows presence and level of intrahepatic and extrahepatic biliary dilatation
- Sensitivity 70–95%, specificity 80–100% for obstructive jaundice
- Very specific for gallstones
- Endoscopic ultrasound, new gadget more accurate than combined CT and ECRP.

CT Scan:
  - Useful in obese or ↑ bowel gas
  - Better to visualize lower end of CBD
  - Staging and assessment of surgical resection of tumors
- *Endoscopic retrograde cholangiogram (ERCP):*
  - Diagnose choledocholithiasis
  - Biopsy possible
  - Therapeutic—sphincterotomy, stone removal, stricture dilatation
- *Percutaneous transhepatic cholangiogram (PTC):*
  - Not commonly done
  - Allow biliary drainage and stenting

Ref: Wylie and Churchill and Davidson's.

30. What are the anesthetic concerns in an obstructive jaundice? (Must know)

Ans. *Cardiovascular dysfunction:*
- Impaired myocardial contractility (bile salts in circulating blood)
- Blunts the response to catecholamines-hypotension (bile salts interfere with the binding of catecholamines to membrane receptors)
- Vasodilatation (↓ ability to mobilize blood from splanchnic vasculature during hemorrhage)
- Bradycardia (vagotonic effect).

Renal:

Acute renal failure due to:
- Myocardial depression
- Hypovolemia
- Nephrotoxic—bile salts, endotoxins.

Sepsis due to:
- Associated cholangitis
- Entry of endotoxins from intestines to portal blood (due to absence of bile salts in intestines)
- ↓ Kupffer cell activity (due to retention of bile salts in liver).

  Prevention: Preoperative antibiotics and oral bile salts.

Coagulopathy:
- Vitamin K deficiency—↓ absorption of vitamin K from intestines due to absence of bile salts in intestines

  ↓ Factor II, VII, IX and X

  ↓ prothrombin time

  Correction: Preoperative vitamin K 10 mg OD × 3 days
- Prolonged biliary obstruction—liver injury

  ↓ synthesis of coagulation factors indicates poor prognosis

  Correction: Fresh frozen plasma.

Multiple vitamin deficiency:
- Vitamin A, D, E and K (due to absence of bile salts in intestines)

  A—Night blindness

  D—Osteoporosis

  E—Leg cramps

  K—Easy bruising
- Hemorrhagic gastritis and stress ulcer
- Impaired wound healing

- Altered drug handling
- Long-standing obstruction—liver dysfunction.

Ref: Barash 6th Edition.

31. Describe the inferences of the LFTs.

Ans. Liver function tests (LFTs)

- *Indices of hepatocellular damage:*
  - Transaminases SGOT/SGPT 0–35 IU/L
    AST/ALT
    Extrahepatic/mainly in liver
    In advanced liver cell injury, they may be N or ↓ due to ↑ loss of parenchymal tissue
  - Lactate dehydrogenase (LDH)—poor diagnostic specific specificity
  - Glutathione-S-transferase (GST) sensitive indicator
- *Indices of obstructed blood flow:*
  - Alkaline phosphatase ↑↑ 35–100 IU/L
    Obtained from plasma membrane of bile duct cells
    Extrahepatic success—bones, intestine, liver, placenta
  - 5-nucleotidase—specific for liver disease
  - Gamma-glutamyl transferase (GGT) most sensitive indicator of biliary tract disease, but poor specificity. It is a membrane bound.
- *Indices of hepatic synthetic function:*
  - Prothrombin time
  - Serum albumin
    Long half-life 20 days
    So not a good indicator for acute or mild liver damage
- *Indices of hepatic blood flow:*
  - Indocyanine green

The patient is posted for laparotomy

Ref: Barash 6th Edition.

32. What preoperative investigations will you do?

Ans.

- Complete blood count (CBC)
  Hb may be decrease—concealed blood loss, hemolysis ↑ TLC, ↑ DLC—infection
  Platelet count
  Clotting studies—BT, PT, PTTK
- Urine analysis
  Bilirubin and bile salts present
- S. proteins
- Blood glucose
- Blood urea ↓ synthesis in liver disease
- S. electrolytes
- KFT: BUN, S. creatinine
- Viral markers—HBV, HCV
- Chest X-ray
- ECG.

33. What are the risk factors for operative mortality in obstructive jaundice patients?

Ans.

- Hematocrit < 30%
- S. bilirubin > 11 mg%
- Azotemia
- Hypoalbuminemia
- Cholangitis.

34. What is the preoperative preparation of this patient?

Ans.

- Short-acting anxiolytic
- Oral H_2 antagonist
- Vitamin K 10 mg OD × 3 days FFP, if required
- Broad-spectrum antibiotics
- Oral bile salts
- Rehydration
- Adequate 1 mL/kg/hr
- If bilirubin > 8 mg
- IV fluid 1–2 mL/kg/hr

35. What are the anesthetic goals in this case of obstructive jaundice?

Ans. *Maintain hepatic blood flow:*

Avoid:

- Sympathetic stimulation, Hypotension, Hypocapnia, Hypoxemia
- Pressure effects—caused by surgical retraction, tumors, laparoscopy
- Hepatic venous congestion produced by
  - Head down position
  - IPPV with PEEP
  - Right heart failure

  Hepatotoxic drugs—halothane, acetaminophen

Maintain Renal Function:

- *Preoperatively:*
  - Avoid NSAIDs and aminoglycosides
  - Prophylactic antibiotics
  - Give oral bile salts to normalize gut flora
  - Stenting to reduce hyperbilirubinemia
- *Intraoperatively:*
  - Avoid hypotension and hypoxemia
  - Avoid dehydration
  - Mannitol/furosemide/low dose of dopamine.

36. What are the anticipated pharmacokinetic and pharmacodynamic alterations in obstructive jaundice?

Ans.

- Careful titration of drug is essential
- Cerebral uptake of benzodiazepines increases
- IV infusions or multiple intermittent IV doses can result in prolonged pharmacological effects
- Although clearance of thiopentone is independent of hepatic blood flow, increased response to standard dose may be seen due to decrease in plasma-protein binding
- Plasma clearance of narcotics is lowered and so action may be prolonged.

Induction of general anesthesia:

Principles: Due to major pharmacokinetic abnormalities, all drugs should be titrated carefully to achieve the desired effect. Careful titration of the induction agent minimizes hemodynamic disturbance.

The initial dose of nondepolarizing drug (rocuronium, atracurium, pancuronium), but not vecuronium may be higher than normal patients.

Maintenance of anesthesia

- Avoid arterial hypotension and low cardiac output states.
- Isoflurane, sevoflurane and desflurane maintains hepatic blood flow and oxygen supply.
- Fentanyl neither decreases the hepatic oxygen nor blood supply in moderate doses.
- Maintain normocapnia.

37. What intraoperative monitoring will you do in this case?

Ans. *Routine*: Pulse oximetry, ECG, NIBP, $EtCO_2$.

Recommended: Urine output, core temperature
NMJ monitoring

Long and major cases:

- IBP, CVP
- S. electrolytes
- Hb, PT, APTT, TEG

38. How will you manage these patients postoperatively?

Ans.

- If NMJ recovery complete and vitals stable → extubate → O_2 enriched air
- If not, continue PPV
- Correct fluid and electrolytes
- Maintain hemodynamics, urine output
- Adequate analgesia.

39. How will you manage postoperative pain?

Ans.

- If coagulation profile normal—lower thoracic or upper lumbar epidural 0.0625% bupivacaine with fentanyl 2 μg/mL.
- If abnormal IV PCA (patient controlled analgesia).

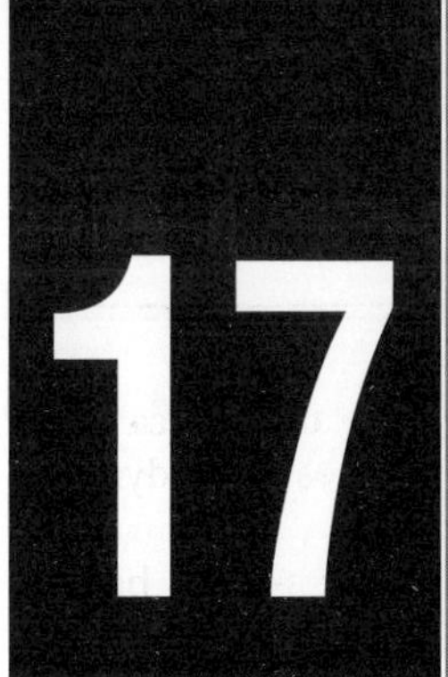

Diabetes Mellitus: Anesthetic Considerations

Ashok Kumar Saxena

Case

A hindu female patient of 61 years, resident of Dilshad Garden shows the following history:

- Chief complaints:
  - Fracture ulcer left foot × 2 month
  - Fracture discharge from ulcer × 20 days
  - Fracture pins and needle sensation × 1 year
- History of present illness:
  - Pins and needle sensation—Left foot → both feet (Associated heaviness)
  - Ulcer following trauma—Papule → pustule → ulcer
- Discharge yellow, foul smelling, blood stained
- No cough/coryza/burning micturition/diarrhea/fainting episodes
- Past history
- Diagnosed 20 years back
  - Tab Glibenclamide × 20 years
  - Insulin 14U subcutaneous BD
- 7 years back → Loss of vision, photocoagulation
- 3 years back → Similar ulcer right foot → amputation of 2nd toe
- *Personal history:* Nonsmoker, Nonalcoholic, house wife with good hygiene
- *Social history:* Middle class with unemployed son
- *Treatment history:* On diabetic diet: 1200 Kcal
  Insulin Mixtard (NPH+Regular) - 42 U BBF
  - 22 U BD

On examination:

- Awake, conscious, oriented, restless and anxious
- Obese, BMI - 30 kg/m^2, xanthomas, brown pigmentation of legs
- P$^+$, Ic$^-$, clubbing$^+$, cyanosis$^-$, Lymphadenopathy$^+$
- Pedal edema - Left foot, nonpitting

- Left inguinal lymph nodes - 3 × 2 cm in size
- Discrete, firm, mobile, tender, erythematous
- PR - 80/min (sitting)
  - 100/min (standing)

  Regular

  Normal volume, character, wall thickness

  All peripheral pulses palpable including dorsalis pedis on affected side, No radiofemoral delay
- BP - 140/80 (sitting), right brachial artery
  - 120/60 (standing)

Local examination:

- *Inspection:* Single irregular ulcer, 4–5 cm in size, extending from base of 2nd metatarsal to 5th metatarsal, inflamed, edematous, sloping edge, red floor with granulation tissue
- *Palpation:* Tender, sloping edge with irregular margins, indurated base, depth 3 mm, not bleeding on touch, mobile, warm surrounding skin, peripheral pulses palpable.

PNS examination:

- Bulk—normal
- Tone—normal
- Reflexes—left knee jerk sluggish, rest normal
- Sensory—↓ pinprick and Vibration {L2–L5 dermatomes}
  Pain/Touch normal
- Power 5/5 in all 4 limbs.

ANS examination:

- Orthostatic hypotension—present
- Deep breath test—positive
- Tachycardia with atropine—present
- Tachycardia during standing—present
- Handgrip test—positive
- Valsalva could not be performed

Investigations

- Hb—10.2 mg/dL
- FBS—242 mg/dL, PP BS—320 mg/dL
- Blood urea—49 mg/dL
- Na^+: 130 mEq/L, K^+: 3.7mEq/L
- S creatinine—1.2 mg/dL
- HbA_{1C}—7%
- Urine—Microalbuminuria
- ECG-NAD, X-ray chest—NAD
- X-ray cervical spine—NAD
- Fundus examination—proliferative retinopathy.

1. What is diabetes mellitus?

Ans. It is clinical syndrome characterized by hyperglycemia due to absolute or relative deficiency of insulin accompanied by absolute or relative excess of glucagon.

2. How can you classify diabetes mellitus?

Ans. Diabetes mellitus (DM) can be classified into four major types (Table 1):

Table 1 | Classification of diabetes mellitus

Class	*Pathogenesis*	*Prevalence*
Type 1	Absolute insulin deficiency • Immune mediated-Idiopathic forms of β-cell dysfunction • Islet cell antibody • Viral: Coxsackie, mumps	0.4% young onset
Type 2	Insulin resistance • Impaired stimulation of glycogen synthesis in muscle by liver due to defective glucose transporter	6.6%—adult >8%—after 65 years
Type 3	Wide range of specific type of diabetes • Genetic defects in β-cell function-MODY • Genetic defects in insulin action • Diseases of exocrine pancreas, etc. • *Endocrinopathies*: Acromegaly, Cushing's syndrome • *Drugs*: Steroids, beta-agonists	
Type 4	Gestational diabetes • Occurs at 24–30 weeks • 30–50% develop type 2 DM with in 10 years	4.0% of all pregnancies

3. What are the risk factors for type 2 DM?

Ans. *Risk factors for type 2 diabetes mellitus:*

- Family history of diabetes (i.e. parent or sibling with type 2 diabetes)
- Obesity (BMI >25 Kg/m^2)
- Habitual physical inactivity
- Race/ethnicity (e.g. African American, Latino, Native American, Asian American, Pacific Islander)
- Previously identified IFG or IGT
- History of GDM or delivery of baby >4 kg (>9 lb)
- Hypertension (blood pressure >140/90 mm Hg)
- HDL cholesterol level <35 mg/dL (0.90 mmol/L) and/or a triglyceride level >250 mg/dL (2.82 mmol/L)
- Polycystic ovary syndrome or acanthosis nigricans
- History of vascular disease.

4. What are the diagnostic criterions for DM?

Ans. Diagnostic criteria for diabetes mellitus (American Diabetes Association 2010)

- Symptoms of diabetes (polyuria, polydipsia, unexplained weight loss) plus a random plasma glucose concentration ≥ 200 mg/dL
  Or
- Fasting (no caloric intake for ≥ 8 hours) plasma glucose ≥ 126 mg/dL
  Or
- 2-hour plasma glucose > 200 mg/dL during an oral glucose tolerance test
  Or
- HbA_{1c} > 6.5%

5. How will you perform oral GTT?

- Seventy-five gram of oral glucose after adequate fasting of at least 12 hours
- In pregnant patients oral GTT done with 50 gm of oral glucose
- Blood sugar levels after 2 hours of ingestion

Normal	*IFG*	*DM*
<7.8 mmol/L	7.8–11.1 mmol/L	>11.1 mmol/L
(140 mg/dL)	(140–200 mg/dL)	(200 mg/dL)

6. What is the relation between whole blood and plasma glucose?

Ans. Venous whole blood glucose + 15% = Plasma glucose

Arterial blood = capillary blood = 7% > venous blood

1 mmol = 18.0 mg glucose

1 mmol/L = 18 mg/dL

7. Explain the synthesis, secretion, and actions of insulin.

Ans. Insulin is produced in the beta cells of the pancreatic islets. It is initially synthesized as a single-chain 86-amino acid precursor polypeptide, preproinsulin. Subsequent proteolytic processing removes the aminoterminal signal peptide, giving rise to proinsulin. Proinsulin is structurally related to insulin-like growth factors I and II, which bind weakly to the insulin receptor. Cleavage of an internal 31-residue fragment from proinsulin generates the C peptide and the A (21 amino acids) and B (30 amino acids) chains of insulin, which are connected by disulfide bonds. The mature insulin molecule and C peptide are stored together and cosecreted from secretory granules in the beta cells.

Glucose is the key regulator of insulin secretion by the pancreatic beta cell, although amino acids, ketones, various nutrients, gastrointestinal peptides, and neurotransmitters also influence insulin secretion. Glucose levels > 3.9 mmol/L (70 mg/dL) stimulate insulin synthesis, primarily by enhancing protein translation and processing. Glucose stimulation of insulin secretion begins with its transport into the beta cell by the GLUT2 glucose transporter. Glucose phosphorylation by glucokinase is the rate-limiting step that controls glucose-regulated insulin secretion. Further metabolism of glucose-6-phosphate via glycolysis generates ATP, which inhibits the activity of an ATP-sensitive K^+ channel. This channel consists of two separate proteins: one is the binding site for certain oral hypoglycemics (e.g. sulfonylureas, meglitinides); the other is an inwardly rectifying K^+ channel protein (Kir6.2). Inhibition of this K^+ channel induces beta cell membrane depolarization, which opens voltage-dependent calcium channels (leading to an influx of calcium), and stimulates insulin secretion. Incretins are released from neuroendocrine cells of the gastrointestinal tract following food ingestion and amplify glucose-stimulated insulin secretion and suppress glucagon secretion. Incretin analogs, such as exenatide, are being used to enhance endogenous insulin secretion (Table 2).

Table 2 | Endocrinologic effects of insulin

Effects on liver	*Effects on muscle*	*Effects on fat*
• Anabolic • Promotes glycogenesis • Increases synthesis of triglycerides, cholesterol, and VLDL • Increases protein synthesis • Promotes glycolysis • Anticatabolic • Inhibits glycogenolysis • Inhibits ketogenesis • Inhibits gluconeogenesis	• Promotes protein synthesis • Increases amino acid transport • Stimulates ribosomal protein synthesis • Promotes glycogen synthesis • Increases glucose transport • Enhances activity of glycogen synthetase • Inhibits activity of glycogen phosphorylase	• Promotes triglyceride storage • Induces lipoprotein lipase, making fatty acids available for absorption into fat cells • Increases glucose transport into fat cells, thus increasing availability of glycerol phosphate for triglyceride synthesis • Inhibits intracellular lipolysis

8. What are the various classes of antidiabetic agents?

Ans. See Table 3.

Table 3 | Different antidiabetic agents with mechanism of action

Oral	*Mechanism of action*	*Examples*	*A1C Reduction (%)*	*Agent-specific advantages*		
Biguanides	Hepatic glucose production, weight loss, glucose, utilization, insulin resistance	Metformin (half life: 6.2 hours)	1–2	Weight loss	Lactic acidosis, diarrhea, nausea	Serum creatinine >1.5 mg/dL (men) >1.4 mg/dL (women), CHF, radiographic contrast studies, seriously ill patients, acidosis
Glucosidase inhibitors	Glucose absorption	Acarbose (half life: 2 hours), Miglitol	0.5–0.8	Reduce postprandial glycemia	GI flatulence, liver function tests	Renal/liver disease
Dipeptidyl peptidase IV (DPP IV) inhibitors	Prolong endogenous GLP-1 and GIP action	Sitagliptin (half life: 8–14 hours) Vildagliptin (half life: 2–3 hours)	0.5–1.0	Does not cause hypoglycemia		Reduce dose with renal disease
Insulin secretagogues—sulfonylureas	Insulin secretion	Chlorpropamide (half life: 36 hours) Glimepiride (half-life: 5 hours) Gliclazide (half life: 10.4 hours)	1–2	Lower fasting blood glucose	Hypoglycemia, weight gain	Renal/liver disease
Insulin secretagogues—nonsulfonylureas	Insulin secretion	Repaglinide (half-life: 1 hour)	1–2	Short onset of action, lowers post-prandial glucose	Hypoglycemia	Renal/liver disease
Thiazolidinediones	Decrease insulin resistance, increases glucose utilization	Rosiglitazone (half-life: 3–4 hours), Pioglitazone (half-life: 3–7 hours)	0.5–1.4	Lower insulin requirements	Peripheral edema, CHF, weight gain, fractures, macular edema; rosiglitazone may increase risk of MI	Congestive heart failure, liver disease
GLP-1 agonist	Insulin, glucagon, slow gastric emptying	Exenatide (half-life: 2.4 hours) subcutaneous injection	0.5–1.0	Weight loss	Injection, nausea, risk of hypoglycemia with insulin secretagogues	Renal disease, agents that also slow GI motility
Amylin agonist	Slow gastric emptying, decrease release of glucagon	Pramlintide (half-life: 48 minutes)	0.25–0.5	Reduce postprandial glycemia, weight loss	Injection, nausea, risk of hypoglycemia with insulin	Agents that also slow GI motility
Medical nutrition therapy and physical activity	Insulin, resistance, insulin secretion	Low-calorie, low-fat diet, exercise	1–2	Other health benefits	Compliance difficult, long-term success low	

9. What all insulin preparations are available?

Ans. See Table 4.

Table 4 | Different types of insulin preparation

Class	Type	Onset	Peak effect	Duration of action
Rapid	Humalog/lispro	15–30 minutes	30–90 minutes	3–5 hours
	Novolog/aspart	10–20 minutes	40–50 minutes	3–5 hours
Short	Regular/Humulin	30 minutes 1 hours	2–5 hours	5–8 hours
Intermediate	Neutral protamine Hagedorn (NPH)	1–2 hours	4–12 hours	18–24 hours
	Lente	1–2.5 hours	3–10 hours	18–24 hours
Long acting	Ultralente	30 minutes 3 hours	10–20 hours	20–36 hours
	Insulin glargine (lantus)	1–1.5 hours	No peak-	20–24 hours
	Insulin Detemir (Levemir) (US)	1–2 hours	6–8 hours	Up to 24 hours

10. What are the newer treatments in research for DM?

Ans. The following are newer modalities for diagnosis:

- Implanted (like a pacemaker) glucose analyzer with electric transmission to a surface (watch) monitor.
- *Scout DS device:* Multiple spectral signatures from fluorophores in epidermis (AGE, NADH, flavoproteins, collagen and elastin) Measures skin scattering from hemoglobin. Being investigated as possible means of noninvasive detection of diabetes.
- *Exhaled breath glucose monitoring:* Altered metabolism →↑ breath acetone + >3000 volatile organic compounds (voc). Investigation of sets of 4 vocs. Acetone, methyl nitrate, ethanol and ethyl benzene, 2-pentyl nitrate, propane, methanol and acetone. Glucose levels can be predicted by noninvasive breath analyses.

Newer insulin innovations:

- Degludec
  - 48+ hr od, flat profile, equivalent glucose lowering compared to glargine. Less hypoglycemia. 0.38–0.45 units/kg
- Insulin patch project
  - Insupatin (infusion site warming device)
  - Heats infusion site to 38.5 for 15 minutes prior to bolus → increased absorption
- Hybrid closed loop
  - Metronic minimed ePID (external physiologic delivery)
  - Uses PID (proportionate-integral-derivative) closed loop controller
- Treat to target technosphere insulin
  - 15 patients with T1D in phase 3 studies
  - ↓HbA_{1c} 0.4% in 45 days. Bolus insulin dose ↑ × 2.5
  - A 2nd dose of 5–10 units taken after meals in 1/3 of patients
- DUROS
  - ITCA implantable device every 3 months/year
  - Formulation stable for 2 years
  - 15 minutes insertion

- Osmotic mini-pump
- Phase 2–48 weeks extension study
  - 24 weeks study initially. 85% continued in extension study
  - ↓HbA_{1c} 1.5%
  - ↓3.5 kg
  - Nausea 10%, diarrhea 3%, skin/injection site problems 7%.

11. What are the GPCR in developmental stage for DM?

Ans.

GPR119 agonist (AS1790091)

- G coupled receptor activation → ↑ insulin secretion via cAMP
- GPR receptors in β-cells and enteroendodermal cells in the small intestine
- PSN 821
  - Small molecule GPR119 agonist
    - ↑ GIP, GLP-1 and PYY

GPR40 agonist (TAK 875)

- G Coupled receptor protein binds to free fatty acid receptor on β-cell → ↑ ER activation → ↑ Ca^{++} → ↑ insulin release
- Phase 2 study
  - 12 weeks 384 completers
  - ↓ HbA_{1c} 0.8%
  - Well tolerated
  - No hypoglycemia.

12. What are the criterions for diagnosis of metabolic syndrome?

Ans. Metabolic syndrome

- At least three of the following:
  - Fasting plasma glucose ≥ 110 mg/dL
  - Abdominal obesity [waist girth > 40 (in men), 35 (in women)]
  - Serum triglycerides ≥ 150 mg/dL
  - Serum high-density lipoprotein cholesterol < 40 mg/dL (men), < 50 mg/dL (women)
  - Blood pressure ≥ 130/85 mm Hg.

13. What are the complications of DM?

Ans. Chronic complications include:

- Microvascular
- Eye disease
- Retinopathy (nonproliferative/proliferative)
- Macular edema
- Neuropathy
- Sensory and motor (mono- and polyneuropathy)
- Autonomic
- Nephropathy
- Macrovascular
- Coronary artery disease
- Peripheral arterial disease
- Cerebrovascular disease
- Other
- Gastrointestinal (gastroparesis, diarrhea)

- Genitourinary (uropathy/sexual dysfunction)
- Dermatologic
- Infectious
- Cataracts
- Glaucoma
- Periodontal disease

Acute complications are:

- Diabetic keto acidosis
- Non-ketotic hyperglycemic hyperosmolar coma.

14. Describe the diagnosis and management of diabetic ketoacidosis and hyperglycemic hyperosmolar state.

Ans. See Tables 5 and 6.

Table 5 | Laboratory values in diabetic ketoacidosis (DKA) and hyperglycemic hyperosmolar state (HHS) (Representative ranges at presentation)

	DKA	*HHS*
Glucose, [a]mmol/L (mg/dL)	13.9–33.3 (250–600)	33.3–66.6 (600–1200)
Sodium, mEq/L	125–135	135–145
Potassium[a]	Normal to slightly	Normal
Magnesium[a]	Normal[b]	Normal
Chloride[a]	Normal	Normal
Phosphate[a]		Normal
Creatinine	Slightly	Moderately
Osmolality (mOsm/mL)	300–320	330–380
Plasma ketones[a]	++++	+/–
Serum bicarbonate, [a] mEq/L	<15 mEq/L	Normal to slightly
Arterial pH	6.8–7.3	>7.3
Arterial PCO_2, [a] mm Hg	20–30	Normal
Anion gap[a] [Na – (Cl + HCO_3)]		Normal to slightly

[a] Large changes occur during treatment of DKA.
[b] Although plasma levels may be normal or high at presentation, total-body stores are usually depleted.

Table 6 | Manifestations of diabetic ketoacidosis

Symptoms	*Physical findings*
Nausea/vomiting	Tachycardia
Thirst/polyuria	Dehydration/hypotension
Abdominal pain	Tachypnea/Kussmaul respirations/respiratory distress
Shortness of breath	Abdominal tenderness (may resemble acute pancreatitis or surgical abdomen)
Precipitating events	Lethargy/obtundation/cerebral edema/possibly coma
Inadequate insulin administration	
Infection (pneumonia/UTI/gastroenteritis/sepsis)	
Infarction (cerebral, coronary, mesenteric, peripheral)	
Drugs (cocaine)	
Pregnancy	

Management of DKA:

- Confirm diagnosis (plasma glucose, positive serum ketones, metabolic acidosis).
- Admit to hospital; intensive-care setting may be necessary for frequent monitoring or if pH <7.00 or unconscious.
- *Assess:*
  - Serum electrolytes (K^+, Na^+, Mg^{2+}, Cl^-, bicarbonate, phosphate)
  - Acid-base status—pH, HCO_3^-, PCO_2^-, b-hydroxybutyrate
  - Renal function (creatinine, urine output)
- *Replace fluids:* 2–3 L of 0.9% saline over first 1–3 hours (10–15 mL/kg/hour); subsequently, 0.45% saline at 150–300 mL/h; change to 5% glucose and 0.45% saline at 100–200 mL/h when plasma glucose reaches 250 mg/dL (14 mmol/L).
- *Administer short-acting insulin:* IV (0.1 units/kg) or IM (0.3 units/kg), then 0.1 units/kg per hour by continuous IV infusion; increase 2- to 3-fold if no response by 2–4 hours. If initial serum potassium is < 3.3 mmol/L (3.3 mEq/L), do not administer insulin until the potassium is corrected to > 3.3 mmol/L (3.3.mEq/L).
- *Assess patient:* What precipitated the episode (noncompliance, infection, trauma, infarction, cocaine)? Initiate appropriate work-up for precipitating event (cultures, CXR, ECG).
- Measure capillary glucose every 1–2 hours; measure electrolytes (especially K^+, bicarbonate, phosphate) and anion gap every 4 hours for first 24 hours.
- Monitor blood pressure, pulse, respirations, mental status, fluid intake and output every 1–4 hours.
- *Replace K^+:* 10 mEq/h when plasma K^+ < 5.5 mEq/L, ECG normal, urine flow and normal creatinine documented; administer 40–80 mEq/h when plasma K^+ < 3.5 mEq/L or if bicarbonate is given.
- Continue above until patient is stable, glucose goal is 150–250 mg/dL, and acidosis is resolved. Insulin infusion may be decreased to 0.05–0.1 units/kg per hour.
- Administer intermediate or long-acting insulin as soon as patient is eating. Allow for overlap in insulin infusion and subcutaneous insulin injection.

Treatment of HHS: Fluid replacement should initially stabilize the hemodynamic status of the patient (1–3 L of 0.9% normal saline over the first 2–3 hours). Because the fluid deficit in HHS is accumulated over a period of days to weeks, the rapidity of reversal of the hyperosmolar state must balance the need for free water repletion with the risk that too rapid a reversal may worsen neurologic function. If the serum sodium > 150 mmol/L (150 mEq/L), 0.45% saline should be used. After hemodynamic stability is achieved, the IV fluid administration is directed at reversing the free water deficit using hypotonic fluids (0.45% saline initially then 5% dextrose in water, D_5W). The calculated free water deficit (which averages 9–10 L) should be reversed over the next 1–2 days (infusion rates of 200–300 mL/h of hypotonic solution). Potassium repletion is usually necessary and should be dictated by repeated measurements of the serum potassium. In patients taking diuretics, the potassium deficit can be quite large and may be accompanied by magnesium deficiency. Hypophosphatemia may occur during therapy and can be improved by using KPO_4 and beginning nutrition.

As in DKA, rehydration and volume expansion lower the plasma glucose initially, but insulin is also required. A reasonable regimen for HHS begins with an IV insulin bolus of 0.1 units/kg followed by IV insulin at a constant infusion rate of 0.1 units/kg per hour. If the serum glucose does not fall, increase the insulin infusion rate by twofold. As in DKA, glucose should be added to IV fluid when the plasma glucose falls to 13.9 mmol/L (250 mg/dL), and the insulin infusion rate should be decreased to 0.05–0.1 units/kg per hour. The insulin infusion should be continued until the patient has resumed eating and can be transferred to a SC insulin regimen. The patient should be discharged from the hospital on insulin, though some patients can later switch to oral glucose-lowering agents.

15. Why to avoid precipitous falls in blood glucose?

Ans.

- *Extreme hyperglycemia:* Brain accumulates idiogenic osmoles (Glucose, polyols, free amino acids) to prevent cerebral osmotic dehydration
- As the movement of these osmoles across BBB is very slow relative to water, hence rapid reduction in B glucose leaves brain hyperosmolar relative to plasma leading to develop of → Osmotic cerebral edema

16. How to manage hypoglycemia in a diabetic patient?

Ans.

- Most frequent and dangerous complication of insulin therapy
- Exacerbated by simultaneous administration of alcohol, OHA, ACE inhibitors, MAO inhibitors, and nonselective beta blockers
- Plasma glucose level less than 50 mg/dL
- *Adrenergic symptoms:* Sweating, tachycardia, palpitations, restlessness, pallor
- *Neuroglycopenic:* Fatigue, confusion, headache, somnolence, convulsions, coma
- *Awake patient:* Sweating, tachycardia, palpitations, restlessness, pallor, disoriented speech
- *Patient under anesthesia:* Signs of sympathetic stimulation, dilated pupils.
- *Treatment:* If conscious—Sugar (sugar cubes, glucose tablets, soft drinks)
- *If unconscious:* Glucose 0.5 mg/kg IV or glucagon 0.5–1.0 mg IV/IM/SC.

17. Why cardiovascular assessment is important in a diabetic patient?

Ans. Diabetic patients need a detailed cardiovascular examination because

- *Coronary A disease:*
  - High risk for cardiac ischemia
  - In type 2 DM. MI as common as in nondiabetics with past history of MI.
  - Silent MI due to symptom denervation
  - Standard ECG—poor predictive value
  - 15–60% of diabetics without CAD symptoms have abnormal exercise electrocardiography
- *Arterial HT:* Present in 29–54% diabetics
- *Cardiac autonomic neuropathy:*
  - Involves 20–40% of diabetics with HT
  - Independent of age and duration of diabetes
  - ↑ intraoperative CVS morbidity

18. What are the anesthetic considerations in a diabetic patient posted for surgery?

Ans. DM is a complex disorder involving all the systems. Its effects on the various body systems are:

Cardiovascular system:

- Premature atheroma formation
- ↑ chances of CAD (Male-double risk; female-triple risk)
- ↑ incidence of silent MI (especially with history of early satiety, lack of sweating, lack of pulse rate change with inspiration or orthostatic maneuvers and impotence)
- HT and its sequelae
- ↓ threshold for arrhythmias
- Cardiac dysautonomia may present with:
  - Sudden hypotension on induction
  - Absence of tachycardia and HT with intubation
- Sudden cardiorespiratory arrest
- Diabetic cardiomyopathy

Nervous system:
- ↑ chances of CVA
- Peripheral neuropathy—↑ incidence of nerve injury and nerve ischemia
  - Care at positioning and transport
  - Use of nerve blocks
  - Avoid epinephrine containing LA solutions
- ANS dysfunction
  - Postural hypotension
  - Gastroparesis—↑ preoperative fasting, rapid sequence induction
  - Loss of signs of hypoglycemia
  - Blunted response to atropine and beta-blockers
  - *Urinary stasis:* Avoid unnecessary bladder catheterization

Respiratory system:
- ↓ Ventilatory response to $PaCO_2$ and PaO_2
- More chances of respiratory tract infections
- ↑ susceptibility to ventilatory depressant drugs
- ↓ FVC and FEV (Due to glycosylation of tissue proteins in connective tissues)
- ↓ 2,3 DPG → ↓ release of O_2 to tissues
- DM affects O_2 transport by causing glucose to covalently bind to Hb molecular and alters allosteric interactions between beta chains

  Airway

  Stiff joint syndrome-restricted neck movements: Due to nonenzymatic glycosylation of proteins and abnormal cross-linkage of collagen.

  The prayer sign: Patient is unable to approximate the palmar surfaces of the phalangeal joints despite maximal effort.
  - Palm print test
  - Degree of interphalangeal joint involvement can also be assessed by scoring the ink impression made by the palm of dominant hand.

Renal system:
- More chances of ARF in perioperative period, due to
  - Intrinsic renal disease
  - Hemodynamic impairement
  - Urosepsis
- *UTI:* Most common postoperative complication in diabetics undergoing surgery
- *Renal failure:* Incidence 7%, most common major complication.

Other systems:
- *Proliferative retinopathy:* Vitreous hemorrhage on laryngoscopy and intubation
- *Infection:* Poor wound healing
  - Trophic ulcers
  - More chances of sepsis
- Associated acute complications
  - DKA
  - NKHS
  - Hypoglycemia

  Increased risk for intraoperative hypothermia.

19. What are the goals of anesthetic management?

Ans.
- To maintain glycemic control
- To avoid further deterioration of pre-existing end organ damage
- To shift patient soon on preoperative glycemic control drugs.

20. What are the aims of preoperative assessment?

Ans. The preoperative assessment aim to:

- Diagnose type of DM and its duration
- Preoperative evaluation and treatment of end organ damage which is responsible for 5-fold increase in preoperative mortality associated with DM
- Assessment of blood sugar control and to obtain a reasonable control with change to short acting drugs
- Limit hospital stay and decrease cost
- Quantification of risk.

21. How will you assess the patient in the preoperative period?

Ans. A detailed history and clinical examination will be done and a set of investigations will be done (Table 7).

Table 7 | Preoperative assessment of a diabetic patient

	History/Examination	*Investigation*
Blood sugar control	• Hypo/hyperglycemic episodes • Hospitalization • Medical compliance	• BS-F and PP • HbA_{1C}
Nephropathy	• History of HT • History of recurrent UTI • History of swelling over face and body	• Urine R/M, albumin • Microalbuminuria • Kidney function tests
Cardiac status	• History of angina/MI • Dyspnea/swelling of feet • Exercise tolerance	• ECG • Chest X-ray • ECHO
PVD	• History of intermittent claudication • Blanching of feet • Nonhealing ulcers	
Retinopathy	• History of visual disturbance • Increasing power of lenses	• Fundus exam
Stiff joint syndrome	• Short stature • Prayer sign • Loss of palmar creases • Tight waxy skin • Alteration in palm print	• X-ray cervical spine (lateral)
Metabolic and electrolyte	• Severe infection/starvation • Compliance • Signs of DKA/hypoglycemia	• ABG • S electrolytes • Ketones-urinary
ANS	• Early satiety • Vomiting • Abdominal distention • Loss of sweating • Orthostatic syncope • Palpitations • Impotence • Nocturnal diarrhea	• Postural changes in BP • HR variability • Valsalva quotient • Sustained handgrip test • Absence of tachycardia with atropine

22. What are the various autonomic function tests?

Ans: See Table 8.

Table 8 | Test for autonomic dysfunction

Clinical examination	*Technique*	*Normal value*
Parasympathetic		
HR response to a Valsalva maneuver	The seated subject blows into a mouthpiece (while maintaining a pressure of 40 mm Hg) for 15 seconds. The Valsalva ratio is the ratio of the longest R-R interval (which comes shortly after release) to the shortest R-R interval (which occurs during the maneuver)	Ratio of >1.21
HR response to standing	HR is measured as the subject moves from a resting supine position to standing. A normal tachycardic response is maximal around the 15th beat after rising. A relative bradycardia follows that is most marked around the 30th beat after standing. The response to standing is expressed as a 30:15 ratio and is the ratio of the longest R-R interval around the 30th beat to the shortest R-R interval around the 15th beat	Ratio of >1.04
HR response to deep breathing	The subject takes six deep breaths in 1 minute. The maximum and minimum heart rates during each cycle are measured, and the mean of the differences (maximum HR - minimum HR) during three successive breathing cycles is taken as the maximum-minimum HR	Mean difference >15 beats/min
Sympathetic		
BP response to standing	The subject moves from resting supine to standing, and standing SBP is subtracted from supine SBP	Difference <10 mm Hg
BP response to sustained handgrip	The subject maintains a handgrip of 30% of the maximum handgrip squeeze for up to 5 minutes. BP is measured every minute, and the initial DBP is subtracted from the DBP just before release	Difference >16 mm Hg

23. What orders will you advice in the preoperative period?

Ans. Consent

- NPO orders
- Anxiolytic/tablet Gabapentin/Pregabalin
- *Aspiration prophylaxis:* 10 mg metoclopramide to facilitate gastric emptying of solids.
- Stop long acting insulin night before surgery
- Morning sample of BS, SE to be sent
- Monitoring IV fluids according to regimen
- To arrange for dextrostix, regular insulin, etc.
- Gentle transfer of patient
- To be taken up as 1st case.

24. What is the effect of various anesthetic drugs on the blood sugar values?

- *Etomidate:* Inhibitory effect on adrenal steroid genesis and decrease glycemic response to surgery
- *Midazolam:* Decrease ACTH and cortisol secretion; decrease sympathoadrenal activity; but stimulates GH secretion. Net effect is decreased glycemic response to surgery
- *α-2 adrenergic agonists:* Decrease sympathetic outflow from hypothesis, inhibits release of ACTH with stimulation of GH release. Glycemic control improved as a result of decreased sympathoadrenal activity. Decreasing plasma C peptide concentration indicating decrease in endogenous insulin secretion
- *Propofol:* Decrease lipid load resulting from propofol infusion may further lead to impairment of metabolism in diabetic patients. Unlikely to be relevant during short anesthesia/induction. Important if prolonged ICU sedation.

25. What are the perioperative goals of insulin replacement?

Ans. Insulin infusion rate:

- 0.02 U insulin/kg/hr or 1.4U/hr (in a 70 kg patient)
- Typically 1 U of insulin lowers glucose approximately by 25–30 mg/dL
- Insulin infusion for CABG @ 0.06 U/kg/hr
- Patients on steroid/severe infection/on vasopressor @ 0.04 U/kg/hr.

Carbohydrate requirement: Insulin infusion accompanied by D 5 ½ NS with 20 mEq KCl @100–150 mL/hr to provide carbohydrate atleast 150 gm/day to inhibit hepatic glucose production and protein catabolism.

Aim:

- To maintain BS at 120–180 mg/dL
- Management of insulin in preoperative period depends on the type of insulin that patient takes and timing of dosing.
- If patient takes subcutaneous insulin each night at bedtime: 2/3rd of this dose (NPH and regular)—night before surgery: 1/2 of the morning NPH dose to be given on day of surgery (morning dose of regular insulin withheld)
- If patients takes glargine at bedtime, take 1/2–3/4 usual dose night before surgery: for patients taking glargine in morning, take 1/2–3/4 usual dose in morning of surgery.
- Oral hypoglycemics to be discontinued 24–48 hours preoperatively.

Intraoperative insulin regimen: There is an inpatient insulin regime which is as described.

Inpatient insulin algorithm (Russell T Wall, et al)
Standard drip: Regular insulin 100 units/100 mL 0.9% NaCl via infusion device.

Initiating the infusion:
Algorithm 1: Start here for most patients.
Algorithm 2: Start here if status post (s/p) CABG, status post (s/p) solid organ transplant or islet cell transplant, receiving glucocorticoids, vasopressors or diabetics receiving > 80 units/day of insulin as an outpatient.

Algorithm 1		*Algorithm 2*		*Algorithm 3*		*Algorithm 4*	
BG	*Units/hour*	*BG*	*Units/hour*	*BG*	*Units/hour*	*BG*	*Units/hour*
< 60 = Hypoglycemia (See below for treatment)							
< 70	Off	< 70	Off	< 70	Off	< 70	Off
70–109	0.2	70–109	0.5	70–109	1	70–109	1.5
110–119	0.5	110–119	1	110–119	2	110–119	3
120–149	1	120–149	1.5	120–149	3	120–149	-5
150–179	1.5	150–179	2	150–179	4	150–179	7
180–209	2	180–209	3	180–209	5	180–209	9
210–239	2	210–239	4	210–239	6	210–239	12
240–269	3	240–269	5	240–269	8	240–269	16
270–299	3	270–299	6	270–299	10	270–299	20
300–329	4	300–329	7	300–329	12	300–329	24
330–359	4	330–359	8	330–359	14	> 330	28
> 360	6	> 360	12	> 360	16		

Moving up: An algorithm failure is defined as BG outside the goal range for 2 hours (see above goal), and the level does not change by at least 60 mg/dL within 1 hour.

Moving down: When BG is < 70 mg/dL for two checks or if BG decreases by > 100 mg/dL in an hour.

Tube feeds or TPN: Decrease infusion by 50% if nutrition (tube feeds or TPN) is discontinued or significantly reduced. Reinstitute hourly BG checks every 4 hours.

Patient monitoring: Check capillary BG every hour until it is within goal range for 4 hours, then decrease to every 2 hours for 4 hours, and if it remains at goal, may decrease to every 4 hours.

26. Describe the sliding scale for insulin therapy.

Ans. Sliding scale (Table 9).

Table 9 | Sliding scale of insulin therapy

Glucose	*Insulin*
150–200 mg/dL	2 U regular subcutaneous
201–250 mg/dL	4 U
251–300 mg/dL	6 U
301–350 mg/dL	8 U
>350 mg/dL	10 U

Sliding scale is not used in the perioperative management of diabetes.

27. What are the various regimens for the perioperative control of blood sugar? What are the advantages and disadvantages?

Ans. There are various regimens for the perioperative management of diabetes.

- Tight control regimen/**Michael Roizen regimen**

  Aim: To keep BS in 79–120 mg/dL

  Indications: Pregnancy, CPB, Neurological surgeries, those require postoperative ICU care.

  Advantages:
  - Improve wound healing
  - Prevent wound infection
  - Improves neurological outcome after global or focal CNS ischemic insult
  - Improves weaning from cardiopulmonary bypass

  Disadvantages:
  - No monitoring of K^+
  - More chances of hypoglycemia
  - Difficult inward settings
  - Meticulous frequent monitoring

  Method:
  - Night before surgery do preprandial glucose.
  - Start 5% D @ 50 mL/hr. (in 70 kg body weight)
  - 'Piggyback' to dextrose infusion, an infusion of regular insulin (50 U insulin in 250 mL of 0.9% NS)
  - Before attaching this piggyback line flush the line with 60 mL of infusion mixture and discard the flushing solution. This approach saturates insulin binding sites of the tubing
  - Set infusion rate @ Plasma Glucose/150 U/h or @ Plasma Glucose/100—if on steroids/sepsis/obesity
  - 4 hourly blood sugar monitoring

- Intraoperatively monitor plasma glucose every 1–2 hourly for 24 hours period
- If hypoglycemia <50, give 15 mL of 50% dextrose intravenous
- This regimen accomplishes its goals except in 'brittle' diabetics given high doses of steroids

- **Tight control regimen 2**
  - *Aim:* Same as for tight control regimen 1
  - Obtain a 'feedback mechanical pancreas' and set the controls for desired plasma glucose regimen.
  - Institute two appropriate intravenous lines.
  - This regimen may supersede all others in many intensive care units if cost of mechanical pancreas can be reduced and if control of hyperglycemia is shown to make a meaningful difference perioperatively.
- **Alberti regimen**
  Used in: Type 1 diabetes or insulin controlled type 2 diabetes
  - Stabilize blood sugar 2–3 days prior to surgery
  - Shift to short acting insulin on day before surgery
  - Omit morning dose of insulin
  - Start GKI (10, 10, 10) after checking BS and K^+ levels @ 100–125 ml/hr
  - 2–3 hourly blood sugar level charting

Blood sugar	*Infusion*
<5 mmol/L (90 mg/dL)	10%D + 5U Insulin + 10 K^+
5–10 mmol/L (90–180)	10 + 10 + 10
10–20 mmol/L (180–360)	10 + 15 + 10
>20 mmol/L (>360)	10 + 20 + 10

  Advantages: Simple, inherent safety
  Disadvantages: Fixed insulin concentration, need to change the bag everytime, waterload, hyponatremia, hyperglycemia
  Postoperatively:
  - GKI @100–125 mL/hr, check blood sugar 4 hourly, till patient starts orally
  - After starting orally stop GKI, give regular insulin
  - Dose 20% extra—if steroids intake or infection present
  - No lactate containing fluids
- **Hirsch's variable rate infusion regimen**
  Aim: To maintain between 120–180 mg/dL
  - Mix 50 U insulin in 500 mL NS (10 mL=1 unit, 1 unit/hr=10 mL/hr)
  - Infuse @ 0.5-1.0 U/hr or 0.01–0.02 U/kg/hr
  - Check blood sugar (hourly during surgery)

<80	Turn off infusion. Give 25 mL of 50% dextrose and recheck in 30 min
80–120	↓ Insulin infusion by 0.3 U/hr
120–180	No change in infusion
180–240	↑ Infusion by 0.3 U/hr
>240	↑ Infusion by 0.5 U/hr

- **Vellore regimen**
  - On the day of surgery OHA and insulin omitted
  - Blood sugar taken at 6 am on the day of surgery
  - 8 am: Start 5% dextrose with 5 U insulin @ 100 mL/hr
  - *Intraoperatively:* For every 50 mg/dL increase in blood glucose concentration more than 100 mg/dL, 1U of insulin was added to the injection port of a 100 mL measured volume set containing 5% dextrose in water
  - Monitor blood glucose hourly (Table 10).

Table 10 | Hourly blood glucose monitoring

Blood glucose	*Insulin*
< 75 mg/dL over 15 min	No insulin, 100 mL of 5% D
75–100 over 1 hour	No insulin, 100 mL of 5% D
100–125	1 U in 100 mL of 5% D over 1 hour
125–180	2 U in 100 mL of 5% D over 1 hour
180–250	3 U in 100 mL of 5% D over 1 hour
>250	4 U in 100 mL of 5% D over 1 hour
If potassium is less than 3 mmol/L and 10 mmol of KCl to the insulin dextrose drip	

28. How to prevent insulin adsorption on tubing/glass bottles?

Ans.

- Add albumin/polygelline
- Add patients own blood
- Flushing with 60 mL of infusion mixture—saturates binding sites
- Use concentrated insulin in small volumes
- 50 mL syringe with infusion pumps.

29. What is the effect of stress response on sugar control?

Ans.

- Glucagon, epinephrine, GH, steroids, ↓ Insulin
- Insulin resistance in postoperative period
- Consequences:
  - Osmolar diuresis-dehydration
  - Disrupts autoregulation of vascular beds
  - Impaired wound healing
  - Decreased chemotaxis and impaired phagocytosis
  - More acute complications.

30. How can you classify surgeries on the basis of risk involved?

Ans.

Minor	<30 minutes	Unlikely to interfere with diabetes treatment	For example, cystoscopy
Intermediate	30 minutes–2 hours	Might interfere with surgery on day of surgery	Laminectomy, internal fixation of fractures
Major	>2 hours	Likely to interfere with management and diet	Cholecystectomy, bowel resection

31. What are the advantages and disadvantages of regional anesthesia?

Ans. *Advantages:*

- Awake patient, intraoperative hypoglycemia (early recognition of hypoglycemia) can be noticed
- ↓ risk of aspiration
- ↓ PONV chances
- Rapid return to diet and insulin/OHA
- ↓ chances of thromboembolism
- Metabolic effects of anesthetic agents avoided
- Epidural anesthesia block catecholamine release irrespective of the segmental level, but prevents the increase in blood glucose and control bodies only if block height T6/T8

Disadvantages:

- Risk of nerve injuries, higher adrenaline use increases risk of ischemic injury
- LA requirement is low—↑ sensitivity
- Risk of infection
- Epidural abscess
- Contraindicated in presence of peripheral neuropathy.

32. What are the indications and technique of lumbar sympathetic block?

Ans. *Indications:* In diabetic gangrene, Buerger's disease, Raynaud's phenomenon, reconstructive vascular surgeries.

- Fusion of L1 and L2 ganglia; and ganglia (size 5–15 mm) aggregate at L2-L3 and L4-L5 discs
- LSB produces pain relief:
  - Interruption of pre- and postgangrene symptom effort influences function of primary afferent neurons
  - Visceral afferent from deep visceral stress in the leg that travel with symptom nerves may be blocked.

Technique:

- Prone position, fluoroscopy, anteroposterior and lateral views
- *Paramedian (Classic Mandl's) approach:* 5–8 cm lateral to spinous process of L2-L4, redirected, passes below and medial to inferior border of transverse process at 10° to sagittal plane: contact confines to anterolateral border of L2-L4 in tight linear fashion and Hugging.
  [1st needle—Inferior 1/3 of L2; 2nd needle—superior 1/3 of L3; 3rd needle-L4]
- *Lateral (Reid's) approach:* 10–14 cm lateral to superior border of spinous process of L4 and L5 at 60° to sagittal plane.

33. What are the postoperative complications in a diabetic patient?

Ans.

- Hypoglycemia
- Hyperglycemia—DKA, NKHC
- Infections
- Delayed wound healing
- Perioperative MI ↑ risk watch till 72 hours
- Problems due to autonomic neuropathy, postural hypotension, atonic bleeding, urinary retention
- PONV
- Pain
- Restoration of routine OHA/insulin.

34. Why is glycemic control important in ICU and what are the guidelines?

Ans.

- Insulin resistance develops in critical illness
- Tightly controlled between 80 and 110 mg/dL by continuous infusion of insulin, irrespective of underlying diabetes → significantly decreases ICU mortality
- Prevents ARF development
- ↓ critical illness polyneuropathy
- ↓ incidence of infections and sepsis
- Improves deranged lipid profile—exerts anti-inflammatory effects.

35. What are the first line drugs for the management of diabetic neuropathy?

Ans. Diabetic neuropathy establishes itself after 6–7 years of manifestation of diabetes mellitus.

Drugs:

Alpha2-delta ligands like:

- Gabapentin in the dose of 300–2100 mg/day
- Pregabalin 75–600 mg/day.

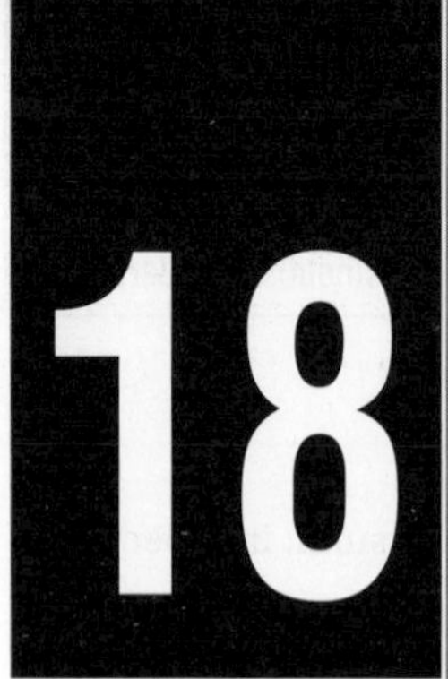

A Patient with Lung Cyst Posted for Pneumonectomy

Anupam Goswami

PATHOPHYSIOLOGY: CYSTS AND BULLAE

Thin-walled, air-filled cavities in the lungs. May represent end-stage emphysematous lung changes or may be congenital and isolated findings. Repeated pneumothoraces from spontaneous rupture, infection, and/or dyspnea are the usual indications for surgery. The degree of functional impairment depends on the condition of the remaining lung, the size of the airspace, and the amount of compression of the surrounding healthy lung tissue by the cyst. With a compliant bulla during controlled ventilation a large portion of the applied tidal volume will be wasted in this additional dead space. Positive pressure ventilation should be used with caution and nitrous oxide must always be avoided, in case the bulla ruptures leading to a tension pneumothorax. Once the chest is opened, the risk of a tension pneumothorax disappears. Intubation with a DLT in a spontaneously breathing awake or anesthetized patient is recommended. Positive pressure ventilation with rapid small tidal volumes at pressures less than 15 cm H_2O can be used during induction and maintenance of anesthesia.

Patients with Cysts and Bullae

Two clinical groups: The first have apical blebs and are usually young with excellent pulmonary reserve, and the second have emphysematous blebs, are older, and have advanced chronic obstructive pulmonary disease (COPD) often with CO_2 retention, may benefit by avoiding thoracotomy.

Video-assisted thoracoscopic resection of bullae and blebs is usually attempted in both groups, with emphysematous group frequently requiring open thoracotomy.

Perioperative Risks

- N_2O expansion of bullae
- Pneumothorax
- Bronchospasm

- Postoperative pulmonary infection—acute bronchitis or pneumonia
- Pulmonary embolism.

Chronic Obstructive Pulmonary Disease

Chronic Bronchitis

- Acquired and virtually always secondary to smoking.
- Chronic productive cough with periodic exacerbation. Enlargement of mucous secreting glands of airway with excessive sputum production. Expiratory airway obstruction. Derangement in V/Q relationships. Chronic hypoxia/hypercarbia with right heart failure. Perioperative risks are bronchospasm, airway stimulation at light levels of anesthesia, laryngospasm from secretions and hyper-reactivity, hypoxia and hypercarbia.
- *Assessment*
  - *Airway:* Difficulty often, due to truncal obesity (corticosteroids), redundant soft tissue in airway, short fat neck.
  - *Cardiovascular effect:* Exercise intolerance, RHF, pulmonary HTN, RV heave dependent edema. *Tests:* ECG, ECHO, PA-catheterization.
  - *Respiratory effect:* Smoking, exercise intolerance, sputum production, airways obstruction, cyanosis. Tests: PFT, DLCO, ABG.
- *Preoperative preparation:* Smoking cessation, antibiotics in acute exacerbations (prophylaxis inefficacious). Glucocorticoids of uncertain benefits, trial appropriate in acute exacerbations. Bronchodilators, when response can be demonstrated by PFT or signs and symptoms.
- *Monitoring:* Arterial line—ABG. PA—catheter for large fluid shift.
- *Preinduction/induction:* Avoid stimulating the airway while in lighter anesthetic plane to avoid bronchospasm. Regional anesthesia preferred.
- *Maintenance:* Frequent suctioning of endotracheal tube. Limit narcotic (perioperative CO_2 retention). Adjuvant regional anesthesia for procedures that affect respiratory mechanics (intercostal nerve blocks, epidural analgesia).
- *Extubation:* Intratracheal bronchodilator in responsive patients prior to extubation.
- *Postoperative problems:* Secretions, mucous plugging, atelectasis, pneumonia, prolonged mechanical ventilation.

Emphysema

- Acquired disease related to smoking usually. Specific occupational exposure like coal mining has also been implicated. Genetic disease due to α_1-antitrypsin deficiency is rare.
- Destruction of interalveolar septae and loss of pulmonary elastic recoil leads to formation of bullae and development of irreversible expiratory airflow obstruction.
- "Pink puffer" with dyspnea, hyperinflation, distant breath sounds, low diffusing capacity. Often have elements of chronic bronchitis and asthma. Hypoxia, hypercarbia, cor-pulmonale are late developments. Mucociliary clearence is often worsened after inhalational anesthetics. Diaphragmatic mechanics impaired by anesthetics, sedatives, NM blockers, conduction block , and supine positioning.
- *Assessment*
  - *Airway:* None unless tumor present in airway. Effects: cor-pulmonale (late)—severe dyspnea, signs of pulmonary hypertension, hepatosplenomegaly, pedal edema, cyanosis, pleural effusion, usually without pulmonary edema, DVT in legs. *Tests:* CXR, ABG
  - *Cardiovascular effects:* Pulmonary emboli—shortness of breath, arrhythmias, DVT in legs. *Tests:* Chest X-ray (CXR), V/Q scan, pulmonary angiogram.

- *Respiratory effect:* Bronchospasm—recent increase in dyspnea, exercise intolerance, increased respiratory rate, expiratory time, accessory muscle use. *Test*: Spirometry pre- and post-bronchodilator.
- *Effect:* Pneumonia—fever, dyspnea, increased sputum, signs of pulmonary consolidation. *Test:* CXR.
- *Preoperative preparation:* Optimize bronchodilation, eradicate any underlying bacterial infection, smoking cessation.
- *Monitoring:* Be cognizant of potential for increased gradient between $PEtCO_2$ and $PaCO_2$.
- *Preinduction/induction:* Careful about airway reactivity. Avoid N_2O to prevent bulla expansion.
- *Extubation:* Residual anesthetics compromise ventilatory response to CO_2 leading to postoperative respiratory failure. Patient may be semiconscious and combative due to hypoxia and hypercarbia on emergence. Evaluate whether postoperative ventilation may be safer.
- *Adjuvants:* β-adrenergic agonist, atropinic agents for airway reactivity.
- *Postoperative period:* Residual anesthetic effects leading to postoperative respiratory failure. Analgesics may depress ventilatory function, but unrelieved incisional pain following abdominal/thoracic surgery may impair breathing.

Right Ventricular Dysfunction

Present in 50% of COPD patients. Poorly tolerant of sudden increases in RV afterload, such as the change from spontaneous to controlled ventilation. Cor-pulmonale in 40% patients with an FEV_1<1 L,70% with an FEV_1<0.6 L. Pneumonectomy candidates with a preoperative FEV_1 of less than 40% should have transthoracic echocardiography to assess right-sided heart function. Elevation of right-sided heart pressures places these patients in a very high-risk group.

Common Types of Lung Surgeries and their Indications: An Overview

1. Wedge resection—malignancy most common. Others are TB, benign neoplasms, bronchiectasis.
2. Lobectomy—same indications as wedge resection.
3. Pneumonectomy—most common indication-malignancy.
4. Lung volume reduction surgery (LVRS) and bullectomy—severe respiratory, failure secondary to emphysema.
5. Drainage of empyema and decortication—secondary to TB, pneumonia, intercostal drain insertion.
6. Repair of bronchopleural fistula.
7. Pleurectomy and pleurodesis—due to recurrent pneumothorax and pleural effusions.

Common Nonpulmonary Surgeries Performed by a Thoracotomy: An Overview

1. Esophagectomy.
2. Closed mitral commissurotomy.
3. Removal of certain mediastinal tumors.
4. Removal of chest wall tumors.
5. Chest wall and diaphragmatic trauma.

Problems of Thoracotomy

- Problems due to existing lung disease
- Compromised cardiovascular function
- Problems of infection
- Problems of secretions
- Problems of increased airway resistance and decreased lung compliance
- Problems of positioning
- Problems of opening the pleura
- Problems of one lung ventilation (OLV)
- Problems of development of pulmonary edema
- Problems of massive blood loss
- Problems of inadequate pain relief
- Problems of mismanagement of pleural drain/waterseal drainage.
- *Problems of lung secretions:* Stagnation of secretions particularly in patients with COPD. Collapse, infection and atelectasis of the dependent lung areas.
- *Causes of increased airway resistance and decreased lung compliance:* Usually, elderly patients. Existing lung disease. COPD associated (as most patients are smokers) decreased mucociliary function.
- *Problems of positioning the patient for surgery*
  - Lateral decubitus, patient anesthetized and controlled ventilation: Controlled ventilation favors the upper lung because it is more compliant than the lower lung.
  - Paralysis of the dependent hemidiaphragm, accumulation of abdominal contents on the dependant side, use of supports to maintain lateral position all add to further decrease in FRC and compliance of the dependant lung.
- *Problems of opening the pleura*
  - Pulmonary collapse.
  - Paradoxical respiration/Pendelluft.
  - Mediastinal displacement.
  - *Reflex disturbance:* All these may be avoided by the use of IPPV.
- *Problems of one lung ventilation:* OLV invariably creates a shunt that may cause hypoxia. The correct choice and positioning of endobronchial tubes is crucial. Requires high technical skill.

Evaluation of a Patient Posted for Lung Resection before Anesthesia

- Routine assessment for major surgery
- Focused and detailed assessment of respiratory and cardiovascular systems
- Routine blood counts, glucose, urea, creatinine, electrolytes
- Spirometry
- ECG—to identify patterns of right atrial and ventricular hypertrophy and changes associated with COPD
- Chest X-ray
- Arterial blood gases.

Specific Evaluation for Lung Resectability

- Clinically fit, good exercise tolerance, normal spirometry—accept for surgery.
- Major medical problems, poor exercise tolerance, grossly impaired spirometry—reject for surgery.
- Reduced exercise tolerance, abnormal spirometry, with or without moderate coexisting disease—assess risk benefit ratio for surgery.

Pulmonary Function Tests for Lung Resectability

- Accepted values for preoperative FEV_1 are:
  - Pneumonectomy > 55%,
  - Lobectomy > 40%,
  - Wedge resection > 35%. (All values are percentages of predicted).
- The predicted postoperative value for pulmonary function tests is preoperative value × (5 – number of lobes resected)/5.
- Estimated postoperative FEV_1 < 800 mL or FVC < 15 mL/kg suggest a need for postoperative ventilation.
- A postoperative goal of achieving FEV_1 > 35 % of predicted value should be targeted.
- Exercise pulse oximetry is a valuable prognostic indicator.
- Failure to cover 300 m or a fall in SpO_2 > 4% in a "six minute walk test" indicate poor prognosis.

Pulmonary Function Testing for Pneumonectomy

Should proceed in 3 phases:

Phase 1: Evaluation of total lung function:

- *Consists of:*
  - Spirommetry/He dilution or body plethysmography
  - Arterial blood gases.
- *Increased risk is present, if:*
  - FEV1 < 50% of FVC
  - FEV1 < 2 L
  - MBC < 50% of predicted
  - Hypercapnia during breathing room air
  - PaO_2 < 50 mm Hg
  - RV/TLC > 50% of predicted.

Phase 2: Evaluation of single lung function (should be performed, if any 1 of phase 1 findings are less than stated limits)

- Consists of:
  - Spirometry
  - Individual split function tests.
- The percentage contribution of each lung to total FEV_1 is assumed to be proportional to the percentage of total pulmonary blood flow it receives, thus, postoperative FEV_1 = % blood flow to remaining lung × total FEV_1.
- Increased risk is present if—predicted postoperative FEV_1 < 0.85 L or blood flow to diseased lung > 70%.

Phase 3: Mimics postoperative condition (to be performed if phase 2 findings are not acceptable)

- Consists of:
  - Temporary occlusion of unilateral main stem bronchus by bronchial blocker, then measuring spirometry of remaining lung (must provide supplemental oxygen).
  - Temporary occlusion of right or left pulmonary artery.
- Increased risk present, if:
  - Mean PAP > 40 mm Hg after occlusion of pulmonary artery of the diseased side.
  - $PaCO_2$ > 60 mm Hg.
  - PaO_2 < 45 mm Hg.
  - Severe breathlessness.

Preparing the Patient for Surgery

- ***Preparation involves:*** To stop smoking. Dilatation of the airways. Loosening of secretions. Removal of secretions. Increasing motivation and education regarding postoperative care.
- ***Premedication:*** Sedatives avoided, antisialogogues may be used.

Types of Tube that may be used for Ventilation

- Ordinary endotracheal tubes.
- Double lumen endobronchial tubes (DLTs).
- *Single lumen endobronchial tubes:* Gordon Green tubes (rarely used nowadays).
- *Endobronchial blockers:* Univent or Arndt endobronchial blocker.

Advantages of using DLTs

- Protects the dependant lung from blood and secretions
- Allows independent control of ventilation in each lung
- Improves surgical access and prevents lung trauma.

Types and Selection of DLT

- *Types:*
  - Carlen's
  - Robertshaw (red rubber)
  - Single use PVC (Bronchocath/Sher-I-Bronch).
- *Selection:* The largest DLT which passes through the glottis should be used. A left-sided tube is generally used.

Placement

Assess risk/benefits of using a DLT. Check Y-connectors. Start intubation with concavity of the endobronchial part facing anteriorly. When the tip is past the glottis, rotate the tube by 90° toward the side of the bronchus to be intubated, to bring the oropharyngeal curve into the sagittal plane. Gently advance the tube until resistance is felt to further placement (about 29 cm at the teeth). Follow a preset protocol for correct tube placement confirmed by fiber optic bronchoscopes (FOB).

Steps of DLT Placement

Protocol for DLT placement—Clinical and bronchoscope.

MANAGEMENT OF ONE LUNG VENTILATION

Initiating OLV

Start with ideal settings during two lungs ventilation. Increase FiO_2 to 1 and begin OLV with tidal volume of 10 mL/kg body weight Clamp Y-connector of non-dependent lung and open sealing cap on that lumen. Observe peak airway pressure. An increase of 30–40% is normal. Change tidal volume and ventilator parameters to keep peak airway pressure below 30 cm water. Observe SpO_2 and $EtCO_2$ closely. Check with the surgeon that the lung is collapsing and the mediastinum has not collapsed. Adjust respiratory rate to maintain $PaCO_2$ of 40 mm Hg.

Hypoxia

Hypoxia is a frequent complication of OLV, occurring after a few minutes of initiation. Keep FiO_2 at 1.0 and maintain adequate cardiac output. Confirm correct positioning of DLT. If partial collapse of dependent lung is suspected add 5–10 cm water PEEP on the dependent lung. If hypoxia still persists, partially inflate non-dependent lung with 5–10 cm water CPAP. If hypoxia continue to persist, add intermittent oxygen breaths through the CPAP system. Early ligation of pulmonary artery branch in pneumonectomy prevents hypoxia. If these maneuvers do not correct hypoxia return to two lung ventilation.

TECHNIQUE AND STEPS OF ANESTHESIA

- GA with IPPV (mandatory)
- Two IV lines
- Two suction catheters for two lungs
- Adequate relaxation and analgesia
- Suppression of reflexes
- Drainage of secretions—lung isolation and patient position.

Steps

- Antisialogogue as premedications
- Induction—intravenous
- IPPV with intubation + opioids/inhalational agents
- Collapse of diseased lung—by using lung isolation techniques (DLT or endobronchial blocker)
- Testing of bronchial stump suture for leaks
- Closure of chest with water seal drainage.

Perioperative Monitoring Parameters

- Standard anesthetic monitoring
- Invasive arterial blood pressure
- Central venous pressure
- Pulmonary artery catheterization
- Transesophageal echocardiography
- Arterial blood gases.

Postoperative Pain Management Strategies

- Intraoperative opioids
- Regional nerve blocks
- Thoracic epidural analgesia
- Thoracic paravertebral catheter
- Oral/rectal analgesics
- Interpleural regional analgesia.

Strategies of Postoperative Care

- Identify and treat serious postoperative complications
- Intensive and aggressive respiratory care regime

- Remove secretions
- Diagnose and treat infections
- Dilating airways
- Chest physiotherapy.

STRATEGIES FOR POSTOPERATIVE MECHANICAL VENTILATION

Problems of Postoperative Ventilation after Pulmonary Surgery

- Added risk of infection
- Problems of continuing air leaks from lung surfaces
- Bronchial suture lines are vulnerable to effects of IPPV
- Trauma following repeated endotracheal suction
- Flow limitation causing hemodynamic collapse with the application of positive-pressure ventilation owing to dynamic hyperinflation of the lungs.

Strategies

- Ventilate preferably using SIMV
- Ensure normocapnia
- Use non-toxic FiO_2 of 0.5
- Add PEEP, if patient cannot maintain oxygenation with above FiO_2
- Titrate PEEP to achieve adequate PaO_2 or at least > 60 mm Hg
- During weaning gradually decrease PEEP to less than 10 cm H_2O, then reduce SIMV rate to 1 breath/min
- Extubate when PaO_2 is adequate and conventional bedside tests to predict success in weaning have improved.

Possible Postoperative Complications

- Hypoxemia due to decreased FRC in relation to closing capacity (CC) leading to increased venous admixture increasing alveolar arterial oxygen gradient
- Increased physiological dead space
- Pneumonia
- Atelectasis
- Lobar collapse
- Aspiration
- Bronchopleural fistula (usually after 2 weeks)
- Pulmonary embolism.

BIBLIOGRAPHY

1. Andrew B Lumb. Nulls applied respiratory physiology. 6th edn; 2005.
2. Miller's Textbook of Anesthesia, 7th edn; 2010.

19

Thyroid Swelling

Subrata Pahari, Koel Mitra

Thyroid diseases are very common. So an anesthesiologist should know what he/she is going to encounter and be well-equipped by proper preanesthetic preparation, intraoperative management and postoperative management to prevent and manage complications when faced.

CASE SUMMARY

A 45-year-old female presented with diffuse swelling in her neck since 15 years that gradually increased in size. Her history of present illness was—dysphagia, weight loss, paroxysmal palpitation and heat intolerance for past 4 years.

- No history of pain, discharge, fever or change in voice.
- She is a known hypertensive on treatment with tablet atenolol 50 mg.
- No history of diabetes mellitus, COPD or any other comorbidity.
- No similar family history.

Personal History

Married with 2 children, last child birth 25 years back. Postmenopausal, nonsmoker, no history of addiction. Bladder and bowel normal.

On Examination

General survey—Thin built, facies—anxious, eyes normal, body weight—48 kg, height-5 ft 1". Pallor/cyanosis/jaundice/clubbing/oedema.

Pulse—70/min regular, all peripheral pulses palpable. No radioradial or radiofemoral delay. BP— 130/80 mm Hg.

Airway-Mouth opening >3 fingers. Neck movement within normal range. Mallampati class II. Dentition—normal.

Examination of the Neck

Inspection: A diffuses globular swelling in front of the neck between the 2 sternocleidomastoids extending up to the sternoclavicular junction. Moves with deglutition and protrusion of tongue. No visible scarring or pulsation or neck veins on the swelling.

PALPATION

From front—neck well-exposed and slightly hyperextended. Temperature—not raised. Texture-nodular. Overlying skin not fixed. Movable side-to-side but not above downwards. All borders are palpable we get below the swelling size—5 × 3 cm.

Palpation by Lahey's method: To palpate the right lobe it is pressed against the right hand and palpation done with opposite hand. In case of a small swelling it is palpated with the thumb while asking the patient to deglute.

Palpation from the back by slightly flexing the neck.

Kocker test: Slight compression on the lateral lobe produces stridor due to obstruction of the trachea.

Percussion—on manubrium sterni (in case of retrosternal extension it is dull). Auscultation—No bruit over the swelling.

Special Examination: Eye Signs

1. *Eyelid retraction (Dalrymple sign):* Eyelids are retracted above the upper sclerocorneal margin and white portion of the eye ball is seen.
2. *Lid-lag (Von Graefe's sign):* When the patient is asked to follow an object downward, the eyelids fail to follow the downward moving globe and upper globe is seen as lid retraction.
3. *Joffroy's sign:* There is absence of wrinkling of forehead when patient tries to look upwards with the face tilted downward.
4. *Möbius sign:* Difficulty in convergence.
5. *Stellwag's sign:* Absence of blinking.

Hands—warm moist (check for tremor by asking to extend both hands in front), no tremor. Systemic examination—(with special reference to CVS)—all within normal limits.

1. What is your diagnosis? How did you come to your diagnosis? (Must know)

Ans. Probably this neck swelling is due to the enlargement of the thyroid gland. The typical midline neck swelling that moves with deglutition and her signs and symptoms are classic for hyperthyroidism.

2. What is the anatomy of the thyroid gland? (Must know)

Ans. The thyroid gland consists of two lateral lobes connected by an isthmus. It is closely attached to the thyroid cartilage and to the upper end of the trachea and thus moves with deglutition. It is often palpable in normal woman. The gland is rich in blood supply from superior and inferior thyroid arteries.

Embryologically, it originates from the base of the tongue and descends to the middle of the neck. Remnants of thyroid tissue can sometimes be found at the base of the tongue (lingual thyroid) and along the line of descent.

The thyroid consists of follicles lined by cuboidal epitheloid cells. Inside the cell is the colloid which is an iodinated glycoprotein, thyroglobulin synthesized by the follicular cells. Each follicle is surrounded by basement membrane between which are parafollicular cells containing calcitonin secreting C cells.

3. How are the thyroid hormones synthesized in the body? (Must know)

Ans. Iodine is absorbed from the GI tract and appears in the plasma as inorganic iodide. The ability of the thyroid gland to concentrate iodide is known as *Iodide Trapping*. After entering the thyroid gland inorganic iodide is oxidized and subsequently incorporated into tyrosine residues to form monoiodotyrosine and di-iodotyrosine. Once iodide is bound to these compounds it is no longer diffusible. The precursors of the thyroid hormones are stored in the thyroid gland until coupling of monoiodotyrosine and di-iodotyrosine form tri-iodotyrosine (T3) and thyroxine (T4). The proteolytic action of thyroid-stimulating hormone (TSH) is responsible for the release of the physiological active thyoid gland hormones into circulation. T4 consists of 95% of the hormone released and the rest is T3. Approximately 100 mcg of thyroid hormone is released per day. T4 undergoes peripheral conversion to the more active T3. These hormones are released in combination with carrier proteins—thyroid binding globulin (TBG), proalbumin and albumin.

4. What is the role of hypothalamic-pituitary axis in thyroid function? (Must know)

Ans. The synthesis and release of thyroid hormones are regulated by thyroid-stimulating hormone (TSH) from the anterior pituitary. The secretion and release of TSH in turn is regulated by a negative feedback mechanism involving the circulating level of thyroid hormones and thyrotropin releasing hormone (TRH) from the hypothalamus.

5. What are the actions of the thyroid hormones? (Must know)

Ans. Thyroid hormones act on almost all cells of the body with effect on growth and development. Many of the actions of thyroid hormones are mediated by their binding to nuclear receptors that have a preferential affinity for T3.

Thyroid hormone regulates cellular glucose utilization by increasing glucose absorption from the GI tract, glycogenolysis and gluconeogenesis and also stimulates insulin secretion. It mobilizes fatty acids and lowers serum cholesterol and also increases protein catabolism.

CVS—Direct effect on the heart by increasing the heart rate, contractility with resultant increase in cardiac output.

Respiratory system: Thyroid hormone increases O_2 consumption and CO_2 production with compensatory increase in the respiratory rate and tidal volume.

Thyroid hormone is important for the development of the brain and skeletal maturation.

Increase in cellular metabolism and production of metabolic end products results in vasodilatation and enhanced tissue blood flow.

6. What are the causes of hyperthyroidism?

Ans.

Common causes: Graves disease, toxic nodular goiter and thyroiditis.

Rare causes: Neonatal hyperthyroidism, inappropriate secretion of TSH, exogenous iodide.

Very rare: Thyroid cancer, choriocarcinoma.

7. What are the causes of hypothyroidism?

Ans.

Primary hypothyroidism:

a. *Thyroid gland dysfunction:*
   - Chronic thyroiditis
   - Previous subtotal thyroidectomy
   - Previous radio-iodine therapy

b. *Thyroid hormone deficiency:*
   - Antithyroid drugs
   - Dietary iodine deficiency

Secondary hypothyroidism:
- Hypothalamic dysfunction (TRH deficiency)
- Anterior pituitary dysfunction.

8. What specific things you will seek in the history and examination of a patient with thyroid swelling?

Ans.

a. *History:* Residence in iodine deficiency area, taking of any medicines, their doses and duration.
   - Pressure effects on the esophagus—dysphagia
   - Pressure effects on the recurrent laryngeal nerve—hoarseness.

b. *Retrosternal extension:* Dysphagia, dyspnea
   - Unable to 'get under the swelling'
   - SVC obstruction—dilated veins in the neck and upper part of the chest
   - Elicitation of Pemberton's sign usually not practiced now a days due to its danger and advent of CT scan and MRI.

c. Intratracheal extension/invasion—dyspnea
   - Hemoptysis

d. *Thyroid hormone status:* Signs and symptoms of hypo- or hyperthyroidism

System involved	*Hyperthyroidism*	*Hypothyroidism*
General	Weight loss, malaise, muscle weakness, heat intolerance, palmar erythema, proximal muscle wasting, sweating	Malaise, cold intolerance, myalgia, arthralgia, dry coarse skin, loss of eye brows, hypothermia, myotonia, anemia, edema
CNS	Irritability, anxiety, hyperkinesis, tremor	Poor memory, depression, psychosis, mental slowness, dementia, poverty of movement, ataxia, slow relaxation of reflexes, deafness
CVS	Palpitation, angina, breathlessness, hypertension, cardiac failure, tachycardia, tachyarrhythmia, atrial fibrillation	Hypertension, bradycardia, heart failure, pericardial and pleural effusion
GI	Increased apetite, vomiting, diarrhea	Constipation, obesity
Genitourinary	Oligomenorrhea, loss of libido	Menorrhagia, loss of libido
Eye	Blurred or double vision, exopthalmos, lid lag, conjunctival edema. Eye signs are present mainly in Graves' disease	

Examination

General Examination

- Built
- Skin over tibia
- CVS
- *Pulse:* Tachycardia even in sleep, irregularity
- *BP:* Hypertension, wide pulse pressure.
- Rule out valvular lesions.
- *CNS:* Tremors in hands and fingers in outstretched hand.
- Fine tremors in tongue

Local Examinations

- Movement with deglutition
- Texture of the gland
- Auscultation over the gland for systolic bruit due to increased vascularity.

9. What is Graves' disease?

Ans. It is an autoimmune disease associated with diffuse enlargement and increased vascularity of the thyroid gland caused by Ig G antibody mimicking TSH. It is associated with exophthalmos and pretibial myxoedema. It can be associated with other autoimmune conditions.

10. What investigations will you recommend for this patient? (Must know)

Ans.

a. *Routine blood tests:* Total blood count, serum sugar, urea, creatinine and electrolytes, calcium, coagulation profile alkaline phosphatase.
b. *CXR:* To assess the size of the goiter and to detect tracheal deviation or compression. Lateral thoracic inlet views may also help to assess retrosternal prolongation.
c. *ECG:* To detect tachyarrhythmia and atrial fibrillation.
d. *CT Scan or MRI:* To determine the extent of the gland and location of tracheal narrowing or tracheal invasion.
e. *Nasal endoscopy:* Performed by otolaryngologist to document vocal cord function. This is important for the anesthetist to assess the laryngeal inlet and any deviation from normal.
f. *Flow volume loop analysis:* Flow-volume loops are generated by inhaling to total lung capacity (TLC) and exhaling to residual volume (RV). Fixed lesions of the upper airway, e.g. large goiter will produce plateaus in both inspiratory and expiratory cycle.

11. How will you test thyroid function? (Must know)

Ans.

a. Total serum T4—Normal 50-200 µg/L
   - Elevated in 90% hyperthyroid patients
   - Low in 85% hypothyroid patients
b. Serum T3—1-3 µg/L
c. Free T4 (10-30 pmol/L); Free T3 (3-8 pmol/L)—increased in hyperthyroidism and may be decreased in primary hypothyroidism.
d. Resin—tri-iodothyronine uptake (RT3)—Normal 30-40%. Distinguishes between thyroid gland dysfunction and altered TBG concentration.
e. Radioactive iodine (I^{131} uptake)—Normal 10-25% in 24 hours. Detects hyper or hypothyroidism.
f. TSH—0.3-3.5 mU/L. Increased in primary hypothyroidism. Decreased in hyperthyroidism.
g. *Thyroid scan:* Distinguishes between benign and malignant growth of the thyroid gland.
h. *USG:* Distinguishes between cystic and solid nodules of the gland.
i. Antibody to thyroid tissue—Hashimoto's thyroiditis.

12. How will you make the patient euthyroid? (Must know)

Ans. Treatment of hyperthyroidism

Drugs	*Dose*	*Mechanism of action*	*Side effects*
Carbimazole	Initial 15–40 mg daily. Maintenance—5–15 mg daily Takes 6–8 weeks time	Prevents synthesis of T3 and T4 by blocking oxidation of iodide to iodine	Rash, pruritus, arthralgias, bone marrow depression, agranulocytosis, crosses placenta-fetal hypothyroidism
Propylthiouracil	Initial 200–400 mg/day Maintenance—50–150 mg/day Takes 6–8 weeks time	Blocks iodination of tyrosine residues present in thyroglobulin. Inhibits conversion of T4-T3	Thrombocytopenia, aplastic anemia, agranulocytosis, hepatitis, nephritis, crosses placenta-fetal hypothyroidism
Iodide/Iodine	Lugol's solution—5 gm iodine solution in 10 gm. KI—0.1–.03 mL TDS	Large dose of iodide inhibits hormone production. Marked reduction of thyroid vascularity over 10–14 days	Hypersensitivity reaction, crosses placenta-fetal hypothyroidism
β blockers Propranolol [metoprolol, atenolol, nadolol]	40–80 mg TDS higher dose may be needed due to increase metabolism	Block peripheral adrenargic manifestation of thyroid hormone. Propranolol block peripheral conversion of T4 to T3	Negative inotropy and chronotropy, bronchospasm
Radioiodine (RAI)	Iodine 131 in ana empirical dose (usually 200–500 MBq)	Accumulates in the thyroid and destroys the gland by local radiation. It takes several months to fully effective	Contraindicated in pregnancy and breastfeeding. Immediate worsening of hyperthyroidism may occur but later hypothyroidism may develop
Steroids Dexamethasone Hydrocortisone	2 mg/6 hourly 50 mg/6 hourly	Reduce thyroid hormone	Hyperglycemia, gastric ulceration, bleeding

13. Treatment of hypothyroidism. (Must know)

Ans. Replacement therapy with levothyroxine is given for lifetime. Starting dose depends upon the severity of deficiency, age and fitness of the patient especially cardiac performance. Treatment initiates with 50-100 mcg/day as single dose, titrated to clinical improvement and by monitoring TSH.

Elderly or patient with IHD the initial dose is 25 mcg/day. If necessary beta blockers are to be added and serial to be done. Clinical improvement begins after 2 weeks and takes 6 months for complete resolution of symptoms.

14. What are the indications of thyroidectomy?

Ans. Indications are:
- Proven or suspected thyroid malignancy
- *Obstructive symptoms:* Dyspnea/dysphagia/hoarseness
- Retrosternal goiter even in the absence of obstructive symptoms.
- *Hyperthyroidism:* Unresponsive to treatment.
- Recurrent hyperthyroidism.

15. Anesthetic considerations in a patient of hyperthyroidism for subtotal thyroidectomy. (Must know)

a. When is the patient ready for elective surgery?

Ans. Elective surgery should be deferred until the patients have been rendered euthyroid. Importance should be placed on relief of symptoms. The patient should demonstrate a return of normal heart rate, pulse pressure and sinus rhythm. Tremors, anxiety, palpitations, dyspnea and heat intolerance should be relieved.

b. How would you premedicate the patient?

Ans. The goals of premedication in a hyperthyroid patient are to allay anxiety and to prevent activation of the SNS. Benzodiazepines, e.g. oral diazepam or central adrenergic blocker clonidine are appropriate. Sedative premedication may be prescribed if the airway is not involved.

Inj. Atropine is not recommended as it causes tachycardia and interferes with normal heat regulation. All antithyroid medications should be continued till the morning of surgery.

c. How would you monitor the patient? (Must know)

Ans. Monitoring should include noninvasive blood pressure (NIBP), pulse oxymetry, ECG, end-tidal carbon dioxide ($ETCO_2$) and core temperature, invasive BP monitoring where excessive blood loss is expected. Monitoring should be started before the administration of anesthesia.

If the patient is currently in or has a history of congestive heart failure (CHF) or myocardial dysfunction/ ischemia or renal impairment then the placement of invasive blood pressures, central venous pressure or a pulmonary artery catheter is necessary.

d. How would you induce this patient for anesthesia? (Must know)

Ans. Induction and intubation can proceed with standard technique if airway obstruction is not suspected. Any intravenous induction agent can be used except ketamine. Thiopentone is an attractive choice due to some antithyroid activity though insignificant.

Intubation with a reinforced ET tube is safe for the thyroid surgery to maintain a patent airway. Smaller size tube may be required.

If difficult intubation is anticipated from patient's history, clinical examination and investigations (CXR, CT scan) then inhalational induction or awake fiber optic intubation should be planned.

Inhalational induction using halothane or sevoflurane will maintain spontaneous respiration and airway patency. Isoflurane and desflurane may be too irritating to the airway for inhalational induction. Intubation should be attempted only after deep plane of anesthesia is achieved.

Patients with features of severe obstruction may require awake fiber optic intubation, anesthetizing the glossopharyngeal, superior laryngeal and recurrent laryngeal nerves. Judicious use of small amount of anxiolytic agents may be necessary to prevent precipitation of thyroid storm.

e. What precautions will you take during positioning? (Must know)

Ans. Thyroid surgery requires hyperextension of the head, care should be taken to support the head adequately to prevent strain on the cervical spinal ligaments and spine injury. In patients with restricted neck movement, the limit of comfortable neck extension should be assessed before and this position should be maintained during intubation and surgery. Chest should be auscultated after positioning of head.

Fixation of ET tube—properly secured.

Arms should be adducted by the patient's side, when at right angles to the body care should be taken to prevent hyperextension at the shoulder joint which can stretch the brachial plexus.

Eye protection with eye drops, eye pads is important especially for patients with proptosis.

f. How will you maintain anesthesia? (Must know)

Ans. Adequate depth of anesthesia should be maintained to avoid exaggerated sympathetic response to surgical stimulation. Isoflurane and sevoflurane can safely be used (Hyperthyroidism has not been seen to increase MAC of volatile anesthetics in animal studies). N_2O and potent short acting opioids can be used.

Appropriate selection of neuromuscular blocking drug is necessary. Pancuronium has the ability to increase heart rate thereby should be avoided. Muscle relaxants that provide greater cardiovascular stability—vecuronium, rocuronium should be used.

If there is coexisting muscle disease (muscle weakness) the initial dose of muscle relaxant should be reduced and subsequent doses carefully titrated. A nerve muscle stimulator is essential.

For the treatment of intraoperative hypotension a direct acting vasopressor (phenylephrine) is preferred.

Reversal is as usual with anticholinesterase and anticholinergic drugs. Glycopyrrolate is better than atropine due to its less chronotropic effect.

g. What are the possible intraoperative problems? (Must know)

Ans. Increased airway resistance is due to:

- Kinking of the endotracheal tube or obstruction of tube by secretion
- Surgeon may manipulate trachea during dissection of the gland.
- Accidental extubation due to hyperextension of the head, as the tube may migrate outwards.
- Chance of disconnection of the tube and the circuit under draping (as surgery occurs at the head end)
- Thyroid crisis—it can occur intraoperatively but more likely to occur 6–18 hours postoperatively.

h. What precautions should be taken during extubation? (Must know)

Ans. If tracheomalacia is suspected the fiber optic bronchoscope can be used to assess for airway collapse and vocal cord movement as the endotracheal tube and bronchoscope together are slowly pulled back. If tracheal collapse is noted the endotracheal tube with the bronchoscope is immediately readvanced.

Vocal cord assessment after thyroid surgery must be done by direct laryngoscopy and asking the patient to phonate 'e'. If there is any doubt about the patient's ability to protect the airway the endotracheal tube is to be left in place.

i. What are the regional anesthetic techniques for thyroid surgery? (Good to know)

Ans. Unilateral and bilateral deep cervical plexus block or superficial cervical plexus block with local supplementation has been described for thyroid surgery.

The block should performed under full monitoring with or without sedation but small amount of amnestic or anxiolytic agent is necessary to prevent thyroid storm.

Advantages of regional anesthesia include—the ability to assess spontaneous respiration and the voice as indicators of recurrent laryngeal nerve (RLN) integrity during the surgery.

Early postoperative pain control with little or no need for systemic analgesia.

Disadvantages: Deep cervical plexus block carries risk of phrenic nerve block leading to diaphragmatic impairment.

- Vertebral artery puncture.
- Epidural subarachnoid spread.

Local anesthetic containing epinephrine should be used with caution or avoided entirely.

Contraindications: Thyrotoxicosis, very large swelling with distorted anatomy and suspected malignancy.

Complications: Local anesthetic toxicity, hematoma, pneumothorax and requires excellent patient cooperation.

j. What are the possible postoperative problems and their management? (Must know)

Ans.

1. *Hemorrhage:* Postoperative bleeding can cause compression and rapid airway obstruction. signs of swelling or hematoma formation that is compromising the patient's airway should be immediately decompressed by removal of surgical clips or sutures. The suture remover should be kept at patient's bed side. Initially patient may be seated at 45° angle to facilitate venous drainage. Early intubation may be necessary before development of airway edema.

2. *Laryngeal edema:* It can occur as a result of traumatic tracheal intubation or in those who develop hematoma that can cause obstruction to venous and lymphatic drainage of the airway. It can usually be managed with steroids and humidified O_2. Racemic epinephrine through nebulization can be used to decrease laryngeal edema. If dyspnea worsens the patient should be intubated.
3. *Recurrent laryngeal nerve (RLN) palsy:* Trauma to the recurrent laryngeal nerve can be caused by ischemia, traction, entrapment or transection of the nerve during surgery and may be unilateral or bilateral. Unilateral vocal cord palsy will present with respiratory difficulty, hoarse voice or difficulty in phonation while bilateral palsy will result in paramedian position of the true cords and respiratory stridor. Bilateral RLN palsy requires immediate intubation and the patient may subsequently need a tracheostomy.
4. *Hypocalcemia:* Secondary to inadvertent excision of parathyroid tissue manifests within the first 3 days postoperatively. Acute airway obstruction in the immediate postoperative period is uncommon. The patient will complain of circumoral numbness and tingling of the hands and feet. If calcium is not supplemented the patient can develop stridor and airway obstruction secondary to muscle weakness. Severe hypocalcemia leads to seizure and tetany. (e.g. Carpopedal spasm, positive chvostek sign, etc.).
5. *Tracheomalacia:* Following tumor resection the airway should be examined by fiber optic bronchoscopy to detect tracheomalacia and determine whether or when tracheal extubation is appropriate. A rigid bronchoscope should be available to re-establish the airway if collapse occurs. Cardiopulmonary bypass should be on stand-by during the case.
   The possibility tracheomalacia should be considered in those patients who have had sustained tracheal compression by large goiter or tumors. A cuff leak just prior to extubation is reassuring but equipment should be available for immediate reintubation if it occurs. Absence of air leak around the tube at the end of surgery alert the possibility of tracheomalacia.
6. *Thyroid storm:* It is a life-threatening condition of exacerbation of hyperthyroid state precipitated by acute stress such as infection, surgery and trauma. It can occur intraoperatively but is more likely to occur 6–18 hours postoperatively.
   C/F:
   a. Temperature elevation with diaphoresis.
   b. Marked tachycardia may manifest as sinus tachycardia, atrial fibrillation or other ventricular dysrhythmia (ECG)
   c. Cerebral dysfunction ranging from agitation restlessness, confusion, seizures and coma.
   d. GI disturbances-vomiting and diarrhea.

   Differential Diagnosis: Malignant hyperthermia, heat stroke, pheochromocytoma.
   Management:
   a. Intravenous administration of cold crystalloid solution.
   b. Inj esmolol—continuous infusion 50–200 μg/kg/min
      OR
      Propranolol 0.5–3 mg IV every 2 mins up to 6–10 mg
      Advantage—prevents the peripheral conversion of T4–T3.
   c. When hypotension is persistent—inj hydrocortisone100–200 mg IV 6–8 hourly.
   d. Propylthiouracil—100 mg every 6 hrs per oral or by NGT.
   e. KI per oral or NaI 100–200 mg IV 8 hourly.
   f. Treatment of any suspected infection.

16. Discuss in brief the anesthetic considerations of a hypothyroid patient? (Must know)
Ans.

1. There is increased risk of hypothermia, hypoglycemia, hyponatremia, anemia, hypovolemia and adrenocortical insufficiency.

Preoperative investigations necessary are—Hb%, serum electrolytes, blood sugar, ECG and CXR, echocardiograph.

2. There is increased sensitivity to sedatives usually little or no sedative premed is needed.
3. Reduced anesthetic requirement anesthetic drugs should be used judiciously. Ketamine has the advantage of sympathetic stimulation. Fentanyl can be used in small titrated doses. N_2O is useful to reduce the requirement of volatile anesthetics as these patients are sensitive to their myocardial depressant effects. Intermediate duration nondepolarizing agents are preferable than long acting pancuronium.
4. Difficult airway patients may have large tongue, airway edema or enlarged thyroid gland making laryngoscopy and intubation difficult.
5. Reduced ventilator response to hypoxia/hypercarbia. So these should be avoided.
6. Gastroparesis is not uncommon in these patients. So, RSI may be considered.
7. Exaggerated hypotension is common and should be treated with judicious fluid replacement and ephedrine. Dopamine and epinephrine can be used for severe hypotension.
8. Monitoring Temperature, SpO_2, ECG, end tidal CO_2 ($ETCO_2$), NIBP, blood sugar and serum electrolytes.
   Invasive BP monitoring and CVP and CO monitoring are necessary when undergoing major surgery and in those with cardiovascular involvement.
   Neuromuscular monitoring with peripheral nerve stimulator is necessary as these patients have increased incidence of myasthenia and other muscular dystrophy.
9. Warming measures are instituted to prevent hypothermia.
10. Delayed recovery is common and postoperative ventilation may be required.
11. Regional anesthesia is preferable and should be used whenever possible. Due to possibility of reduced drug metabolism care should be taken with the dose of local anesthetic agent.

17. What is myxedema coma? (Must know)

Ans. The condition is mostly seen in elderly patients and tends to occur more often in women, has a high mortality rate.

Factors which trigger these conditions include drugs (sedatives, narcotics, anesthetics), infection, trauma, stroke, heart failure.

C/F: Spontaneous hypothermia, loss of deep tendon reflexes, hypoventilation, cardiovascular collapse, coma, death.

Treatment: Intravenous tri-iodothyronine, fluid resuscitation, glucose supplementation, hydrocortisone 100 IV 6–8 hourly.

Maintenance of temperature—gradual rewarming.

O_2 inhalation, if necessary intubation and ventricular support.

Adequate monitoring of CVS and temperature.

18. What are the implications of pregnancy in hyperthyroidism? (Must know)

Ans. During pregnancy, the increase in TBG causes increased total serum thyroid hormones, so free T4 and T3 levels should be used to determine the thyroid status.

Both propylthiouracil and methimazole cross the placenta and can affect fetal thyroid function. Propylthiouracil is less teratogenic than methimazole. In pregnancy in hyperthyroid patients the target T4 level is at or slightly higher than upper normal limit. This can be achieved by the lowest effective dose of antithyroid drugs. Aim is to ensure normal thyroid status in the fetus. Iodide is contraindicated in pregnancy as it causes fetal hypothyroidism so is radioactive iodine.

During pregnancy USG monitoring is necessary to assess fetal development and to check the presence of fetal goiter. The condition generally improves in 2nd and 3rd trimester allowing reduction or discontinuation of antithyroid drugs but it can exacerbate in the postpartum period.

Pre-eclampsia and preterm delivery are the major complications in mothers suffering from hyperthyroidism.

Women on thyroxine therapy for hypothyroidism should have their dose increased by up to 50% during pregnancy. Avoiding maternal and also fetal hypothyroidism is extremely important because of potential damage of fetal neural development and an increase risk of miscarriage.

19. How do you manage a patient with uncontrolled hyperthyroidism presenting for emergency surgery? (Must know)

Ans. When the surgery is emergent measures are to be taken to prevent thyroid storm. Reduction of hyperadrenergic state with continuous esmolol infusion or intravenous propranolol till heart rate is under control. Propranolol also prevents the peripheral conversion of T4–T3.

Antithyroid drugs should be given to prevent thyroid hormone synthesis. Propylthiouracil prevents the peripheral conversion of T4.

Intravenous dexamethasone or hydrocortisone be administered. They also prevent the peripheral conversion of T4.

In premedication use of anxiolytics are essential. Atropine is contraindicated.

Intraoperative sympathetic stimulation is to be prevented. Avoid—ketamine, pancuronium, and adrenaline. Adequate pain relief is necessary. Therapy should also be directed at correcting systemic decompensation. Fluids and electrolytes must be replaced.

Preoperative monitoring of HR, temp, invasive BP, $ETCO_2$, SpO_2, ECG, ABG. Invasive monitoring may be needed to guide the administration of vasopressor and inotropes when hypotension is unresponsive to fluids.

Postoperative intensive monitoring and good analgesia.

20. What are the special considerations in case of a huge goiter? (Must know)

Ans. The additional considerations in these cases:

Difficult ventilation/difficult intubation. Even if these patients can be well ventilated in awake state and do not have any respiratory obstruction they often cannot be ventilated just after induction and muscle relaxation due to loss of tone and the huge growth pressing down and totally occluding the trachea. So, awake fiber optic intubation/awake intubation may be planned, if not possible then inhalational induction followed by laryngoscopy and intubation and then muscle relaxation after securing the airway may be done.

Huge blood loss, injury to vital structures in the neck during surgery.

Tracheomalacia: Postoperative extubation to be done carefully if at all possible as confirmed by FOB.

21. What are the special considerations in case of a retrosternal goiter? (Must know)

Ans. Usually presents with features of mediastinal compression—dyspnea/dysphagia/hoarseness/SVC syndrome. They may also cause cerebral hypoperfusion, RLN palsies, horners syndrome, pleural and pericardial effusions. These cases are to be dealt carefully as cardiopulmonary bypass may be required for maintenance of oxygenation and perfusion dusion excision of the mediastinal mass.

BIBLIOGRAPHY

1. Adam L, Davies S. Anaesthesia for thyroid surgery. Anaesthesia tutorial of the week 162; 2009.
2. Anaesthetic management of patient with hyperthyroidism; Anaesthesiology. 1974;(Vol 41).
3. Barash P, Cullen B, Stoelting R. Clinical anaesthesia. 4th edn. 2006.
4. Farling PA . Thyroid Disease. BJA. 2000;85(1):15-28.
5. Goldman D. Surgery in patients with endocrine dysfunction. Med Clin. North Am. 1987;71:502-4.

6. Kaplan MM, Muier DA. Treatment of hyperthyroidism with radioactive iodine. Endocrinol metabolic clinic. North America. 1998:27(1).
7. Kumar P, Clark M. Clinical Medicine 6th edn. 2005.
8. Malhotra S, Sodhi V. Anaesthesia for thyroid and parathyroid surgery. Continuing Education in Anaesthesia critical care and pain. 2007;7(2).
9. Nicoloff J. Thyroid storm and myxedema coma. Med Clin. North Am. 1985;69:1005-12.
10. Spanknabul K, Chabot JA. Thyroidectomy using local anaesthesia. Journal of American College of Surgeons. 2005;201(3):375-85.
11. Stoelting RK, Miller RD. Anaesthesia and coexisting disease. 4th edn. Churchill Livingstone, 2002.
12. Tiegens S, Leimung M. Thyroid storm. Med Clin North Am. 1995;79:169-78.

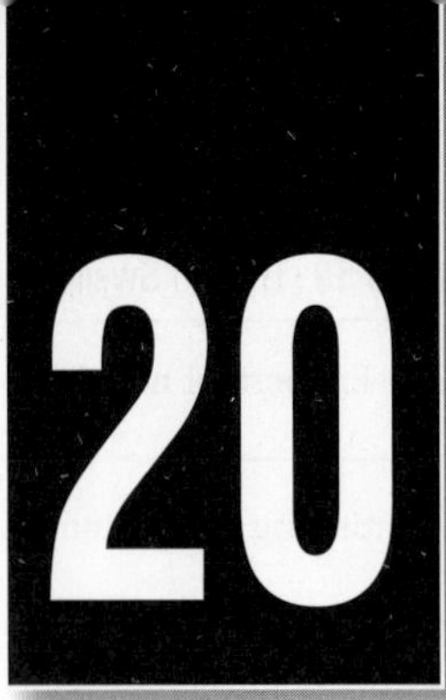

Abdominal Sepsis with Septic Shock, Posted for Exploratory Laparotomy for Source Control: An Approach

Sanghamitra Mishra

CASE

You are the on duty anesthesiologist. You are given a call to examine and plan for the anesthetic, for a patient who has just arrived in the emergency department and to undergo immergency laparotomy.

1. What is your case? (Must know)

Ans. The patient, Munilal Sharma, 48-year-old male, a caterer by profession, a resident of Khurda Odisha, has been admitted today (05.10.2013) half an hour ago at 9.30 pm with chief complaint of drowsiness, fever, nil urine for last 12 hours.

He was apparently alright 6 days back. To start with he had high fever with chills and rigor associated with right upper quadrant pain. He was given some medicine by the local doctor and his pain and fever subsided. But he gradually lost his appetite and generalized pain abdomen, following which, he stopped taking food and there was no bowel movement for last 3 days. The fever relapsed patient became bed ridden. Gradually he became drowsy and has not passed urine for last 12 hours.

There is no significant past, family, medication or addiction history.

On examination, patient is drowsy, disoriented and irritable. His pulse rate is 156/min, regular, palpable in all peripheral sites, but thready with associated cold extremities. There is no pallor, lymphadenopathy or pedal edema. There is mild ecterus. His temperature is 102°F. Examination of chest reveils normal heard sounds, but breath sound diminished over both lower lungs field. Respiration rate is 28/min, regular and thoracoabdominal pattern. Attached monitor shows poor pulse signal with a SpO_2 of 85%, BP of 86/46/58 mm Hg over right upper arm and normal ECG pattern. Examination of abdomen revealed absent bowel sound and generalized guarding. Preliminary investigation report yet to reach. Bed side glucose monitoring is 186 mg%. ABG shows PaO_2 of 66 with FiO_2 0.5.$PaCO_2$ of 28, Na 131, K 5.2, Cl 103, Hb 11 gm% and lactate of 3.2 mmol/L.

2. What are the five group of patients, where, speed and appropriateness of therapy administered in the initial golden hours of diagnosis are likely to influence outcome? (Must know)

Ans.
1. Stroke
2. Poly trauma
3. Acute myocardial infarction
4. Severe sepsis
5. Septic shock.

3. What is the definition of SIRS, sepsis, severe sepsis and septic shock as per surviving sepsis guidelines 2012? (Must know)

Ans. SIRS (Systemic inflammatory response syndrome) is defined as presence of two or more of the following criteria:
- Temperature >38°C or <36°C
- Heart rate >90 beats min^{-1}
- Ventilatory frequency >20 bpm or $PaCO_2$ < 4.3 kPa
- WBC <4 × 10^9 $liter^{-1}$ or >12 × 10^9 $liter^{-1}$ or >10% immature forms
- Sepsis is defined as the presence (probable or documented) of infection together with systemic manifestations of infection.
- Severe sepsis is defined as sepsis plus sepsis-induced organ dysfunction or tissue hypoperfusion.
- Septic shock is defined as sepsis-induced hypotension persisting despite adequate fluid resuscitation.

4. How do you define sepsis-induced tissue hypoperfusion? (Must know)

Ans. Sepsis induced tissue hypoperfusion is defined in SSC (surviving sepsis campaign) as:
1. Hypotension [systolic blood pressure (SBP) < 90 mm Hg or mean arterial pressure (MAP) <70 mm Hg or a SBP decrease > 40 mm Hg or less than two standard deviations below normal for age in the absence of other causes of hypotension] persisting after initial fluid challenge.

Or

2. Blood lactate concentration ≥ 4 mmol/L.

5. When do you diagnose sepsis-induced tissue hypoperfusion and organ dysfunction?

Ans. When the following findings are present in association with documented or suspected infection sepsis-induced tissue hypoperfusion or organ dysfunction has been said to occur:
- Sepsis-induced hypotension
- Lactate above upper limits of laboratory normal value
- Urine output < 0.5 mL/kg/hr for more than 2 hours despite adequate fluid resuscitation
- Acute lung injury with PaO_2/FiO_2 < 250 in the absence of pneumonia as infection source
- Acute lung injury with PaO_2/FiO_2 < 200 in the presence of pneumonia as infection source
- Creatinine > 2.0 mg/dL (176.8 μmol/L)
- Bilirubin > 2 mg/dL (34.2 μmol/L)
- Platelet count < 100,000 μL
- Coagulopathy (international normalized ratio > 1.5).

6. How do you define sepsis-induced hypotension? How it differs from therapeutic target/threshold, referred in sepsis bundles to consider for the use of vasopressors? (Must know)

Ans. Sepsis-induced hypotension is defined as a systolic blood pressure (SBP) < 90 mm Hg or mean arterial pressure (MAP) < 70 mm Hg or a SBP decrease > 40 mm Hg or less than two standard deviations below normal for age in the absence of other causes of hypotension. An example of a therapeutic target or typical threshold for the reversal of hypotension is seen in the sepsis bundles for the use of vasopressors. In the bundles, the MAP threshold is ≥ 65 mm Hg.

7. What are the possible signs/laboratory findings of systemic inflammation that should be sought for every 'septic-looking' patients ? (Must know)

Ans. *General variables*

- Fever (> 38.3°C)
- Hypothermia (core temperature < 36°C)
- Heart rate > $90/min^{-1}$ or more than two standard deviations above the normal value for age
- Tachypnea
- Altered mental status
- Significant edema or positive fluid balance (> 20 mL/kg over 24 hours)
- Hyperglycemia (plasma glucose > 140 mg/dL or 7.7 mmol/L) in the absence of diabetes.

Inflammatory variables

- Leukocytosis (WBC count > 12,000 μL^{-1})
- Leukopenia (WBC count < 4000 μL^{-1})
- Normal WBC count with greater than 10% immature forms
- Plasma C-reactive protein more than two standard deviation above the normal value
- Plasma procalcitonin more than two standard deviation above the normal value.

Hemodynamic variables

- Arterial hypotension (SBP < 90 mm Hg, MAP < 70 mm Hg, or an SBP decrease > 40 mm Hg in adults or less than two standard deviation below normal for age).

Organ dysfunction variables

- Arterial hypoxemia (PaO_2/FiO_2 < 300)
- Acute oliguria (urine output < 0.5 mL/kg/hr for at least 2 hours despite adequate fluid resuscitation)
- Creatinine increase > 0.5 mg/dL or 44.2 μmol/L
- Coagulation abnormalities (INR > 1.5 or aPTT> 60 s)
- Ileus (absent bowel sounds)
- Thrombocytopenia (platelet count < 100,000 μL^{-1})
- Hyperbilirubinemia (plasma total bilirubin > 4 mg/dL or 70 μmol/L).

Tissue perfusion variables

- Hyperlactatemia (> 1 mmol/L)
- Decreased capillary refill
- Mottling.

8. Which all are the most probable areas, where the anesthesiologists are frequently involved in the care of severely septic patients ? (Useful to know)

Ans. The areas are:

- The emergency department
- Operating theater
- ICU.

9. What are the points one should keep in mind while selecting antibiotics in severe sepsis and septic shock? (Must know)

Ans.

- Antimicrobial drugs are best given through intravenous route
- In sufficient dosage to achieve therapeutic concentration.

- The choice of agents should be based on the:
  - Clinical history
  - Physical examination
  - Likely pathogen(s)
  - Optimal penetration of antimicrobial drugs into infected tissues
  - Local pattern of sensitivity to antimicrobial agents.
- Broad spectrum agents should be used initially with one or more agents active against all likely bacterial/fungal/viral pathogens.
- Administration of effective intravenous antimicrobials within the first hour of recognition of septic shock (grade 1B) and severe sepsis without septic shock (grade 1C) as the goal of therapy.
- Antimicrobial regimen should be reassessed daily for potential de-escalation (grade 1B).
- Use low procalcitonin levels or similar biomarkers to discontinue empiric antibiotics in patients who initially appeared septic, but have no subsequent evidence of infection (grade 2C).
- Use combination empirical therapy for neutropenic patients with severe sepsis (grade 2B) and for patients with difficult-to-treat, multidrug-resistant bacterial pathogens such as *Acinetobacter* and *Pseudomonas spp.* (grade 2B). For patients with severe infections associated with respiratory failure and septic shock, use combination therapy with an extended spectrum beta-lactam and either an aminoglycoside or a fluoroquinolone for *P. aeruginosa* bacteremia (grade 2B). A combination of beta-lactam and macrolide for patients with septic shock from bacteremic *Streptococcus pneumoniae* infections (grade 2B).
- Empiric combination therapy should not be administered for more than 3–5 days. De-escalation to the most appropriate single therapy should be performed as soon as the susceptibility profile is known (grade 2B).
- Duration of therapy typically 7–10 days; longer courses may be appropriate in patients who have a slow clinical response, (undrainable foci of infection, bacteremia with *S. aureus*; some fungal and viral infections or immunologic deficiencies, including neutropenia) (grade 2C).
- Antimicrobial agents should not be used in patients with severe inflammatory states determined to be of noninfectious cause (UG).

10. What is the role of culture and what is the guideline for it in case of aseptic patient? (Must know)

Ans.

- Cultures of different samples as clinically appropriate should be done before antimicrobial therapy, if no significant delay (> 45 minutes) in the start of antimicrobial(s) occurs (grade 1C).
- At least 2 sets of blood cultures (both aerobic and anaerobic bottles) be obtained before antimicrobial therapy with at least 1 drawn percutaneously and 1 drawn through each vascular access device, unless the device was recently (<48 hours) inserted (grade 1C). Quantitative cultures of catheter and peripheral blood may also be useful for determining whether the catheter is the source of infection.

  Ref: Blot F, Schmidt E, Nitenberg G, et al. Earlier positivity of central venous-versus peripheral-blood cultures is highly predictive of catheter-related sepsis. J Clin Microbiol. 1998;36:105-9.
- The volume of blood drawn with the culture tube should be ≥ 10 mL.

  Ref: Mermel LA, Maki DG. Detection of bacteremia in adults: Consequences of culturing an inadequate volume of blood. Ann Intern Med. 1993;119:270-2.

11. What diagnostic tests, will you advice for suspected invasive candidiasis? (Must know)

Ans.

- 1,3 β-D-glucan assay (grade 2B)
- Mannan and anti-mannan antibody assays (grade 2C).

12. What do you mean by SOD and SDD? What are the guidelines in SSC-2012? (Useful to know)

Ans. SOD and SDD means selective oral decontamination and selective digestive decontamination respectively.

In 2012-SSC guideline, it has been suggested that selective oral decontamination (SOD) with oral chlorhexidine gluconate (CHG) and selective digestive decontamination (SDD) should be introduced and investigated and can then be instituted in health care settings and regions where this methodology is found to be effective to reduce incidence of VAP (grade 2B).

13. What are the clinical targets (goal) for early golden hour (6 hours) resuscitation (early goal directed therapy), once diagnosis of severe sepsis or septic shock is made? (Must know)

Ans. The recommended clinical target one has to reach within 6 hours of resuscitation are:

- CVP 8–12 mm Hg
- MAP ≥ 65 mm Hg
- Urine output ≥ 0.5 mL/kg/hr
- Superior vena cava oxygenation saturation ($ScvO_2$) or mixed venous oxygen saturation (SvO_2) 70% or 65%, respectively.

Another suggested clinical target is normalization of elevated lactate level.

14. What are surviving sepsis campaign (SSC) bundles? (Must know)

Ans. The SSC bundle has been divided into 2 parts.

A. *Tasks to be completed within 3 hours:*
   - Measure lactate level
   - Obtain samples for blood cultures prior to administration of antibiotics
   - Administer broad spectrum antibiotics
   - Administer 30 mL/kg crystalloid for hypotension or lactate level more than 4 mmol/L.

B. *Tasks to be completed within 6 hours:*
   - Use vasopressors (for hypotension not responding to initial fluid resuscitation) to maintain a mean arterial pressure (MAP) of 65 mm Hg
   - In the event of persistent arterial hypotension despite volume resuscitation (septic shock) or initial lactate 4 mmol/L (36 mg/dL):
     - Measure central venous pressure (CVP)*
     - Measure central venous oxygen saturation ($ScvO_2$)*
   - Remeasure lactate if initial lactate was elevated*.

15. Which is the vasopressor of choice in septic shock and severe sepsis ? (Must know)

Ans. Norepinephrine.

16. What is the role of phenylephrine in septic shock? (Useful to know)

Ans. With its almost pure α-adrenergic effects, phenylephrine is the adrenergic agent least likely to produce tachycardia, but it may decrease stroke volume and is therefore not recommended for use in the treatment of septic shock except in circumstances where norepinephrine is:

- Associated with serious arrhythmias
- Cardiac output is known to be high
- As salvage therapy when other vasopressor agents have failed to achieve target MAP (65 mm Hg)

Ref: Morelli A, Ertmer C, Rehberg S, et al. Phenylephrine versus norepinephrine for initial hemodynamic support of patients with septic shock: A randomized, controlled trial. Crit Care. 2008;12:R143.

Note: * Achieve the targets of CVP, $ScvO_2$ and normal lactate level.

17. How does epinephrine affects lactate clearance in severe sepsis and septic shock? (Nice to know)

Ans. Epinephrine may increase aerobic lactate production via stimulation of skeletal muscles' β2-adrenergic receptors and thus may prevent the use of lactate clearance to guide resuscitation.

18. When does the role of dobutamine infusion and PRBC transfusion arise, during early goal directed therapy in patients with severe sepsis and septic shock? (Must know)

Ans. During the first 6 hours of resuscitation, if $ScvO_2$ is less than 70% or SvO_2 equivalent of less than 65% persists with what is judged to be adequate intravascular volume repletion in the presence of persisting tissue hypoperfusion, then dobutamine infusion (to a maximum of 20 μg/kg/min) or transfusion of packed red blood cells to achieve a hematocrit of greater than or equal to 30% in attempts to achieve the $ScvO_2$ or SvO_2 goal are options.

19. In early goal directed therapy for severe sepsis and septic shock, the usual CVP target is 8–12 cm of H_2O. But what are the conditions, where you target for a higher CVP of 12–15? (Must know)

Ans. The conditions are:
- Mechanically ventilated patients
- Known pre-existing decreased ventricular compliance
- Increased abdominal pressure
- Pre-existing clinically significant pulmonary artery hypertension.

20. What are the recommendations for using steroid in septic shock? (Must know)

Ans.
- Intravenous hydrocortisone, the only steroid is recommended at a dose of 200 mg per day, in adult septic shock patients, if adequate fluid resuscitation and vasopressor therapy are not able to restore hemodynamic stability (grade 2C).
- ACTH stimulation test is not suggested to be used to identify the subset of adults with septic shock who should receive hydrocortisone (grade 2B).
- Tapering of steroid therapy is suggested, when vasopressors are no longer required for resuscitation of septic shock patients (grade 2D).
- It is recommended that corticosteroids should not be administered for the treatment of sepsis in the absence of shock (grade 1D).
- When hydrocortisone is used for septic shock, it is suggested that continuous infusion rather than repetitive bolus injections be used (grade 2D).

21. What is the recommended threshold for red cell transfusion in severe sepsis, once tissue hypoperfusion is resolved? In which group of patients one should target for a higher hematocrit? (Must know)

Ans.
- The red cell transfusion threshold, in sepsis, when tissue hypoperfusion is resolved is 7 gm%. One should target for a Hb level of 7–9 gm%. The transfusion threshold of 7 gm/dL contrasts with early goal-directed resuscitation protocols that use a target hematocrit of 30% in patients with low $ScvO_2$ during the first 6 hours of resuscitation of septic shock.
- A higher level than 7–9 gm% is targeted in the following group of patients
  - Myocardial ischemia
  - Severe hypoxemia
  - Acute hemorrhage
  - Ischemic coronary artery disease
  - Tissue hypoperfusion.

22. What is the recommendation for transfusion of FFP in case of coagulation abnormalities associated with sepsis? (Must know)

Ans. It is suggested that fresh frozen plasma should not be used to correct laboratory clotting abnormalities in the absence of bleeding or planned invasive procedures (grade 2D).

23. What is the recommendation for platelet transfusion in sepsis? (Must know)

Ans. In patients with severe sepsis, administer platelets prophylactically when counts are:
- <10,000/mm³ (10×10^9/L) (in the absence of apparent bleeding)
- < 20,000/mm³ (20×10^9/L) (if the patient has a significant risk of bleeding) and at
- ≥50,000/mm³ (50×10^9/L) (for active bleeding, surgery, or invasive procedures) (grade 2D).

24. What are the mechanical ventilation and other guidelines for ARDS associated with severe sepsis and septic shock? (Must know)

Ans.
- It is recommended to target a tidal volume of 6 mL/kg predicted body weight in patients with sepsis-induced ARDS (grade 1A).
- It is recommended that plateau pressures should be measured in patients with ARDS and initial upper limit goal for plateau pressures in a passively inflated lung be ≤30 cm H_2O (grade 1B).
- It is recommended that positive end-expiratory pressure (PEEP) should be applied to avoid alveolar collapse at end expiration (atelectrauma) (grade 1B).
- It is suggested that strategies based on higher rather than lower levels of PEEP should be used for patients with sepsis-induced moderate or severe ARDS (grade 2C).
- It is suggested that recruitment maneuvers should be used in sepsis patients with severe refractory hypoxemia ($PaO_2/FiO_2 \leq 100$ mm Hg) (grade 2C).
- It is suggested that prone positioning should be used in sepsis-induced ARDS patients with a PaO_2/FiO_2 ratio ≤ 100 mm Hg in facilities that have experience with such practices (grade 2B).
- It is recommended that mechanically ventilated sepsis patients should be maintained with the head of the bed elevated to 30–45 degrees to limit aspiration risk and to prevent the development of ventilator-associated pneumonia (grade 1B).
- It is suggested that noninvasive mask ventilation (NIV) should be used in that minority of sepsis-induced ARDS patients in whom the benefits of NIV have been carefully considered and are thought to outweigh the risks (grade 2B).
- It is recommended that a weaning protocol should be in place and mechanically ventilated patients with severe sepsis should undergo spontaneous breathing trials regularly to evaluate the ability to discontinue mechanical ventilation when they satisfy the following criteria:
  - Arousable
  - Hemodynamically stable (without vasopressor agents)
  - No new potentially serious conditions
  - Low ventilator and end-expiratory pressure requirements
  - Low FiO_2 requirements which can be met safely delivered with a face mask or nasal cannula.

  If the spontaneous breathing trial is successful, consideration should be given for extubation (grade 1A).
- Recommendation is there against the routine use of the pulmonary artery catheter for patients with sepsis-induced ARDS (grade 1A).
- A conservative (CVP <4 or PAWP <8 mm Hg) rather than liberal fluid strategy is recommended for patients with established sepsis-induced ARDS who do not have evidence of tissue hypoperfusion (grade 1C).
- In the absence of specific indications such as bronchospasm, it is recommended that beta 2-agonists should not be used for treatment of sepsis-induced ARDS (grade 1B).

25. What are the role of diagnostic imaging in case of severe sepsis and septic shock? (Must know)

Ans. The role of diagnostic imaging studies are to:
- Confirm the site of infection
- Exclude alternative pathology
- Guide radiological or surgical source control procedures.

26. What are the source control measures in case of severe sepsis and septic shock? (Must know)

Ref: Marshall JC, Al Naqbi A. Principles of source control in the management of sepsis. Crit Care Clin. 2009;25:753-68, viii–ix.

Ans. Source control measures should include:
- Drainage procedure (percutaneously under image-guidance or by an open surgical approach, for well circumscribed infection)
- Debridement procedures (physical removal of nonviable solid tissue usually by an open surgical approach)
- Definitive correction of anatomical abnormalities which has led to ongoing contamination of previously sterile tissue

A surgeon with experience in dealing with complex infections in critically ill patients must be involved in the decision-making process regarding a particular source control procedure.

27. For the above mentioned patient the attending surgeon requests you to take the patient for an exploratory laparotomy. What are the SSC-2012 guidelines as far as source control measures are concerned in a septic patient?

Ans.
- A specific anatomical diagnosis of infection requiring consideration for emergent source control be sought and diagnosed or excluded as rapidly as possible, and intervention be undertaken for source control within the first 12 hours after the diagnosis is made, if feasible (grade 1C).
- When infected peripancreatic necrosis is identified as a potential source of infection, definitive intervention is best delayed until adequate demarcation of viable and nonviable tissues has occurred (grade 2B).
- When source control in a severely septic patient is required, the effective intervention associated with the least physiologic insult should be used (e.g. percutaneous rather than surgical drainage of an abscess) (UG).
- If intravascular access devices are a possible source of severe sepsis or septic shock, they should be removed promptly after other vascular access has been established (UG).

Ref: O'Grady NP, Alexander M, Dellinger EP, et al. Guidelines for the prevention of intravascular catheter-related infections. Clin Infect Dis. 2002;35:1281-307.

28. As an anesthesiologist, what are the important points you should keep in mind while a septic patient is posted for diagnostic imaging? (Must know)

Ans. First of all an unstable septic patient if possible should not be shifted while undergoing resuscitation. Point of care USG and mobile CT scan should be used if available.

If at all it is necessary to shift the patient for diagnostic imaging all important therapeutic measures should be continued throughout the procedure, namely:
- Intravenous fluid resuscitation
- Antimicrobial therapy
- Mechanical ventilation.

Expert interpretation of all imaging studies should be sought to assist in planning the optimal management strategy.

29. In surviving sepsis campaign, 2012—International Guidelines for Management of Severe Sepsis and Septic Shock, what are the major categories of recommendations given? (Useful to know)

Ans. Major categories are as follows:

Ref: Surviving Sepsis Campaign: International Guidelines for Management of Severe Sepsis and Septic Shock: 2012, Critical Care Medicine. 2013;41(2):580-637.

A. *Initial resuscitation and infection issues*
- Initial resuscitation
- Screening for sepsis and sepsis performance improvement
- Diagnosis
- Antimicrobial therapy
- Source control
- Infection prevention.

B. *Hemodynamic support and adjunctive therapy*
- Fluid therapy of severe sepsis
- Vasopressors
- Inotropic therapy
- Corticosteroids.

C. *Supportive therapy of severe sepsis*
- Blood product administration
- Immunoglobulins
- Selenium
- History of recommendations regarding use of recombinant activated protein C
- Mechanical ventilation of sepsis-induced acute respiratory distress syndrome
- Sedation, analgesia, and neuromuscular blockade in sepsis
- Glucose control
- Renal replacement therapy
- Bicarbonate therapy
- Deep vein thrombosis prophylaxis
- Stress ulcer prophylaxis
- Nutrition
- Setting goals of care.

D. *Pediatric considerations in severe sepsis*
- Initial resuscitation
- Antibiotics and source control
- Fluid resuscitation
- Inotropes/vasopressors/vasodilators
- Extracorporeal membrane oxygenation
- Corticosteroids
- Protein C and activated protein concentrate
- Blood products and plasma therapies
- Mechanical ventilation
- Sedation/analgesia/drug toxicities
- Glycemic control
- Diuretics and renal replacement therapy
- DVT prophylaxis
- Stress ulcer prophylaxis
- Nutrition.

30. What are the recommendations for sedation, analgesia, and neuromuscular blockade in sepsis? (Useful to know)

Ans.

- Continuous or intermittent sedation is recommended to be minimized in mechanically ventilated sepsis patients, targeting specific titration endpoints (grade 1B)
- Neuromuscular blocking agents (NMBAs) are not recommended in the septic patient without ARDS due to the risk of prolonged neuromuscular blockade following discontinuation. If NMBAs must be maintained, either intermittent bolus as required or continuous infusion with train-of-four monitoring of the depth of blockade should be used (grade 1C)
- A short course of NMBA of not greater than 48 hours is suggested for patients with early sepsis-induced ARDS and a $PaO_2/FiO_2 < 150$ mm Hg (grade 2C).

31. What are the recommendations for glucose control in sepsis? (Must know)

Ans.

- A protocolized approach is recommended for blood glucose management in ICU patients with severe sepsis commencing insulin dosing when 2 consecutive blood glucose levels are >180 mg/dL. This protocolized approach should target an upper blood glucose ≤180 mg/dL rather than an upper target blood glucose ≤ 110 mg/dL (grade 1A)
- Blood glucose value is recommended to be monitored every 1–2 hours until glucose values and insulin infusion rates are stable and every 4 hours thereafter (grade 1C)
- Glucose levels obtained with point-of-care testing of capillary blood is recommended to be interpreted with caution, as such measurements may not accurately estimate arterial blood or plasma glucose values (UG).

32. What are the guidelines for renal replacement therapy in sepsis? (Useful to know)

Ans.

- Continuous renal replacement therapies and intermittent hemodialysis are suggested to be equivalent in patients with severe sepsis and acute renal failure (grade 2B)
- Use of continuous therapies to facilitate management of fluid balance in hemodynamically unstable septic patients is recommended (grade 2D).

33. What are the guidelines regard sodium bicarbonate therapy? (Must know)

Ans. Sodium bicarbonate therapy is not recommended for the purpose of improving hemodynamics or reducing vasopressor requirements inpatients with hypoperfusion-induced lactic acidemia with pH ≥7.15 (grade 2B).

34. What are the guidelines for deep vein thrombosis prophylaxis in sepsis? (Must know)

Ans.

- Daily pharmacoprophylaxis against venous thromboembolism (VTE) is recommended in patients with severe sepsis (grade 1B).

  This should be accomplished with daily subcutaneous low-molecular weight heparin (LMWH) (grade 1B versus twice daily UFH, grade 2C versus three times daily UFH).

  If creatinine clearance is <30 mL/min, use dalteparin (grade 1A) or another form of LMWH that has a low degree of renal metabolism (grade 2C) or UFH (grade 1A).
- Patients with severe sepsis are suggested to be treated with a combination of pharmacologic therapy and intermittent pneumatic compression devices whenever possible (grade 2C).
- Pharmacoprophylaxis is not recommended in septic patients who have a contraindication for heparin use (e.g. thrombocytopenia, severe coagulopathy, active bleeding, recent intracerebral hemorrhage) (grade 1B), but mechanical prophylactic treatment, such as graduated compression stockings or intermittent compression devices (grade 2C) are suggested, unless contraindicated. When the risk decreases pharmacoprophylaxis is suggested (grade 2C).

35. What is the comparative guideline between H_2 blocker or proton pump inhibitor use for stress ulcer prophylaxis in sepsis? (Useful to know)

Ans.

- Stress ulcer prophylaxis using H_2 blocker or proton pump inhibitor is recommended for patients with severe sepsis/septic shock who have bleeding risk factors (grade 1B)
- When stress ulcer prophylaxis is used, proton pump inhibitors rather than H_2RA is suggested (grade 2D)
- Patients without risk factors are not recommended for prophylaxis (grade 2B).

36. What are the nutrition guidelines in sepsis? (Must know)

Ans.

- Oral or enteral (if necessary) feedings are suggested, as tolerated, rather than either complete fasting or provision of only intravenous glucose within the first 48 hours after a diagnosis of severe sepsis/septic shock (grade 2C)
- Mandatory full caloric feeding in the first week should be avoided, rather low dose feeding (e.g. up to 500 calories per day), advancing only as tolerated is suggested (grade 2B)
- Intravenous glucose and enteral nutrition is suggested as against total parenteral nutrition (TPN) alone or parenteral nutrition inconjunction with enteral feeding in the first 7 days after a diagnosis of severe sepsis/septic shock (grade 2B)
- Nutrition with no specific immunomodulating supplementation is suggested in patients with severe sepsis rather than nutrition providing specific immunomodulating supplementation, (grade 2C).

37. What are the goals of care in severe sepsis and septic shock? (Nice to know)

Ans.

- Discuss goals of care and prognosis with patients and families (grade 1B)
- Incorporate goals of care into treatment and end-of-life care planning, utilizing palliative care principles where appropriate (grade 1B)
- Address goals of care as early as feasible, but no later than within 72 hours of ICU admission (grade 2C).

38. In the near future what are the rapid, non-culture-based molecular diagnostic methods going to replace standard diagnostic method for sepsis such as culture? And where these methods are considered to be beneficial? (Nice to know)

Ref: Tissari P, Zumla A, Tarkka E, et al. Accurate and rapid identification of bacterial species from positive blood cultures with a DNA based microarray platform: An observational study. Lancet. 2010;375:224-30.

Ans. *The future diagnostic methods are:*

- Polymerase chain reaction
- Mass spectroscopy
- Microarrays.

These methods are possibly beneficial for:

- A quicker identification of pathogens
- Major antimicrobial resistance determinants
- For difficult-to-culture pathogens
- In clinical situations where empiric antimicrobial agents have been administered before culture samples.

39. What are the risk factor for candidemia, where you should consider for empirical antifungal therapy? (Must know)

Ans. Risk factors for candidemia are:

- Immunosuppressed
- Neutropenic state

- Prior intense antibiotic therapy
- Colonization in multiple sites.

40. What should be the usual duration of antibiotic therapy in septic shock and severe sepsis? When should one opt for a longer duration of therapy? (Must know)

Ans. The duration of therapy should be 7–10 days. Longer courses may be appropriate in patients who have a:

- Slow clinical response
- Undrainable foci of infection
- Bacteremia with *S. aureus*
- Some fungal and viral infections
- Immunologic deficiencies, including neutropenia.

41. What foci of infections are amenable to source control measure? (Must know)

Ans. Foci of infection readily amenable to source control measures include:

- Intra-abdominal abscess
- Gastrointestinal perforation
- Cholangitis
- Pyelonephritis
- Intestinal ischemia
- Necrotizing soft tissue infection
- Other deep space infection, such as an empyema or septic arthritis.

Ref: Boyer A, Vargas F, Coste F, et al. Influence of surgical treatment timing on mortality from necrotizing soft tissue infections requiring intensive care management. Intensive Care Med. 2009;35:847-53.

42. What are the recommendations for fluid therapy in severe sepsis and septic shock? (Must know)

Ans.

- Crystalloids are the initial fluid of choice in the resuscitation of severe sepsis and septic shock (grade 1B).
- Hydroxyethyl starches should not be used for fluid resuscitation of severe sepsis and septic shock (grade 1B).
- Albumin can be used when patients require substantial amounts of crystalloids (grade 2C).
- Initial fluid challenge in patients with sepsis-induced tissue hypoperfusion with suspicion of hypovolemia should be used to achieve a minimum of 30 mL/kg of crystalloids (a portion of this may be albumin equivalent). More rapid administration and greater amounts of fluid may be needed in some patients (grade 1C).
- Fluid challenge technique should be applied wherein fluid administration is continued as long as there is hemodynamic improvement either based on dynamic (e.g. change in pulse pressure, stroke volume variation) or static (e.g. arterial pressure, heart rate) variables (UG).

43. What are the principles of anesthetic management of a septic patient requiring surgery for control of septic foci? (Must know)

Ans. *Preoperative preparation include:*

- Timely administration of appropriate intravenous antimicrobial therapy
- Resuscitation, aimed at optimizing major organ perfusion (before organ failure develops), is based on judicious use of fluids, vasopressors, and inotropes.

Ref: Russell JA, Walley KR, Gordon AC, et al. Dieter Ayers for the Vasopressin and Septic Shock Trial Investigators. Interaction of vasopressin infusion, corticosteroid treatment, and mortality of septic shock. Crit Care Med. 2009;37:811-8.

Intraoperative anesthesia management requires:

- Careful induction and maintenance of anesthesia
- Optimizing intravascular volume status
- Avoidance of lung injury during mechanical ventilation
- Ongoing monitoring of arterial blood gases, lactate concentration, hematological and
- Renal indices, and electrolyte levels.

Postoperative care overlaps with ongoing management of the severe sepsis syndrome patient in the intensive care unit. These patients are by definition, high risk, already requiring multiple supports, and require experienced and skillful decision-making to optimize their chances of a favorable outcome.

BIBLIOGRAPHY

1. Blot F, Schmidt E, Nitenberg G, et al. Earlier positivity of central venous-versus peripheral-blood cultures is highly predictive of catheter-related sepsis. J Clin Microbiol. 1998;36:105-9.
2. Boyer A, Vargas F, Coste F, et al. Influence of surgical treatment timing on mortality from necrotizing soft tissue infections requiring intensive care management. Intensive Care Med. 2009;35:847-53.
3. Marshall JC, Al Naqbi A. Principles of source control in the management of sepsis. Crit Care Clin. 2009;25:753-68, viii–ix.
4. Mermel LA, Maki DG. Detection of bacteremia in adults: Consequences of culturing an inadequate volume of blood. Ann Intern Med. 1993;119:270-2.
5. Morelli A, Ertmer C, Rehberg S, et al. Phenylephrine versus norepinephrine for initial hemodynamic support of patients with septic shock: A randomized, controlled trial. Crit Care. 2008;12:R143.
6. O'Grady NP, Alexander M, Dellinger EP, et al. Guidelines for the prevention of intravascular catheter-related infections. Clin Infect Dis. 2002;35:1281-307.
7. Russell JA, Walley KR, Gordon AC, et al. Dieter Ayers for the Vasopressin and Septic Shock Trial Investigators. Interaction of vasopressin infusion, corticosteroid treatment, and mortality of septic shock. Crit Care Med. 2009;37:811-8.
8. Surviving Sepsis Campaign: International Guidelines for Management of Severe Sepsis and Septic Shock: 2012, Critical Care Medicine. 2013;41(2):580-637.
9. Tissari P, Zumla A, Tarkka E, et al. Accurate and rapid identification of bacterial species from positive blood cultures with a DNA based microarray platform: An observational study. Lancet. 2010;375:224-30.

21

Transurethral Resection of the Prostate Syndrome in Patient with Hypertension and Ischemic Heart Disease

Baljit Singh, Indira Malik

1. Describe the anatomy of coronary circulation.

Ans. There are two main coronary arteries: The right coronary artery (RCA) and the left coronary artery (LCA). The RCA arises from the right sinus of Valsalva, runs anteriorly and then follows the right atrioventricular groove to reach the area where the interventricular septum (IVS) meets the atrioventricular groove. In 84% people, it terminates as the posterior descending artery (PDA) which is the sole supply of the posterosuperior IVS. It also gives a branch to the sinus node in 60% and the atrioventricular (AV) node in 85% people.

The LCA arises from the left sinus of Valsalva as the left main coronary artery (LMCA). It courses anteriorly and to the left, where it divides into the left anterior descending (LAD) and circumflex arteries (LCx). The LAD passes along the anterior interventricular groove and its major branches are the diagonals which supply the free wall of the LV. The septal branches supply the major portion of the IVS. The LCx arises at a sharp angle from the LMCA and courses towards the crux of the heart in the AV groove. If it gives rise to the PDA, the circulation is called left dominant. Here the left coronary supplies the entire IVS and AV node. In up to 40% people it also supplies the sinoatrial (SA) node. Up to 4 obtuse marginal branches arise from the LCx and supply the lateral wall of the LV.

All these epicardial arteries create small vessels that supply the outer third of the myocardium and penetrating vessels that anastomose with the subendocardial plexus. Significant collateral circulation does not exist at the microcirculatory level. Coronary artery disease (CAD) most commonly affects the epicardial muscular arteries with rare intramyocardial lesions.

Venous drainage of the myocardium is mainly to the coronary sinus (96%); remainder goes directly to the right atrium (RA).

2. How much is the normal coronary blood flow?

Ans. The normal coronary blood flow is 225 mL/min, which is 4–5% of the cardiac output. It is maximum during diastole.

Coronary perfusion pressure (CPP) = Aortic diastolic pressure – LVEDP

Blood flow falls to a low value during systole, especially in the subendocardial area because of compression of left ventricular muscle around the intramuscular vessels and small pressure gradient between aorta and left ventricle.

- Subendocardial autoregulation is hampered at 40 mm Hg.
- Subepicardial autoregulation is impaired at 25 mm Hg.

3. What is coronary reserve?

Ans. Myocardial ischemia causes intense coronary vasodilation. After a 10–30 seconds occlusion, restoration of perfusion pressure is accompanied by a marked increase in blood flow. This may be 5–6 times the resting flow. This is called reactive hyperemia. Oxygen extraction declines during hyperemia. The presence of high coronary flows when venous oxygen content is high suggests that mediators other than oxygen are responsible for this vasodilation. The difference between the resting coronary blood flow and peak flow during reactive hyperemia represents the autoregulatory coronary flow reserve, i.e. the further capacity of the arteriolar bed to dilate in response to ischemia. This coronary reserve is greater at higher perfusion pressures and lower MvO_2. It has been generally accepted that the coronary resistance vessels are maximally dilated when CPP is sufficiently reduced to cause myocardial ischemia.

4. What are the determinants of myocardial oxygen supply/demand ratio?

Ans.

a. Heart rate
b. Myocardial contractility
c. Wall stress (chamber pressure × radius/wall thickness)

Determinants of myocardial O_2 supply:

- Oxygen content = Hb × 1.34 × saturation (%) + 0.003 × pO_2
- *Coronary blood flow:* Depends on metabolic factors, autonomic factors, hormonal factors, endothelial modulation, anatomic factors, hematocrit and hypothermia.
- Flow in stenotic coronaries depends upon the length and degree of stenosis, presence or absence of collaterals, pattern of stenosis, coexisting diseases like diabetes and hypertension.

5. How is myocardial contractility assessed?

Ans.

- *Quantitative:* The contractile state of the heart is a dynamic intrinsic characteristic that is not influenced by preload or afterload. It can be approximated in a load independent fashion using the slope of the end systolic pressure-volume loops.
- *Qualitative:* Visual assessment of contractility when the pericardium is open. Transesophageal echocardiography (TEE) is a good means for qualitative estimation of LV contractility.

6. Describe the pathophysiology of myocardial ischemia.

Ans. Although the large epicardial arteries are capable of constriction and relaxation, in healthy persons they act as conduits and are referred to as conductance vessels, while the intramyocardial vessels are called resistance vessels. Abnormal constriction of either the epicardial or the intramyocardial vessels causes ischemia. The normal coronary circulation is dominated by the heart's requirements for oxygen. This is met by the ability of the coronary vascular bed to vary its resistance considerably while the myocardium extracts a high and relatively fixed percentage of oxygen. The resistance vessels adapt to physiological alterations in BP to maintain blood flow at levels appropriate to cardiac needs (autoregulation). By reducing the lumen of the vessels, atherosclerosis limits appropriate increase in perfusion while the demand is augmented in conditions like exercise or excitement. If the luminal reduction is severe, even basal myocardial perfusion is hampered. Coronary spasm, emboli, congenital abnormalities may also cause ischemia. Two or more causes of ischemia may coexist, such as increase in demand due to LVH and decrease in supply due to atherosclerosis and anemia.

7. Enumerate the risk factors for ischemic heart disease (IHD).

Ans. The high-risk factors for ischemic heart disease are:
- High levels of plasma LDL
- Low levels of plasma HDL
- Cigarette smoking
- Hypertension
- Diabetes mellitus
- Males/postmenopausal females.

8. What are the clinical manifestations of IHD.

Ans. The IHD manifests as myocardial ischemia:

In patients with known CAD, the most important risk factors to be assessed preoperatively are:

i. Amount of myocardium at risk
ii. Ischemic threshold, i.e. heart rate at which ischemia occurs
iii. Ventricular function, i.e. ejection fraction
iv. Stability of symptoms
v. Current medical therapy

Myocardial ischemia may present as:

a. *Stable coronary syndrome (stable angina pectoris):* Chest pain from myocardial ischemia is most commonly associated with physical exertion but may occur after meals or with emotion, i.e. whenever the myocardial oxygen demand exceeds the supply.

   Chronic stable angina often results from obstruction to the coronary blood flow by a fixed atherosclerotic lesion in one of the major epicardial vessels. However, even in the absence of such lesions, myocardial ischemia may occur due to coronary vasospasm, vasculitis, trauma or LV hypertrophy. In patients with chronic stable angina, a reproducible amount of exercise predictably precipitates angina. This angina threshold is an important guide to perioperative management. The level of exercise producing symptoms as described by the NYHA predicts both the risk of an ischemic event and operative mortality. Angina at rest implies a subtotal obstruction by atherosclerotic plaque which may be ruptured, coronary vasospasm or severe AS coexisting with CAD. Stable angina often responds to medical therapy and PCI.

b. *Acute coronary syndrome (unstable angina pectoris):* Also called as 'crescendo angina, preinfarction angina or unstable coronary syndrome.' It usually presents as rest angina of more than 20 minutes duration, within the first week of onset, new onset angina markedly limiting activity within two weeks of onset; increasing angina which is more frequent, occurs with less exercise and of longer duration. These symptoms indicate rapid growth, rupture or embolization of an existing plaque. These patients have a higher incidence of myocardial infarction (MI) and sudden death.

c. *Myocardial ischemia without angina:* It may be manifested by fatigue, rapid onset of pulmonary edema, arrhythmias, syncope or an 'angina equivalent' characterized as indigestion or jaw pain. Silent ischemia is more common in elderly and diabetic patients. Perioperative myocardial ischemia occurs in about 20% patients with risk factors for CAD, before noncardiac surgery, 25% during surgery and 40% postoperatively.

d. *Prior MI:* Patients who have suffered a preoperative MI more than 1 month previously; no longer appear to benefit from the delay of noncardiac surgery. However, a history of heart failure or arrhythmias helps to predict perioperative problems. Perioperative infarctions occur most often in the first 3 postoperative days and have 50–70% mortality. The risk of perioperative MI in patients who have undergone CABG previously is 1.2%.

9. What is the gradation of angina?

Ans. Angina is graded according to the NYHA classification:

Grade I: No symptoms with ordinary physical activity
Grade II: Symptoms with ordinary physical activity
Grade III: Symptoms with less than ordinary physical activity
Grade IV: Symptoms at rest

10. What is the normal oxygen extraction ratio?

Ans. Normal oxygen extraction ratio is 70%.

11. Explain coronary steal phenomenon.

Ans. Coronary steal occurs when the perfusion pressure for a vasodilated vascular bed is lowered by vasodilation in a parallel vascular bed, both being distal to a stenosis. There are two kinds of coronary steal: collateral and transmural.

Collateral steal is one in which one vascular bed distal to an occluded vessel is dependent on collateral flow from a vascular bed supplied by a stenotic artery.

Normally, vasodilator reserve is less in the subendocardium. In the presence of a stenosis, flow may become pressure dependent in the subendocardium whereas autoregulation is maintained in the subepicardium.

The term 'steal' is most appropriate when the vasodilatation is caused by a pharmacological agent like adenosine or dipyridamole which produce' luxury' perfusion in the vascular bed with coronary reserve.

12. What is coronary collateral anastomosis?

Ans. Coronary collaterals are anastomotic connections without an intervening capillary bed, between coronary arteries or branches of the same artery. In patients with CAD, well developed collaterals play a major role in preventing death and myocardial infarction. Individual differences in the capability to develop a sufficient collateral circulation is a determinant of the vulnerability of the myocardium in CAD. Human collaterals are tortuous and corkscrew shaped on angiography. Collaterals do not constrict in response to α receptor activation but dilate in response to β receptor stimulation. They also constrict in response to PGF2α and angiotensin II and vasopressin. Relaxation in response to nitroglycerin (NTG) is enhanced.

13. Define critical stenosis.

Ans. It is usually defined as a coronary constriction sufficient to prevent an increase in flow over resting values in response to increased myocardial oxygen demand. This is a greater degree of obstruction than an angiographically significant stenosis which is usually defined as a reduction in cross-sectional area of 75%. It can be demonstrated experimentally by blunting or abolishing reactive hyperemia.

14. Define dynamic coronary stenosis.

Ans. Patients with CAD have variable exercise tolerance during the day and between days. There is variation overtime in the severity of obstruction to blood flow imposed by coronary stenosis. Most stenoses are eccentric and have a remaining arc of compliant tissue. Even 10% shortening of the muscle in the compliant region can cause dramatic changes in lumen caliber.

15. What are the risk factors for unstable angina?

Ans. The risk factors can be classified as below.

Major

- Acute MI (< 7 days)
- Recent MI (7–30 days)

- Unstable angina
- Decompensated CHF
- Significant arrhythmias

Intermediate

- Current or prior angina pectoris
- Prior MI
- CHF
- Advanced age (> 70 years)
- Severely limited exercise tolerance
- Chronic renal insufficiency (creatinine > 2 mg/dL)

Minor

- Familial history of coronary artery disease
- Polyvascular status
- Uncontrolled systemic hypertension
- Hypercholesterolemia
- Smoking
- ECG abnormalities (arrhythmia, LVH, bundle branch block)
- Postinfarction (> 3 months), asymptomatic without treatment
- Post CABG or PTCA > 3 months and < 6 years, and no symptoms of angina on anti-anginal therapy

16. How is risk stratification done for perioperative ischemia according to the type of surgery?
Ans. *Major* vascular (reported cardiac risk often > 5%)

- Aortic and other major vascular surgery
- Peripheral vascular surgery.

Intermediate (reported cardiac risk generally 1–5%)

- Intraperitoneal and intrathoracic surgery
- Carotid endarterectomy
- Head and neck surgery
- Orthopedic surgery
- Prostate surgery.

Minor (reported cardiac risk generally <1%)

- Endoscopic procedures
- Superficial procedure
- Cataract surgery
- Breast surgery
- Ambulatory surgery.

17. What problems are anticipated in patients presenting for TURP?
Ans. Patients presenting for TURP most often belong to the geriatric age group and may be further classified as:

- Elderly (65–74 years)
- Aged (75–84 years)
- Very old (> 85 years).

They are likely to be suffering from various comorbid conditions like hypertension, CAD, diabetes mellitus, neurological and musculoskeletal disorders. These patients are also vulnerable to hypothermia, cardiovascular collapse due to blood loss or following subarachnoid block and altered mentation.

18. How will you evaluate cardiac function based on history and physical examination?
Ans.
- *Exercise capacity:* Poor exercise tolerance in the absence of pulmonary or other systemic disease indicates an inadequate cardiac reserve.
- Duke activity status index and approximate metabolic equivalents (1 METs = Oxygen consumption of 3.5 mL/kg/min).
  - *1–4 METs:* Light home activities, walk around the house, eating, dressing, bathing, using toilet, walking 1–2 blocks, and gardening.
  - *5–9 METs:* Climb a flight of stairs (20 steps 6 inches height), walk uphill, running short distance, golf, tennis, dancing, mountain walk, moderate cycling.
  - *>/= 10 METs:* Swimming, basketball, running rapidly.
  - *4 METs:* Good exercise capacity.

19. What are the tests for evaluating patients with known or suspected IHD?
Ans.
- *Noninvasive cardiological investigation:* Exercise ECG or Stress ECG—its utility is somewhat limited. Mean sensitivity and specificity are 68% and 77%, respectively, for detection of single vessel disease and 81% and 66% for multivessel disease. ECG is recorded both during and after the exercise which is usually done on a treadmill. Performance is usually symptom limited, the test is discontinued if there is evidence of chest discomfort, severe shortness of breath, dizziness, severe fatigue, ST segment depression > 0.2 mV or 2 mm, fall in systolic BP > 10 mm Hg or development of ventricular tachyarrhythmias. The ischemic ST segment response is generally defined as flat depression of the ST segment > 0.1 mV below baseline, lasting 0.08 sec. Upsloping or junctional ST segment changes are not considered characteristic of ischemia and do not constitute a positive test. T wave abnormalities, conduction disturbances and ventricular arrhythmias are also not diagnostic. Negative test, i.e. where 85% of the minimum predicted heart rate is not achieved are not diagnostic.
- *Pharmacological stress testing:* Dipyridamole Thallium Myocardial Imaging (sensitivity and specificity: 85–90%), Thallium Scintigraphy. (useful when exercise stress testing is not possible)
- *Dobutamine stress echocardiography:* Negative predictive value: 100%
- Coronary angiography
- CT and MRI for coronary artery circulation.
- *Positron emission tomography:* Regional myocardial blood flow and metabolism

20. What are the recommendations for ECG and noninvasive stress testing?
Ans.
A. *12 lead ECG:* Recommendations
  - *Class I:*
    - Vascular surgical procedure with at least 1 clinical risk factor
  - *Class IIa:*
    - Intermediate risk surgery with CAD, peripheral vascular disease, cerebrovascular disease
  - *Class III:*
    - Asymptomatic patient with low-risk surgical procedure

B. *Noninvasive stress testing:* Recommendations
  - *Class I:*
    - Active cardiac lesions need noncardiac surgery
  - *Class II a:*
    - 3 or more clinical risk with poor functional capacity need vascular surgery

- *Class II b:*
  - 1–2 risk factor and MET $< 4 \rightarrow$ intermediate risk surgery
  - 1–2 risk factor and MET $\geq 4 \rightarrow$ vascular surgery
- *Class III (Test not useful):*
  - No risk factor with intermediate risk surgery
  - Low-risk noncardiac surgery

21. When will the supplemental preoperative evaluation be done?
Ans.

Class I: Patients with suspected or proven CAD:
- High-risk results noninvasive testing
- Angina pectoris unresponsive to adequate medical therapy
- Unstable angina pectoris
- Nondiagnostic or equivocal noninvasive test in a high-risk patient

Class II:
- Intermediate-risk results during noninvasive testing
- Nondiagnostic or equivocal noninvasive test in a low-risk patient for a high-risk surgery
- Urgent surgery in a patient convalescing from acute MI
- Perioperative MI

Class III:
- Low-risk surgery in a patient with known CAD and low-risk results on noninvasive testing
- Screening for CAD without appropriate noninvasive testing
- Asymptomatic after coronary revascularization, with excellent exercise capacity (7 METs)
- Mild stable angina in patients with good LV function, low-risk noninvasive test results
- Not a candidate for coronary revascularization because of co-morbid illness
- Prior normal coronary angiogram within 5 years
- Severe LV dysfunction (LVEF $< 20\%$) and not candidate for revascularization
- Unwilling for coronary revascularization.

22. What are the recommendations for preoperative coronary revascularization?
Ans.
Class I:
1. Coronary revascularization before noncardiac surgery is useful in patients with stable angina, who have significant left main coronary artery stenosis (Level of evidence: A)
2. Coronary revascularization before noncardiac surgery is useful in patients with stable angina who have 3-vessel disease (Survival benefit is greater when LVEF $< 50\%$) (Level of Evidence: A)
3. Coronary revascularization before noncardiac surgery is useful in patients with stable angina who have 2-vessel disease with significant proximal LAD stenosis and either EF less than 0.50 or demonstrable ischemia on noninvasive testing (Level of Evidence: A)
4. Coronary revascularization before noncardiac surgery is recommended for patients with high-risk unstable angina or non-ST segment elevation MI (Level of Evidence: A)
5. Coronary revascularization before noncardiac surgery is recommended in patients with acute ST-elevation MI (Level of Evidence: A)

Class IIa: In patients in whom coronary revascularization with PCI is appropriate for mitigation of cardiac symptoms and who need elective surgery.

23. Summarize the plan for evaluating a patient with IHD scheduled for TURP.

Ans. See Flow chart 1

Flow chart 1 ACC/AHA 2007 Guideline for evaluating patient with IHD for noncardiac surgery

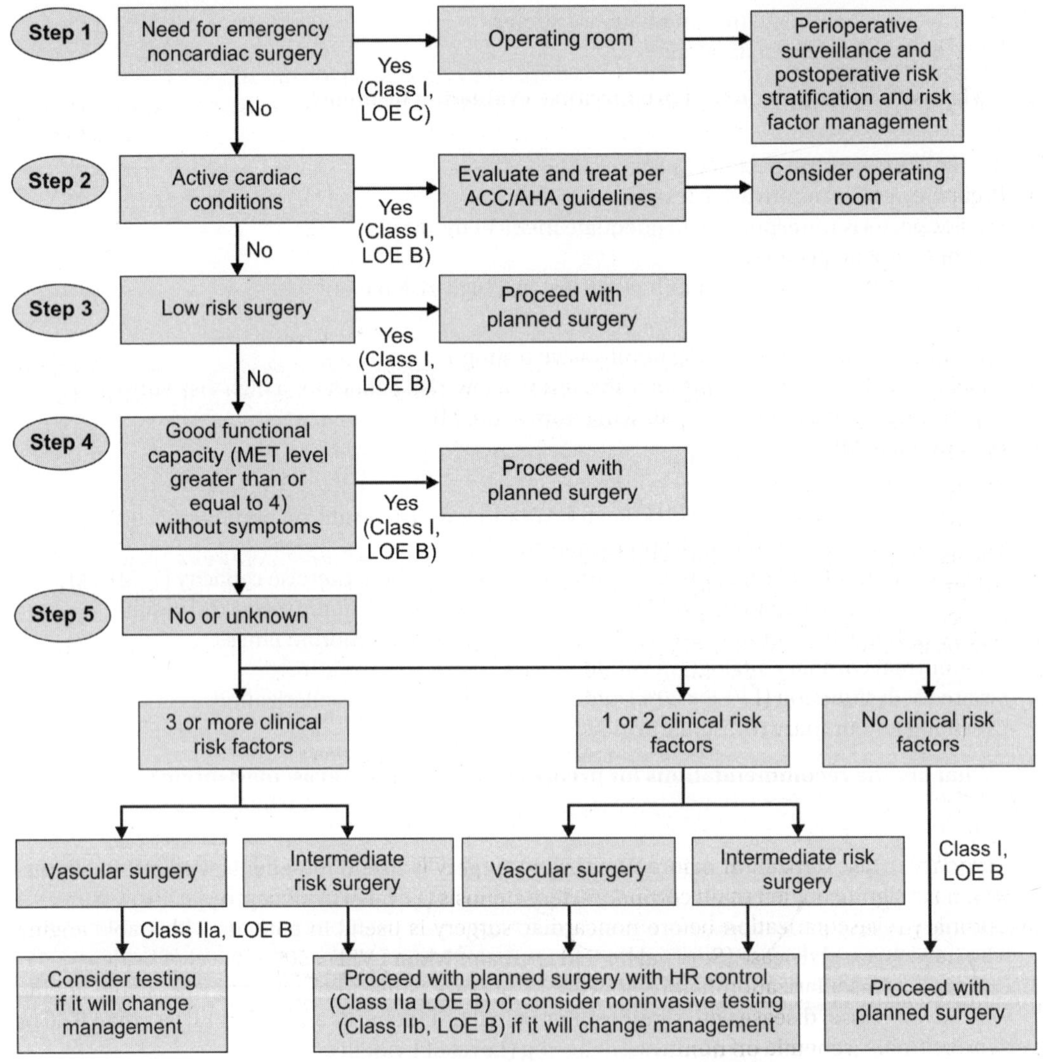

24. What investigations are required in the preoperative work-up of this patient?

Ans.

- Complete hemogram (Hb, TLC, DLC, platelet count, ESR)
- Renal function tests (Blood urea, creatinine)
- Serum electrolyte
- Blood sugar
- Urine R/E, culture sensitivity
- Blood grouping and cross-match
- Chest X-ray
- ECG

- Echocardiography
- PSA, serum alkaline phosphatase.

25. How will you prepare the patient for surgery?

Ans.

- Optimization of pre-existing conditions
- Continue all anti-hypertensive and anti-angina medications till the morning of surgery.
- It is better not to stop aspirin if it is being given as a therapeutic measure like post-acute coronary syndrome/post-stenting. If it is being given prophylactically, it may be stopped 5–7 days before.
- Advice regarding fasting status
- Preoperative anxiolysis
- H_2 blocker
- Arrangement of blood

Perioperative betablocker therapy

Class I

1. Beta blockers should be continued in patients undergoing surgery who are receiving beta blockers to treat angina, symptomatic arrhythmias, hypertension, or other ACC/AHA class I guideline indications (level of evidence: C).
2. Beta blockers should be given to patients under vascular surgery who are at high cardiac risk owing to the finding of ischemia on preoperative testing (level of evidence: B).

Class IIb

1. The usefulness of beta blockers is uncertain for patients who are undergoing either intermediate risk procedures or vascular surgery, in whom preoperative assessment identifies a single clinical risk factor (level of evidence: C).
2. The usefulness of beta blockers is uncertain in patients undergoing vascular surgery with no clinical risk factors who are not currently taking beta blockers (level of evidence: B).

Class III: Beta blockers should not be given to patients undergoing surgery who have absolute contradictions to beta blockade (level of evidence: C).

Perioperative statin therapy

Class I: For patients currently taking statins and scheduled for noncardiac surgery, statins should be continued (level of evidence: B).

Class IIa: For patients undergoing vascular surgery with or without clinical risk factors, statin use is reasonable (level of evidence: B).

Class IIb: For patients with at least 1 clinical risk factor, who are undergoing immediate risk-procedures, statins may be considered (level of evidence: C).

Perioperative calcium channel blockers

- Calcium channel blockers significantly reduce death/MI
- The majority of these benefits are attributable to diltiazem.
- Dihydropyridines and verapamil do not decrease the incidence of myocardial ischemia, although verapamil decreases the incidence of supraventricular tachycardia.

Risks associated with perioperative antiplatelet agents

- Aspirin should be stopped for at least 7 days prior to surgery when the risks of bleeding are high (major surgery) than the risk of withdrawing it or where the risks of even minor bleeding are significant (retinal or intracranial surgery).

- Patients receiving clopidogrel or ticlopidine should have a 5–7 day interval between stopping the drug and elective surgery.
- Abciximab to be stopped 7 days before, eptifibatide and tirofiban 8 hours preoperatively.

26. What would be your choice of anesthesia?

Ans. The two options for anesthesia are:

- Regional anesthesia
- General anesthesia

Regional anesthesia may be:

a. Combined spinal epidural block
b. Subarachnoid block
c. Epidural block.

Combined spinal epidural block: This is the most preferred choice as it gives the advantages of spinal as well as the epidural block without the commonly observed side effects of either. The spinal block ensures early onset of action and dense motor blockade while the indwelling epidural catheter ensures extension of the anesthesia, if required and also postoperative analgesia. Also the fall in blood pressure is less marked that the spinal block as the dose of the local anesthetic injected in the subarachnoid space is very low.

Subarachnoid block

This is another commonly used technique because of the following advantages:

- Technically easier to perform
- Lower incidence of PDPH
- Better relaxation of pelvic floor muscles
- Dense motor blockade
- Sacral sparing is minimal
- Early diagnosis of TURP syndrome—as the patient is conscious
- Decreased blood loss
- Improved postoperative pain control
- Low incidence of MI, DVT
- Homeostasis of neuroendocrine system and immune response better preserved after regional than general anesthesia.

However, subarachnoid block may cause precipitous drop in blood pressure in elderly patients suffering from hypertension and CAD due to sudden peripheral vasodilation and inadequate intravascular volume. The sudden fall in pressure may lead to ischemic manifestations.

Epidural anesthesia

Epidural anesthesia as the sole anesthetic technique is less preferred because of:

- Sacral segments inadequately blocked
- Less dense block
- Late onset
- Less predictable
- Technically difficult in elderly patients.

ASRA Guidelines: To be read from published 2010 guidelines

27. What is the level of regional anesthesia required?

Ans.

- Level of blockade should be up to the T_{10} dermatome to ensure that there is no discomfort due to bladder distention.
- S_3 level may be adequate in 25% patients, if the bladder is not allowed to overfill.

28. How would you monitor this patient?

Ans.

- *ECG:* Lead II and V5 simultaneously monitored detects ischemia in 90% cases
- NIBP
- Pulse oximetry
- Temperature
- Serum electrolytes
- Blood loss
- Patient responsiveness
- Pulmonary artery catheter (PAC) in severely compromised cardiac patients.
- *TEE:* Till induction of general anesthesia, it cannot be inserted and is expensive requiring skilled personnel. Earliest indication of ischemia will be diastolic dysfunction which can be detected by TEE.
- Blood glucose estimation
- ST segment monitoring
- Troponin

Recommendations for perioperative use of pulmonary artery catheters

Class IIb: Reasonable in patients at risk of major hemodynamic disturbances.

Decision based on 3 parameters: Patient disease, expected intra- and postoperative fluid shifts and practice setting whether experienced in interpretation of PAC based derivatives (level of evidence: B).

Class III: Routine use in patient at low-risk of developing hemodynamic disturbances is not recommended (level of evidence: A).

Intraoperative and postoperative use of ST-segment monitoring:

Class IIa: Useful to monitor patients with known CAD or those undergoing vascular surgery with computerized ST-segment analysis (level of evidence: B).

Class IIb: May be considered in patients with single or multiple risk factors for CAD who are undergoing noncardiac surgery (level of evidence: B).

Surveillance for perioperative MI

Class I: Postoperative troponin measurement is recommended in patients with ECG changes or chest pain typical of ACS (level of evidence: C).

Class IIb: Not well-established in patients who are clinically stable and have undergone vascular and intermediate risk surgery (level of evidence: C).

Class III: Not recommended in asymptomatic stable patients who have undergone low-risk surgery (level of evidence: C).

29. Enumerate the problems due to the surgical procedure?

Ans.

- TURP syndrome
- Bladder perforation
- Bleeding and coagulation abnormalities
- Hypothermia
- Transient bacterial septicemia
- Problems due to the lithotomy position.

30. What are the physiologic changes in lithotomy?

Ans.
- ↓ FRC/VC—Atelectasis and hypoxia, accentuated by Trendelenburg position and old age
- Elevation of legs ↑venous return →↑overload →↑BP
- ↓ venous return after lowering of legs → hypotension
- Exaggeration of hypotension with subarachnoid block.

31. What are the irrigating fluids commonly used?

Ans.

Distilled water (osmolality = 0)
- Advantages—Improved visibility
- Disadvantages—Hemolysis, hemoglobinemia, hemoglobinuria, hyponatremia

Glycine 1.5% (osmolality = 200 mOsm/L)
- Advantages—less TURP syndrome
- Disadvantages—transient postoperative visual impairment, hyperammonemia, hyperoxaluria

Sorbitrol 3.3% (osmolality = 165)
- Advantages—less TURP syndrome
- Disadvantages—hyperglycemia, lactic acidosis, osmotic diuresis

Mannitol (osmolality = 275)
- Advantages—isosmolar, not metabolized
- Disadvantages—osmotic diuresis, acute intravascular volume expansion

32. What are the characteristics of ideal irrigating fluid?

Ans. The fluid used must be clear, isotonic/nearly isotonic, cheap, nonhemolytic, electrically inert, rapidly excreted, no metabolism and nontoxic.

33. What is TURP syndrome?

Ans.
- It is a general term used to describe a wide range of neurologic and cardiopulmonary symptoms that occur when irrigating fluid is absorbed during TUR procedure, especially TURP.
- The main problems are due to rapid intravascular fluid expansion, hyponatremia, hypo-osmolality along with problems of irrigating solution.

34. What is the presentation of TURP syndrome?

Ans. See Flow chart 2
- Clinical manifestations:
  - *Mild:* Restlessness, nausea, shortness of breath, dizziness
  - *Severe:* Seizures, coma, hypertension, bradycardia, cardiovascular collapse.
- During regional anesthesia:
  - Dizziness, nausea, tightness in chest, breathlessness or lethargy
  - Restlessness, retching, confusion
  - ↑BP, ↓HR, cyanosis, hypotension
  - Tonic-clonic seizures, coma, arrest
- During GA
  - Rise followed by fall in BP, ST changes, nodal rhythm, widen QRS, delayed recovery.

Flow chart 2 Pathophysiology of TURP syndrome

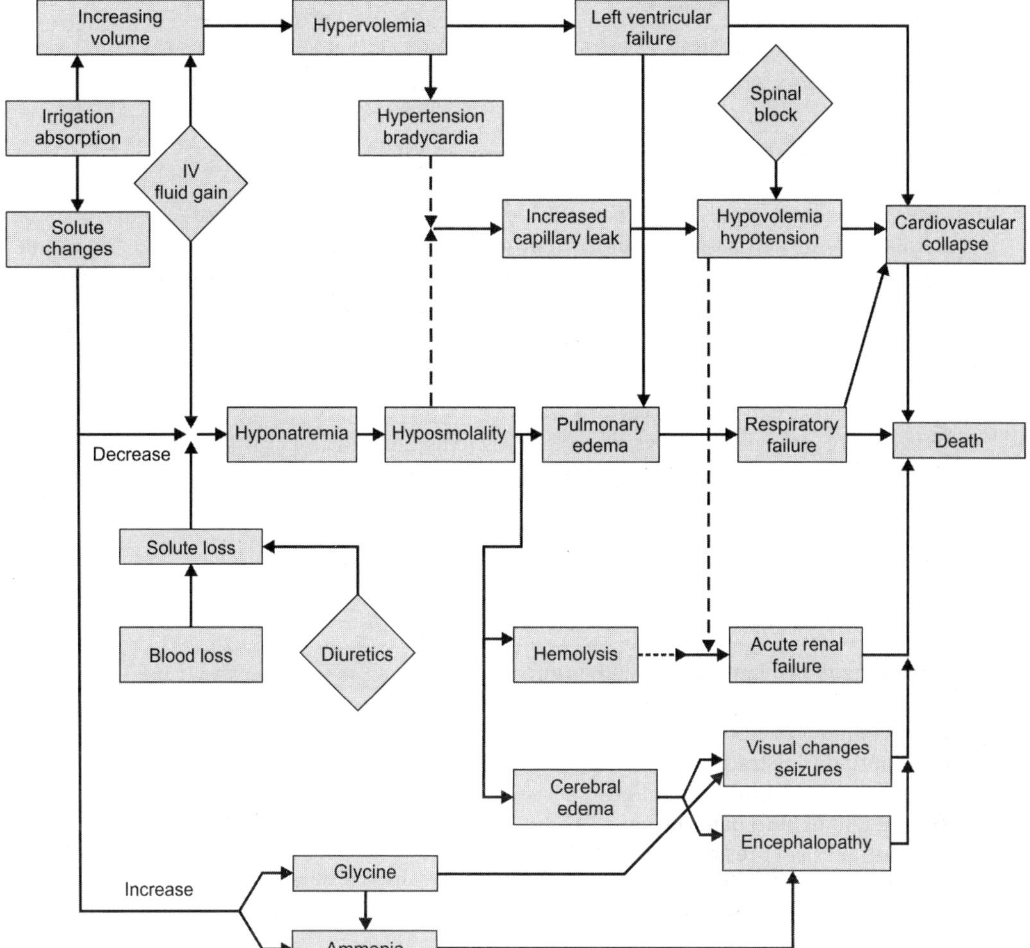

35. What is the pathophysiology of hyponatremia and how does it present?

Ans. Hyponatremia occurs due to absorption of sodium free irrigation fluid. The amount of fluid absorbed during the procedure is directly related to the number and size of venous sinuses opened, duration of resection, hydrostatic pressure of the irrigating fluid and venous pressure at the irrigant blood interface. To prevent excessive absorption of irrigation fluid, it has been recommended that:

- The resection time be limited to < 1 hour
- The bag of irrigating fluid should be suspended no more than 30 cm above the operating table at the beginning of resection and 15 cm in the final stages of resection.

Serum Na	CNS changes	ECG changes
120 Meq/L	Confusion, restlessness	Possible widening of QRS complex
115 Meq/L	Somnolence, nausea	Wide QRS complex and elevated ST segment
110 Meq/L	Seizures, coma	Ventricular tachycardia/fibrillation

36. What are the causes and clinical manifestations of TURP blindness?

Ans.

- Blindness associated with TURP occurs due to retinal dysfunction consequent to hyperglycinemia. Glycine acts as an inhibitory neurotransmitter in the brain, spinal cord and retina.
- *Clinical features:* Blurred vision, haloes around light, papillary dilation, unresponsive pupils
- Transient blindness in OT/PACU
- Recovery 8–48 hrs—after surgery.

37. Why is the pathophysiology of hyperammonemia?

Ans.

- Due to excessive absorption of glycine containing irrigation fluid
- Glycine → glyoxylic acid + ammonia (by oxidative deamination)
- Ammonia → urea (by arginine), blood ammonia levels as high as 834 μM/L have been documented. Hyperoxaluria has also been observed.
- *Clinical features:* Nausea, vomiting followed by coma (> 500 mmol/L)
- Prophylactic arginine can prevent this complication
- CNS depression is transient and recovers within 24–48 hours.

38. How would you prevent TURP syndrome?

Ans. TURP can be prevented with the following measures:

- Correct fluid and electrolyte imbalances
- Cautious administration of IV fluids
- Reduce surgical time (< 60 mins)
- Max-height of fluid bag = 60 cm
- Max-intravesical pressure = 15 cm of H_2O
- Vaporization technique
- Use of vasoconstrictor at operative site.

39. How would you measure fluid absorption?

Ans. Volume absorbed = preoperative Na ÷ postoperative Na × extracellular fluid – extracellular fluid

- Volumetric method
- CVP measurement
- Ethanol concentration in exhaled breath when ethanol labeled fluid irrigation

40. How will you manage a case of TURP syndrome?

Ans.

- Ensure oxygenation and circulatory support
- Terminate surgery, as soon as possible and change the irrigating fluid to NS
- Consider invasive monitoring if cardiovascular collapse occurs
- Send blood for electrolyte, creatinine, glucose, ABG
- Obtain 12 lead ECG

- *Treat mild symptoms (Na > 120):* Fluid restriction, loop diuretics
- *Treat severe symptoms (Na < 120):* 3% sodium chloride IV (< 100 mL/hr)
- Discontinue 3% sodium chloride when serum Na > 120
- The rate of correction should not exceed 12 Meq/L/24 hr
- Supportive therapy
- Hyposmolality rather than hyponatremia is the major detrimental factor since blood-brain barrier is impermeable to sodium but permeable to water.

41. How would you diagnose and manage bladder perforation?

Ans.

- In conscious patients
  - Decreased return of irrigating fluids
  - Pain abdomen
  - Pallor
  - Sweating
  - Nausea and vomiting
  - Abdominal rigidity
- Management
  - Oxygen inhalation
  - Fluids
  - Vasopressors
  - Intubation and ventilation
  - Laparotomy

42. What is the source of bleeding in TURP patients?

Ans. Bleeding depends upon:

- Weight of resected tissue (15 mL/gm)
- Surgical time (2–5 mL/min)
- Number of open prostatic sinuses
- Unrecognized arterial bleeding
- Associated infection
- Increased fibrinolysis due to release of urokinase

Assessment of blood loss

- Visual method is grossly inadequate
- Serial hemoglobin/hematocrit

43. What is the cause of hypothermia?

Ans.

- Prolonged and continuous irrigation with large amount of cold irrigating fluid.
- Reduced thermoregulatory capacity (decrease of 1°C/hr of surgery)
- Geriatric patients are more prone to hypothermia.

Prevention: Irrigation solution should be warm.

44. Describe postoperative care.

Ans.

- Monitor the patient in postanesthesia care unit
- Monitor vitals and CNS in general

- Continue routine analgesic—usually NSAIDS/opioids suffice
- Close monitoring for the occurrence of septicemia, characterized by fever, chills, hypotension and tachycardia

So, broad spectrum antibiotics must be considered in perioperative period.

BIBLIOGRAPHY

1. Dorsh. Understanding Anesthetic Equipment. 6th end, 2009.
2. Fleisher LA, Beckman JA, Brown KA, et al. ACC/AHA Guidelines 2007. Guidelines on perioperative cardiovascular evaluation and care for noncardiac surgery: Executive summary: A report of the ACC/AHA task force on practice guidelines. J Am Coll Cardiol. 2007;50:1707-32.
3. Joel A Kaplan. Kaplan's cardiac anaesthesia: The Echo era, 6th edn, 2011.
4. Miller's Text book of Anaesthesiology. RD Miller, 7th edn.
5. Paul G Barash, Clinical Anaesthesia. 6th edn.
6. Yao and Artusio's Anaesthesiology Problem Oriented Patient Management, 7th edn.

22

A 65-Year-Old Male Hypertensive Patient Posted for Elective Herniorrhaphy

Rahul Guha Biswas, Chandan Kumar Mandal

HYPERTENSION

An adult is considered to be hypertensive when the systemic blood pressure is 140/90 mm Hg or more on at least two occasions measured at least 1–2 weeks apart.

Classification of Hypertension for Adults

Category	*Systolic blood pressure (mm Hg)*	*Diastolic blood pressure (mm Hg)*
Normal	<120	<80
Prehypertension	120–139	80–89
Stage 1 hypertension	140–159	90–99
Stage 2 hypertension	≥160	≥100

- Adolescent 100/75 mm Hg
- Early childhood 85/55 mm Hg
- Infant 70/45 mm Hg.

Systolic hypertension is a marker of macrovascular disease and large arterial stiffening (atherosclerosis) and diastolic hypertension is a consequence of microvascular disease involving typically vessels less than 1 mm in size (arteriosclerosis).

1. Why HTN is so important?

Ans. Hypertension (HTN) is a significant risk factor for the development of ischemic heart disease and a major cause of congestive heart failure, cerebrovascular accident (stroke), arterial aneurysm, and end-stage renal disease.

2. What are the causes of HTN?

Ans. Systemic hypertension is characterized as essential or primary hypertension when a cause for the increased blood pressure cannot be identified. It is termed secondary hypertension when an identifiable cause is present.

3. What is essential hypertension?

Ans. Essential hypertension, which accounts for more than 95% of all cases of hypertension, is characterized by a familial incidence and inherited biochemical abnormalities.

4. What is the pathophysiology of essential hypertension?

Ans. Pathophysiologic factors implicated in the genesis of essential hypertension include increased sympathetic nervous system activity in response to stress, overproduction of sodium-retaining hormones and vasoconstrictors, high sodium intake, inadequate dietary intake of potassium and calcium, increased renin secretion, deficiencies of endogenous vasodilators such as prostaglandins and nitric oxide (NO), and the presence of medical diseases such as diabetes mellitus and obesity.

The final common pathway in the pathophysiology of essential hypertension is salt and water retention. Hypertension, insulin resistance, dyslipidemia, and obesity often occur concomitantly, and an estimated 40% of persons with hypertension also manifest hypercholesterolemia. Alcohol and tobacco use, obstructive sleep apnea is associated with essential hypertension.

5. What are the features of poorly controlled hypertension?

Ans. A history of ischemic heart disease, angina pectoris, left ventricular hypertrophy, congestive heart failure, cerebrovascular disease, stroke, peripheral vascular disease, or renal insufficiency suggests end-organ disease due to chronic, poorly controlled essential hypertension.

6. What are the laboratory investigations for essential hypertension?

Ans. Blood urea nitrogen and serum creatinine assays to quantify renal function. Hypokalemia in the presence of essential hypertension suggests primary aldosteronism. Fasting blood glucose concentrations should be evaluated because 50% of hypertensive patients manifest glucose intolerance. An ECG is useful for detecting evidence of ischemic heart disease or left ventricular hypertrophy.

7. What are the causes of secondary HTN?

Ans. Secondary HTN has a demonstrable cause but accounts for less than 5% of all cases of systemic hypertension. Renovascular hypertension due to renal artery stenosis is the most common cause of secondary hypertension.

- Renovascular disease
- Hyperaldosteronism
- Aortic coarctation
- Pheochromocytoma
- Cushing's syndrome
- Renal parenchymal disease
- Pregnancy-induced hypertension.

Other Causes of Secondary Hypertension (Table 1)

Table 1 | Isolated systolic, systolic and diastolic hypertension

Systolic and diastolic hypertension
- Renal
  - Renal transplantation
  - Renin-secreting tumors
- Endocrine
  - Acromegaly
  - Hyperparathyroidism
- Obstructive sleep apnea
- Postoperative hypertension
- Neurologic disorders
  - Increased intracranial pressure
  - Spinal cord injury
  - Guillain-Barre syndrome
  - Dysautonomia
- Drugs
  - Glucocorticoids
  - Mineralocorticoids
  - Cyclosporine
  - Sympathomimetics
  - Tyramine and monoamine oxidase inhibitors
  - Nasal decongestants

Sudden withdrawal from antihypertensive drug therapy (central acting and β-adrenergic antagonists)

Isolated Systolic Hypertension
- Aging with associated aortic rigidity
- Increased cardiac output
  - Thyrotoxicosis
  - Anemia
  - Aortic regurgitation
- Decreased peripheral vascular resistance
  - Arteriovenous shunts
  - Paget's disease

8. What are the treatments of essential hypertension?

Ans.
- Decreasing blood pressure by lifestyle modification and pharmacologic therapy is intended to decrease morbidity and mortality
- Standard goal of therapy
- Decrease systemic blood pressure to lower than 140/90 mm Hg, but in the presence of diabetes mellitus or renal disease, the goal is lower than 130/80 mm Hg.

Lifestyle modification:
- Weight reduction or prevention of weight gain
- Moderation of alcohol intake
- Increased physical activity
- Maintenance of recommended levels of dietary calcium and potassium
- Moderation in dietary salt intake
- Smoking cessation.

Pharmacologic therapy: Initiation of drug therapy should occur in tandem with lifestyle modification. After drug therapy is started, patients are seen every 1–4 weeks to titrate the antihypertensive drug dose and then every 3–4 months once the desired degree of blood pressure control has been achieved.

Lifestyle Modification

↓↓

Not at goal blood pressure (< 140/90 mm Hg) (< 130/80 mm Hg for those with diabetes mellitus or chronic kidney disease)

↓

Initial drug choice

↓

Without compelling indication		With compelling indication
↓		↓
Stage 1 hypertension	Stage 2 hypertension	Drugs for compelling indication
(SBP≥140–159 or DBP≥90–99 mm Hg) Thiazide type Diuretics for most May consider ACEI, ARB, BB, CCB Or combination	(SBP≥160 or DBP≥100 mm Hg) Two drug combination for most (usually Thiazide type Diuretics and ACEI, ARB, BB, CCB)	

(ACEI = Angiotensin converting enzyme inhibitor
ARB = Angiotensin receptor blocker
BB = Beta blocker
CCB = Calcium channel blocker)

DRUGS FOR COMPELLING INDICATION

Compelling indications for specific classes of antihypertensive drugs (Table 2).

Table 2 | Classes of antihypertension drugs

Comorbid condition	*Class of antihypertensive drugs*
Postmyocardial infarction	ACE inhibitor Aldosterone antagonist β-blocker
Heart failure	ACE inhibitor Aldosterone antagonist ARB β-blocker Diuretic
High risk of coronary artery disease	ACE inhibitor β-blocker Calcium channel blocker Diuretic
Diabetes	ACE inhibitor ARB β-blocker Calcium channel blocker Diuretic
Chronic kidney disease	ACE inhibitor ARB
Recurrent stroke prevention	ACE inhibitor Diuretic

9. What are the treatments of secondary hypertension?

Ans.

1. Surgical
2. Pharmacologic therapy

Surgical therapy: Surgical therapy is reserved for identifiable causes of secondary hypertension, and includes correction of renal artery stenosis via angioplasty or direct repair and adrenalectomy for adrenal adenoma or pheochromocytoma.

Pharmacologic therapy: For patients in whom renal artery revascularization is not possible, blood pressure control may be accomplished with ACE inhibitors alone or in combination with diuretics. Renal function and serum potassium concentration must be carefully monitored when ACE inhibitor therapy is initiated in these patients. Primary aldosteronism in women is treated with an aldosterone antagonist such as spironolactone, but amiloride is used in men for this purpose because spironolactone may cause gynecomastia.

10. What is hypertensive crisis?

Ans. Hypertensive crises typically present with a blood pressure of higher than 180/120 and can be categorized as either hypertensive urgency or a hypertensive emergency, based on the presence or absence of impending or progressive target organ damage.

11. What is hypertensive emergency?

Ans. Patients with evidence of acute or ongoing target organ damage (encephalopathy, intracerebral hemorrhage, acute left ventricular failure with pulmonary edema, unstable angina, dissecting aortic aneurysm, acute myocardial infarction, eclampsia, microangiopathic hemolytic anemia, or renal insufficiency) require prompt pharmacologic intervention to lower the systemic blood pressure.

12. What is the goal of therapy in hypertensive emergency?

Ans. The goal of treatment in hypertensive emergencies is to decrease the diastolic blood pressure promptly but gradually. A precipitous decrease in blood pressure to normotensive levels may provoke coronary or cerebral ischemia. Typically, mean arterial pressure is reduced by about 20% within the first 60 minutes and then more gradually. Thereafter, the blood pressure can be reduced to 160/110 over the next 2–6 hours as tolerated by the absence of symptomatic hypoperfusion of target organs.

13. What is hypertensive urgency?

Ans. Hypertensive urgencies are situations in which BP is severely elevated, but the patient is not exhibiting evidence of target organ damage. These patients can present with headache, epistaxis, or anxiety. Selected patients may benefit from oral antihypertensive therapy because noncompliance with or unavailability of prescribed medications is often the factor responsible for this problem.

14. What is the treatment for hypertensive emergency?

Ans. The initial choice of pharmacologic therapy for a hypertensive emergency lies in an analysis of the patient's comorbidities and the symptoms and signs at presentation.

Treatment of Hypertensive Emergencies (Table 3)

Table 3 | Treatment of hypertensive emergencies

Etiology/Manifestation	*Primary agents*	*Cautions*	*Comments*
Encephalopathy and intracranial hypertension	Nitroprusside, labetalol, fenoldopam, nicardipine	Cerebral ischemia may result from lower blood pressure due to altered autoregulation Risk of cyanide toxicity Nitroprusside increases intracranial pressure	Lower blood pressure may lessen bleeding in intracerebral hemorrhage Elevated BP often resolves spontaneously
Myocardial ischemia	Nitroglycerin	Avoid β-blockers in acute congestive heart failure	Include morphine and oxygen therapy
Acute pulmonary edema	Nitroglycerin, nitroprusside, fenoldopam	Avoid β-blockers in acute congestive heart failure	Include morphine, loop diuretic, and oxygen therapy
Aortic dissection	Esmolol, vasodilators Trimethaphan	Vasodilators may cause reflex tachycardia	*Goal:* Lessening of pulsatile force of left ventricular contraction
Renal insufficiency	Fenoldopam, nicardipine	Tachyphylaxis occurs with fenoldopam	May require emergent hemodialysis Avoid ACE inhibitors and ARBs
Preeclampsia and eclampsia	Methyldopa, hydralazine Magnesium sulfate Labetalol, nicardipine	Lupus-like syndrome with hydralazine Risk of flash pulmonary edema Calcium channel blockers may reduce uterine blood flow and inhibit labor	Definitive therapy is delivery ACE inhibitors and ARBs are contraindicated during pregnancy due to teratogenicity
Pheochromocytoma	Phentolamine, phenoxybenzamine, propranolol	Unopposed α-adrenergic stimulation following β-blockade worsens hypertension	
Cocaine intoxication	Nitroglycerin, nitroprusside, phentolamine	Unopposed α-adrenergic stimulation following β-blockade worsens hypertension	

Discuss Relevance of Commonly used Antihypertensive Drugs to Anesthesiologist

Mechanism of action	*Examples*	*Relevance to anesthetist*
Diuretics	Thiazide, frusemide	Electrolyte disturbance mainly hypokalemia
Vasodilator	Hydralazine, diazoxide	Tachycardia
Central sympathetic depression	Clonidine, methyldopa	Rebound hypertension if withdrawn
Beta blocker	Metoprolol, labetalol	Avoid in asthmatics, overt CHF, PVD
Alpha blocker	Phenoxabenzamine, phentolamine	Tachycardia
CCB	Amlodipine, nifedipine,	Precipitous hypotension
ACEI	Captopril, ramipril	Potentiate hypotension with anesthetic drugs

CHF—Congestive heart failure; PVD—Peripheral vascular disease

Discussion the Anesthetic Management in a Hypertensive Patient

1. Preoperative evaluation
2. Induction and maintenance of anesthesia
3. Postoperative management.

- *Preoperative evaluation:*
  - Determine adequacy of blood pressure control
  - Review pharmacology of drugs being administered to control blood pressure
  - Evaluate for evidence of end-organ damage
  - Continue drugs used for control of blood pressure.
- *Induction and maintenance of anesthesia:*
  - Anticipate exaggerated blood pressure response to anesthetic drugs
  - Limit duration of direct laryngoscopy
  - Administer a balanced anesthetic to blunt hypertensive responses
  - Consider placement of invasive hemodynamic monitors
  - Monitor for myocardial ischemia.
- *Postoperative management:*
  - Anticipate periods of systemic hypertension
  - Maintain monitoring of end-organ function.

Preoperative Evaluation

The incidence of hypotension and evidence of myocardial ischemia during maintenance of anesthesia is increased in patients who are hypertensive prior to induction of anesthesia.

The magnitude of blood pressure decreases during anesthesia is greater in hypertensive than in normotensive patients. However, intraoperative increases in blood pressure commonly occur in patients with a history of hypertension, whether or not the blood pressure is controlled preoperatively.

Patients with White coat syndrome who manifest anxiety-related hypertension are likely to have exaggerated pressor responses to direct laryngoscopy and are more likely than others to develop perioperative myocardial ischemia or to require antihypertensive therapy during the perioperative period.

End-organ damage (angina pectoris, left ventricular hypertrophy, congestive heart failure, cerebrovascular disease, stroke, peripheral vascular disease, renal insufficiency) should be evaluated preoperatively.

Important to review the pharmacology and potential side effects of the drugs. Many of these drugs interfere with autonomic nervous system function. Preoperatively, this may manifest as orthostatic hypotension. During anesthesia, exaggerated decreases in blood pressure seen with blood loss, positive pressure ventilation or sudden changes in body position could reflect impaired vascular compensation due to these autonomic inhibitory effects. Administration of vasopressors, such as phenylephrine and ephedrine, results in predictable and appropriate blood pressure responses in these patients.

Risk of rebound hypertension is there especially with β-adrenergic antagonists and clonidine, if they are abruptly discontinued.

Antihypertensive agents that act independent of the autonomic nervous system such as ACE inhibitors are not associated with rebound hypertension.

Decreased anesthetic requirements parallel the sedative effects produced by clonidine.

Hypokalemia (<3.5 mEq/L) despite potassium supplementation is a common preoperative finding in patients being treated with diuretics, but this drug-induced hypokalemia does not increase the incidence of cardiac dysrhythmias.

Hyperkalemia can be seen patients being treated with ACE inhibitors who are also receiving potassium supplementation or have renal dysfunction.

Angiotensin-converting enzyme inhibitors: There is a risk that hemodynamic instability and hypotension will occur during anesthesia in patients receiving ACE inhibitors. Three systems exist to maintain normal blood pressure. Following blunting of autonomic responses by induction of anesthesia and blunting of the renin-angiotensin-aldosterone system by an ACE inhibitor, the only remaining system to support blood pressure is the vasopressin system, and so blood pressure is likely to be volume dependent. Maintenance of intravascular fluid volume is crucial during surgery in patients on long-term treatment with these drugs. Surgical procedures involving major fluid shifts have been associated with hypotension in patients being treated with ACE inhibitors. This hypotension has been responsive to fluid infusion and administration of sympathomimetic drugs. Hypotension resistant to such measures may require administration of vasopressin or a vasopressin agonist. Careful titration of anesthetic drugs may prevent or limit the hypotension attributable to ACE inhibitors. It may be prudent to discontinue ACE inhibitors 24–48 hours preoperatively in patients at high risk of intraoperative hypovolemia and hypotension. The major disadvantage of drug discontinuation is the potential loss of blood pressure control.

Angiotensin receptor blockers: Angiotensin receptor blockers (ARBs) effectively treat hypertension by preventing angiotensin II from binding to its receptor. As with ACE inhibitors, blockade of the renin-angiotensin-aldosterone system by ARBs increases the potential for hypotension during anesthesia. The hypotensive episodes experienced by patients treated with ARBs may be refractory to conventional vasoconstrictors such as ephedrine and phenylephrine, necessitating use of vasopressin or one of its analogs. For these reasons, it is recommended that ARBs be discontinued on the day before surgery.

15. How would you anesthetize this patient?

Ans. *Premedication:* Alprazolam (0.5 mg) or lorazepam (1–2 mg) or nitrazepam (5–10 mg) night before and 2 hours before on the day of surgery.

Induction of Anesthesia

Induction of anesthesia with rapidly acting intravenous drugs may produce an exaggerated decrease in blood pressure due to peripheral vasodilatation in the presence of a decreased intravascular fluid volume.

Direct laryngoscopy and tracheal intubation can produce significant hypertension in patients with essential hypertension, even if these patients have been rendered normotensive preoperatively.

Evidence of myocardial ischemia is likely to occur in association with the hypertension and tachycardia that accompany laryngoscopy and intubation.

Patients at high risk for developing myocardial ischemia may benefit from maneuvers that suppress tracheal reflexes and blunt the autonomic responses to tracheal manipulation such as deep inhalation anesthesia or injection of an opioid, lidocaine, β-blocker, or vasodilator.

In addition, the duration of laryngoscopy is important in limiting the pressor response to this painful stimulus. Direct laryngoscopy that does not exceed 15 seconds in duration helps minimize blood pressure changes.

Maintenance of Anesthesia

The hemodynamic goal during maintenance of anesthesia is to minimize wide fluctuations in blood pressure.

Intraoperative hypertension:
Causes:
- The most likely intraoperative blood pressure change is hypertension produced by painful stimulation, i.e. light anesthesia
- Infiltration with vasopressors by surgeons
- Airway problem (ventilator malfunction, hypoventilation)
- Endobronchial intubation
- Hypercarbia
- Unusual or uncommon conditions like pheochromocytoma, hyperthyroidism, and malignant hyperthermia, raised ICP, fluid overload.

Management:
- First confirm that blood pressure change is real. (check BP cuff/pressure transducer level)
- Check for ventilator malfunction, deepen plane of anesthesia, inform surgeons and interrupt surgery if necessary, recheck drug errors or delivery of anesthesia (if any)
- Volatile anesthetics are useful in attenuating sympathetic nervous system activity responsible for pressor responses. Volatile anesthetics produce dose-dependent decreases in blood pressure, reflecting decreases in systemic vascular resistance and myocardial depression. There is no evidence that one volatile anesthetic drug is preferable to another to control intraoperative hypertension
- Antihypertensive medication by bolus or by continuous infusion is an alternative to the use of a volatile anesthetic for blood pressure control intraoperatively
- There is no evidence that a specific neuromuscular blocker is best for patients with hypertension. Pancuronium can modestly increase blood pressure, but there is no evidence that this pressor response is exaggerated in the presence of essential hypertension.

Intraoperative hypotension:
Cause: Most common cause is hypovolemia due to blood loss.
Management:
- Hypotension during maintenance of anesthesia may be treated by decreasing the depth of anesthesia and/or by increasing fluid infusion rate.
- Sympathomimetic drugs such as ephedrine or phenylephrine may be necessary to restore vital organ perfusion pressures until the underlying cause of hypotension can be ascertained and corrected creasing fluid infusion rates.
- Intraoperative hypotension in patients being treated with ACE inhibitors or ARBs is responsive to administration of intravenous fluids, sympathomimetic drugs, and/or vasopressin.
- Cardiac rhythm disturbances that result in loss of sequential atrioventricular contraction such as junctional rhythm and atrial fibrillation can also create hypotension and must be treated promptly.

Monitoring: Influenced by the complexity of the surgery.

Electrocardiography is particularly useful in recognizing the occurrence of myocardial ischemia during periods of intense painful stimulation such as laryngoscopy and tracheal intubation.

Invasive monitoring with an intra-arterial catheter and a central venous or pulmonary artery catheter may be useful if extensive surgery is planned and there is evidence of left ventricular dysfunction or other significant end-organ damage.

Transesophageal echocardiography is an excellent monitor of left ventricular function and adequacy of intravascular volume replacement.

Recovery: Coughing on the ET tube during emergence will increase BP. Adequate opioid should be given. These patients should be extubated in deeper plane of anesthesia if airway is safe.

Role of regional anesthesia: Spinal and epidural anesthesia can cause unpredictable and profound arterial hypotension in poorly controlled hypertensive patient. Well controlled hypertensive patients have more predictable response.

Local blocks, e.g. brachial plexus block or ankle block should always be considered in hypertensive patients as the potential hazards of general anesthesia are thereby avoided.

Emergency surgery: Aim for intraoperative BP should be around 140/90 mm Hg but avoid swings > ±20% from baseline blood pressure. Urine output should be closely monitored.

Postoperative Management

Postoperative hypertension is common in patients with essential hypertension. This hypertension requires prompt assessment and treatment to decrease the risk of myocardial ischemia, cardiac dysrhythmias, congestive heart failure, stroke, and bleeding.

Hypertension that persists despite adequate treatment of postoperative pain may necessitate administration of an intravenous antihypertensive medication such as labetalol. Gradually, conversion can be made to the patient's usual regimen of oral antihypertensive medication.

16. What are the common causes of postoperative hypertension?

Ans. Pain, emergence excitement, hypercarbia, intolerence to ET tube, full bladder, hypervolemia, peripheral vasoconstriction due to hypothermia.

BIBLIOGRAPHY

1. Aronson S, Fontes ML. Hypertension: a new look at an old problem. Curr Opin Anesth. 2006;19:59-64.
2. Barash PG, Cullen BF, Stoelting RK (Eds). Clinical anesthesia, 5th edn. Philadelphia: Lippincott Williams & Wilkins; 2006.pp.481-9.
3. Braunwald E. Heart disease, 6th edn. Philadelphia: WB Saunders; 2001.pp.950-5.
4. Coriat P, Richters C, Douraki T, et al. Influence of chronic angiotensin-converting enzyme inhibition on anesthetic induction. Anesthesiology. 1994;81:299-307.
5. Cucchiara RF, Benefiel DJ, Matteo RS, et al. Evaluation of esmolol in controlling increases in heart rate and blood pressure during endotracheal intubation in patients undergoing carotid endarterectomy. Anesthesiology. 1986;65:528-31.
6. Fleisher LA, Barash PH. Preoperative cardiac evaluation for noncardiac surgery. Anesth Analg. 1992;74:586-98.
7. Fleisher LA. Preoperative evaluation of the patient with hypertension. JAMA. 2002;287:2043-6.
8. Franklin SS. Systolic blood pressure: it's time to take control. Am J Hypertens. 2004;17:49S-54S.
9. Gold MI, Sacks DJ, Grosnoff DB, et al. Use of esmolol during anesthesia to treat tachycardia and hypertension. Anesth Analg. 1989;68:101-4.
10. Helfman SM, Gold MI, Delisser EA, et al. Which drug prevents tachycardia and hypertension associated with tracheal intubation: lidocaine, fentanyl, or esmolol? Anesth Analg. 1991;72:482-6.
11. Kapnoudhis P, Vaghadia H, Jenkins LC, et al. Esmolol versus fentanyl for preventing haemodynamic response to intubation in cardiovascular disease. Can J Anaesth. 1990; 37:S145.
12. Kasper DL, Braunwald E, Fauci AS, et al. (Eds). Harrison's principles of internal medicine, 16th edn. New York: McGraw-Hill; 2005.pp.1465-75.
13. Lee KW, Blann AD, Lip GY. High pulse pressure and nondipping circadian blood pressure in patients with coronary artery disease: relationship to thrombogenesis and endothelial damage/dysfunction. Am J Health. 2005;18:104-15.

14. Lovett JK, Howard SC, Rothwell PM. Pulse pressure is independently associated with carotid plaque ulceration. J Hypertens. 2003;21:1669-76.
15. Martin DE, Rosenberg H, Aukburg SJ, et al. Low-dose fentanyl blunts circulatory responses to tracheal intubation. Anesth Analg. 1982;61:680.
16. Prichard BN, Walder RJ. The syndrome associated with the withdrawal of beta-adrenergic receptor blocking drugs. Br J Clin Pharmacol. 1982;13 (Suppl 2):337S-43S.
17. Prys-Roberts C, Greene LT, Meloche R, et al. Studies of anaesthesia in relation to hypertension. II: haemodynamic consequences of induction and endotracheal intubation. Br J Anaesth. 1971;43:531
18. Sear JW, Jewkes C, Tellez JC, et al. Does the choice of antihypertensive therapy influence haemodynamic responses to induction, laryngoscopy and intubation? Br J Anaesth. 1994;73:303-8.
19. Seventh Report of the Joint National Committee on Prevention, Detection, Evaluation and Treatment of High Blood Pressure. Hypertension. 2003;42:1206-52.
20. Sladen RN. Perioperative hypertension. IARS review course lectures, Cleveland: International Anesthesia Research Society; 2002.pp.100-14.
21. Song D, Singh H, White PF, et al. Optimal dose of nicardipine for maintenance of hemodynamic stability after tracheal intubation and skin incision. Anesth Analg. 1997;85:1247-51.
22. Stoelting RK. Blood pressure and heart rate changes during short-duration laryngoscopy for tracheal intubation: influence of viscous or intravenous lidocaine. Anesth Analg. 1978;57:197.
23. Zipes DP, Libby P, Bonow RO, et al. (Eds). Heart disease, 7th edn. Philadelphia: WB Saunders; 2005. pp.968-73.

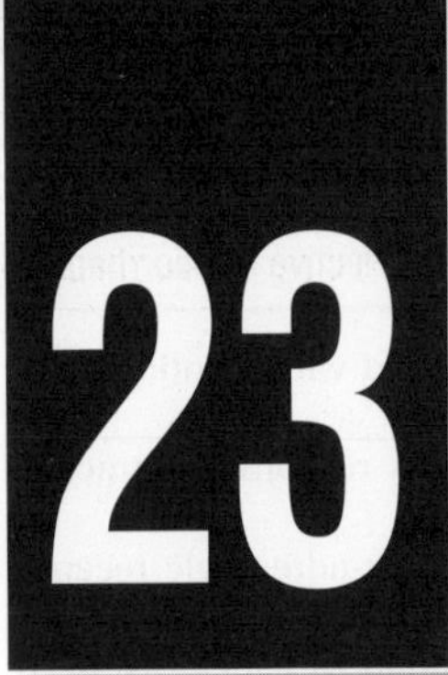

Renal Transplant Anesthesia

Kanak Kanti Kundu

CASE SUMMARY

A 32-year-old male presenting with generalized swelling of whole body with reduced urine output not responding to dialysis with serum creatinine level of 4.5 mg/dL and serum potassium level of 5.5 mEq/L. He has been planned for renal transplant.

1. How is renal transplant anesthesia different from other speciality anesthesia?

Ans. The main differences are as follows:

- Requires a thorough understanding of the metabolic and systemic abnormalities in end stage renal disease
- Familiarity with transplant medicine
- Expertise in managing and optimizing these patients for the best possible outcome
- Also, the associated co-morbid conditions increase the complexity of anesthesia, pain management perioperative morbidity and mortality.

Hence, a good perioperative management of these patients includes a multidisciplinary collaboration with well-planned anesthetic strategies.

2. Discuss in short the evolution of renal transplant surgery?

Ans. It was since the beginning of the 20th century that the endeavor to replace diseased organ began.

In 1950s, Dr Rene Kuss performed the first kidney transplantation that functioned in humans. The kidney worked without immunosuppression but was rejected 2 months later.

In 1954, Dr Joseph Murray performed the first successful kidney transplantation using a kidney from an identical twin.

Later in 1959, Dr Roy Calne first used Azathioprine. Dr Thomas Starlz used its combination with steroids. He also introduced antilymphocyte globulin.

Dr Folkert Belzer (1968) and Dr Jeffrey Collins (1969) developed organ preserving solutions.

Ref: Onaca N, Goldstein RM, Levy MF, et al. Regional Transplant Institute: an update on liver, kidney, and pancreas transplantation. Proceedings from Baylor University Medical Center. 2003;16:297–301.

Ref: Surman OS. The ethics of partial-liver donation. N Engl J Med. 2002;346:1038.

3. How will you classify donors?

Ans. They may be (a) cadaveric donors (nonheart beating or brain dead with beating heart) (b) living donors (related or unrelated).

Related may be identical twins or nonidentical.

Ref: Kälble T, Alcaraz A, Budde K, Humke U, Karam G, Lucan M, et al. Guidelines on Renal Transplantation European Association of Urology 2010.

4. Which is more advantageous—cadaveric or live donor and why?

Ans. Living donors are a better choice due to:

- Better results (both long- and short-term) compared to deceased donor grafts
- Consistent early function and easier management
- Avoidance of long waiting time for transplantation
- Less aggressive immunosuppressive regimens
- Emotional gain to donor
- Increases globally the kidney transplant rate.

Ref: Abouna GM. Ethical issues in organ and tissue transplantation. Exp Clin Transplant. 2003;1(2):125-38.

Ref: Banasik M. Living donor transplantation—the real gift of life. Procurement and the ethical assessment. Ann Transplant. 2006;11(1):4-6.

5. What are the exclusion criterion for living donors?

Ans. Absolute contraindications

- Age < 18 years
- Uncontrolled hypertension
- Diabetes mellitus
- Proteinuria (> 300 mg/24 hours)
- Abnormal GFR for age
- Microscopic hematuria
- High-risk of thromboembolism
- Medically significant illness (chronic lung disease, recent malignant tumor, heart disease)
- History of bilateral kidney stones
- HIV positive

Relative contraindications

- Active chronic infection (e.g. tuberculosis, hepatitis B/C, parasites)
- Obesity
- Psychiatric disorders

Ref: Kälble T, Alcaraz A, Budde K, Humke U, Karam G, Lucan M, et al. Guidelines on Renal Transplantation European Association of Urology, 2010.

6. What are the kidney donor selection and refusal criterion?

Ans. A diagnosis of brain death is required in a comatose subject who may potentially be a deceased organ donor. The potential donor must be evaluated for any transmissible pathological condition and the quality of any organ(s) being considered for transplantation. However, a short ischemia time is mandatory, as well as careful donor selection, particularly because older donors have more comorbidity.

The potential donor must be checked for:

Infectious Diseases

Infections to be checked for in potential donor

- Human immunodeficiency virus-1, -2 (HIV-1, HIV-2)
- Hepatitis C

- Hepatitis B surface antigen (HBsAg), anti-HBc; acute hepatitis (liver enzymes)
- Cytomegalovirus (CMV)
- Epstein-Barr virus (EBV), only in pediatric recipients
- Active syphilis
- Viral infection, sepsis, tuberculosis, infections of unknown etiology
- Family history of (or clinical signs that may be caused by) Creutzfeldt-Jacob disease

However, special exceptions exists for infections like HIV or hepatitis.

HCV-positive Donor

- In an HCV-positive recipient, transplant is allowed following informed consent
- In an HCV-negative recipient, there is a high-risk of disease transmission. However, transplant may be possible in emergency situations following informed consent.

HBsAg-positive Donor

- In an HBsAg-positive recipient (if HDV antigen is negative), transplant is allowed after informed consent
- In an HBsAg-negative recipient with high anti-HBs antibody titer and HBc positivity, transplant is allowed after informed consent
- In an HBsAg-negative recipient with intermediate/high anti-HBs antibody titer alone (HBc-antibody negative), transplantation may carry a higher risk but is allowed after informed consent
- In an HBsAg-negative recipient with undetectable anti-HBs antibody, transplant is allowed only in a life-saving situation, when HDV antigen is negative and following informed consent.

HBc-antibody-positive Donor

In liver transplantation, there is a high-risk (50%) of transmitting hepatitis B from an anti-HBc antibody positive donor to the recipient. In this situation, liver transplantation is allowed after informed consent.

Kidneys, heart and lungs carry a low, but not absent, risk of hepatitis B transmission, so kidney transplant is allowed in an HBsAg-positive recipient, or an HBsAg-negative recipient with anti-HBs antibody titer ≥10 mIU/mL, following informed consent.

In an HBsAg-negative recipient with no anti-HBsAg antibody, only life-saving transplants are allowed, after informed consent.

Malignant Tumors

A previous history of malignancy is not usually a contraindication for organ donation. However, there are some absolute contraindications that make a donor unsuitable for transplant. These are:

- Active cancer or
- History of metastatic cancer (with a few exceptions, such as testicular cancer)
- Cancers with high recurrence rates, such as advanced breast carcinoma, melanoma, leukemia, or lymphoma.

When a potential donor has experienced a brain hemorrhage of unknown etiology, metastasis must be excluded as a cause of intracranial bleeding.

However, a prior history of neoplasia is no longer an absolute contraindication for organ donation. Nonmelanoma low-grade skin cancer and selected CNS tumors that have not undergone surgical manipulation may also be acceptable. The following tumors are not contraindications to donation:

- Basal cell carcinoma
- Nonmetastatic spinocellular carcinoma of the skin
- Cervical carcinoma *in situ*
- Carcinoma *in situ* of the vocal cords.

Vascular Conditions and Renal Function

Important risk factors for organ failure are a prolonged history of diabetes mellitus or serious hypertension with retinal vascular damage. Factors for excluding potential donors or for considering a donor as a single—rather than a multiorgan donor include:

- Previous myocardial infarction
- Coronary bypass and angina
- Severe systemic vascular disease
- Events of long-lasting hypotension
- Oliguria
- Long-lasting intensive care stay.

Renal Functions

A donor's renal function should be evaluated at admission using creatinine clearance (Cockcroft-Gault formula), which corrects the serum creatinine value for age, body weight and sex. The urinary tract can also be assessed by 24 hours proteinuria and ultrasound kidney imaging, particularly in elderly donors. In many transplant centers, a calculated creatinine clearance level of 50 mL/min is at the lower range for kidneys usable for two recipients, independent of the histology of the organ, but according to the history of the donor, while other centers evaluate glomerular sclerosis and arteriolar sclerosis from renal biopsy.

Acute renal failure is not itself a contraindication.

Marginal Donors

The following criteria need to be considered in a marginal organ:

- Age over 70 years without other risk factors.
- Age between 60 and 70 years, with a history of diabetes mellitus, hypertension, clinical proteinuria up to 1 gm/24 h, or retinal vascular changes.
- Calculated creatinine clearance of 50 mL/min—the organs are still valuable for a single graft.
- Calculated creatinine clearance < 50 mL/min—the organs should be used as dual graft or discarded if histologically abnormal.
- Approximately 5-20% of glomerulosclerosis at biopsy with at least 25 glomeruli taken from both kidneys—the organs are still valuable for a single or double graft.
- More than 20% glomerulosclerosis—an individual decision has to be made based on renal function.

Ref: European best practice guidelines for renal transplantation (part 1). Transplantation Section II: Evaluation and selection of donors. Nephrol Dial Transplant. 2000;15(Suppl 7):39-51.

Ref: Scheinkestel CD, Tuxen DV, Cooper DJ, et al. Medical management of the (potential) organ donor. Anesth Intensive Care. 1995;23(1):51-9.

Ref: Penn I. Precautions to be taken to prevent transmission of neoplastic diseases in the grafting process. In: Organ and Tissue Transplantation in the European Union. London: Graham and Trotman; 1994.pp.33-41.

Ref: Cockcroft DW, Gault MH. Prediction of creatinine clearance from serum creatinine. Nephron. 1976;16(1):31-41.

Ref: Karpinski J, Lajoie G, Cattran D, Fenton S, Zaltzman J, Cardella C, et al. Outcome of kidney transplantation from high-risk donors is determined by both structure and function. Transplantation. 1999;67(8):1162-7.

7. Which kidney is usually recommended for donation and why?

Ans. Removal of the left kidney from a living donor is recommended because of the longer length of the left renal vein and easier surgical exposure. However if donors vascular supply reveals an abnormality then risk assessment should be done. It is recommended that the donor should always be left with the better kidney.

Ref: Berardinelli L. Technical problems in living donor transplantation. Transplant Proc. 2005;37(6):2449-50.

Ref: Desai MR, Ganpule AP, Gupta R, et al. Outcome of renal transplantation with multiple versus single renal arteries after laparoscopic live donor nephrectomy: a comparative study. Urology. 2007;69(5):824-7.

8. What are the different approaches for harvesting the kidney?

- *Open:* Classical transperitoneal, extraperitoneal, dorsal lumbar.
- *Laparoscopic:* Transperitoneal or retroperitoneoscopic
- Robotic hand assisted donor nephrectomy.

Before starting the incision, the donor's diuresis is increased, usually by giving mannitol, 25 gm. Arterial spasm may be prevented with externally applied papaverine.

Laparoscopic kidney removal is a less traumatic technique, entails less pain, a shorter hospital stay and may encourage more people to consider donation.

Ref: Sasaki TM, Finelli F, Bugarin E, Fowlkes D, Trollinger J, Barhyte DY, et al. Is laparoscopic donor nephrectomy the new criterion standard? Arch Surg. 2000;135(8):943-7.

Ref: Horgan S, Benedetti E, Moser F. Robotically assisted donor nephrectomy for kidney transplant. Am J Surg. 2004;188:45-51.

9. How shall you evaluate the donor for anesthetic fitness?

Ans. Evaluation of a potential donor may be performed by an independent physician and consists of a:

- Complete history and physical examination
- Routine laboratory testing
- Serological evaluation for Epstein-Barr virus (EBV), herpes virus, cytomegalovirus (CMV), human immunodeficiency virus (HIV) and hepatitis B and C viruses (HBV, HCV).
- Routine evaluation should also include urinalysis and culture, together with 24-hour urine collection for creatinine clearance and protein excretion.

A borderline hypertensive blood pressure should be measured on at least three, and as many as 10, separate occasions.

- Renal angiography is indicated only if spiral computed tomography (CT) scan with three-dimensional reconstruction or MRI angiography with reconstruction are not available.
- 5 hours glucose tolerance test for potential donors for siblings with diabetes
- 24 hours urine specimen must be free of proteinuria.

A history of thromboembolism or thrombophlebitis places a potential donor at increased risk of pulmonary embolism and contraindicates donation, as does advanced heart disease or a history of malignant neoplasia.

- Obesity is a relative contraindication for any potential donor > 30% above ideal body weight.

Ref: Kälble T, Alcaraz A, Budde K, Humke U, Karam G, Lucan M, et al. Guidelines on Renal Transplantation European Association of Urology, 2010.

10. What are the special anesthetic considerations while retrieving kidney from living donor?
Ans. The patient is placed in either a right or a left lateral position with the table flexed and the kidney rest elevated.

Invasive monitoring is not required, and one or two large peripheral intravenous lines suffice. Some centers have 2 U of blood (frequently autologous) available in the operating room in case of injury to major vascular structures, which would require emergency exploratory laparotomy. To maintain good diuresis and to optimize graft function, fluid administration is generous (10–20 mL/kg/hr), even though blood loss is minimal in most cases. The preferred type of fluid is isotonic crystalloids.

The anesthetic technique in these healthy patients is not different from that used for other laparoscopic procedures.

Nitrous oxide is contraindicated because it causes bowel distention and worsens surgical exposure. Similarly, the potential complications seen during any laparoscopic procedure (e.g. pneumothorax, subcutaneous emphysema) can be encountered during this procedure.

The first phase of the procedure consists of mobilization of the colon followed by the upper portion of the kidney, with subsequent identification and dissection of the ureter, renal vein, and artery. Division of the adrenal vein also is performed.

The surgeon may request administration of furosemide or mannitol (or both) during the operation to maintain adequate urine output.

Shortly before the renal vessels are clamped, intravenous heparin (3000–5000 IU) is administered.

After complete mobilization of the kidney and clamping of the vascular structures, the kidney is retrieved by either a hand-assisted or nonhand-assisted technique through a small periumbilical or infraumbilical incision under direct laparoscopic vision.

If heparin has been given, protamine may be administered to normalize coagulation.

After the kidney is removed, the surgical field is inspected again for bleeding.

Closure, as in all laparoscopic cases, is rapid, and care should be taken to maintain reversibility of neuromuscular blocking agents at the conclusion of the procedure.

Postoperative pain is usually mild to moderate and can be managed easily in most cases with supplemental intravenous opioids in the immediate postoperative period.

Ref: El-Galley R, Hammontree L, Urban D, et al. Anesthesia for laparoscopic donor nephrectomy: Is nitrous oxide contraindicated? J Urol. 2007;178:225-7.

Ref: Ratner LE, Smith P, Montgomery RA, et al. Laparoscopic live donor nephrectomy: Pre-operative assessment of technical difficulty. Clin Transpl. 2000;14(2):427-32.

Ref: Buell JF, Hanaway MJ, Potter SR, et al. Hand-assisted laparoscopic living-donor nephrectomy as an alternative to traditional laparoscopic living-donor nephrectomy. Am J Transplant. 2002;2:983-8.

11. What are the kidney storage solutions?
Ans. Commonly used ones are:

- Celsior solution
- UV (University of Wisconsins)
- HTK (Histidine-Tryptophane-ketoglutarate)

However for living donors in whom a long cold ischemia time is not expected, perfusion with crystalloid solution (Ringer Lactate) is sufficient.

There are two methods of kidney preservation:

1. Initial flushing with cold preservative (4 degrees) followed by ice storage
2. Continuous pulsatile hypothermic machine perfusion (clinical relevance for non heart beating donors and marginal donors).

Ref: Agarwal A, Murdock P, Fridell JA. Comparison of histidine-tryptophan ketoglutarate solution and University of Wisconsin solution in prolonged cold preservation of kidney allografts. Transplantation. 2006;81(3):480-2.

Ref: Booster MH, van der Vusse GJ, Wijnen RM, Yin M, Stubenitsky BM, Kootstra G. University of Wisconsin solution is superior to histidine tryptophanketoglutarate for preservation of ischemically damaged kidneys. Transplantation. 1994;58(9):979-84.

Ref: De Boer J, De Meester J, Smits JM, Groenewoud AF, Bok A, van der Velde O, et al. Eurotransplant randomized multicenter kidney graft preservation study comparing HTK with UW and Euro-Collins. Transpl Int. 1999;12(6):447-53.

12. What should be the ideal duration of organ preservation?

Ans. It should be as short as possible. Elderly kidneys (>55 years) are more sensitive to ischemia. Organ preservation mainly relies on hypothermia which:

- Reduces metabolic rate
- Conserves store of ATP
- Prevents formation of oxygen free radicals during reperfusion phase.

Typically, kidneys can be stored in cold preservation solution for up to 24–30 hours before transplantation, although the ischemia time does have an impact on outcome.

13. What should ideally be the cold and warm ischemia time?

Ans. The cold ischemia time in a living donor should be restricted to 20–30 minutes while the warm ischemia time should not exceed 3–5 minutes.

Ref: Baxi V, Jain A, Dasgupta D. Anesthesia for renal transplantation: an update. Indian Journal of Anaesthesia. 2009;53(2):139-47.

14. What are the clinical problems in chronic kidney disease related to anesthesia?

Ans. Kidneys are essential for adjusting body fluid volumes, electrolyte composition, acid base balance and hemoglobin concentration.

They receive about 25% of cardiac output and function as filters for toxins and drugs in the circulation. Chronic renal failure or more appropriately chronic kidney disease (CKD) refers to a decline in the glomerular filtration rate (GFR) caused by a variety of diseases such as

- Diabetes mellitus (40%)
- Hypertension (27%)
- Chronic glomerulonephritis (13%)
- Cystic kidney disease (3.5%)
- Interstitial nephritis (4%)
- Other diseases such as obstructive uropathy, lupus nephritis and human immunodeficiency virus.

CKD may be categorized as (by the Cockcroft-Gault equation)

- Mild (GFR of 60–89 mL/min/1.73m^2),
- Moderate (GFR of 30–59 mL/min/1.73 m^2),
- Severe (GFR of 15–29 mL/min/1.73 m^2), or
- End-stage renal disease (ESRD). Hemodialysis or peritoneal dialysis is typically initiated as the GFR falls to less than 15 mL/min/1.73 m^2. The progression of renal disease from one stage to the next results in deleterious effects on multiple organ systems.

Hemodialysis or peritoneal dialysis is typically initiated as the GFR falls to less than 15 mL/min/1.73 m^2.

Ref: Kasper DL, Braunwald E, Fauci AS. Harrison's principles of internal medecine, 16th edn. New York: McGraw-Hill; 2005.p.1654.

Ref: Cockcroft DW, Gault MH. Prediction of creatinine clearance from serum creatinine. Nephron. 1976;16(1): 31-41.

CARDIOVASCULAR SYSTEM

Causes 50% mortality in CKD. Damage starts early in form of—IHD, DCM, CCF, LVF with pulmonary hypertension, hemorrhagic uremic pericarditis. Accelerated arteriosclerosis is promoted by diabetes and dyslipidemias, while hypertension and cardiomyopathy is usually due to:

- *Volume overload:* Resulting from ECF expansion, high blood flow through AV fistula and anemia.
- *Pressure overload:* Resulting from hypertension and administration of erythropoietin.
- *Increased* levels of rennin angiotensin

  Goal is to achieve a blood pressure of < 130/80 mm Hg.

Ref: US Renal Data System.USRD2003 annual data report: atlas of end stage renal disease in the United States. Bethesda, MD: National Institute of Diabetes and Digestive and Kidney Diseases; 2003.

HEMATOLOGICAL SYSTEM

Normocytic normochromic anemia due to:

- Impaired erythropoiesis secondary to decreased erythropoietin synthesis and release
- Decreased red cell lifespan
- Increased hemolysis and bleeding
- Repeated loss during hemodialysis
- Aluminum toxicity
- Uremia induced bone marrow suppression
- Iron, folate and vitamin and B_6 and B_{12} deficiencies.

  Hb value ranges between 5 and 7 gm/dL and hematocrit around 15–20%.

Management

See Table 1.

Table 1 | Management guidelines for correction of anemia of chronic renal disease

Erythropoietin	
Starting dosage	50–150 units/kg per week IV or SC (once, twice, or three times per week)
Target hemoglobin (Hb)	11–12 gm/dL
Optimal rate of correction	Increase Hb by 1–2 gm/dL over 4-week period
Darbepoetin alfa	
Starting dosage	0.45 µg/kg administered as a single IV or SC injection once weekly 0.75 µg/kg administered as a single IV or SC injection once every 2 weeks
Target Hb	≤12 gm/dL
Optimal rate of correction	Increase Hb by 1–2 gm/dL over 4-week period
Iron	
1. Monitor iron stores by percent transferrin saturation (TSat) and serum ferritin.	
2. If patient is iron-deficient (TSat <20%; serum ferritin <100 µg/L), administer iron, 50–100 mg IV twice per week for 5 weeks; if iron indices are still low, repeat the same course.	
3. If iron indices are normal yet Hb is still inadequate, administer IV iron as outlined above; monitor Hb, TSat, and ferritin.	
4. Withhold iron therapy when TSat > 50% and/or ferritin > 800 ng/mL (>800 gm/L).	

Use of packed, washed irradiated RBC is recommended however with the risk of hyperkalemia.

Ref: Kasper DL, Braunwald E, Fauci AS. Harrison's principles of internal medecine, 16th edn. New York: McGraw-Hill, 2005.p.1659.

Ref: Collins AJ, Brenner RM, Ofman JJ. Epoetin alpha use in patients with ESRD: an analysis of recent US prescribing patterns and hemoglobin outcomes. American Journal of Kidney Diseases. 2005;46:481-8.

Ref: Eknoyan G. The importance of early treatment of the anaemia of chronic kidney disease. Nephrol Dial Transplant. 2001;16(Suppl 5):S45-9.

RESPIRATORY SYSTEM

Hypoxemia and hypocapnia may result from pulmonary congestion due to volume overload.

Intraperitoneal fluids used in peritoneal dialysis causes diaphragmatic splinting leading to basal atelectasis and shunting.

Uremic lung is a radiological identity characterized by perihilar congestion.

ELECTROLYTES AND ACID BASE STATUS

Inability of kidney to excrete water electrolytes and free acids lead to metabolic acidosis, hyponatremia, hyperchloremia and hyperkalemia.

For every 0.1 unit change in pH, potassium increases by 0.6 mEq/L.

Hence electrolyte correction is mandatory before any procedures.

Ref: Gennari FJ, Segal AS. Hyperkalemia: An adaptive response in chronic renal insufficiency. Kidney Int. 2002;62(1):1-9.

ENDOCRINE SYSTEM

As GFR falls, phosphate excretion falls leading to reduced absorption of calcium from gastrointestinal tract and vitamin D deficiency. Hyperactivity of parathyroid glands attempts to maintain calcium. This secondary hyperparathyroidism however leads to osteomalacia, osteosclerosis and osteitis fibrosa cystica (uremic osteodystrophy). The result is bone demineralization making these patients susceptible to spontaneous pathological fractures.

Ref: Goodman WG. Calcium and phosphorus metabolism in patients who have chronic kidney disease. Medical Clinics of North America. 2005;89:631-47.

Glucose metabolism and insulin removal from circulation is also impaired. Hence many hypoglycemic drugs require dose reduction and metformin is contraindicated.

Ref: Kasper DL, Braunwald E, Fauci AS. Harrison's principles of internal medicine, 16th edn. New York: McGraw-Hill, 2005.p.1659.

COAGULATION

Accumulation of endogenous toxic products like guanininosuccinate, phenol and phenolic acids leads to platelet dysfunction and decreased levels of platelet factor III. PT and PTT remain normal but bleeding time is prolonged. Treatment includes platelet transfusion, cryoprecipitate, desmopressin acetate or conjugated estrogen.

Ref: Mannucci PM, Remuzzi C, Pusineri F. DDAVP shortens the bleeding time in uremia. New England Journal of Medicine. 1983;308:8.

Ref: Jubelirer SJ. Hemostatic abnormalities in renal disease. Am J Kidney Dis. 1985;5(5):219-25.

CENTRAL NERVOUS SYSTEM

The manifestations include malaise, fatigue and inability to concentrate, pruritus progressing to myoclonus, seizures, coma and death.

- Dialysis dysequilibrium syndrome resulting from changes in ECF volume, electrolyte composition and cerebral edema is characterized by dehydration, vomiting and hypotension.

- Dementia affects patients on long-term dialysis and may be due to aluminum toxicity.

Ref: Baxi V, Jain A, Dasgupta D. Anaesthesia for renal transplantation: an update. Indian Journal of Anaesthesia. 2009;53(2):139-47.

GASTROINTESTINAL SYSTEM

Anorexia, nausea, vomiting, gut bleeding and diarrhea and hiccups are common. Delayed gastric emptying time, increased acidity and gastric volume necessitate use of H_2 blockers and proton pump inhibitors.

Ref: Kasper DL, Braunwald E, Fauci AS. Harrison's principles of internal medecine, 16th edn. New York: McGraw-Hill; 2005.p.1659.

DERMATOLOGICAL

Uremic pruritus results from deposition of pigmented metabolites/urochromes or urea itself and improves with dialysis.

Ref: Kasper DL, Braunwald E, Fauci AS. Harrison's principles of internal medecine, 16th edn. New York: McGraw-Hill; 2005.p.1659.

PROBLEMS OF DIALYSIS

Mainly lead to:

- Excessive or persistent heparinization
- Abnormal fluid shifts
- β_2 microglobulinemia
- Dialysis dysequilibrium syndrome
- Hepatitis
- HIV
- Leukopenia and hypocomplementemia
- Poor care of AV fistulae leading to local gangrene, sepsis and the need for amputation of the limb
- Peritoneal dialysis on the other hand can cause peritonitis and sub-acute intestinal obstruction.

Ref: Malhotra V, Sudheendra V, Diwan S. Anesthesia and The Renal and Genitourinary Systems. Miller's Anesthesia, 6th edn. Churchill Livingstone; 2005.pp.2181-7.

Ref: Baxi V, Jain A, Dasgupta D. Anaesthesia for renal transplantation: an update. Indian Journal of Anaesthesia. 2009;53(2):139-47.

15. What are the effects of CKD on pharmacokinetics and pharmacodynamics of anesthetic drugs?

Ans. Lipid soluble, unionized drugs are extensively reabsorbed by renal tubular cells. Termination of their action is not dependent on renal excretion.

Lipid insoluble or highly ionized drugs in the physiologic range are eliminated in urine. Their duration of action may be extended in patients with impaired renal function.

Ref: Malhotra V, Sudheendra V, Diwan S. Anesthesia and The Renal and Genitourinary Systems. Miller's Anesthesia, 6th edn. Churchill Livingstone; 2005.pp.2181-7.

Premedication Drugs

- Atropine and glycopyrrolate are eliminated 20–50% by kidney. Hence a single dose causes no toxic effect
- H_2-histamine receptor antagonists (ranitidine, famotidine) unaltered by ESRD

- Metoclopromide (<20% elimination) there is significant reduction in clearance (16.7 L/h compared with 52.5 L/h) and prolongation of the terminal half life (13.9 h compared with 2.8 h).
- Benzodiazepines have decreased plasma protein binding, increased volume of distribution and increased systemic clearance secondary to increased free unbound fraction (1.4–7.9%) of diazepam in patients with CKD. CKD does not alter the distribution, elimination, or clearance of unbound midazolam. After a single oral dose (2.5 mg) lorazepam there is prolonged action due to decreased urinary excretion of its metabolites.

Ref: Bateman DN, Gokal R. Metoclopromide in renal failure. Lancet. 1980;1:982.

Ref: Ochs HR, Greenblatt DJ, Divoll M. Diazepam kinetics in patients with renal insuffiency or hyperthyroidism. Br J Clin Pharmacol. 1981;12:829-32.

Ref: Vinik Ronald H, Reves JG, Greenblatt, David J, Abernethy, Darrell R, et al. The pharmacokinetics of midazolam in chronic renal failure patients. Anesthesiology. 1983;59:390-4.

Ref: Verbeeck R, Tjandramaga TB, Verberckmoes R, et al. Biotransformation and excretion of lorazepam in patients with chronic renal failure. Br Jr Clin Pharmacol. 1976;3:1033–9.

Induction Agents

Decreased albumin levels causes increased fraction of drug in the plasma.

Altered blood brain barrier due to uremia causes increased levels of unbound drug into the CNS. Hence, dose adjustment needed as per:

- Volume status
- Acidic pH
- Increased sensitivity of the nervous system to these drugs.

Thiopental

Distribution and elimination remains unchanged.

Propofol

The pharmacokinetics and pharmacodynamics are unchanged by chronic kidney disease but higher dose is required to reach clinical end point of hypnosis and BIS of 50 due to hyperdynamic circulation high plasma volume resulting from anemia.

Ketamine

Unaltered but is undesirable due to its hypertensive effects.

Etomidate

Well tolerated and preserves hemodynamic stability. And associated steroid suppression is also not relevant in patients receiveing steroids for immunosuppression as it is short lived.

Ref: Burch PG, Stanski DR. Decreased protein binding and thiopental kinetics. Anesthesiology. 1983;59:215-9.

Ref: Goyal P, Puri GD, Pandey CK. Evaluation of induction doses of Propofol: comparison between end stage renal disease and normal renal function patients. Anaesth Intensive Care. 2002;30:584-7.

Ref: Ickx B, Cockshott ID, Barvais L, Byttebier G, De Pauw L, Vandesteene A, et al. Propofo infusion for induction and maintenance of anaesthesia in patients with end-stage renal disease. Br J Anaesth. 1998; 81(6):854-60.

OPIOIDS

Morphine—since metabolites have renal excretion hence accumulation results in CNS and respiratory depression.

Meperedine—also excreted via kidneys thereby causing convulsions.

Fentanil—metabolized in the liver. Only 7% excreted unchanged in urine, hence safe for short-term use. However long-term use causes accumulations.

Sufentanil—unaltered.

Remifentanil—metabolites excreted through kidney but is insignificant because of it low potency (1/4000th of parent compound).

Ref: Dean M. Opioids in renal failure and dialysis patients. J Pain Symptom Manage. 2004;28:497-504.

Ref: Bower S, Sear JW. Disposition of alfentanil in patients receiving a renal transplant. J Pharm Pharmacol. 1989;41(9):654-7.

Ref: Chauvin M, Lebrault C, Levron JC, et al. Pharmacokinetics of alfentanil in chronic renal failure. Anesth Analg. 1987;66(1):53-6.

Ref: Hoke JF, Shlugman D, Dershwitz M, Michalowski P, Malthouse-Dufore S, Connors PM, et al. Pharmacokinetics and pharmacodynamics of remifentanil in persons with renal failure compared with healthy volunteers. Anesthesiology. 1997;87(3):533-41.

Ref: Szeto HH, Inturrisi CE, Houde R, Saal S, Cheigh J, Reidenberg MM. Accumulation of normeperidine, an active metabolite of meperidine, in patients with renal failure of cancer. Ann Intern Med. 1977;86(6):738-41.

Ref: Angst MS, Buhrer M, Lotsch J. Insidious intoxication after morphine treatment in renal failure: delayed onset of morphine-6-glucuronide action. Anesthesiology. 2000;92(5):1473-6.

MUSCLE RELAXANTS

Succinylcholine

Within 3–5 minutes after its administration of, an increase in potassium of approximately 0.5–1.0 mEq/L occurs that lasts less than 10–15 minutes hence to be used if plasma potassium concentration is < 5.5 mEq/L and repeated doses are avoided. Plasma cholinesterase is below normal in > 20% ESRD patients.

Ref: Thapa S, Brull SJ. Succinylcholine induced hyperkalemia in patients with renal failure: an old question revisited. Anesth Analg. 2000;91:237-41.

NONDEPOLARIZING AGENTS

- *Vecuronium and Rocuronium:* The duration of action may be prolonged due to an increase in the distribution volume.
- *Cis-Atracurium:* Undergoes Hofmann elimination, an organ-independent elimination pathway occurring in plasma and tissue, which is not altered in patients with chronic kidney disease.
- *Mivacurium:* Effect prolonged by approximately 50% in patients with renal failure.
- *Pancuronium:* Not suitable for use because of the kinetics of distribution and elimination. The kidneys excrete the majority of pancuronium and its active metabolites.
- Prolonged duration of action of nondepolarizing agents is primarily due to delayed clearance hence careful monitoring of the degree of neuromuscular blockade is recommended.

Drug	*Renal excretion*	*Normal t1/2*	*Anephric t1/2*
Pancuronium	85%	132 min	258 min
Rocuronium	10%	42 min	58 min
Vecuronium	40–50%	54 min	84 min
Atracurium	10–40%	18 min	24 min
Cisatracurium	16%	34 min	No effect
Mivacurium	<5%	1.8 min	3.6 min
Succinylcholine	<25%	1 min	1 min

Ref: Beauvoir C, Peray P, Daures JP, et al. Pharmacodynamics of vecuronium in patients with and without renal failure: a meta-analysis. Can J Anaesth 1993;40(8):696-702.

Ref: Bevan DR, Donati F, Gyasi H, et al. Vecuronium in renal failure. Can Anaesth Soc J. 1984; 31(5):491-6.

Ref: Cooper RA, Mirakhur RK, Wierda JM, Maddineni VR. Pharmacokinetics of rocuronium bromide in patients with and without renal failure. Eur J Anaesthesiol Suppl. 1995;11:43-4.

Ref: Szenohradszky J, Fisher DM, Segredo V, Caldwell JE, Bragg P, Sharma ML, et al. Pharmacokinetics of rocuronium bromide (ORG 9426) in patients with normal renal function or patients undergoing cadaver renal transplantation. Anesthesiology. 1992;77(5):899-904.

Volatile Anesthetic

Sevoflurane and enflurane: Biodegraded to inorganic fluorides of concentration ≥50 μmol/L which is the peak value for nephrotoxicity. There is evidence of transient impairment of renal concentrating ability and renal tubular injury in patients receiving sevoflurane and enflurane. FDA recommends the use of sevoflurane with fresh gas flows rates atleast 1 L/min for exposures up to 1 hour and atleast 2 L/min for exposures greater than 1 hr.

Fluoride levels after Isoflurane and Halothane increase by 3–5 μmol/L and 1–2 μmol/L, respectively. Hence, the risk of nephrotoxicity is remote.

Desflurane is resistant to biodegradation and so even a prolonged exposure to desflurane (7.0 MAC hrs) has been associated with normal renal function.

Ref: Gentz BA, Malan TP. Renal toxicity of sevoflurane: a storm in a teacup? Drugs. 2001;61:2155-62.

Ref: Goldberg ME, Cantillo J, Larijani GE, Torjman M, Vekeman D, Schieren H. Sevoflurane versus isoflurane for maintenance of anesthesia: are serum inorganic fluoride ion concentrations of concern? Anesth Analg. 1996;82(6):1268-72.

Ref: Eger 2nd EI, Koblin DD, Bowland T, Ionescu P, Laster MJ, Fang Z, et al. Nephrotoxicity of sevoflurane versus desflurane anesthesia in volunteers. Anesth Analg. 1997;84(1):160-8.

Anticholinesterase Drugs

Renal excretion accounts for approximately 50% of the clearance of neostigmine and approximately 75% of elimination of edrophonium and pyridostigmine.

Renal failure allows some protection against residual NM blockade because renal elimination half times of anticholinesterase drugs is prolonged.

Ref: Stoelting RK, Dierdorf SF. Anesthesia and co-existing diseases, 4th edn. Philadelphia: Churchill Livingstone; 2002.pp.347-8.

16. How are the organ matching and allocations done?

Ans. Initial testing is done to determine major blood group compatibility. Cadaveric kidney should be ABO identical to the recipient while a live donor kidney may be either ABO identical or compatible. However, it is possible to place an ABO-incompatible organ in a recipient using various protocols like plasmapheresis and immunoabsorption to overcome rejection as the Rh system is not expressed in the graft tissue. The human major histocompatibility complex is a cluster of genes on chromosome 6 that encode human leukocyte antigens (HLA). Before transplant, HLA antigens are identified by DNA based methods in all donors and recipients. Outcome is best with a perfect HLA matched donor and recipient. A crossmatching test determines if the recipient has serum antibodies directed against donor HLA lymphocyte antigens. These may arise as a result of exposure through pregnancies or blood transfusions in past. A positive crossmatch may cause rejection of graft. Currently, the methods to reduce allosensitization are use of immunoglobulins and plasmapheresis.

Ref: Danovitch GM. Handbook of kidney transplantation, 4th edn. Philadelphia: Lippincott Williams and Wilkins; 2005.pp.43-71.

17. Which are the drugs used for immunosuppression and discuss briefly their pharmacology?

Ans. Different centers in the world use several regimens of immunosupressants to decrease the incidence of graft rejection (Table 2). Their use is divided in three phases:

- First phase (induction therapy) started before and during first week post transplant and involves marked immune suppression. They are:
  Thymoglobulin, OKT3, Daclizumab, or Basiliximab.
- Second phase (maintenance therapy) involving drug administration continuously for three to six months to prevent acute graft rejection and induce tolerance.
- Third phase involves long-term immunosupression maintained for the rest of the life.
  Interaction of these agents with anesthetic drugs is not clinically significant. E.g. Steroids.

Table 2 | **Maintenance immunosuppressive drugs**

Agent	*Pharmacology*	*Mechanisms*	*Side effects*
Glucocorticoids	Increased bioavailability with hypoalbuminemia and liver disease; prednisone/ prednisolone generally used	Binds cytosolic receptors and heat shock proteins. Blocks transcription of IL-1,-2,-3,-6, TNF-α, and IFN-γ	Hypertension, glucose intolerance, dyslipidemia, osteoporosis
Cyclosporine (CsA)	Lipid-soluble polypeptide, variable absorption, microemulsion more predictable	Trimolecular complex with cyclophilin and calcineurin → block in cytokine (e.g. IL-2) production; however, stimulates TGF-β production	Nephrotoxicity, hypertension, dyslipidemia, glucose intolerance, hirsutism/hyperplasia of gums
Tacrolimus (FK506)	Macrolide, well absorbed	Trimolecular complex with FKBP-12 and calcineurin → block in cytokine (e.g. IL-2) production; may stimulate TGF-β production	Similar to CsA, but hirsutism/hyperplasia of gums unusual, and diabetes more likely
Azathioprine	Mercaptopurine analog	Hepatic metabolites inhibit purine synthesis	Marrow suppression (WBC > RBC > platelets)
Mycophenolate mofetil (MMF)	Metabolized to mycophenolic acid	Inhibits purine synthesis via inosine monophosphate dehydrogenase	Diarrhea/cramps; dose-related liver and marrow suppression is uncommon
Sirolimus	Macrolide, poor oral bioavailability	Complexes with FKBP-12 and then blocks p70 S6 kinase in the IL-2 receptor pathway for proliferation	Hyperlipidemia, thrombocytopenia

18. Discuss briefly the anesthetic management in a renal transplant recipient?

Ans. *Preoperative considerations:* Recipients involving cadaveric donor organs are often scheduled as urgent or emergency procedures. However, a well-preserved kidney provides enough time to prepare the recipient and if necessary dialyze to normalize electrolyte and volume imbalance.

Routine tests include:

- CBC
- Platelet count
- Electrolytes
- Serum glucose
- BUN, serum creatinine
- PT, PTT, INR
- Liver function tests
- Urine analysis
- ECG
- Chest radiograph and
- 2D echocardiogram.

Evaluation of cardiac function is of central importance. To help detect coronary artery disease and perhaps to lower the risk of adverse effects with transplantation, all patients and especially diabetic patients with ESRD are evaluated for the presence and/or absence of coronary artery disease. Besides routine ECG, echocardiogram and treadmill test, dobutamine stress echocardiogram is being increasingly used as the initial noninvasive test, given the superiority of this test compared with other examinations and the potential adverse effects of catheterization.

Ref: Steinman TI, Becker BN, Frost AE, Olthoff KM, Smart FW, Suki WN, et al. Guidelines for the referral and management of patients eligible for solid organ transplantation. Transplantation. 2001;71(9):1189-204.

Ref: Kasiske BL, Cangro CB, Hariharan S, Hricik DE, Kerman RH, Roth D, et al. The evaluation of renal transplantation candidates: clinical practice guidelines. Am J Transplant. 2002;1(Suppl 2): 1-95.

Ref: Holley JL, Fenton RA, Arthur RS. Thallium stress testing does not predict cardiovascular risk in diabetic patients with end-stage renal disease undergoing cadaveric renal transplantation. Am J Med. 1991;90(5):563-70.

- Dialysis if indicated is done within 24 hrs of the operation. Overzealous ultrafiltration is best avoided. Volume status is roughly estimated by their dry weight. Loss of more than 2 kg during dialysis suggests significant intravascular depletion.

DRUGS MODIFICATIONS

- Antihypertensives drugs should be continued until the time of surgery.
- Oral hypoglycemic agents should be held on the morning of the surgery. Sliding scale insulin regimen may be used intraoperatively if blood glucose levels are high.
- Antibiotic prophylaxis includes a first generation cephalosporin or if penicillin allergic, vancomycin.
- Induction of immunosupression is started before entering operating theater.

Intraoperative Management

- Successful use of regional anesthesia has been reported by some centers after due considerations of:
  - Uremic bleeding tendency
  - Effect of residual heparin given during dialysis
  - Altered platelet function
  - Decrease in coagulation factors and
  - Duration of surgery.

The advantages of combined spinal-epidural technique are rapid onset and good muscle relaxation from spinal and supplemental analgesia through epidural during and after surgery. Most centers however use balanced general anesthesia to provide stable hemodynamics, excellent muscle relaxation and predictable depth of anesthesia.

- Standard ASA monitors are adequate, although, patients with more advanced co-morbid conditions require extensive monitoring such as continuous arterial pressure or CVP monitoring. Those with the most severe co-morbid conditions, such as symptomatic CAD or history of congestive heart failure, should be monitored with a pulmonary artery catheter or transesophageal echocardiography.
- Strict asepsis should be maintained at all times.
- The status of hemodialysis shunts or fistulae should be monitored during positioning and intraoperatively. Assesment of the area over the fistula for infection, redness, edema, soreness, warmth and palpation of distal pulses should be routinely done. To establish and document the patency of the fistula, palpation for a thrill or vibration and auscultation over the fistula for a swishing noise or bruit is mandatory. The fistula may have to be covered with soft gamgee rolls to prevent any trauma intraoperatively.
- Also, great care should be taken while transferring these patients on to the operation table as they are prone to patholological fractures.
- Risk of aspiration during induction of anesthesia necessitates rapid sequence induction while maintaining cricoid pressure.
- The induction drugs should be given slowly to minimize drug-induced hypotension. Attenuation of sympathetic nervous system by antihypertensives, diabetic autonomic neuropathy, disruption of blood brain barrier, increased levels of unbound drug and increased sensitivity of central nervous system makes the patient vulnerable to hypotension on induction. Propofol, thiopentone, or etomidate can all be used in routine circumstances.
- Short acting beta adrenergic blocker esmolol and short acting opioids like fentanyl, remifentanil have been effective for blunting the hemodynamic response to intubation.
- Succinylcholine can be safely used in patients with chronic renal failure. If preoperative potassium is high normal or if there is underlyingmetabolic acidosis, additional increase of 0.5–1.0 mEq/L may occur with succinylcholine administration and hence should be avoided. When choosing a nondepolarizing agent for maintenance, it is better to use ones that are independent of renal clearance mechanisms (cisatracurium, atracurium, mivacurium).
- The choice of inhaled anesthetic includes desflurane, isoflurane and sevoflurane. The metabolism of sevoflurane has been implicated in renal toxicity with production of fluoride ions and compound A formed by breakdown of sevoflurane by sodium or barium hydroxide. However, studies have shown that fresh gas flows more that 4 L/min did not change renal function indices.
- Fentanyl, sufentanil, alfentanil and remifentanil are suitable for perioperative pain control, while morphine and pethidine are best avoided.

Ref: Baxi V, Jain A, Dasgupta D. Anaesthesia for renal transplantation: an update. Indian Journal of Anaesthesia. 2009;53(2):139-47.

Ref: Yost C Spencer, Neimenn CU. Miller's Anesthesia, 6th edn. Churchill Livingstone; 2005.p.2159.

19. How will you manage the fluid status of the patient intraoperatively? What will be your choice of fluid?

Ans. Postdialysis patients have intravascular volume depletion. To decrease the incidence of postoperative acute tubular necrosis, a liberal hydration policy is employed intraoperatively.

Goal

- The systolic blood pressure is maintained between 130 and 160 mm Hg.
- CVP between 10 and 15 mm Hg
- Mean pulmonary artery pressure of 18–20 mm Hg to optimize cardiac output and renal blood flow.

Crystalloids solutions are usually preferred to correct fluid and electrolyte imbalance, however in situations of severe hypovolemia, colloids may be used. Over the last few decades, there has been a shift in practice from using natural colloids such as blood, albumin and fresh frozen plasma to synthetic colloids. Most anesthesiologists avoid potassium-containing fluids during renal transplantation with the belief that it may worsen hyperkalemia in case of impaired graft function. Balanced crystalloids should be alternated with normal saline (0.9%) as large volumes of saline could lead to hyperchloremic acidosis. Hypotension may occur after unclamping the iliac vessels and reperfusion of the graft. It is critical that patient is well hydrated, as renal function is critically dependent on renal perfusion. It is especially important in pediatric recipients because reperfusion of an adult size kidney graft may divert a significant amount of their own blood volume.

Vasopressors with alpha agonist activity should be avoided as they can compromise blood flow to the transplanted organ. Immediate graft function has been associated with a blood volume greater than 70 mL/kg and a plasma volume greater than 45 mL/kg. CVP may decline 25–50% 1–2 hours after revascularization despite aggressive fluid management. This decline is similar in recipients of cadaveric as well as living related donor kidney and the cause may be multifactorial:

- Redistribution of fluids
- Changes in vascular permeability
- Increased nitric oxide levels.

Increased hydration works by atrial distention and subsequent release of atrial natriuretic peptide and increased renal perfusion. Transfusion when required should be preferably with packed cells that are saline washed, irradiated and cytomegalovirus negative.

Ref: Luciani J, Frantz P, Thibault P, Ghesquierre F, Conseiller C, Cousin MT, et al. Early anuria prevention in human kidney transplantation. Advantage of fluid load under pulmonary arterial pressure monitoring during surgical period. Transplantation. 1979;28(4):308-12.

Ref: Carlier M, Squifflet JP, Pirson Y, et al. Maximal hydration during anesthesia increases pulmonary arterial pressures and improves early function of human renal transplants. Transplantation. 1982;34(4):201-4.

Ref: Thomsen HS, Lokkegaard H, Munck O. Influence of normal central venous pressure on onset of function in renal allografts. Scand J Urol Nephrol. 1987;21(2):143-5.

Ref: Dawidson IJ, Sandor ZF, Coorpender L, Palmer B, Peters P, Lu C, et al. Intraoperative albumin administration affects the outcome of cadaver renal transplantation. Transplantation. 1992;53(4):774-82.

Ref: Dawidson IJ, Ar'Rajab A. Perioperative fluid and drug therapy during cadaver kidney transplantation. Clin Transpl; 1992.pp.267-84.

20. Is there any special significance of urine output monitoring in these cases? What other parameters can be used?

Ans. Yes, it is an indirect measurement of the graft condition after transplantation.

Immediate urine production is seen in over 90% of living donor kidney and between 40–70% of cadaveric transplants. A decrease in urine production at the latter stages of closure of surgical wound, a decrease in urine output strongly suggests mechanical impingement of the graft, vessel or ureter. The urinary catheter should be irrigated to ensure that clot or tissue has not affected its patency.

Intraoperative ultrasound can be used to examine the flow in arterial and venous anastomosis.

Ref: Baxi V, Jain A, Dasgupta D. Anaesthesia for renal transplantation: an update. Indian Journal of Anaesthesia. 2009;53(2):139-47.

21. Is there any role of diuretics in post transplant stage?

Ans. Loop diuretics, mannitol and occasionally dopamine may be used to enhance urine production. Mannitol induces osmotic diuresis and also has a protective effect on the tubular cells of the transplanted kidney from ischemic injury. Loop diuretics block the Na/K channels present in the thin ascending limb of Henle, while low dose dopamine is commonly used to stimulate dopaminergic receptors in the kidney vasculature to induce vasodilatation and increased urine output. However, the utility of this approach is questioned in that a newly transplanted, denervated kidney may not respond to low dose dopamine like normal kidneys do.

Ref: Kadieva VS, Friedman L, Margolius LP. The effect of dopamine on graft function in patients undergoing renal transplantation. Anesth Analg. 1993;76:362-5.

Ref: Tiggeler RG, Berden JH, Hoitsma AJ, et al. Prevention of acute tubular necrosis in cadaveric kidney transplantation by the combined use of mannitol and moderate hydration. Ann Surg. 1985;201(2):246-51.

Ref: van Valenberg PL, Hoitsma AJ, Tiggeler RG, Berden JH, van Lier HJ, Koene RA. Mannitol as an indispensable constituent of an intraoperative hydration protocol for the prevention of acute renal failure after renal cadaveric transplantation. Transplantation. 1987;44(6):784-8.

22. Discuss in short the outines of the postoperative care in this patient?

Ans.

- Renal transplant recipients should be reversed and extubated only when the established criterion for extubation is fulfilled and there is no concern for airway protection.
- In general, renal transplant patients are postoperatively nursed in a high-dependency unit. They rarely require intensive care unit admission unless there is fluid overload, a cardiac event or sepsis.
- Strict monitoring of fluid input output is essential.
- Re-exploration of the wound should not be delayed if kinking of the vascular attachments or obstruction of the ureter along its course is suspected.
- Postoperative pain is usually mild to moderate after renal transplant. Patient controlled analgesia with opioids and intercostals nerve blocks have been successfully used. Nonsteroidal anti-inflammatory drugs inhibit prostaglandins synthesis which are integral for renal blood flow and glomerular filtration rate autoregulation. Hence, these drugs are absolutely contraindicated.

Ref: Knowles P, Hancox D, Letheren M. An evaluation of intercostals nerve blocks for analgesia following renal transplantation. Eur J Anaesthsiol. 1998;15:457-61.

Ref: Williams M, Milner QJ. Postoperative analgesia following renal transplantation—current practice in the UK. Anaesthesia 2003;58(7):712-3.

23. What are the anesthetic complications in this patient?

Ans. The major postoperative anesthetic complications are:

- Vomiting and pulmonary inhalation
- Delayed respiratory depression
- Pulmonary edema
- Hypotension
- Hypertension
- Cardiac arrhythmias which can lead to cardiac arrest.

Cardiovascular complications are responsible for 33% of all mortality (most common cause of death) with 50% showing arterial hypertension. Factors that lead to increased risk in recipients include age greater than 60 years are coronary artery disease and diabetes mellitus.

Ref: Divarkar D, Bailey Lynn RR. Long term complications following renal transplantation. NZ J Med. 1991;104:352.

Ref: Matas AJ, Humar A, Gillingham KJ, Payne WD, Gruessner RW, Kandaswamy R, et al. Five preventable causes of kidney graft loss in the 1990s: a single-center analysis. Kidney Int. 2002; 62(2):704-14.

24. Now if this post-transplant patient is posted for a nonrenal surgery, what are the points which needs to be assessed before the surgery?

Ans.

- Information regarding the current disease for which he is undergoing the surgery
- Indication for the transplant (renal or systemic)
- Effects on other systems (reversible or irreversible)
- Status and function of the transplanted kidney
- Any comorbidities if present
- Current medications.

Ref: Fischer SP, Bader AM, Sweitzer BJ. Preoperative Evaluation Miller's Anesthesia, 7th edn. Churchill Livingstone; 2010.pp.1038-9.

25. How will you assess the transplanted kidney in a post transplant patient?

Ans. The following questions need to be answered:

- Interval since the transplant
- Organ source (live or cadaveric)
- Previous episodes of rejections
- Any history of fever, infections or contact (chickenpox, HIV, CMV)
- Immunosuppressive therapy, route or any recent changes in doses
- Compliance with therapy
- Need for dialysis, frequency, interval since last dialysis.

Ref: Fischer SP, Bader AM, Sweitzer BJ. Preoperative Evaluation Miller's Anesthesia, 7th edn. Churchill Livingstone; 2010.pp.1038-9.

26. How will you manage a case of trauma in a post transplant patient?

Ans.

- Resuscitate like a normal patient
- Note that they have increased risk of poor wound healing, sepsis, DVT, renal failure and peritonitis hence take adequate precautions.

27. What special considerations to be taken into account in pregnancy?

Ans.

- A minimum gap of 1 year should be kept between transplant and pregnancy
- Cell mediated immunity is compromised but humoral immunity remains unaffected.

In these patients the level of immunosuppressants should be monitored as there is hemodilution. They may also cross the placenta and compromise the immunity of the fetus. The common immunosuppressive treatment used during pregnancy is cyclosporine, with or without azathioprine and prednisone

- Mycophenolate mofetil (MMF), which, like sirolimus, is contraindicated due to teratogenicity
- Regional anesthesia is preferred as it reduces stress response
- Avoid methergin
- Increased risk of infection hence checking for bacterial urinary tract infection with monthly urine cultures and always treating bacteriuria, whether symptomatic or asymptomatic
- Antibiotics agents should be chosen from the penicillin and cephalosporine families to avoid fetal and renal toxicity
- Breastfeeding is not suggested because of the baby's risk of ingesting immunosuppressive agents
- A close follow-up of the mother in the first three postpartum months is recommended, including weekly renal function tests
- Delay vaccinations until the infant is 6 months old.

Ref: Bar J, Ben-Rafael Z, Pados A, Orvieto R, Boner G, Hod M. Prediction of pregnancy outcome in subgroups of women with renal disease. Clin Nephrol. 2000;53(6):437-44.

Ref: Sifontis NM, Coscia LA, Costantinescu S, Lavelanet AF, Moritz MJ, Armenti VT. Pregnancy outcomes in solid organ transplant recipients with exposure to micophenolate mofetil or sirolimus. Transplantation. 2006;82(12):1698-702.

Ref: Armenti VT, Moritz MJ, Davison JM. Drug safety issues in pregnancy following transplantation and immunosuppression: effects and outcomes. Drug Saf. 1998;19(3):219-32.

28. What are the factors related to pregnancy which affect kidney graft survival?

Ans. Factors that may affect a kidney graft during pregnancy

- Hemodynamic changes
- Hypertension
- Impairment of renal function (5–10)
- Rejection (11)
- Urinary tract infections.

Ref: EBPG Expert Group on Renal Transplantation. European best practice guidelines for renal transplantation. Section IV: Long term management of the transplant recipient. IV.10. Pregnancy in renal transplant recipients. Nephrol Dial Transplant. 2002;17(Suppl 4):50-5.

Ref: Hou S. Pregnancy in chronic renal insufficiency and end-stage renal disease. Am J Kidney Dis. 1999; 33(2):235-52.

Ref: First MR, Combs CA, Weislttel P, Miodovnik M. Lack of effect of pregnancy on renal allograft survival or function. Transplantation. 1995;59(4):472-8.

BIBLIOGRAPHY

1. Abouna GM. Ethical issues in organ and tissue transplantation. Exp Clin Transplant. 2003;1(2):125-38.
2. Agarwal A, Murdock P, Fridell JA. Comparison of histidine-tryptophan ketoglutarate solution and University of Wisconsin solution in prolonged cold preservation of kidney allografts. Transplantation. 2006;81(3):480-2.
3. Angst MS, Buhrer M, Lotsch J. Insidious intoxication after morphine treatment in renal failure: delayed onset of morphine-6-glucuronide action. Anesthesiology. 2000;92(5):1473-6.
4. Armenti VT, Moritz MJ, Davison JM. Drug safety issues in pregnancy following transplantation and immunosuppression: effects and outcomes. Drug Saf. 1998;19(3):219-32.
5. Banasik M. Living donor transplantation—the real gift of life. Procurement and the ethical assessment. Ann Transplant. 2006;11(1):4-6.
6. Bar J, Ben-Rafael Z, Pados A, Orvieto R, Boner G, Hod M. Prediction of pregnancy outcome in subgroups of women with renal disease. Clin Nephrol. 2000;53(6):437-44.
7. Bateman DN, Gokal R. Metoclopromide in renal failure. Lancet. 1980;1:982.
8. Baxi V, Jain A, Dasgupta D. Anaesthesia for renal transplantation: an update. Indian Journal of Anaesthesia. 2009;53(2):139-47.
9. Beauvoir C, Peray P, Daures JP, et al. Pharmacodynamics of vecuronium in patients with and without renal failure: a meta-analysis. Can J Anaesth. 1993;40(8):696-702.
10. Berardinelli L. Technical problems in living donor transplantation. Transplant Proc. 2005;37(6):2449-50.
11. Bevan DR, Donati F, Gyasi H, et al. Vecuronium in renal failure. Can Anaesth Soc J. 1984;31(5):491-6.
12. Booster MH, van der Vusse GJ, Wijnen RM, Yin M, Stubenitsky BM, Kootstra G. University of Wisconsin solution is superior to histidine tryptophanketoglutarate for preservation of ischemically damaged kidneys. Transplantation. 1994;58(9):979-84.
13. Bower S, Sear JW. Disposition of alfentanil in patients receiving a renal transplant. J Pharm Pharmacol. 1989;41(9):654-7.
14. Buell JF, Hanaway MJ, Potter SR, et al. Hand-assisted laparoscopic living-donor nephrectomy as an alternative to traditional laparoscopic living-donor nephrectomy. Am J Transplant. 2002;2:983-8.
15. Burch PG, Stanski DR. Decreased protein binding and thiopental kinetics. Anesthesiology. 1983;59:215-9.
16. Carlier M, Squifflet JP, Pirson Y, et al. Maximal hydration during anesthesia increases pulmonary arterial pressures and improves early function of human renal transplants. Transplantation. 1982;34(4):201-4.

17. Chauvin M, Lebrault C, Levron JC, et al. Pharmacokinetics of alfentanil in chronic renal failure. Anesth Analg. 1987;66(1):53-6.
18. Cockcroft DW, Gault MH. Prediction of creatinine clearance from serum creatinine. Nephron. 1976;16(1):31-41.
19. Collins AJ, Brenner RM, Ofman JJ. Epoetin alpha use in patients with ESRD: an analysis of recent US prescribing patterns and hemoglobin outcomes. American Journal of Kidney Diseases. 2005;46:481-8.
20. Cooper RA, Mirakhur RK, Wierda JM, Maddineni VR. Pharmacokinetics of rocuronium bromide in patients with and without renal failure. Eur J Anaesthesiol Suppl. 1995;11:43-4.
21. Danovitch GM. Handbook of kidney transplantation, 4th edn. Philadelphia: Lippincott Williams and Wilkins; 2005.pp.43-71.
22. Dawidson IJ, Ar'Rajab A. Perioperative fluid and drug therapy during cadaver kidney transplantation. Clin Transpl; 1992.pp.267-84.
23. Dawidson IJ, Sandor ZF, Coorpender L, Palmer B, Peters P, Lu C, et al. Intraoperative albumin administration affects the outcome of cadaver renal transplantation. Transplantation. 1992;53(4):774-82.
24. De Boer J, De Meester J, Smits JM, Groenewoud AF, Bok A, van der Velde O, et al. Eurotransplant randomized multicenter kidney graft preservation study comparing HTK with UW and Euro-Collins. Transpl Int. 1999;12(6):447-53.
25. Dean M. Opioids in renal failure and dialysis patients. J Pain Symptom Manage. 2004;28:497-504.
26. Desai MR, Ganpule AP, Gupta R, et al. Outcome of renal transplantation with multiple versus single renal arteries after laparoscopic live donor nephrectomy: a comparative study. Urology. 2007;69(5):824-7.
27. Divarkar D, Bailey Lynn RR. Long term complications following renal transplantation. NZ J Med. 1991;104:352.
28. EBPG Expert Group on Renal Transplantation. European best practice guidelines for renal transplantation. Section IV: Long term management of the transplant recipient. IV.10. Pregnancy in renal transplant recipients. Nephrol Dial Transplant. 2002;17(Suppl 4):50-5.
29. Eger 2nd EI, Koblin DD, Bowland T, Ionescu P, Laster MJ, Fang Z, et al. Nephrotoxicity of sevoflurane versus desflurane anesthesia in volunteers. Anesth Analg. 1997;84(1):160-8.
30. Eknoyan G. The importance of early treatment of the anaemia of chronic kidney disease. Nephrol Dial Transplant. 2001;16(Suppl 5):S45-9.
31. El-Galley R, Hammontree L, Urban D, et al. Anesthesia for laparoscopic donor nephrectomy: Is nitrous oxide contraindicated? J Urol. 2007;178:225-7.
32. European best practice guidelines for renal transplantation (part 1). Transplantation Section II: Evaluation and selection of donors. Nephrol Dial Transplant. 2000;15(Suppl 7):39-51.
33. First MR, Combs CA, Weislttel P, Miodovnik M. Lack of effect of pregnancy on renal allograft survival or function. Transplantation. 1995;59(4):472-8.
34. Fischer SP, Bader AM, Sweitzer BJ. Preoperative Evaluation Miller's Anesthesia, 7th edn. Churchill Livingstone; 2010.pp.1038-9.
35. Gennari FJ, Segal AS. Hyperkalemia: An adaptive response in chronic renal insufficiency. Kidney Int. 2002;62(1):1-9.
36. Gentz BA, Malan TP. Renal toxicity of sevoflurane: a storm in a teacup? Drugs. 2001;61:2155-62.
37. Goldberg ME, Cantillo J, Larijani GE, Torjman M, Vekeman D, Schieren H. Sevoflurane versus isoflurane for maintenance of anesthesia: are serum inorganic fluoride ion concentrations of concern? Anesth Analg. 1996;82(6):1268-72.
38. Goodman WG. Calcium and phosphorus metabolism in patients who have chronic kidney disease. Medical Clinics of North America. 2005;89:631-47.
39. Goyal P, Puri GD, Pandey CK. Evaluation of induction doses of Propofol: comparison between end stage renal disease and normal renal function patients. Anaesth Intensive Care. 2002;30:584-7.
40. Hoke JF, Shlugman D, Dershwitz M, Michalowski P, Malthouse-Dufore S, Connors PM, et al. Pharmacokinetics and pharmacodynamics of remifentanil in persons with renal failure compared with healthy volunteers. Anesthesiology. 1997;87(3):533-41.
41. Holley JL, Fenton RA, Arthur RS. Thallium stress testing does not predict cardiovascular risk in diabetic patients with end-stage renal disease undergoing cadaveric renal transplantation. Am J Med. 1991;90(5):563-70.

42. Horgan S, Benedetti E, Moser F. Robotically assisted donor nephrectomy for kidney transplant. Am J Surg. 2004;188:45-51.
43. Hou S. Pregnancy in chronic renal insufficiency and end-stage renal disease. Am J Kidney Dis. 1999; 33(2):235-52.
44. Ickx B, Cockshott ID, Barvais L, Byttebier G, De Pauw L, Vandesteene A, et al. Propofo infusion for induction and maintenance of anaesthesia in patients with end-stage renal disease. Br J Anaesth. 1998; 81(6):854-60.
45. Jubelirer SJ. Hemostatic abnormalities in renal disease. Am J Kidney Dis. 1985;5(5):219–25.
46. Kadieva VS, Friedman L, Margolius LP. The effect of dopamine on graft function in patients undergoing renal transplantation. Anesth Analg. 1993;76:362-5.
47. Kälble T, Alcaraz A, Budde K, Humke U, Karam G, Lucan M, et al. Guidelines on Renal Transplantation European Association of Urology 2010.
48. Karpinski J, Lajoie G, Cattran D, Fenton S, Zaltzman J, Cardella C, et al. Outcome of kidney transplantation from high-risk donors is determined by both structure and function. Transplantation. 1999;67(8):1162-7.
49. Kasiske BL, Cangro CB, Hariharan S, Hricik DE, Kerman RH, Roth D, et al. The evaluation of renal transplantation candidates: clinical practice guidelines. Am J Transplant. 2002;1(Suppl 2): 1-95.
50. Kasper DL, Braunwald E, Fauci AS. Harrison's principles of internal medecine, 16th edn. New York: McGraw-Hill; 2005.p.1654.
51. Kasper DL, Braunwald E, Fauci AS. Harrison's principles of internal medecine, 16th edn. New York: McGraw-Hill, 2005.p.1659.
52. Knowles P, Hancox D, Letheren M. An evaluation of intercostals nerve blocks for analgesia following renal transplantation. Eur J Anaesthsiol. 1998;15:457-61.
53. Luciani J, Frantz P, Thibault P, Ghesquierre F, Conseiller C, Cousin MT, et al. Early anuria prevention in human kidney transplantation. Advantage of fluid load under pulmonary arterial pressure monitoring during surgical period. Transplantation. 1979;28(4):308-12.
54. Malhotra V, Sudheendra V, Diwan S. Anesthesia and The Renal and Genitourinary Systems. Miller's Anesthesia, 6th edn. Churchill Livingstone; 2005.pp.2181-7.
55. Mannucci PM, Remuzzi C, Pusineri F. DDAVP shortens the bleeding time in uremia. New England Journal of Medicine. 1983;308:8.
56. Matas AJ, Humar A, Gillingham KJ, Payne WD, Gruessner RW, Kandaswamy R, et al. Five preventable causes of kidney graft loss in the 1990s: a single-center analysis. Kidney Int. 2002; 62(2):704-14.
57. Ochs HR, Greenblatt DJ, Divoll M. Diazepam kinetics in patients with renal insuffiency or hyperthyroidism. Br J Clin Pharmacol. 1981;12:829-32.
58. Onaca N, Goldstein RM, Levy MF, et al. Regional Transplant Institute: an update on liver, kidney, and pancreas transplantation. Proceedings from Baylor University Medical Center. 2003;16:297–301.
59. Penn I. Precautions to be taken to prevent transmission of neoplastic diseases in the grafting process. In: Organ and Tissue Transplantation in the European Union. London: Graham and Trotman; 1994.pp.33-41.
60. Ratner LE, Smith P, Montgomery RA, et al. Laparoscopic live donor nephrectomy: Pre-operative assessment of technical difficulty. Clin Transpl. 2000;14(2):427-32.
61. Sasaki TM, Finelli F, Bugarin E, Fowlkes D, Trollinger J, Barhyte DY, et al. Is laparoscopic donor nephrectomy the new criterion standard? Arch Surg. 2000;135(8):943-7.
62. Scheinkestel CD, Tuxen DV, Cooper DJ, et al. Medical management of the (potential) organ donor. Anesth Intensive Care. 1995;23(1):51-9.
63. Sifontis NM, Coscia LA, Costantinescu S, Lavelanet AF, Moritz MJ, Armenti VT. Pregnancy outcomes in solid organ transplant recipients with exposure to micophenolate mofetil or sirolimus. Transplantation. 2006;82(12):1698-702.
64. Steinman TI, Becker BN, Frost AE, Olthoff KM, Smart FW, Suki WN, et al. Guidelines for the referral and management of patients eligible for solid organ transplantation. Transplantation. 2001;71(9):1189-204.
65. Stoelting RK, Dierdorf SF. Anesthesia and co-existing diseases, 4th edn. Philadelphia: Churchill Livingstone; 2002.pp.347-8.
66. Surman OS. The ethics of partial-liver donation. N Engl J Med. 2002;346:1038.
67. Szenohradszky J, Fisher DM, Segredo V, Caldwell JE, Bragg P, Sharma ML, et al. Pharmacokinetics of rocuronium bromide (ORG 9426) in patients with normal renal function or patients undergoing cadaver renal transplantation. Anesthesiology. 1992;77(5):899-904.

68. Szeto HH, Inturrisi CE, Houde R, Saal S, Cheigh J, Reidenberg MM. Accumulation of normeperidine, an active metabolite of meperidine, in patients with renal failure of cancer. Ann Intern Med. 1977;86(6):738-41.
69. Thapa S, Brull SJ. Succinylcholine induced hyperkalemia in patients with renal failure: an old question revisited. Anesth Analg. 2000;91:237-41.
70. Thomsen HS, Lokkegaard H, Munck O. Influence of normal central venous pressure on onset of function in renal allografts. Scand J Urol Nephrol. 1987;21(2):143-5.
71. Tiggeler RG, Berden JH, Hoitsma AJ, et al. Prevention of acute tubular necrosis in cadaveric kidney transplantation by the combined use of mannitol and moderate hydration. Ann Surg. 1985;201(2):246-51.
72. US Renal Data System.USRD2003 annual data report: atlas of end stage renal disease in the United States. Bethesda, MD: National Institute of Diabetes and Digestive and Kidney Diseases; 2003.
73. van Valenberg PL, Hoitsma AJ, Tiggeler RG, Berden JH, van Lier HJ, Koene RA. Mannitol as an indispensable constituent of an intraoperative hydration protocol for the prevention of acute renal failure after renal cadaveric transplantation. Transplantation. 1987;44(6):784-8.
74. Verbeeck R, Tjandramaga TB, Verberckmoes R, et al. Biotransformation and excretion of lorazepam in patients with chronic renal failure. Br Jr Clin Pharmacol. 1976;3:1033–9.
75. Vinik Ronald H, Reves JG, Greenblatt, David J, Abernethy, Darrell R, et al. The pharmacokinetics of midazolam in chronic renal failure patients. Anesthesiology. 1983;59:390-4.
76. Williams M, Milner QJ. Postoperative analgesia following renal transplantation—current practice in the UK. Anaesthesia 2003;58(7):712-3.
77. Yost C Spencer, Neimenn CU. Miller's Anesthesia, 6th edn. Churchill Livingstone; 2005.p.2159.

24

Hypertensive Diseases in Pregnancy

Sampa Dutta Gupta, Maupali Ghosh, Samarendra Samui

CASE SUMMARY

A 25 years old female primigravida 36 weeks gestation with history of pregnancy induced hypertension since 20 weeks of gestational age (on tablet amlodipine), presented with headache and pain in upper abdomen for last 4–5 days in her routine antenatal checkup. On physical examination heart rate 88/min, BP 160/100 mm Hg, edema over ankles, chest-B/clear, heart sounds—audible, urine protein—positive. The patient was normotensive, nonproteinuric and asymptomatic on routine antenatal check-up 2 weeks ago. Now the patient is posted for elective CS.

1. How will you classify hypertensive disordered in during pregnancy?

Ans. According to Working Group of National High Blood Pressure Education Program 2000, hypertensive diseases of pregnancy is classified as:

- Gestational hypertension
- Pre-eclampsia
- Eclampsia
- Pre-eclampsia superimposed on chronic hypertension
- Chronic hypertension.

Ref: Cunningham F Gary, Leveno Kenneth J, Bloom Steven L, Hauth John C, Rouse Dwight J, Spong Catherine Y Williams. Obstetrics, 23rd edn. The McGraw-Hill Companies, Inc. 2010;34:706-49.

2. Define gestational hypertension, pre-eclampsia and eclampsia.

Ans. *Gestational hypertension*

- BP ≥ 140/90 mm Hg for first time in pregnancy
- No proteinuria
- BP returns to normal < 12 weeks postpartum
- Final diagnosis made only postpartum
- May have other signs or symptoms of pre-eclampsia, e.g. epigastric discomfort or thrombocytopenia.

Pre-eclampsia:

Minimum criteria:

- BP ≥ 140 mm Hg after 20 weeks of gestation
- Proteinuria ≥ 300 mg/24 hours or 1 + dipstick.

Increased certainty of pre-eclampsia:
- BP ≥ 160/100 mm Hg
- Proteinuria 2.0 g/24 hours or 2 + dipstick
- Serum creatinine >1.2 mg/dL unless known to be previously elevated
- Platelets < 100,000/mm^3
- Microangiopathic hemolysis (↑LDH)
- ↑AST or ALT
- Persistent headache or other cerebral or visual disturbance
- Persistent epigastric pain.

Eclampsia: Seizures that cannot be attributed to other causes in a women with pre-eclampsia.

Superimposed pre-eclampsia on chronic hypertension:
- New onset proteinuria ≥ 300 mg/24 hours in hypertensive patient but no proteinuria before 20 weeks of gestations
- A sudden increase in proteinuria or BP or platelet count < 100,000 μL in women with hypertension and proteinuria before 20 weeks of gestations.

Chronic hypertension:
- BP ≥ 140 mm Hg before pregnancy or diagnosed before 20 weeks of gestations not attributable to gestational trophoblastic diseases

Or

- Hypertension first diagnosed after 20 weeks gestation and persistent after 12 weeks postpartum.

Ref: Cunningham F Gary, Leveno Kenneth J, Bloom Steven L, Hauth John C, Rouse Dwight J, Spong Catherine Y. Williams Obstetrics, 23rd edn. The McGraw-Hill Companies, Inc. 2010;34:706-49.

3. What are the features of severe pre-eclampsia?

Ans.
- Sustained systolic blood pressure (SBP) > 160 mm Hg or diastolic blood pressure (DBP) > 110 mm Hg (measured twice, at least six hours apart)
- Proteinuria ≥ 5 g/24 hours or ≥ 3 + on two random urine samples at least 4 hours apart
- Oliguria urine output < 500 mL in 24 hours
- CNS disturbance (altered vision, headache and altered consciousness)
- Pulmonary edema or cyanosis
- Liver dysfunction
- Hepatic rupture
- Epigastric/right upper quadrant pain (stretching of hepatic capsule)
- Thrombocytopenia, HELLP syndrome (may occur without proteinuria)
- Evidence of fetal compromise (Intrauterine growth restriction (IUGR), oligohydramnios, nonreassuring fetal testing).

4. What are the risk factors of pre-eclampsia?

Ans.
- *Maternal obstetric factors*: Nulliparity, history of pre-eclampsia, multiple gestation pregnancy, gestational hypertension, molar pregnancy
- *Maternal comorbid conditions*: Chronic hypertension, pregestational vascular/endothelial/renal disease, pregestational diabetes
- *Maternal genetic factors*: Antiphospholipid antibody, Factor V Leiden mutation (protein C resistance), first-degree relative with pre-eclamptic pregnancy
- *Maternal lifestyle factors*: Obesity, smoking
- *Other maternal factors*: African-American race, age 40 years

- *Paternal obstetric factors*: Paternity by male who fathered a previous pre-eclamptic pregnancy in another woman, paternity by a male born from a pre-eclamptic pregnancy.

5. What is the etiology and pathogenesis of pregnancy-induced hypertension (PIH)?

Ans. Pre-eclampsia is a disorder of unknown etiology. It is a systemic disorder with heterogeneous causes that are linked to following:

- Placental implantation with abnormal trophoblastic invasion of uterine vessels
- Immunological maladaptive tolerance between maternal, paternal (placental), and fetal tissues
- Maternal maladaptation to cardiovascular or inflammatory changes of normal pregnancy
- Genetic factors including inherited predisposing genes as well as epigenetic influences.

Pathogenesis: Exact mechanism unknown.

Placenta: The pathogenic focus of the disease.

- Abnormal placentation, ↓Trophoblastic perfusion and uterine ischemia
- Maternal and placental oxidative stress
- Release of cytotoxic substances
- Damage to vascular endothelial cells
  - Triggers vasoconstriction (hypertension)
  - Platelet activation and aggregation
  - Prostacyclin—thromboxane imbalance, ↓NO
  - Activation of Renin—Angiotensin, ↑Aldosterone
- Further endothelial cell damage, disruption of capillary integrity
- Release of trophoblastic material, fibrin deposition, renal glomerular lesion and proteinuria.

Ref: Cunningham F Gary, Leveno Kenneth J, Bloom Steven L, Hauth John C, Rouse Dwight J, Spong Catherine Y. Williams Obstetrics, 23rd edn. The McGraw-Hill Companies, Inc. 2010;34:706-49.

6. What are pathological alterations in pre-eclampsia?

Ans. See Flow chart 1.

Flow chart 1 Pathological alteration in pre-eclampsia

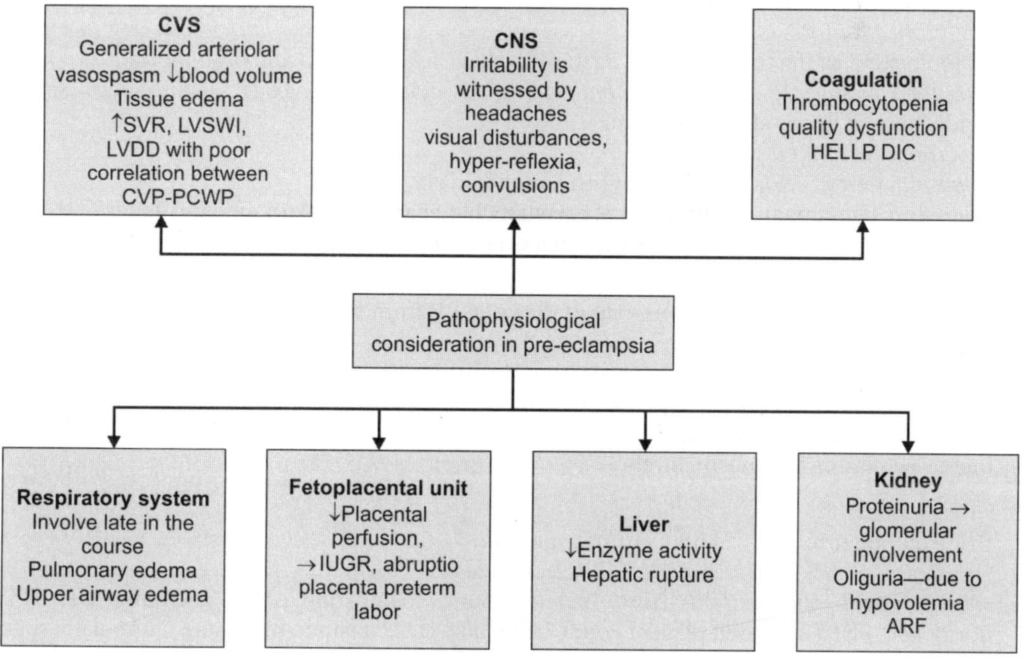

7. What are the latest methods of prevention of PIH in a high-risk patient?

Ans. *Dietary manipulation:* Low-salt diet, calcium supplementation, fish oil supplementation [ω-3 fatty acids, eicosapentaenoic acid (EPA) and docosahexaenoic (DCHA)].

Cardiovascular drugs: Diuretics, antihypertensive drugs.

Antioxidants: Ascorbic acid (vitamin C), tocopherol (vitamin E).

Antithrombotic drugs: Low-dose aspirin, aspirin/dipyridamole, aspirin + heparin, aspirin + ketanserin.

Antiplatelet drugs (low dose Aspirin 50–150 mg/day) effectively inhibits platelet thromboxane A2 biosynthesis with minimal effects on vascular prostacyclin production.

Ref: Cunningham F Gary, Leveno Kenneth J, Bloom Steven L, Hauth John C, Rouse Dwight J, Spong Catherine Y. Williams Obstetrics, 23rd edn. The McGraw-Hill Companies, Inc. 2010;34:706-49.

8. What is HELLP syndrome?

Ans.

- Hemolysis elevated liver enzymes and low platelet count seen in 20% cases of severe pre-eclampsia. It can occur in antepartum and post preterm. Delivery is the only definite treatment of HELLP.
- *Clinical Signs and symptoms:* Epigastric pain, upper abdominal tenderness, systemic HT, proteinuria, nausea and vomiting and jaundice.
- *Complications:* Pulmonary edema, pleural, effusions, cerebral edema, hematuria, oliguria, acute tubular necrosis, panhypopituitirism and disseminated intravascular coagulation (DIC)
- *Management:*
  - Management is same as severe pre-eclampsia. Antiseizure prophylaxis with $MgSO_4$ and correction of coagulation abnormality is done.
  - Assess fetal condition. General anesthesia (GA) is anesthetic of choice for cesarean section.
  - Corticosteroids can be given for fetal lung maturity before 34 weeks, if time permits.

9. What are the usual clinical presentation and diagnostic procedures for evaluation of hypertensive diseases in pregnancy?

Ans. A. *Clinical features include:*

- *Asymptomatic*, at the time they may be found to have hypertension and proteinuria.
- *Symptoms of severe pulmonary embolism (PE)* associated with visual disturbances, severe headache, and upper abdominal pain.
- *Superimposed HELLP syndrome*
- *Eclampsia* may develop before during and after delivery.
- *Eclampsia death* may be due to cerebrovascular events, renal or hepatic failure, HELLP syndrome, DIC, or other complication of hypertension.

Prediction:

- *Roll-over test:* Increase of >20 mm Hg of diastolic BP from left lateral position turn to supine position
- *MAP (mean arterial blood pressure):* >85 mm Hg during 20–28 weeks of gestation.
- *Urinary calcium excretion:* Urinary calcium/blood creatinine ratio >0.04
- Serum uric acid levels >5.9 mg/dL
- Increased plasma fibronectin levels.

B. *Investigations:*

- Urine output, urinalysis, 24 hours urinary protein
- Serum uric acid/Serum creatinine/LFT/electrolytes
- *Hematological investigations:* HB%, platelet count, coagulation profile including PT, PTT, fibrinogen, FDP (Indicated platelet count <1, 00,000, DIC, abruptio placenta). Normal life span of platelets is ↓ from 8–10 to 3–5 days pre-eclampsia.

- Uterine artery Doppler flow studies; ↑resistance to flow, ↑likelihood of pre-eclampsia is six fold
- Plasma fibronectin (early marker)
- Plasminogen activator inhibitor; PAI-1 to PAI-2 ratio.

10. What are the principles of management of severe pre-eclampsia?

Ans.

- *Definitive treatment*: Delivery of fetus
- *Supportive treatment:* It includes general management, control of hypertension, prevention of seizures, correction of intravascular fluid volume, correct clotting abnormalities, maintenance of urine output, and management of associated maternal complication.

11. What is the medical management of PIH?

Ans.

- Antihypertensive agents
- Directly acting vasodilators

Hydralazine: Hydralazine is preferred by most obstetricians as the first-line of treatment for control of hypertension. Hydralazine is given IV in doses of 5–10 mg to lower the diastolic pressure to less than 110 mm Hg. The onset of action is approximately 20 minutes. Hydralazine is a direct vasodilator that lowers MAP and sustained virologic response (SVR), increases CO and HR without affecting PCWP. The slow onset, delayed peak effect, and compensatory tachycardia make hydralazine a less than an ideal agent to prevent the hypertensive response during intubation.

Sodium nitroprusside (SNP): The use of SNP is limited to situations such as acute hypertensive crisis, severe intractable hypertension, and occasionally blunting of hypertensive response to tracheal intubation. It is a potent arteriolar dilator. The recommended dose is 0.5–5 μg/kg/min. Sodium nitroprusside is also a cerebral vasodilator and may increase intracranial pressure. The major concern is the potential for fetal cyanide toxicity. However, SNP has been safely used for the treatment of hypertension, pulmonary congestion, and heart failure without any adverse fetal effects.

Nitroglycerin (NTG): Nitroglycerin is a venodilator and the indications for its use are similar to those for SNP. In patients with severe pre-eclampsia, NTG lowers MAP, PCWP, but has no effect on CVP, SV, and HR. Nitroglycerin can be given prophylactically to blunt the hypertensive response to tracheal intubation. NTG readily crosses the placenta. Dose 0.5 μg/kg/min.

Ganglion Blocking Agents

Trimethaphan: Trimethaphan is a drug with a large molecular weight and therefore has limited placental transfer. It is given as an infusion or bolus doses. Unfortunately, this drug inhibits plasma pseudo cholinesterase and prolongs the action of succinylcholine. Other side effects, such as histamine release and tachyphylaxis, limit the usefulness of this drug.

β-Adrenergic Blocking Agents

Labetalol: The mechanism of hypertension in PIH is mediated by circulating catecholamines, making Labetalol a preferred antihypertensive agent. Labetalol decreases maternal SVR without increasing maternal HR or decreasing cardiac index, uterine blood flow or fetal HR, when it is given in a total dose of < 1 gm/kg. Labetalol crosses the placental barrier and the fetal:maternal ratio is 1:1. Despite the high drug levels in the fetus, labetalol does not cause β blockade and therefore, neonatal hypoglycemia and hypotension are rarely present.

Esmolol: Esmolol is a pure β-receptor antagonist which selectively blocks the β-1 receptors of the heart with a rapid onset and offset of action. It can be given intravenously in a dose of 0.5–1 mg/kg for preventing or blunting the hypertensive response to tracheal intubation.

Calcium-channel Blocking Agents

Nifedipine and nicardipine: Nifedipine has been used for treatment of hypertension in pregnancy for several years. Nifedipine, given orally or sublingually, lowers MAP reliably and safely within 10–30 minutes. After an initial dose of 10 mg sublingually it may be repeated in 30 minutes and subsequently given in a maintenance dose of 10–20 mg every 3–6 hours. Nifedipine lowers BP by decreasing peripheral vascular resistance without compromising cardiac output.

Ref: Cunningham F Gary, Leveno Kenneth J, Bloom Steven L, Hauth John C, Rouse Dwight J, Spong Catherine Y. Williams. Obstetrics, 23rd edn. The McGraw-Hill Companies, Inc. 2010;34:706-49.

Ref: Miller RD, Eriksson LI, Fleisher LA, Wiener-Kronish JP, Young WL, Miller's Anesthesia, 7th edn. Churchill Livingstone; 2009.

12. What are the oral antihypertensive drug treatment in pregnancy?

Ans. See Table 1.

Table 1 | Oral antihypertensive drug treatment in pregnancy

Drug	*Dose*	*Action*	*Contraindications*	*Practice points*
Methyl dopa	250–750 mg tds	Central	Depression	Slow onset of action over 24 hours. Dry mouth, sedation, depression, blurred vision.
Clonidine	75–300 µg tds			Withdrawal effect with clonidine
Labetalol	100–400 mg tds	β blocker with mild alpha vasodilator effect	Asthma, chronic airways limitation	Bradycardia, bronchospasm, headache, nausea, scalp tingling which usually resolves within 24–48 hours (labetalol only)
Oxprenolol	20–160 mg tds	β blocker with ISA	Heart block	
Nifedipine	20 mg bd – 60 mg SR bd	Ca channel antagonist	Aortic stenosis	Severe headache associated with flushing, tachycardia Peripheral edema, constipation
Prazosin	0.5–5 mg tds	α blocker		First dose effect-orthostatic hypotension
Hydralazine	25–50 mg tds	Vasodilator		Flushing, headache, nausea, lupus-like syndrome

Ref: Cunningham F Gary, Leveno Kenneth J, Bloom Steven L, Hauth John C, Rouse Dwight J, Spong Catherine Y. Williams Obstetrics, 23rd edn. The McGraw-Hill Companies, Inc. 2010;34:706-49.

13. Discuss the management of a patient with convulsion in pregnancy at term.

Ans.

- Rule out the causes of convulsion other than pre-eclampsia
- Management of airway
- Resuscitation
- Termination of placenta in convulsion.

How will you manage the convulsion?

Seizures are usually short-lived. If necessary, small doses of barbiturate or benzodiazepine (midazolam, 1-2 mg) or injection thiopental sodium 75 mg instead of long acting sedative diazepam and supplemental oxygen by mask. If seizure persists or patient is not breathing, rapid sequence induction with cricoid pressure and intubation should be performed. Patient may be extubated once she is completely awake, recovered from neuromuscular blockade, and magnesium sulfate has been administered and place monitors. Turn patient to full left or right lateral decubitus and get suction immediately available. Avoid polypharmacy and long-lasting medications so that a neurologic exam can be done as soon as possible.

Monitor the fetus if possible, but recognize that heart rate abnormalities are common and usually resolve soon after the seizure is terminated. Do not intervene unless abruption or cord prolapse has occurred. Consider CT or MRI imaging to rule out a cerebral hemorrhage if seizures are recurrent or focal, if seizures occur despite therapeutic and repeated magnesium dosing, or if there is decreasing level of consciousness when not postictal. Although eclampsia is an indication for delivery, it is not an indication for cesarean delivery, but termination of placenta is the treatment of choice in eclampsia. Consider whether induction is feasible or whether labor is already progressing.

Drug of choice: Magnesium sulfate ($MgSO_4$)

Mechanisms of action:

- Both peripheral and central effects.
- Block calcium influx via N-methyl-D aspartate and reverses cerebral vasoconstriction
- ↓ Presynaptic release of Ach at the neuromuscular junction
- Postjunctional receptors sensitivity ↓
- Mild relaxant effects on vascular and uterine smooth muscle
- Decrease fibrin deposition and increase hepatic and renal circulation

Suggested regimen

Pritchard regimen:

- Only for patients with eclampsia — loading dose of 4g IV (dilute 8 mL of 50% mg with 12 mL of sterile water or use 20 mL 20% solution — given over 3–5 minutes.
- Intramuscular loading dose — administer 10 mL of 50% Mg deeply in the outer quadrant of each buttock using a 3 inch 20 gm needle. The IM does is followed by IV dose in patients with convulsions.
- Maintenance dose — 5 gm (10 mL of 50% solution) deep IM in alternative buttock every 4 hours if patellar reflex is present, urine output has been at least 100 mL during the preceding 4 hours. Respiratory rate is normal. Usually continued for 24 hours after delivery.
- Monitors—hourly urine output, respiratory rate, O_2 saturation, patellar reflexes every 10 minutes for first 2 hours and then every 30 minutes. Check serum magnesium levels every day if infusion is continued for 24 hours.
  - *If seizure persists:* 10 mg diazepam/200 mg of thiopentone slowly infused.

What are the other regimens?

a. *University of Tenesse guideline for IV regimen:*
   Loading dose: Initial IV infusion of 4–6 gm over 15–20 minutes (30 mL of 20% Mg in 100 mL of 5% dextrose)
   Maintenance dose: Continuous infusion of 2–3 gm/hr. Add 20 gm of Mg in 1000 mL of D5 and infuse at a rate of 100 mL/h, obtain a serum mg level 4–6 hours apart and adjust the rate of infusion to keep the level 4.8–9.6 mg/dL. If serum levels are not available, dose is adjusted according to urine output and patellar reflex.
b. Zuspan's regimen — Loading dose — 4 gm IV over 5–10 min. Maintenance — 1–2 gm IV/hr.
c. Sibais regimen — 6 gm IV over 20 min. Maintenance — 2–3 gm IV/hr.

Monitoring and management of magnesium toxicity:
- Renal excretion
- Pre-eclamptics prone to renal failure
- $MgSO_4$ crosses placenta and there can be evidence of decreased beat-to-beat variability in fetal HR, neonatal depression can also occur.
- Magnesium levels must be monitored frequently either clinically (patellar reflexes) or by checking serum levels 6–8 hourly.
- *Therapeutic range:* 4–6 mEq/L.
- *Normal levels:* 1.5–2 mEq/L.
- *Monitoring:* Knee jerk and Mg. Levels (if possible) respiration, urine output (>100 mL in 4 hours).
- *Toxicity:*
  6–8 mEq/L — Nausea, vomiting, diplopia, somnolence and decrease myometrical contractility.
  5–10 mEq/L — Increase PQ interval, wide QRS.
  10 mEq/L — Loss of deep tendon reflexes.
  15 mEq/L — SA and AV blocks respiratory paralysis.
  25 mEq/L — Cardiac arrest.

Treatment: Stop Mg, support ventilation, calcium gluconate 1 gm (10%) over 10 minutes.

How to avoid Mg toxicity?
- Urine flow of at least 100 mL during last 4 hours before administering next dose
- Patellar reflexes present
- No respiratory depression
- Magnesium levels to be measured 2 hours after start of treatment.

Significance of $MgSO_4$ in anesthetic management:
- Clinically significant potentiation of both depolarizing and nondepolarizing
  - Careful titration of doses of muscle relaxants.
  - Neuromuscular monitoring.
- Potentiates sedatives and opioids, ↓ Dose
- Potentiation of calcium channel blockers
- *Postpartum uterine relaxation:* Excessive blood loss
- *Neonatal:*
  Transient loss of fetal beat to beat variability
  ↓ Neonatal skeletal Muscle tone and hypoventilation
  (Ca^{2+} may be given to overcome the problem)

14. What are the acute blood pressure lowering agents other than $MgSO_4$ for severe hypertension in pregnancy?

Ans. See Table 2.

Table 2 | Acute blood pressure lowering agents

	Dose	*Route*	*Onset of action*
Labetalol	20–50 mg	IV bolus over 2 mins	5 mins, repeat after 15–30 min
Nifedipine	5–10 mg capsule 10–20 mg tablet	Oral Oral	10–20 min, repeat after 30 min 30–45 min, repeat after 45 min
Hydralazine	5–10 mg	IV bolus	20 min, repeat after 30 min
Diazoxide	15–45 mg, max 300 mg	IV rapid bolus	3–5 min, repeat after 5 min

Ref: Cunningham F Gary, Leveno Kenneth J, Bloom Steven L, Hauth John C, Rouse Dwight J, Spong Catherine Y. Williams Obstetrics. 23rd edn. The McGraw-Hill Companies, Inc. 2010;34:706-49.

15. Describe the management of oliguria in severe pre-eclampsia.

Ans. Fluid challenge is 500 mL of balanced salt solution over 20 minutes. Repeat once or twice, if urine output remains unchanged or declined, central venous catheter or PA catheter to be instituted before further fluid therapy.

- If patients found in volume depleted state having low filling pressure, hyperdynamic ventricular function and moderate increase in vascular resistance, further volume infusion with an increase in PAOP and decrease in SVR with no change in BP.
- If patients found oliguric with renal artery vasospasm having hyperdynamic ventricular function with high filling pressure (9–18 mm Hg) and normal SVR respond to vasodilator therapy with hydralazine alongwith judicious fluid administration.
- Women found oliguric having elevated ventricular filling pressure respond to low dose dopamine (1–5 μg/min).
- Patients having depressed left ventricular function, increased PAOP and marked increase in SVR needs afterload reduction, relieve vasospasm and improve cardiac output.

Indication of CVP cannulation:

- The correlation between CVP and PAWP is known to be poorly correlated in many pre-eclampsia patients. Central venous pressure monitoring is indicated
- In severe pre-eclampsia for persistent oliguria (<0.05 mL/kg/h) unresponsive to small fluid challenge
- If pulmonary edema develops. Although central venous pressure does not always correlate well with pulmonary arterial wedge pressure, a low CVP is almost never associated with high PCWP.

Indication of PA catheterization:

- Intractable hypertension
- Pulmonary edema
- Persistent oliguria unresponsive to fluid challenge (CVP > 6 mm Hg)
- Noninvasive measurement of cardiac output using impedance measurements and Doppler imaging are now possible, however these techniques are of limited use in the anesthetic management of patient with pre-eclampsia.

16. How will you administer fluid for resuscitation after seizure control prior to administration of anesthesia?

Ans.

- Initial fluid therapy should be restricted to 75–125 mL/hour in severe pre-eclampsia
- Further fluid should be guided by clinical sign like tissue perfusion, urinary output CVP, and cardiac output.
- Fluid is infused to maintain CVP upto 2–4 mm Hg, and 1 L of BSS is infused.
- If further fluid is required then preloading with 25–50 mL of 25% salt poor albumin is used.

17. Describe the Anesthetic management of pre-eclampsia patients.

Ans. *Goal of anesthesia:*

- To reduce maternal and fetal complication
- Seizure control
- BP control
- Monitoring and proper hydration by judicious administration of IV fluid
- Analgesia for labor
- Anesthesia for cesarean section.

18. Explain the anesthetic consideration in severe pre-eclampsia.

Ans.

- *Problems related to anesthesia* are hypertension (antihypertensive drugs), risk of seizures, difficult airway, reduced plasma volume, risk of pulmonary edema, coagulopathy, renal dysfunction, hypoproteinemia, altered liver function.
- *Preoperative considerations:* Physiological anemia rarely permits hematocrit >30%. In pre-eclampsia there is left shift of P50 which decrease the oxygen release to the fetus. Maternal base deficit (–8 mEq/L) may predict fetal acidosis and demise alongwith maternal end organ ischemia and injury.

  Instead of relying on laboratory coagulation profile, examination of women for abnormal coagulation profile like bleeding gums, bleeding from IV sites and other sources should be elicited. Consider D-dimer assay to detect the fibrin degradation product, abnormal platelet consumption and aspirin therapy for optimization.

  Hypovolemic, urine output and creatinine clearance are to be considered for renal function assessment.

  Elevated liver enzymes in association with HELLP syndrome alongwith upper quadrant/epigastric pain should be revealed for liver affection.

  Headache, visual disturbances as a premonitory sign of convulsion and neurodeficit forcerebral edema or cerebral hemorrhage should be elicited. Indications for CT or MRI are controversial.

  Fetal evaluation should be done prior to anaesthesia.
- *Intraoperative monitoring:* Automated noninvasive blood pressure, accurate intake and urine output measurement, examination of deep tendon reflexes and S. magnesium assay in magnesium sulfate recipients.

  Fetal scalp electrodes, if cervix is dilated.

  ECG and cardiac filling pressure monitoring.

19. Describe the anesthetic management.

Ans. *Choice of anesthesia:* Controversy exists over the superiority between regional vs. general anesthesia in pre-eclampsia. Epidural anesthesia would probably be preferred by many anesthesiologists in a severely pre-eclamptic patient in a nonurgent setting. For urgent cases it is reassuring to know that spinal is also safe (if not contraindicated). This allows us to avoid general anesthesia with the potential for encountering a swollen, difficult airway and/or labile hypertension.

Epidural Anesthesia

- Assess coagulation status
- Assess volume status and determined need for invasive hemodynamic monitoring
- Secure an intravenous line and hydrate the patient with 1000 mL of crystalloid or infuse enough fluids to increase CVP to no more than 4 mm Hg or a PCWP of 5–8 mm Hg
- Identified the epidural space and insert a catheter
- Aspirate the catheter for blood and cerebrospinal fluid
- Inject 2–3 mL 0.5% bupivacaine to detect subarachnoid catheter location and wait 3–5 minutes.
- Inject an additional 0.5% bupivacaine in 3–5 mL increments to a total dose of 20–25 mL to raise sensory blockage to at least T4 level.
- Assess hemodynamic changes in between each increment of drugs and give additional IV fluid or vasopressor as needed.

Spinal Anesthesia

- Although controversial, a growing body of data suggests that spinal anesthesia is a reasonable choice for women with severe pre-eclampsia
- Both prospective and retrospective studies suggest the hemodynamic changes associated with spinal and epidural anesthesia are similar in these women
- Profound hypotension can occur with either technique.

General Anesthesia

- Administer aspiration prophylaxis
- Secure an intravenous line and hydrate the patient
- Evaluate the airway
- In the operating room place the patient in the left tilt position and begin preoxygenation with 100% oxygen
- Use increasing doses of labetalol (5, 10, 20 mg) to lower blood pressure to a mean of approx. 105 to 110 mm Hg (diastolic pressure approx. 90–95 mm Hg)
- Rapid sequence induction with cricoid pressure. (fentanyl 100 μg, injection thiopental 5 mg/kg, succinylcholine 1.5 mg/kg)
- Maintenance with N_2O, O_2 and isoflurane and atracurium.
- Treat hypotension at delivery based on hemodynamic changes (i.e. volume versus pressure versus inotropic support)
- Infuse oxytocin immediately after delivery and avoid ergot alkaloid with can cause hypertension
- Reverse neuromuscular blockage and extubate in awake condition.
- Blunt hypertensive response to intubation and extubation—labetalol, NTG, IV esmolol, opoids.

Ref: Noris Mark C. Handbook of Obstetric Anesthesia. Lippincott Williams and Wilkings. 2000;21:395-417.
Ref: Miller RD, Eriksson LI, Fleisher LA, Wiener-Kronish JP, Young WL, Miller's Anesthesia, 7th edn. Churchill Livingstone; 2009.

20. What are the special considerations in the postpartum care of pre-eclamptic patients?
Ans.

- Continuous postpartum monitoring
- Continue $MgSO_4$ for 24 hours.
- Continue antihypertensive agents
- Pain medications to safeguard against convulsions
- Epidural narcotic (morphine) can provide sustained postoperative analgesia
- Maintain IV fluids
- Blood transfusion if excessive blood loss
- Comfortable and quiet environment
- Moist O_2
- Postnatal thromboprophylaxis should be administered to women with pre-eclampsia except where there is a surgical contraindication. Units should have clear protocols to deal with the timing of LMWH administration in regard to the insertion and withdrawal of epidural and spinal cannula.

BIBLIOGRAPHY

1. Cunningham F Gary, Leveno Kenneth J, Bloom Steven L, Hauth John C, Rouse Dwight J, Spong Catherine Y. Williams Obstetrics, 23rd edn. The McGraw-Hill Companies, Inc. 2010;34:706-49.
2. Miller RD, Eriksson LI, Fleisher LA, Wiener-Kronish JP, Young WL, Miller's Anesthesia, 7th edn. Churchill Livingstone; 2009.
3. Noris Mark C. Handbook of Obstetric Anesthesia. Lippincott Williams and Wilkings. 2000;21:395-417.

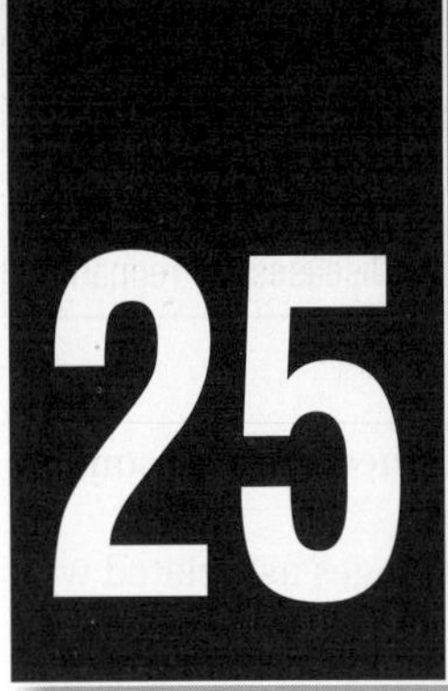

A Patient Suffering from Ischemic Heart Disease, have an Intracoronary Stent, on Beta Blockers, Calcium Channel Blocker and Statin Therapy, Posted for Elective Abdominal Surgery

Minati Choudhury

CASE

A 58-year-old man suffering from ischemic heart disease, have an intracoronary stent in left anterior descending artery two weeks back. He is on anticoagulation and antiplatelet therapy (warfarin, globally and clopidogrel), posted for elective abdominal surgery. He is on beta blocker, calcium channel blocker and statin therapy.

Things you must know regarding the management of such a case..........................

Before proceeding for the management one should remember that any of the noncardiac surgery after percutaneous coronary intervention with an intracoronary stent and anticoagulation and antiplatelet therapy has been associated with adverse cardiac events ranges from simple ST-T changes in the ECG to myocardial infarction, bleeding and death. These patients mostly have a recent history of acute coronary syndrome, due to significant blockade of coronary artery (varied from single vessel disease to triple vessel disease). Patients with drug eluting stent (DES) at high risk of late stent thrombosis and should be placed postoperatively in a monitored setting and all team members should be aware of signs and symptoms of stent thrombosis and the need for urgent intervention if such an event occurs. Antiplatelet therapy should be restarted as soon as possible.

1. **Is an intra-abdominal procedure a high-risk surgery?**

Ans. Apart from abdominal aortic aneurysm other intraperitoneal surgeries carries intermediate risk.

2. What are the preoperative predictors for perioperative cardiac morbidity?

Ans. According to 2002 American College of Cardiology (ACC) and American Heart Association (AHA) guideline update on perioperative cardiovascular evaluation clinical predictors are categorized into major, intermediate, and minor factors as follows:

Major Predictors

Unstable coronary syndromes, decompensated heart failure, significant arrhythmias (high-grade atrioventricular block, symptomatic ventricular arrhythmias, supraventricular arrhythmias with uncontrolled ventricular rate) and associated severe valvular disease.

Intermediate Predictors

Mild angina pectoris (Canadian class I or II), previous MI by history or pathologic waves, compensated or prior heart failure, diabetes mellitus (particularly insulin-dependent), renal insufficiency.

Minor Predictors

Advance age, abnormal ECG (LV hypertrophy, LBBB, ST abnormalities), rhythm other than sinus (e.g. atrial fibrillation), low functional capacity (e.g. inability to climb one flight of stairs with a bag of groceries), history of stroke and uncontrolled systemic hypertension.

3. What is the incidence of perioperative reinfarction?

Ans. It depends on the time interval between MI and operation. Even if in the presence of an intracoronary stent if the previous myocardial infarction occurred within a period of less than six months before surgery, it is associated with a very high-risk of reinfarction rate.

4. Would you recommend that the surgery be postponed for a certain period of time? If so, why?

Ans. As there is a significant decrease in reinfarction rate after 6 months of a MI, it is generally recommended to delay surgery 6 months after a MI. But at time this is difficult to practice as ethics is concerned. Again, the earlier the surgery is performed after stent placement, the more the chance of stent thrombosis.

The best data suggests that, wait 4–6 weeks after stent placement to perform elective surgery.

5. What is the New York Heart Association (NYHA) classification of heart failure?

Ans. It is determined by severity of symptoms including dyspnea and fatigue.

- *Class I:* No symptoms
- *Class II:* Symptoms with ordinary activity
- *Class III:* Symptoms with less than ordinary activity
- *Class IV:* Symptoms at rest.

6. What are the determinants of myocardial oxygen demand? How are they measured clinically?

Ans. The three major determinants are myocardial wall tension which is determined by LV preload and afterload, contractility and heart rate.

7. Which factors determine myocardial oxygen supply?

Ans. Aortic diastolic pressure, LV end-diastolic pressure, patency of coronary arteries.

8. What is the mechanism of myocardial ischemia?

Ans. Myocardial ischemia occurs whenever myocardial oxygen supply cannot match myocardial oxygen demand. Intraoperative ischemia can be precipitated by increases in myocardial oxygen demand caused by tachycardia, hypertension, anemia, hypoxemia, stress, sympathomimetic drugs, discontinuation of β-blockers or stent thrombosis.

9. This patient is on beta blockers, calcium channel blocker and statin therapy. What you are going to do about these drugs?

Ans. Continue with all these drugs along with the routine premedication (This reduces the perioperative adverse cardiac events to a significant level).

10. What are the types of intracoronary stents?

Ans. BMS: Bare metal stent, DES: Drug eluting stent, SES: Sirolimus eluting stent and PES: Pacitaxel eluting stent.

11. How you are going to manage the anticoagulant and antiplatelet agent perioperatively?

Ans.

- Continue dual antiplatelet therapy during and after surgery. This is done if the patient is undergoing a surgery early after stent implantation (6 weeks). Warfarin can be switch over to continuous infusion of heparin or low molecular weight heparin. OR,
- If surgery is scheduled 6 weeks after, discontinue antiplatelet therapy 48 hours before and warfarin 24 hours before; and bridge the patient to surgery with continuous infusion of heparin or low molecular weight heparin. Restart all these agents as soon as the surgery is over.

12. How would you evaluate the patient's cardiac condition? What laboratory tests would you like to have done?

Ans. The initial history, physical examination, and electrocardiographic assessment should focus on identification of potentially serious cardiac disorders (e.g. prior MI, angina pectoris), CHF, and electrical instability (e.g. symptomatic arrhythmias).

Define disease severity, *stability*, and prior *treatment.*

Assessment of functional capacity, comorbid conditions (e.g. diabetes mellitus, peripheral vascular disease, renal dysfunction, chronic pulmonary disease).

The preoperative investigation should also include: Routine hemogram and blood chemistry, International normalization ratio (INR, this should be kept between 1.5 and 2 to reduce the incidence of bleeding as well as stent thrombosis), chest X-ray (to rule out cardiomegaly and congestive cardiac failure), 12-lead ECG (to know new onset of ischemia), transthoracic echocardiography (TTE), which has appeared very helpful in evaluating the perioperative risk of major cardiac complications. TTE data include global LV function, regional wall motion abnormalities (RWMAs), hypertrophy indexes, and Doppler-derived measurements for the valvular functions.

13. How would you premedicate this patient?

Ans. I would like to sedate this patient before surgery to avoid anxiety-induced tachycardia and hypertension that may cause adverse myocardial ischemic events. Appropriate doses of diazepam, lorazepam, or midazolam plus a analgesic is given along with all the antianginal medications.

14. How would you monitor the patient?

Ans.

- *ECG:* Simultaneous leads V_5 and II, multiple-lead ST-segment analysis if available
- *Blood pressure:* Noninvasive automatic Doppler sphygmomanometric technique/invasive arterial line if available.

- Pulse oximeter for arterial oxygenation
- *Temperature:* Esophageal
- *Swan-Ganz catheter:* PCWP, pulmonary artery diastolic pressure (PAD), hemodynamic study only for patients with ventricular dysfunction
- *Central venous pressure (CVP) line:* If the patient has good LV function
- *Foley catheter:* Urine output
- Oxygen analyzer for inspired gas mixture
- End-tidal CO_2 analyzer.

15. How would you monitor ECG? Why V_5?

Ans. The ST segment changes in ECG are most commonly used for detection of intraoperative myocardial ischemia. Leads II and V_5, can detect 96% of ischemic events. Combination of leads II and V_5 was only 80% sensitive, whereas combining leads V_4 and V_5 increased sensitivity to 90% in patients with known CAD undergoing noncardiac surgery with general anesthesia. The sensitivity increased to 96% by combining leads II, V_4, and V_5.

If only one lead can be displayed, V_5 should be used because lead V_5 has the greatest sensitivity, 75% intraoperatively.

16. How would you induce anesthetic?

Ans. Smooth induction is essential to prevent hypotension, hypertension, and tachycardia, which can precipitate myocardial ischemia. Different induction techniques may be employed to achieve this goal. While the patient is being preoxygenated, fentanyl 2–5–8 mcg/kg is given slowly to achieve drowsiness. Then, thiopental in 3–5 mg/kg or midazolam in 1 mg increments is titrated to produce unconsciousness, followed by succinylcholine 1 mg/kg or rocuronium 0.6–1 mg/kg to facilitate tracheal intubation. All the intravenous anesthetic agents are acceptable with the exception of ketamine, which may produce significant hypertension and tachycardia. Induction with volatile anesthetic agent, particularly sevoflurane can be used in case of anticipated difficult intubation/otherwise.

17. What is your opinion regarding etomidate/dexmedetomidine?

Ans. Etomidate has a better hemodynamic profile than other commonly used induction agents, especially in the setting of coronary heart disease. It also attenuates the reaction to the tracheal intubation to a greater extent than thiopental. It is a good choice if the patient has poor LV function. The dose is 0.2–03 mg/kg. Dexmedetomidine is cardio stable, causes a better control of heart rate, need expertise for titration. It is usually used an adjunct to thiopentone induction. The usual dose is: loading dose of 0.5 to 1 μ/kg is administered for 10 minutes followed by a maintenance infusion of 0.3 μ/kg/hr.

18. How you will maintain of anesthesia?

Ans. There is no best myocardial protective agent or technique. The use of inhalational versus intravenous anesthesia in such patients depends upon the attending anesthesiologist. Because I would like to extubate the patient at the end of surgery, I will use nitrous oxide and a combination of low-dose sevoflurane/isoflurane and fentanyl for maintenance of anesthesia.

19. What muscle relaxant would you choose?

Ans. The hemodynamic goals are to avoid hypotension, tachycardia, and hypertension. I will like to use intermediate-acting neuromuscular blocking agents such as vecuronium, cisatracurium, or rocuronium for their cardiostability. A peripheral nerve stimulator can be used to monitor the degree of blockade.

20. Significant depression of ST segment was noticed intraoperatively. How would you treat it?
Ans. ST-depression indicates myocardial ischemia, either from increased myocardial oxygen demand or from decreased oxygen supply. The treatment includes the following:
- *Increase O_2 supply:* Correct hypotension, hypoxemia, and severe anemia
- *Decrease O_2 demand:* Correct hypertension and tachycardia by deepening the level of anesthesia or by using vasodilator, β-blockers, and calcium channel blockers.

If there are no obvious changes in hemodynamics (silent intraoperative ischemia), nitroglycerin infusion may be used to relieve suspected coronary spasm.

21. What is the significance of tight controlling the heart rate intraoperatively?
Ans. Intraoperative tachycardia could cause myocardial ischemia. Therefore, tight control of heart rate intraoperatively could significantly reduce the risk of perioperative myocardial events.

22. How you will manage the perioperative fluid and blood transfusion for this patient?
Ans. Similar to any other similar kind of patient without a stent/anticoagulation. At times there may be increase requirement of platelet transfusion which is not essential routinely in a patient without a stent. If profound bleeding occurs, the ultimate solution is recombinant factor VIIa. However, platelet transfusions or factor VIIa render the patient hyperthrombotic and hypercoagulable and should be reserved for life-threatening bleeding when all other measures of hemostasis have failed.

23. When would you extubate this patient? What could you do to prevent hypertension and tachycardia during extubation and emergence?
Ans. At the end of surgery I would extubate the patient when the patient is awake, breathing adequately, and neuromuscular blockade is fully reversed. To prevent tachycardia and hypertension associated with extubation and emergence, I would give the patient low doses of preventive medication such as 1 mg/kg of lidocaine or esmolol or 0.1 mg/kg of labetalol 2 minutes before extubation.

24. How would you control postoperative pain?
Ans. Patient-controlled intravenous (ketorolac/tramadol/NSAIDS) and/or epidural analgesia.

25. Can you go for regional anesthesia?
Ans. It can be used with caution and in expert hands only when general anesthesia is a contraindication. This is because of the fact that, risk of bleeding/epidural hematoma is always a concern as the patient is on anticoagulant.

Most studies have suggested no difference in infarction rate during general and regional (spinal, epidural, and nerve block, local) anesthesia in a patient with ischemic heart disease.

These facts are good to know...

1. Describe antianginal drugs and their mechanism of action.
Ans. The major antianginal drugs are nitrovasodilators, calcium channel blockers and β-adrenergic antagonists, ACE inhibitors.

Nitrovasodilators (Nitroglycerin, Isosorbide Dinitrate)

In low doses, decreased LV preload (low dose) leading to decreased LV filling pressure and LV diastolic chamber size, systemic and pulmonary venodilatation. In higher doses it causes decrease in systemic blood pressure, systemic vascular resistance.

Coronary circulation: Coronary artery and arteriolar dilation (high dose), reversal/prevention of coronary spasm, stenosis dilation, increased collateral flow, improvement of regional subendocardial ischemia.

β-Adrenergic Antagonists (Propranolol, Esmolol, Atenolol)

- Reductions in myocardial oxygen consumption, improvements in coronary blood flow, prolonged diastolic perfusion period, improved collateral flow, increased flow to ischemic areas
- Overall improvement in supply/demand ratio
- Stabilization of cellular membranes
- Inhibition of platelet aggregation
- Reduced mortality after MI.

Calcium Channel Blockers (Verapamil, Diltiazem, Nifedipine, Nicardipine)

Calcium channel blockers reduce myocardial oxygen demand by depression of myocardial contractility and dilation of coronary and collateral vessels, which improve blood flow.

2. Would the patient have increased risk for perioperative major cardiac complications if the patient's preoperative electrocardiogram (ECG) shows right bundle branch block (RBBB) or left bundle branch block (LBBB)?

Ans. Presence of RBBB or LBBB was not associated with a high incidence of postoperative cardiac complications. Nevertheless, the patients with LBBB may not tolerate certain stress of perioperative noncardiac complications, such as severe sepsis. The presence of LBBB or RBBB may alert the clinician to the possibility of impaired LV functions.

3. Would you recommend further cardiac testing or coronary revascularization before surgery?

Ans. No.

4. How would you classify the cardiac risk according to the type of surgery?

Ans. Surgery-specific risk for noncardiac surgery can be stratified as high, intermediate, and low.

- High-risk surgery (cardiac risk often greater than 5%) includes major emergency surgery, particularly in the elderly; aortic and other major vascular surgery; peripheral vascular surgery; and anticipated prolonged procedures associated with large fluid shifts and/or blood loss
- Intermediate-risk (cardiac risk generally less than 5%) procedures include carotid endarterectomy, head and neck surgery, intraperitoneal and intrathoracic, orthopedic, and prostate surgery
- Low-risk (cardiac risk generally less than 1%) procedures include endoscopic and superficial procedures, cataract surgery, and breast surgery.

5. Are patients with a Q-wave infarction at greater risk of reinfarction than those with a non-Q-wave infarction?

Ans. Recent studies indicate that individuals who survive a non-Q-wave infarction are at greater risk of reinfarction than those who survive a Q-wave infarction. Patients who have not had a transmural wall infarction probably have border zones of that infarction that remain at high-risk for subsequent damage. These border zones might not be present with a clear-cut transmural Q-wave infarction.

6. Is there a role for α-2 agonist in premedication?

Ans. α-2 agonists stimulate prejunctional receptors and decrease norepinephrine release from prejunctional terminals, thereby decreasing noradrenergic central nervous system transmissions, producing sedation, anxiolysis, and analgesia. Clonidine/dexmedetomidine as a premedication reduces hypertension, tachycardia, and norepinephrine may also reduce postoperative myocardial ischemia events in high-risk patients.

7. Would you give prophylactic intravenous nitroglycerin to prevent myocardial ischemia?

Ans. It can be used if there is evidence of ischemia though there are insufficient data about the effects of prophylactic intraoperative intravenous nitroglycerin in these patients.

8. What are the perioperative sign of stent thrombosis? And how will you react is such a situation arises?

Ans. The usual manifestation is ST elevation but pre-emptive signs such as refractory hypotension, new onset atrioventricular block or ventricular arrhythmias should raise a high index of suspicion. If such a diagnosis is entertained, interventional cardiologists should be immediately involved in the care and the patients transferred to a catheterization laboratory for thrombectomy. Occurrence of cardiovascular collapse may require inotropic support or emergency placement of an intra-aortic balloon pump. A defibrillator device should be available in the operating room and during transport to other locations.

9. What are the postoperative predictors of cardiac morbidity?

Ans. Pain, postoperative unintentional hypothermia, hypercoagulability, and anemia are associated with an increased incidence of myocardial ischemia.

The postoperative period can be stressful because of the onset of pain during emergence from anesthesia, fluid shifts, temperature changes, and alteration of respiratory function. Marked changes occur in plasma catecholamine concentration, hemodynamics, ventricular function, and coagulation occurs following the surgery, that can increase the incidence of postoperative morbidity.

10. Is postoperative anemia associated with adverse cardiac outcome?

Ans. Yes. It is well documented that a hematocrit on postoperative day 2 less than 29% is associated with a high degree of ischemia on the first two postoperative days (55%).

11. Is postoperative hypothermia associated with postoperative myocardial ischemia?

Ans. Yes. It is well described in the literature that, unintentional hypothermia [sublingual temperature less than 35°C on arrival to postoperative intensive care unit (ICU)] is associated with a significantly higher incidence of myocardial ischemia (36%) and PaO_2 less than 80 mm Hg (52%) during the early postoperative period. Therefore, aggressive warming and heat conservation are mandatory during and after surgery. It is recommended to continue forced-air warming for the first several hours after surgery in hypothermic patients.

12. How would you make a diagnosis of perioperative MI?

Ans. Abnormalities of wall motion detected by TEE are almost universally present, even when no ST-segment elevation is seen.

Intraoperative hemodynamic compromise (hypotension, arrhythmia) in the absence of volume loss.

Elevation of cardiac enzymes, e.g. creatine kinase (CK-MB), troponin-I (cTn I), troponin-T (cTn T) have some value.

13. How would you manage the patient with suspected perioperative MI?

Ans. Resume therapy with aspirin and β-blockers.

Consult with cardiologist, cardiac surgical and anesthesia team for prompt reperfusion with angioplasty of the remaining vessels and stenting or coronary artery bypass grafting.

Nice to know........................

1. Would you use a pulmonary artery catheter (PAC)?

Ans. A numbers of studies report that PAC is an insensitive monitor for myocardial ischemia and should not be inserted with this as a primary indication.

Few studies that have been reported compare patient outcomes after treatment with or without PACs. This monitoring mode is especially beneficial if there is expectation of massive fluid shifts, patients with a recent MI complicated by CHF; who are undergoing procedures associated with significant hemodynamic stress (abdominal aortic aneurysm/major abdominal malignancy requiring prolonged dissection); and those with systolic or diastolic LV dysfunction, cardiomyopathy, and associated valvular disease.

2. Would you monitor transesophageal echocardiography (TEE)?

Ans. The TEE is a highly sensitive ischemia monitor, which can detect new RWMAs, decreased systolic wall thickening, and ventricular dilation to recognize ischemic events. At the same time TEE examination may divert the anesthesiologists' attention from more important clinical details. Definitely it has a value if one additional anesthetist is present who can manage clinical details.

3. What is the ideal time for elective surgery if the patient is with a DES stent?

Ans. Elective surgery should be deferred for 12 months following DES stent because of likely increase risk of death/myocardial infarction/stent thrombosis.

4. What is the guideline for antithrombotic treatment after insertion of an intracoronary stent?

Ans. General:
- *Bare metal stent:* Clopidogrel for 3–4 weeks and life-long treatment with acetylsalicylic acid.Dual antiplatelet therapy with warfarin is commonly used to prevent stent thrombosis.
- *Drug-eluting stent:* Clopidogrel for 9–12 months and life-long treatment with acetylsalicylic acid.
- *Acute coronary syndrome:* Clopidogrel for 9–12 months and life-long treatment with acetylsalicylic acid irrelevant of stent type.

After late stent thrombosis:
- Acetylsalicylic acid and clopidogrel for several years if cause of the stent thrombosis has not been identified and treated.

Elective noncardiac surgery:
- *Bare metal stent:* Delay surgery for at least 6 weeks. No discontinuation of acetylsalicylic acid.
- *Drug-eluting stent and low-risk of bleeding:* Delay surgery for at least 6 months. Ideal is, do the surgery after 12 months. Continuous treatment with acetylsalicylic acid and clopidogrel.
- *Drug-eluting stent and a great risk of bleeding:* Delay surgery for 9–12 months after stent implantation. Acetylsalicylic acid should be continued perioperatively.

Dental treatment:
- No premature discontinuation of blood platelet inhibitors. With great risk of bleeding, delay dental treatment for at least 6 weeks with bare metal stents and for 9–12 months with drug-eluting stents. Acetylsalicylic acid should be continued perioperatively.

Warfarin in combination with blood platelet inhibition:
- *Strong indication for anticoagulation:* Warfarin in combination with acetylsalicylic acid and clopidogrel.
- *Weaker indication for anticoagulation:* Acetylsalicylic acid and clopidogrel. Warfarin is discontinued during the period with dual platelet inhibition. Use warfarin and acetylsalicylic acid after the treatment period with dual blood platelet inhibitors.

Skin rash after stenting:
- Ticlopidine, 250 mg two times daily, with the same treatment duration as for clopidogrel.

BIBLIOGRAPHY

1. ACC/AHA 2007 Guidelines on Perioperative Cardiovascular Evaluation and Care for Noncardiac Surgery: Executive Summary. A Report of the American College of Cardiology/American Heart Association Task Force on Practice Guidelines (Writing Committee to Revise the 2002 Guidelines on Perioperative Cardiovascular Evaluation for Noncardiac Surgery) Circulation. 2007;116: 1971-96.
2. Brilakis E, Banerjee S, Berger PB. Perioperative management of patient with coronay stent. J Am Coll Cardiol. 2007;22:2145-50.
3. Douketis JD, Berger PB, Dunn AS, Jaffer AK, Spyropoulos AC, Becker RC, Ansell J; American College of Chest Physicians. The perioperative management of antithrombotic therapy: American College of Chest Physicians Evidence-Based Clinical Practice Guidelines (8th edn).Chest. 2008;133(6 Suppl):299S-339S. doi: 10.1378/chest.08-0675.
4. Eagle KA, Berger PB, Calkins H, et al. (Eds). ACC/AHA guideline update for perioperative cardiovascular evaluation for noncardiac surgery—executive summary. A report of the American College of Cardiology/ American Heart Association Task Force on practice guidelines. Anesth Analg. 2002:94:1052-64.
5. Fleisher LA, Barash PG. Preoperative cardiac evaluation for noncardiac surgery: a functional approach. Anesth Analg. 1992:74:586-98.
6. Goldman L. Cardiac risk in noncardiac surgery: an update. Anesth Analg. 1995:80:810–20.
7. Newsome LT, Weller RS, Gerancher JC, et al. Coronary artery stents: II.Perioperative considerations and management. Anesth Analg. 2008;107:570-90.
8. Popescu WM. Perioperative management of the patient with a coronary stent. Current Opinion in Anaesthesiology. 2010;23:109-15.
9. Rohde LE, Polanczyk CA, Goldman L, et al. Usefulness of transthoracic echocardiography as a tool for risk stratification of patients undergoing major noncardiac surgery. Am J Cardiol. 2001;87:505-9.
10. Smith SC Jr, Allen J, Blair SN, et al. ACC/AHA/SCAI 2005 guideline update for percutaneous coronary intervention: a report of the American College of Cardiology/American Heart Association Task Force for Practice Guidelines. www.americanheart.org/presenter.jhtml?identier=3035436 (28.5.2007).
11. Sourgounis A, Lipiecki J, Hamon M. Coronary stents and chronic anticoagulation. Circulation. 2009;119: 1682-8.

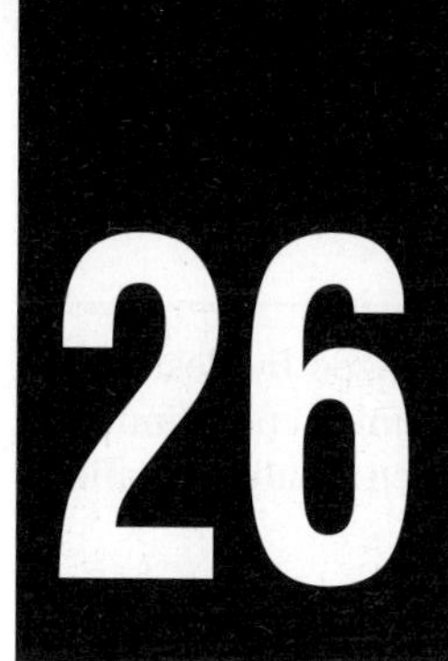

Anesthetic Management of a Patient with Airway Disorder Posted for Upper Abdominal Elective Surgery

Sampa Dutta Gupta, Pooja Banerjee, Rajat Choudhuri

1. What is the case summary?

Ans.

- A 45-year-old male patient posted for an upper abdominal elective surgery has come for preanesthetic evaluation. During preanesthetic check-up, history revealed patient, a chronic smoker, is suffering from chronic cough with sputum production for last 7 years with progressive decrease in disease-free period, no seasonal predilection, complaining of disturbed sleep for last 2 years and respiratory distress on climbing 2 flight of stairs. Not on any regular medication except for occasional use of MDI salmeterol-budesonide, seeking medical advice only during exacerbation, no hospital admission in past.
- Physical examination revealed P = 80/min, BP = 130/84 mm Hg, no pallor, edema, clubbing; Chest—barrel shaped, B/L reduced VBS, rhonchi++; S1, S2—normal, no murmur; interincisor gap—3 fingers, MP grade 2.
- His investigation reports were Hb = 13.2, fbs = 104, S.ur = 30, S.cr = 1.2, PFT: FEV_1 = 60%, FEV_1/FVC = 0.55, CXR: hyperinflated lung fields, ECG = RAD with RV strain pattern, ABG: PaO_2 = 85, $PaCO_2$ = 47.

2. What are the differential diagnoses for this patient?

Ans. According to the case summary, the probable differential diagnoses are:

- Chronic obstructive pulmonary disease (COPD)
- Asthma
- Restrictive lung disease.

3. Define COPD?

Ans.

- Disease state characterized by airflow limitation that is not fully reversible. The airflow limitation is usually both progressive and associated with an abnormal inflammatory response of the lungs to noxious particles or gases.

- COPD includes *emphysema,* an anatomically defined condition characterized by destruction and enlargement of the lung alveoli; *chronic bronchitis,* a clinically defined condition with chronic cough and phlegm; and *small airways disease,* a condition in which small bronchioles are narrowed.

  Ref: Harrison's Principles of Internal Medicine, 18th edn; P2631, Chapter: COPD.

4. What are the variants of COPD?

Ans.

- The COPD includes emphysema and chronic bronchitis.
- *Emphysema:* Abnormal permanent enlargement of the air spaces distal to the terminal bronchioles accompanied by destruction of their walls and without obvious fibrosis.
- *Chronic bronchitis:* Presence of chronic productive cough for 3 months in each of 2 successive years in a patient in whom other causes of chronic cough have been excluded.

Ref: Harrison's Principles of Internal Medicine, 18th edn, Chapter: COPD.

5. How does a patient with emphysema present?

Ans.

- *Symptoms:* These patients are usually not cyanosed but are dyspneic and are sometimes called 'pink puffers.' Pursed lip breathing (this occurs in emphysema and not in chronic bronchitis), i.e. expiration through partly closed lips increases the end-expiratory pressure and keeps airways open, helping to minimize air trapping.
- *Signs:* The signs result from hyperinflation like barrel-shaped chest with increased antero-posterior diameter.
- Use of accessory muscles of respiration and drawing in of the lower intercostal muscles with inspiration.
- *Palpation:* Reduced expansion and a hyperinflated chest.
- *Percussion:* Hyper-resonant with decreased liver dullness.
- *Breath sounds:* Decreased, early inspiratory crackles.
- Wheeze is often absent.
- Signs of right heart failure may occur, but only late in the course of the disease, when they usually indicate a preterminal state.

Ref: Clinical Examination 5th edn, Talley, O'connor.

6. What is the relation of history disturbed sleep at night in patients with COPD?

Ans. The COPD patient desaturate more frequently and more severely during sleep due to rapid/shallow breathing pattern that occurs in all patients during rapid eye movement sleep. In COPD patients, breathing air, causes a significant increase in respiratory dead space/tidal volume ratio (VDS/VT) and fall in alveolar oxygen tension (PaO_2) and PaO_2. This is not sleep apnea/hypoventilation syndrome, the oxygen saturation falls to less than 50% at sometime during the sleep which may cause increase in pulmonary arterial pressure, interstitial edema and respiratory distress during sleep. This tendency to desaturate combined with the postoperative fall in FRC, use of opioid analgesia may lead to severe postoperative hypoxemia during sleep.

Ref: Miller's Anesthesia, 7th edn; Editor-Ronald D. Miller, Associate editors-Lars I. Eriksson, Lee A. Fleisher. Chapter: Anesthesia management of Concurrent Diseases.

7. How does a patient with chronic bronchitis present?

Ans.

- *Symptoms:* Loose cough and sputum (mucoid or mucopurulent) as a result of bronchial hypersecretion and airways obstruction. These patients are sometimes called 'blue bloaters' because of cyanosis present in the latter stages and because of associated edema from right ventricular failure.

- *Signs*
- *Palpation:* Hyperinflated chest with reduced expansion.
- *Percussion:* Increased resonance.
- *Breath sounds:* Reduced with end-expiratory high or low-pitched wheezes and early inspiratory crackles.
- Signs of right ventricular failure.

Clinical Examination 5th edn, Talley, O'connor, Chapter: chest examination.

How would you differentiate emphysema from chronic bronchitis?

	Emphysema pink puffer	*Chronic bronchitis blue bloater*
Cyanosis	Absent	Prominent
Dyspnea	++	+
Hyperinflation	++	+
Cor pulmonale	–	Common
Respiratory drive	High	Low

8. Define bronchial asthma?

Ans.

- This may be defined as paroxysmal recurrent attacks of wheezing (or in childhood of cough) due to airways narrowing which changes in severity over short periods of time.
- How does a patient with bronchial asthma present?

Symptoms: Wheezing, dry or productive cough

Signs: Tachypnea, tachycardia, prolonged expiration, use of accessory muscles of respiration, Hyperinflated chest (increased anteroposterior diameter with high shoulders and, on percussion, decreased liver dullness), inspiratory and expiratory wheezes.

Ref: Harrison's Principles of Internal Medicine, 18th edition.

9. How will you differentiate COPD from asthma?

Ans.

Suggestive features COPD:

- Mid-life onset
- Slowly progressing symptons
- Long history of smoking
- Dyspnea during exercise
- Largely irreversible airflow limitation.

Early onset asthma

- Symptoms vary from day-to-day
- Symptoms at the night/early morning
- Airflow limitation that is largely reversible
- Allergy, rhinitis, eczema.

10. How does a patient with restrictive lung disease present?

Ans. Patients with interstitial lung diseases (ILDs) come to medical attention mainly because of the onset of progressive exertional dyspnea or a persistent nonproductive cough. Hemoptysis, wheezing, and chest pain may be present. Often, the identification of interstitial opacities on chest X-ray focuses the diagnostic approach on one of the ILDs.

Ref: Harrison's Principles of Internal Medicine, 18th edition.

11. Enumerate the causes of restrictive lung disease.

Ans.

A. *Intrinsic restrictive lung disorders:*

- Sarcoidosis
- Idiopathic pulmonary fibrosis
- Interstitial pneumonitis
- Tuberculosis
- Pnuemonectomy
- Pneumonia.

Ref: Fishman's Pulmonary Diseases and Disorders, 4th edn, 2008.pp.664-74.

B. *Extrinsic restrictive lung disorders:*

- Scoliosis, kyphosis
- Ankylosing spondylitis
- Pleural effusion
- Pregnancy
- Gross obesity
- Tumors
- Ascites
- Pain on inspiration—pleurisy, rib fractures.

Ref: Fishman's Pulmonary Diseases and Disorders, 4th edition

C. *Neuromuscular restrictive lung disorders:*

- Generalized weakness—malnutrition
- Paralysis of the diaphragm
- Myasthenia gravis
- Muscular dystrophy
- Poliomyelitis
- Amyotrophic lateral sclerosis.

Ref: Fishman's Pulmonary Diseases and Disorders, 4th edition.

12. What should be the preoperative evaluation of this patient?

Ans. Preoperative evaluation should include:

- History
- Physical examination
- Investigations.

13. What are the investigations to be done in this case?

Ans.

- Complete hemogram, blood sugar
- Serum urea, creatinine
- ECG
- Chest X-ray
- Pulmonary function tests, reversibility
- Arterial blood gas analysis
- Echocardiography

Sputum culture, α_1 antitrypsin levels, if indicated.

14. What are the components of pulmonary function test?

Ans.

- Lung volumes and capacities
- Expiratory flow rates

- Lung elasticity
- Diffusion capacity
- Airway resistance
- Tests for small airway disease
- Gas exchange.

Ref: Fishman's pulmonary disease and disorders. 4th edn, 2008.pp.664-74.

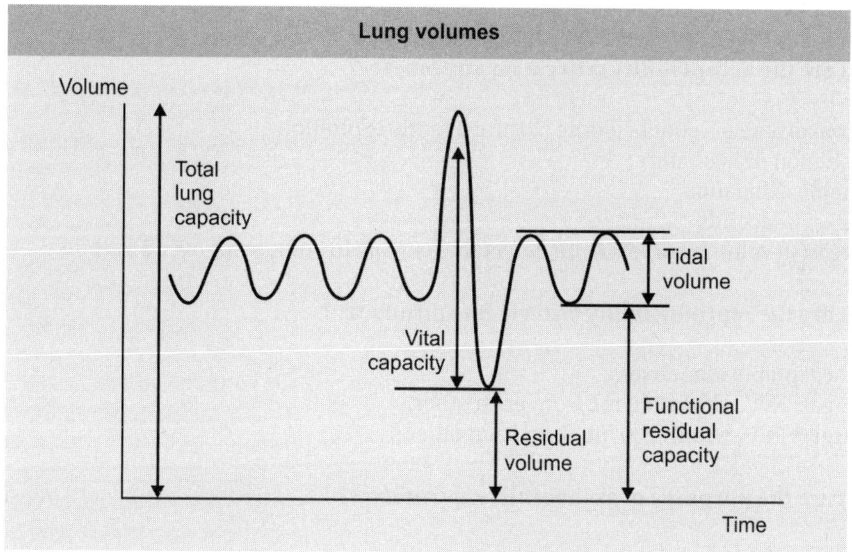

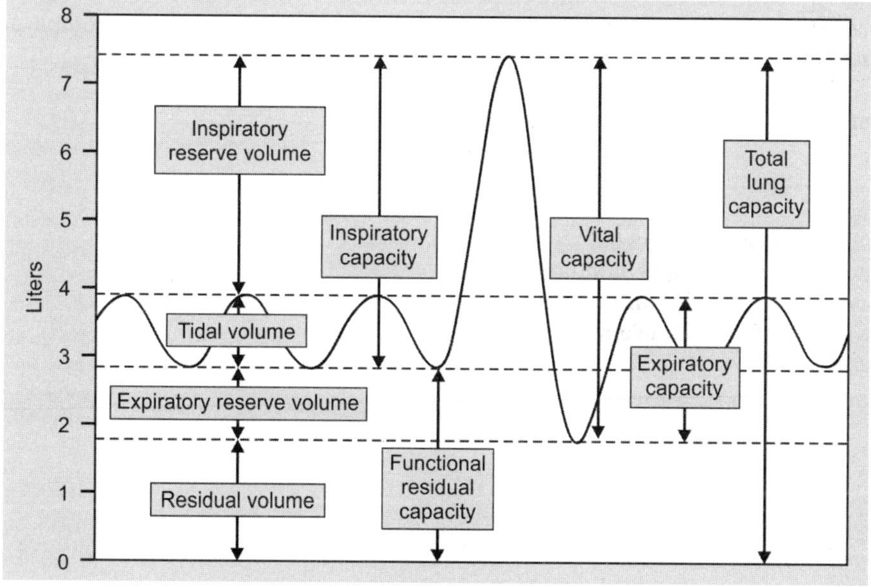

15. What is spirometry?

- Measure of airflow and lung volumes during a forced expiratory maneuver from full inspiration using a spirometer. It is an effort dependent test.
- Spirometric measurement

A. Absolute values	*B. Graphic forms*
1. FEV_1	1. Volume vs time curve
2. FVC	2. Flow rate vs volume loop
3. FEV_1/FVC	

16. What are the acceptability criteria for spirometry?

Ans.

- Free from artifacts—cough, glottic closure in early expiration.
- No hesitation or false start.
- Acceptable exhalation
  - At least 6 seconds
  - Plateau in volume curve, i.e. no detectable change in volume for over 1 second.

17. What are the reproducibility criteria for spirometry?

Ans.

- Three acceptable maneuvers.
- Two largest FVC within 200 mL from each other.
- Two largest FEV_1 within 200 mL from each other.

18. What are the purposes of preoperative spirometry?

Ans.

- To evaluate airway obstruction in patients at risk.
- To institute appropriate preoperative remedial measures
- Intense preoperative respiratory therapy minimizes postoperative pulmonary complications by 50% in COPD.

19. What are the contraindications of spirometry?

Ans.

- Myocardial infarction in last 1 month.
- Pregnancy.
- Recent seizure, syncope, angina.
- Significant hemoptysis, pneumothorax.
- Aneurysm (cerebral, abdominal, thoracic)
- Chest or abdominal pain of any cause
- Dementia.

Ref: Goldman DR. perioperative medicine.

20. How to interpret spirometry findings?

Ans.

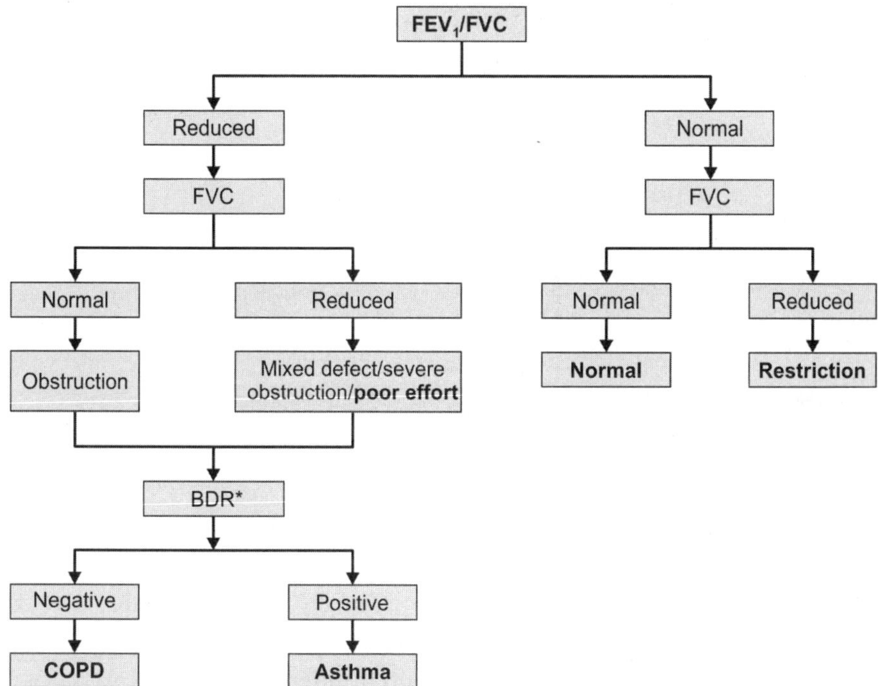

*BDR = Bronchodilator responsiveness

21. How interpretation of PFTs is done?

Ans.

Step 1: Look at the flow-volume loop to determine acceptability of the test, and look for upper airway obstruction pattern.

Step 2: Look at the FEV_1 to determine if it is normal (≥ 80% predicted).

Step 3: Look at FVC to determine if it is within normal limits (≥ 80%).

Step 4: Look at the FEV_1/FVC ratio to determine if it is within normal limits (≥ 70%).

Step 5: Look at FEF 25–75% (Normal (≥ 60%):

- If FEV_1, FEV_1/FVC ratio, and $FEF_{25-75\%}$ all are normal, the patient has a normal PFT.
- If both FEV_1 and FEV_1/FVC are normal, but $FEF_{25-75\%}$ is ≤ 60%, then think about early obstruction or small airways obstruction.
- If FEV_1 ≤ 80% and FEV_1/FVC ≤ 70%, there is obstructive defect, if FVC is normal, it is pure obstruction. If FVC ≤ 80%, possibility of additional restriction is there.
- If FEV_1 ≤ 80%, FVC ≤ 80% and FEV_1/FVC ≥ 70%, there is restrictive defect, get lung volumes to confirm.

Ref: Clinics in chest medicine. 2001;22:703-14.

22. What do you mean by flow volume loop?
Ans.

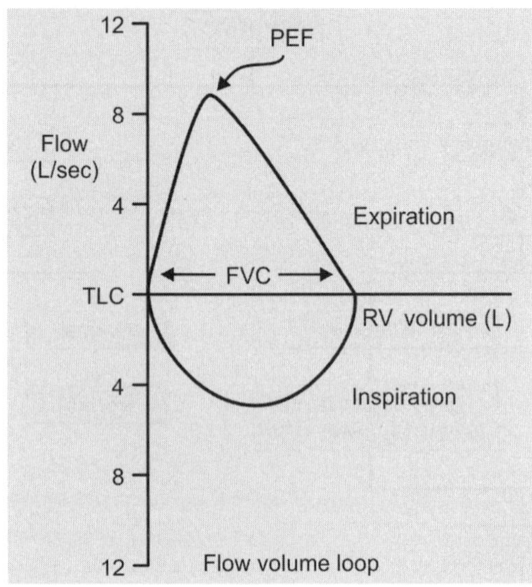

Flow volume loop is a plot of inspiratory and expiratory flow in the vertical axis against volume in the horizontal axis, during the performance of maximally forced inspiratory and expiratory maneuvers.

23. Describe the usefulness of the flow volume loops in different conditions.
Flow volume loop is useful in assessing acceptability of the maneuvers:
- Lack of early peak suggests poor effort.
- Sudden tailing off of expiration curve suggest that the patient stopped blowing too early
- Cough

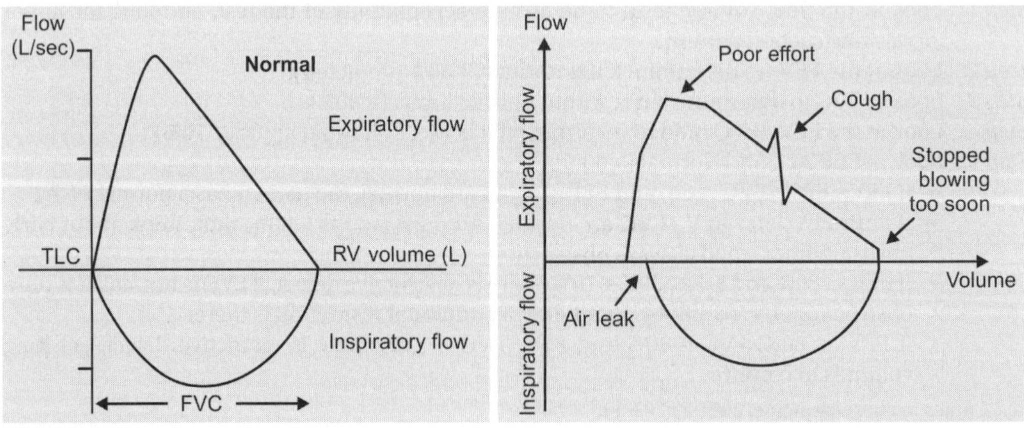

Asthma:
- Peak expiratory flow reduced so maximum height of the loop is reduced
- Airflow reduces rapidly with the reduction in the lung volumes because the airways narrow and the loop become concave

- Concavity may be the indicator of airflow obstruction and may present before the change in FEV_1 or FEV_1/FVC

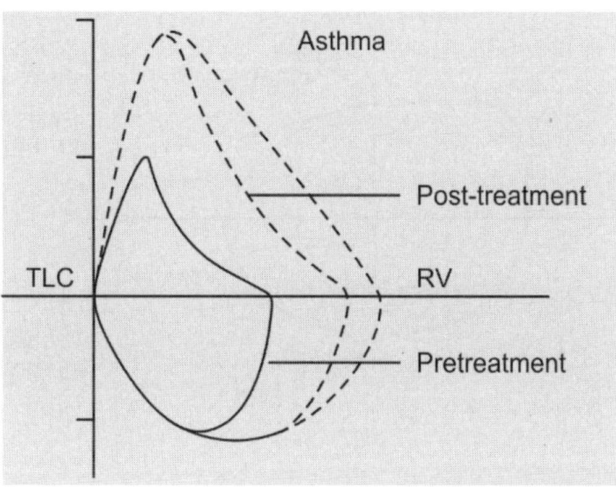

Emphysema:

Airways may collapse during forced expiration because of destruction of the supporting lung tissue causing a reduced flow at low lung volume and a characteristic (dog-leg) appearance to the flow volume curve.

Reversibility:

- Improvement in FEV_1 by 12–15% or 200 mL in repeating spirometry after treatment with Salbutamol 2.5 mg or ipratropium bromide by nebulizer after 15–30 minutes.
- Reversibility is a characteristic feature of bronchial asthma. In chronic asthma, there may be only partial reversibility of the airflow obstruction.
- While in COPD the airflow is irreversible although some cases showed significant improvement.

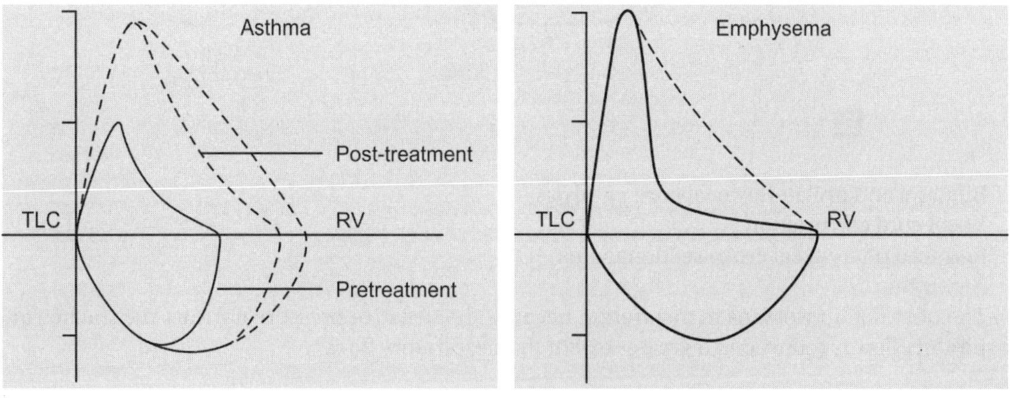

Fixed obstruction:

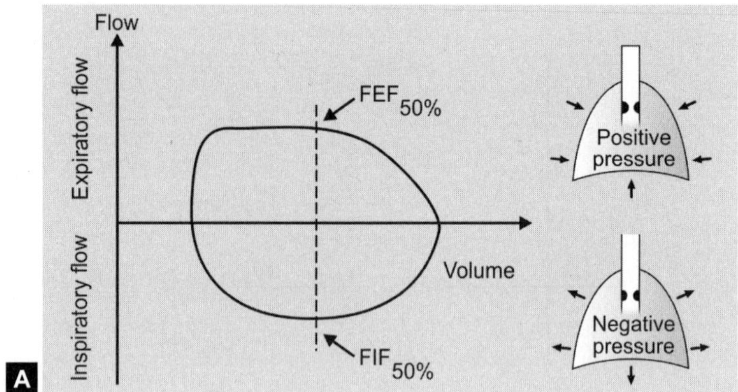

- Postintubation stenosis
- Goiter
- Endotracheal neoplasms
- Bronchial stenosis

Maximum airflow is limited to a similar extent in both inspiration and expiration.

Variable extrathoracic obstruction:

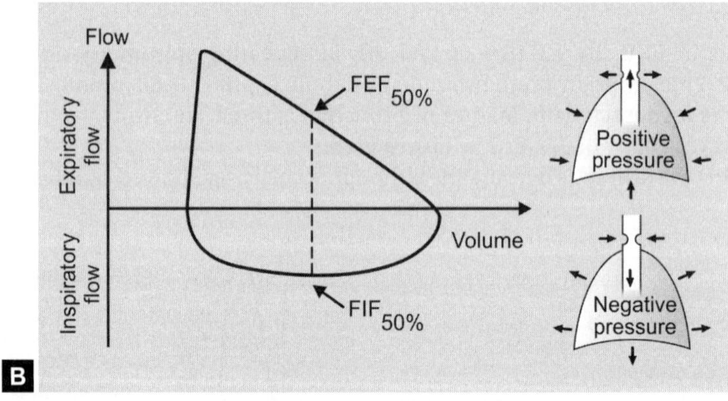

- Bilateral and unilateral vocal cord paralysis
- Vocal cord constriction
- Reduced pharyngeal cross-sectional area
- Airway burns

The obstruction worsens in inspiration because the negative pressure narrows the trachea and inspiratory flow is reduced to a greater extent than expiratory flow.

Variable intrathoracic obstruction:

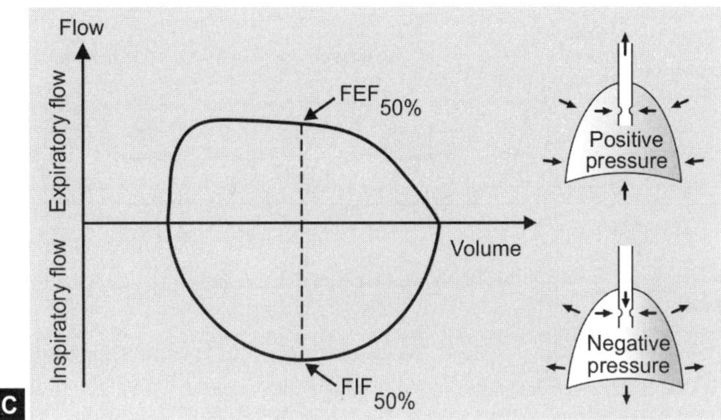

- Tracheomalacia
- Polychondritis
- Tumors of the lower trachea or main bronchus.

The narrowing is maximal in expiration because of increased intrathoracic pressure compressing the airway.

The flow volume loop shows a greater reduction in the expiratory phase.

Flow volume loop in restrictive lung disease:

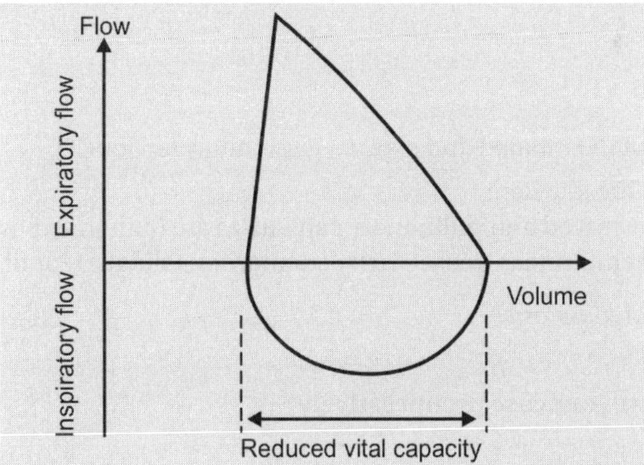

- Full lung expansion is prevented by fibrotic tissue in the lung parenchyma and the FVC is reduced.
- Elastic recoil may be increased by fibrotic tissue leading to increased airflow.
- Both FEV_1 and FVC may be reduced because the lungs are small and stiff, but the peak expiratory flow may be preserved or even higher than predicted leading to tall, narrow and steep flow volume loop in expiratory phase.

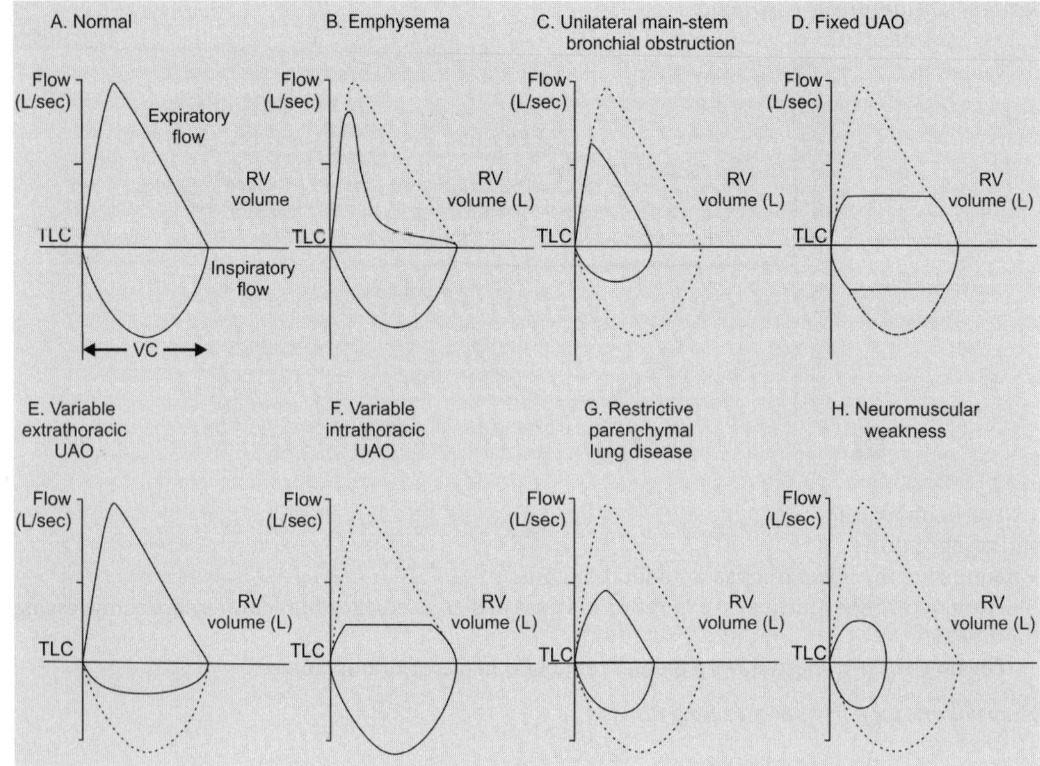

Diffusing capacity:

- DL_{CO}
- Low concentration of CO inhaled and expired gas is analyzed for CO.

Diffusing capacity is reduced when:

- Alveolar walls are destroyed and pulmonary capillaries are obliterated by emphysema
- Alveolar-capillary membrane is thickened by edema, consolidation or fibrosis.

What is your provisional diagnosis?
COPD

24. How will you assess your case preoperatively?

Ans.

- Preoperative assessment of the case:
  - History
  - Examination
  - Investigations
  - Bedside PFT.

25. What are the bedside pulmonary tests?

Ans.

- Sabrasez breath holding time (BHT)—ask patient to hold breath after a deep breath:
  - *BHT > 40 sec:* Normal
  - *BHT 20–30 sec:* Compromised cardiopulmonary reserve

  - *BHT < 20 sec:* Very poor cardiopulmonary reserve
- *Snider's match test:* Max breathing capacity (MBC)—Patient sitting + mouth opened and blow a match stick (Contraindicated in patient who needs therapeutic O_2)
  - *At 22 cm:* MBC > 150 L/min
  - *At 15 cm:* MBC > 100 L/min
  - *At 7.5 cm* MBC > 50 L/min
- *Cough test:* Ask patient to take a deep breath and cough once—recurrent coughing indicates (+) ve test.
- *Expiratory time over trachea:* Forced expiratory time > 4 seconds—reduced maximal expiratory flow.
- Wright's respirometer and peak flow meter
- *Wheeze test:* Ask patient to take 5 deep inspiration/expiration—check for wheeze between shoulder blades.
- Single breath count
- Chest expansion, maximum laryngeal height- at end expiration distance between top of thyroid cartilage and suprasternal notch < 4 cm—accurate sign of COPD.
- *Exercise test:* Stair climbing, 6 MWT, Shuttle Walk test.

26. Current recommendation is to go for combined assessment.

Ans.

- Assess symptoms
- Assess degree of airflow limitation using spirometry
- Assess risk of exacerbations
- Assess comorbidities.

Assessment of symptoms is done by using the COPD assessment test (CAT) or mMRC breathlessness scale:

mMRC dyspnea scale	*CAT score*
• Provide an assessment of the impact of dyspnea on disability	Provides a broader coverage of impact of COPD on patient's daily life and well-being
• More symptoms—mMRC grade ≥2	More symptoms—CAT score ≥10
• In the absence of a CAT score, mMRC scores may be used	Preferred over mMRC

Gold criteria for COPD severity:

Gold stage	*Severity*	*Symptoms*	*Spirometry*
0	At risk	Chronic cough, sputum production	Normal
I	Mild	With or without chronic cough or sputum production	$FEV_1/FVC < 0.7$ and $FEV_1 \geq 80\%$ predicted
IIA	Moderate	With or without chronic cough or sputum production	$FEV_1/FVC < 0.7$ and $50\% \leq FEV_1 \leq 80\%$ predicted
III	Severe	With or without chronic cough or sputum	$FEV_1/FVC < 0.7$ and $30\% \leq FEV_1 \leq 50\%$ predicted
IV	Very severe	With or without chronic cough or sputum	$FEV_1/FVC < 0.7$ and $FEV_1 < 30\%$ predicted or $FEV_1 < 50\%$ predicted with repiratory failure or signs of right heart failure

- Assessment of risk of exacerbations is done by history of exacerbations and spirometry—Two exacerbations or more within the last year or FEV_1 <50% predicted indicate high risk:
- Thus, mMRC ≥ 2 or CAT score ≥ 10, Gold criteria 3 or 4, no. of exacerbations 2 or more—Indicate high-risk patient.
- mMRC < 2 or CAT score < 10, Gold criteria 1 or 2, no. of exacerbations < 2—Indicate low-risk patient.

27. How will you manage and optimize your case preoperatively?

Ans.

Management of stable COPD:

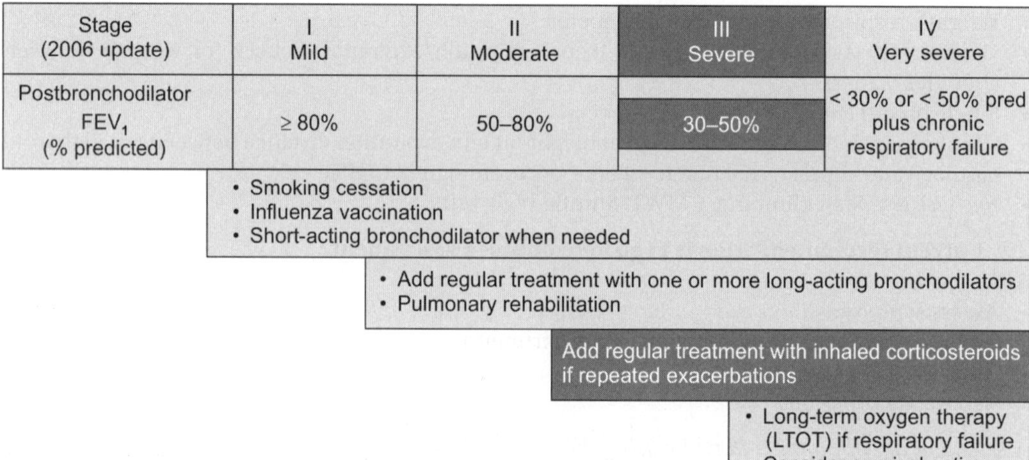

Place of drugs in the management of COPD:

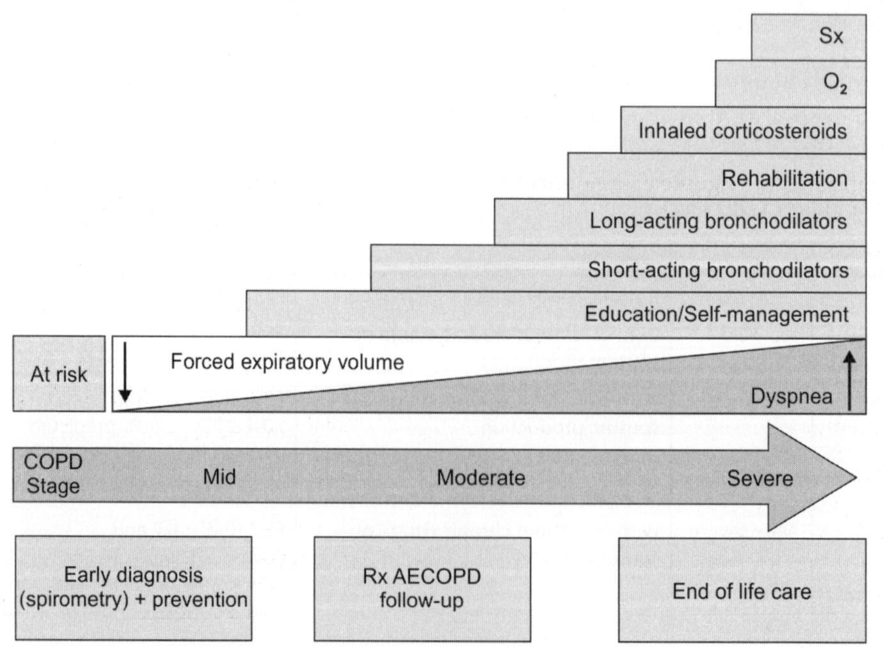

General measures:

- Institute therapy after assessment of symptoms, potential risks, costs, and benefits.
- Only three interventions have been demonstrated to influence the natural history:
  - Smoking cessation
  - Oxygen therapy in chronically hypoxemic patients
  - Lung volume reduction surgery in selected patients with emphysema
- All other current therapies are directed at improving symptoms and decreasing frequency and severity of exacerbations.
- There is suggestive, but not definitive, evidence that the use of inhaled glucocorticoids may alter mortality (but not lung function).
- Therapeutic response should determine continuation of treatment.

Pharmacotherapy:

- Bronchodilators
  - Used to treat symptoms
  - The inhaled route is preferred.
  - Side effects are less than with parenteral delivery.
- Anticholinergic agents
  - Trial of inhaled anticholinergics is recommended in symptomatic patients.
  - Side effects are minor.
  - Improve symptoms and produce acute improvement in FEV
  - Do not influence rate of decline in lung function
- β-agonists
  - Provide symptomatic benefit
  - Long-acting inhaled β-agonists have benefits similar to anticholinergics.
  - Addition of a β-agonist to inhaled anticholinergic therapy provides incremental benefit.
  - Side effects include tremor and tachycardia
- Inhaled glucocorticoids
  - May reduce frequency of exacerbations by 25–30%
  - May slow decline in quality of life
  - Recent meta-analysis showed no effect on mortality
  - No evidence of a beneficial effect for the regular use of inhaled glucocorticoids on the rate of decline of lung function, as assessed by FEV_1
  - Consider a trial in patients with frequent exacerbations (≥2 per year) and those who demonstrate a significant amount of acute reversibility in response to inhaled bronchodilators
  - Risks include increased rates of oropharyngeal candidiasis and loss of bone density.
- Oral corticosteroids
  - Long-term use of oral glucocorticoids is not recommended.
  - Side effects include osteoporosis, weight gain, cataracts, glucose intolerance, and increased risk of infection.
- Exacerbation
  - Assess the severity of both the acute and chronic components of the patient's illness.
  - Attempt to identify and treat the precipitant of the exacerbation.

Anticholinergic agents

- Ipratropium bromide (short-acting anticholinergic) (Atrovent)
  - *Inhaled:* 30-minute onset of action; 4-hour duration
  - *Atrovent:* Metered-dose inhaler (or in nebulized solution); 18 μg per inhalation; 1-2 inhalations qid

- Tiotropium (long-acting anticholinergic) (Spiriva)
  - *Spiriva:* Powder via handihaler; 18 μg per inhalation; 1 inhalation qd
  - Improves symptoms and reduces exacerbations.

β-agonists
- Salmeterol (Serevent):
  - Powder via diskus; 50 μg inhalation every 12 hours
  - Formoterol (Foradil)
- Powder via aerolizer; 12 μg inhalation every 12 hours
  - Albuterol (short-acting) (Ventolin, Proventil)
- Metered-dose inhaler (or in nebulizer solution); 180 μg inhalation every 4–6 hours as needed
- *Combined β-agonist/anticholinergic:* Albuterol/ipratropium
- Metered-dose inhaler (or in nebulized solution); 120 mcg/21 μg per inhalation 1–2 inhalations qid

Inhaled glucocorticoids beclomethasone (QVAR): Metered-dose inhaler; 40–80 μg/spray; 40–160 μg bid
- *Budesonide (Pulmicort):* Powder via Turbuhaler; 200 μg/spray; 200 μg inhaled bid
- *Fluticasone (Flovent):* Metered-dose inhaler; 44, 110 or 220 μg/spray; 88–440 μg inhaled bid
- *Triamcinolone (Azmacort):* Metered-dose inhaler via built-in spacer; 100 μg/spray; 100–400 μg inhaled bid.

Other agents:
- Theophylline
  - Produces modest improvements in expiratory flow rates and vital capacity and a slight improvement in arterial oxygen and carbon dioxide levels in moderate to severe COLD
  - *Dose:* Various dosages and preparations; typical dose 300–600 mg/d, adjusted based on levels
- N-acetyl cysteine
  - Used for its mucolytic and antioxidant properties
  - A prospective trial failed to find any benefit with respect to decline in lung function or prevention of exacerbations.
- Intravenous α_1AT augmentation therapy for patients with severe α_1AT deficiency
  - A randomized, controlled trial of α_1AT augmentation therapy has never proved efficacious in reducing decline of pulmonary function.
- Antibiotics: Long-term suppressive or 'rotating' antibiotics are not beneficial.

Oxygen therapy:
- Supplemental O_2 is the only pharmacologic therapy demonstrated to decrease mortality.
- In resting hypoxemia (resting O_2 saturation < 88% or < 90% with signs of pulmonary hypertension or right heart failure), the use of O_2 has been demonstrated to significantly affect mortality.
- Supplemental O_2 is commonly prescribed for patients with exertional hypoxemia or nocturnal hypoxemia.
  - Rationale for supplemental O_2 in these settings is physiologically sound, but benefits are not well substantiated.

Long-term oxygen therapy (LTOT) in COPD:
(O_2 for 15 hrs a day or longer)
- Improves survival
  Indications:
  - $pO_2 < 55$

- pO_2 55–59 with PH, cor pulmonale, polycythemia, edema from right heart failure or impaired mental state.
- Desaturation during sleep, exercise and high altitude

Ref: www.goldcopd.org/guidelines-copd-diagnosis-and-management.html

- General medical care
  - Annual influenza vaccine
  - Polyvalent pneumococcal vaccine is recommended, although proof of efficacy in patients with COLD is not definitive.
- Pulmonary rehabilitation
  - Improves health-related quality of life, dyspnea, and exercise capacity
  - Rates of hospitalization are reduced over 6–12 months
- Lung volume reduction surgery
  - Offers both a mortality benefit and a symptomatic benefit in certain patients with emphysema
- Patients with upper lobe–predominant emphysema and a low postrehabilitation exercise capacity are most likely to benefit.

28. What are the effects of smoking on different organ system?

Ans.

- Long-term smoking has deleterious effects on vascular disease of peripheral, cerebral and coronary circulation:
  - Risk factor for development of coronary artery disease. Cardiovascular effects are caused by action of nicotine on sympathetic nervous system, producing tachycardia and hypertension and decreases exercise capacity. Smoking increases the coronary vascular resistance, thus cessation of smoking improves the symptoms of angina.
  - Smoking decreases mucociliary activity, results in hyper-reactive airways and decreases pulmonary immune function. Carbon monoxide converts the hemoglobin to carboxy hemoglobin which may cause reduction in available oxygen by as much as 25%. Effect of smoking on respiratory tract leads to 6 fold increase in respiratory morbidity.
  - Cessation of smoking is suggested prior to anesthesia. Half-life of carboxy hemoglobin is short.
  - Therefore abstinence for 12 hours leads to increase in arterial oxygen content. Abstinence for 6 weeks results in reduced bronchoconstriction and secretion in tracheobronchial tree.

Ref: Miller's Anaesthesia 8th edn, Chapter 59—Anesthesia for Thoracic Surgery, Peter D. Slinger, Javier H. Campos.

Smoking cessation:

- All patients with COPD should be strongly urged to quit and educated about the benefit of cessation and risks of continuation.
- Combining pharmacotherapy with traditional supportive approaches enhances considerably the chances of successful smoking cessation.
  - Bupropion
  - Varenicline
  - Nicotine replacement (gum, transdermal, inhaler, nasal spray, lozenge)
  - Recommendation is for all smokers considering quitting to be offered pharmacotherapy in the absence of any contraindication.

Preoperative preparation of this case should include:

- Stop smoking
  - Improve mucociliary function, decrease sputum production and airway reactivity—2 months
  - Reduce CO levels—12 hours

- Bronchodilators
- Control of infection
- *Chest physiotherapy, hydration:* Familiarize patient with deep breathing exercises and respiratory therapy equipment that are likely to be used postoperative
- Improve oxygenation
- Steroids
- Diuretics, digitalis.

29. Which patients should receive perioperative steroids? What are equivalent doses of steroids?

Ans.

- Long-term steroids >10 mg prednisolone daily
- Patients on steroids >10 mg daily, in last 3 months
- Patients on high dose inhalation steroids
- Prednisolone 5 mg is equivalent to
- Betamethasone 750 micrograms
- Cortisone acetate 25 mg
- Dexamethasone 6 mg
- Hydrocortisone 20 mg
- Methylprednisolone 4 mg

Ref: Clinical Guideline for Perioperative Steroid Replacement, NHS.

30. What are the recommendations for perioperative steroids?

Ans.

Dose	*Surgery*	*Recommended dose*
<10 mg/day	Minor/Moderate/Major	Additional steroid cover not required (assume normal HPA response)
>10 mg/day	Minor surgery	25 mg of hydrocortisone at induction and normal medications postoperative
>10 mg/day	Moderate surgery	Usual dose preoperative and 25 mg hydrocortisone IV at induction then 25 mg IV TDS for 1 day then recommence preoperative dosage
>10 mg/day	Major surgery	Usual dose preoperative and 100 mg hydrocortisone at induction then 100 mg IV TDS for 2–3 days

31. Would you use steroids in our patient? What are the dangers?

Ans.

- Problems
  - Impaired wound healing
  - Delayed recovery
  - Increased postoperative infections.

32. What should be the anesthetic management of this patient?

Ans.

- *Premedication of this patient should include:*
  - Steroid hydrocortisone 100 mg IV
  - Salbutamol 2 puffs, ipratropium 2 puffs, budesonide 2 puffs before sending the patient to OT
  - Atropine

  - Decreases airway resistance
  - Decreases secretion-induced airway reactivity
  - Decreases bronchospasm from reflex vagal stimulation
  - But can cause drying of secretions, mucus plugging
- Small dose of benzodiazepine is acceptable
- Avoid H_2 receptor antagonists.

Ref: Miller's Anaesthesia, 8th edn

- *Choice of Anesthesia*

  Points in favor of general anesthesia:
  - Allows control of ventilation, excellent muscle relaxation
  - Ensures oxygenation and CO_2 elimination
  - IPPV overcomes decrease in lung compliance, increased resistance and decreased FRC
  - Comfort to patient in prolonged procedures.

Ref: Anesthesiology 1996;85:460-7.

Points in favor of regional anesthesia:
- Avoids risk of bronchospasm due to intubation
- Excellent intraoperative and postoperative analgesia
- Problems with regional anesthesia:
  - Spontaneous ventilation may lead to hypoventilation
  - Hypercarbia and acidosis can increase PVR
  - Inadequate muscle relaxation, coughing/bucking
  - High levels of spinal/epidural block
    - Increase parasympathetic tone and cause bronchospasm
    - Decrease ERV by ~50%, detrimental for active expiration
    - Hypotension
  - Prolonged procedure, patient discomfort, shivering
  - Heavy sedation may be worse than light GA.

Ref: Anesthesiology 1996;85:460-7.

- My choice of anesthesia

  GA combined with epidural analgesia as it provides:
  - All benefits of GA
  - Excellent analgesia with epidural
  - Reduced requirement of muscle relaxants
  - Lower risk of hypotension
  - Postoperative analgesia without excessive systemic narcotics
  - May facilitate early ambulation
  - Better performance of respiratory therapy maneuvers
  - May reduce postoperative pulmonary complications
  - May reduce risk of DVT.

Induction:
- Avoid thiopentone
  - Thiobarbiturates may cause histamine release
- Prefer oxybarbiturates (methohexitone)
  - Airway instrumentation or other stimulation under light thiopentone anesthesia may provoke bronchospasm

- Ketamine
  - Tachycardia and HT, may increase PVR
  - Agent of choice in unstable/wheezing patient
- Propofol
  - Offers marked protection from bronchospasm
  - But watch for hemodynamic compromise
  - Agent of choice in stable patient.

Ref: Miller's Anaesthesia, 8th Edition.

Intubation:

- Nondepolarizing muscle relaxant—vecuronium, rocuronium are preferred for performing intubation.
- IV plus topical lignocaine prior to laryngoscopy and intubation should be administered.
- Deep plane of anesthesia should be maintained prior to intubation
- LMA avoids tracheal stimulation but is not preferred in this setting
  - Upper abdominal surgery
  - IPPV in a patient with compromised lung function
  - Risk of aspiration high comparable with any other surgery using LMA.

Ref: Miller's Anaesthesia, 8th Edition.

Maintenance:

- IPPV
- Muscle relaxant
  - Atracurium, mivacurium are to be avoided.
  - Vecuronium, pancuronium, rocuronium are preferred.
- Inhaled agent
  - Halothane most potent bronchodilator (< 1.7 MAC)
  - Isoflurane is comparable at higher MACs
  - Irritant smell may provoke bronchospasm.
- Narcotic
  - Fentanyl is preferred.
  - Morphine, pethidine may cause histamine release.

Ref: Miller's Anesthesia, 8th Edition.

Bronchodilation:

- Halothane
  - Suppression of airway reflexes
  - Direct relaxation of airway smooth muscle
  - Dose related
  - Beta-adrenergic receptor stimulation, which is decreased by beta-blocking agents
- Ketamine
  - Indirectly through adrenergic stimulation
  - Not dose related
  - Not predictable.

Ref: Miller's Anaesthesia, 8th Edition.

Monitoring of patients in intraoperative period is done by:

- ECG, HR
- *BP:* NIBP, arterial line

- Pulse oximetry
- $ETCO_2$
- Airway pressure
- Expired tidal and minute volume
- CVP
- Temperature
- Precordial stethoscope
- Hourly urine output.

33. What special monitoring is required in perioperative anesthetic management in patients with cor pulmonale?

Ans. Right ventricular dysfunction occurs in 50% of COPD patients which is poorly tolerant with sudden increase in afterload that occurs during the change from spontaneous to controlled ventilation. As the pulmonary artery pressure remains increased in these patients, the right ventricular function becomes critical with this increased afterload though right ventricular ejection fraction remains normal as in normal patients. These changes progress with repeated recurrent hypoxemia which subsequently progress to cor pulmonale.

Cor pulmonale in adult COPD patients have FEV ranging between 0.6 and 1 liter, i.e. 40% of expected FEV. Goal of oxygen supplementation is to maintain PAO_2 between 60 and 65 mm Hg. Compared to patients with chronic bronchitis, emphysematous COPD patients lead to have a decreased cardiac output and mixed venous oxygen tension while maintaining lower pulmonary artery pressure. Hence CVP monitoring and transthoracic echocardiography is necessary to assess the right sided heart function.

Ref: Cochrane Database Syst Rev. 2004;(3).

34. What may be the causes of increased airway pressure in intraoperative period in this patient? How will you manage?

Ans.

- Light anesthesia, coughing, bucking
- Obstruction in the circuit
- Blocked/kinked tube
- Endobronchial intubation
- Bronchospasm
- Pneumothorax
- Major atelectasis
- Pulmonary edema
- Aspiration pneumonia
- Head down position, bowel packing.

Ref: Smetana GW Cleve Clin J Med. 2009;76(Suppl 4):S60-5.

35. What is the management of a patient with increased airway pressure?

Ans. The following steps are to be undertaken in this setting:

- Check vitals, take the bag in hand
- Ventilate with an Ambu bag
- Check position of ETT, chest movements
- Auscultate the chest
- Percuss the chest
- Ask surgeon to pause surgery
- Suction.

36. What are the probable causes that are suspected in case of intraoperative broncho spasm?
Ans. Differential diagnoses of intraoperative bronchospasm:
- Kinked ETT
- Secretions, blood in ETT
- Pulmonary edema
- Pneumothorax
- Aspiration
- Pulmonary embolism
- Endobronchial intubation
- Coughing and straining on the ETT
- All that wheezes is not asthma!

Ref: Smetana GW. Cleve Clin J Med. 2009;76 (Suppl 4):S60-5.

37. How will you manage intraoperative bronchospasm?
Ans.
- Increase FiO_2
- Deepen anesthesia
  - Most common cause is surgical stimulation under light anesthesia
  - Administer incremental dose of ketamine or propofol
- Relieve mechanical stimulation
  - Endotracheal suction
  - Stop surgery
- Beta-2 agonists – nebulize, or MDI
  - subcutaneous terbutaline, IV adrenaline
- Intravenous aminophylline
- Intravenous corticosteroid indicated if severe bronchospasm.

Ref: Smetana GW. Cleve Clin J Med. 2009;76(Suppl 4):S60-5.

38. What are the causes of hypercarbia in a patient under anesthesia?
Ans. The probable causes of hypercarbia and its management include:
- Hypoventilation
- Compressible volume of typical anesthesia circuit is large enough that wasted ventilation is often 7–10 cc/cm H_2O
  - If Paw is 50, 350–500 mL of set TV may go in distending the circuit
- If respiratory impedance is high, at high airway pressures, attempts to increase MV are often unrewarding
  - Decreased minute ventilation
- Overdistension of some lung units
  - Increase in dead space, especially if hypotension present
- Ventilating manually with the pressure limiting valve almost fully open.
- Soda lime exhausted.

Ref: Smetana GW. Cleve Clin J Med. 2009;76(Suppl 4):S60-5.

39. What are the causes of hypotension in this case in the intraoperative period?
Ans.
- Effects of anesthetic agents
- Hypovolemia
- IPPV
- Pneumothorax

- Severe hypoxia, hypercarbia, acidosis
- Myocardial ischemia
- Arrhythmia
- Dynamic hyperinflation and auto-PEEP.

40. What are the effects of positive pressure ventilation in severe flow limited COPD patients?
Ans.

- Severe COPD patients are flow limited even during tidal volume expiration at rest in comparison to normal patients where flow limitation can occur only during forced expiratory maneuvers.

In normal patients, during normal expiration pressure in the lumen of airway exceeds the intrapleural pressure because of the upstream elastic recoil pressure that is transmitted from the alveoli. The effect of elastic recoil pressure diminishes as air flows downstream in the airway. With forced expiration, the intrapleural pressure becomes equal (equal pressure point) to the intraluminal pressure which then limits the air flow.

Severe flow limited COPD patients have primary problem of loss of elastic recoil and have marked dyspnea on exertion. Flow limitation cause dyspnea because of stimulation of mechanoreceptors in the muscles of respiration, thoracic cage and airway distal to the equal pressure point. Any increase in the work of respiration will aggravate dyspnea.

Application of positive pressure ventilation in severely flow limited patients develop hemodynamic collapse owing tom dynamic hyperinflation of the lung. Even with modest positive airway pressure associated with manual ventilation during bag-mask induction can lead to hypotension because these patients have no increased resistance to inspiration but have a marked resistance to expiration.

Ref: Ram FS. Cochrane Database Syst Rev. 2004;(3).

41. What is dynamic hyperinflation or auto-PEEP?
Ans.

- Dynamic hyperinflation and auto-PEEP

Patients with severe COPD often breathe in a pattern that interrupts expiration before the alveolar pressure has fallen to atmospheric pressure. This incomplete expiration is due to a combination of factors, which include flow limitation, increased work of respiration, and increased airway resistance. This interruption leads to an elevation of the end-expiratory lung volume above the FRC. This positive end-expiratory pressure (PEEP) in the alveoli at rest has been termed *auto-PEEP* or *intrinsic-PEEP*. During spontaneous respiration the intrapleural pressure will have to be decreased to a level that counteracts auto-PEEP before inspiratory flow can begin. Thus, COPD patients can have an increased inspiratory load added to their already increased expiratory load.

Auto-PEEP becomes even more important during mechanical ventilation. It is directly proportional to tidal volume and inversely proportional to expiratory time. The presence of auto-PEEP is not detected by the manometer of standard anesthesia ventilators. It can be measured by end-expiratory flow interruption, a feature available on the newer generation of intensive care ventilators. Auto-PEEP has been found to develop in most COPD patients during one-lung anesthesia.

Ref: Miller's Anaesthesia, 8th edition.

42. What is to be done if there is development of auto-PEEP?
Ans.

- Apnea test is done to confirm auto-PEEP. (end expiratory pause)
- Management
  - Tidal volume is reduced.
  - Respiratory rate is reduced.

  - Peak inspiratory flow rate is to be increased.
  - Patient may require an ICU ventilator
  - Aggressive treatment of bronchospasm needs to be done.

Ref: Cleveland Clinic Journal of Medicine September 2005, vol. 72(9)801-9.

43. How will you manage this patient in the postoperative period?

Ans. Important postoperative measures should include:

- Institute lung volume expansion maneuvers.
- Voluntary deep breathing
- Incentive spirometry
- Continuous positive airway pressure (CPAP)
- Maximal analgesia with:
  - Neuraxial opioid
  - Intercostal nerve blocks
  - PCA
- Ambulate as early as possible to prevent pulmonary morbidity and other complications (such as DVT and PTE).

Ref: Smetana GW, Cleve Clin J Med. 2009;76(Suppl 4):S60-5.

44. What are the probable postoperative pulmonary complications?

Ans.

- Decreased FRC
- Large incision
- Postoperative pain
- Splinting of the diaphragm
- Decreased sputum clearance
- Atelectasis, pneumonia
- Mechanical ventilation, prolonged ICU/hospital stay
- Delayed ambulation
- DVT, PE
- Cor pulmonale.

Ref: Smetana GW. Cleve Clin J Med. 2009;76(Suppl 4):S60-5.

45. What are the criterias to predict postoperative pulmonary complication (POPC)?

Ans.

- *Patient-related:* Age >60 years, ASA>II, congestive heart failure, pre-existing pulmonary ds (COPD) functionally dependent, cigarette smoking
- *Procedure-related:* Emergency surgery, abdominal/thoracic/head-neck/neuro/vascular/aortic aneurysm surgery, prolonged anesthesia (>2.5 hours), GA
- *Test predictors:* Albumin < 3.5 g/dL

Ref: Smetana GW. Cleve Clin J Med. 2009;76(Suppl 4):S60-5.

FEW ALGORITHM RELATED TO THE MANAGEMENT

Long-term Oxygen Therapy

Supplemental long-term oxygen therapy (LTOT) improves survival, exercise, sleep and cognitive performance in hypoxemic patients. Reversal of hypoxemia supersedes concerns about carbon dioxide (CO_2) retention. Arterial blood gas (ABG) assessment is the preferred method to determine oxygen need because it includes acid-base information. Arterial oxygen saturation as measured by pulse oximetry (SpO_2) is adequate for trending. Physiological indications for oxygen include a arterial oxygen tension (PaO_2) v7.3 kPa (55 mm Hg). The therapeutic goal is to maintain SpO_2 w90% during rest, sleep and exertion.

A flow chart for prescribing long-term oxygen therapy (LTOT):

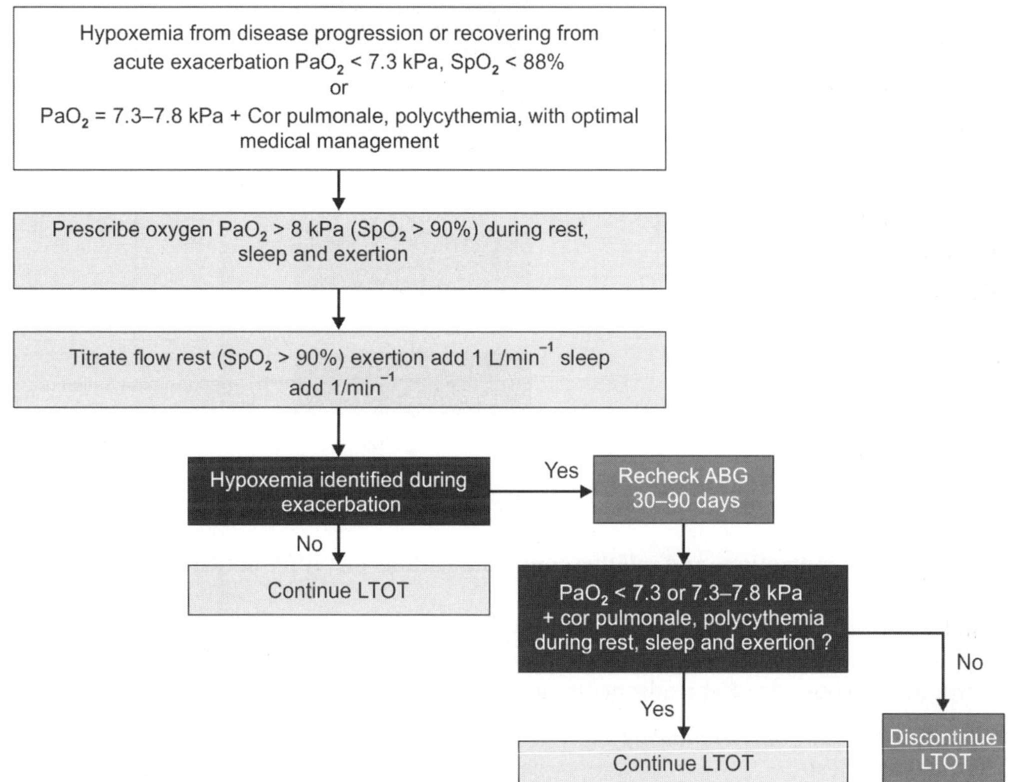

Exacerbation of COPD—inpatient oxygen therapy:

During a severe exacerbation, ABGs should be monitored for PaO_2, arterial carbon dioxide tension ($PaCO_2$) and pH. The SpO_2 should be monitored for trending and adjusting oxygen settings. The goal of inpatient oxygen therapy is to maintain PaO_2 8 kPa (60 mm Hg) or SpO_2 90% in order to prevent tissue hypoxia and preserve cellular oxygenation.

Algorithm to correct hypoxemia in an acutely ill chronic obstructive pulmonary disease patient in pre-or postoperative settings:

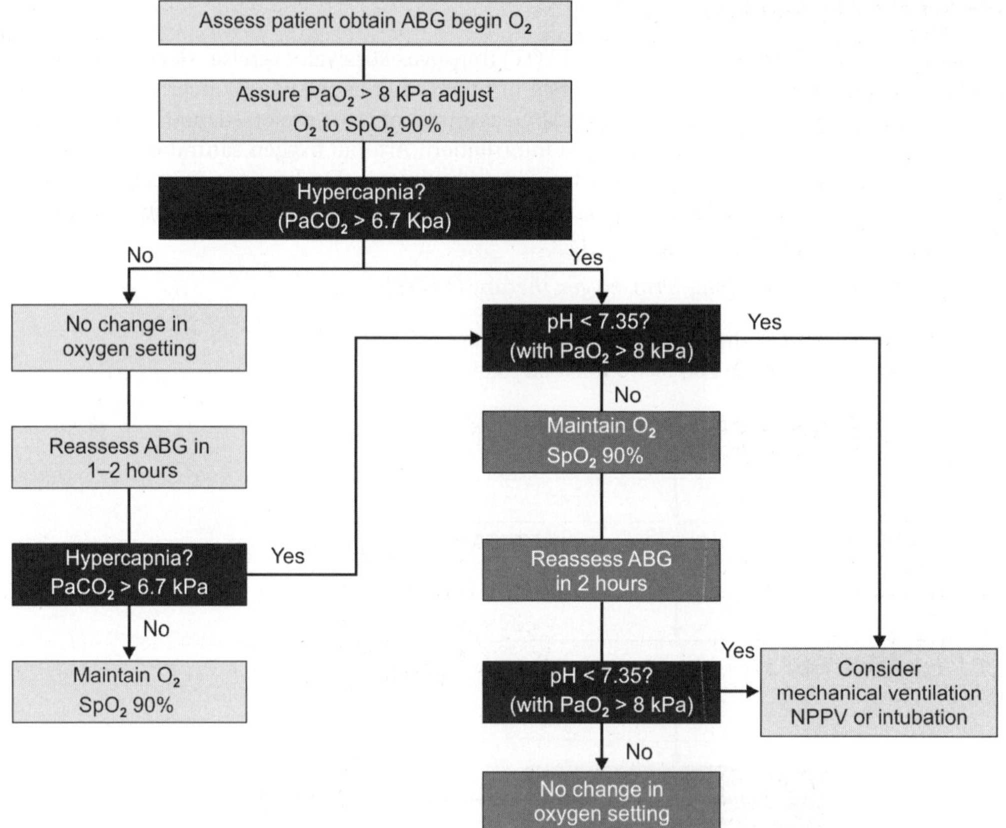

46. What are the indications and relative contraindications for NPPV in COPD.

Selection criteria

- Moderate to severe dyspnea with use of accessory muscles and paradoxical abdominal motion.
- Moderate to severe acidosis (pH ≤ 7.35) and hypercapnia ($PaCO_2$ > 6.0 kPa, 45 mm Hg).
- Respiratory frequency > 25 breaths per minute.

Exclusion criteria (any may be present)

- Respiratory arrest.
- Cardiovascular instability (hypotension, arrhythmias, myocardial infarction).
- Somnolence, impaired mental status, uncooperative patient.
- High aspiration risk; viscous or copious secretions.
- Recent facial or gastroesophageal surgery.
- Craniofacial trauma, fixed nasopharyngeal abnormalities.
- Burns.
- Extreme obesity.

The NPPV is by far the most popular mode of providing noninvasive ventilation. It is typically administered as a combination of continuous positive airway pressure (CPAP) plus pressure support ventilation (PSV). The ABG improve because of an increase in alveolar ventilation without significant modifications in the alveolar ventilation/perfusion mismatching and gas exchange in the lungs.

The ABGs are fundamental for the correct assessment and guidance of therapy. Once baseline ABGs are obtained, if the pH is v7.35 in the presence of hypercapnia, NPPV should be delivered in a controlled environment such as intermediate ICUs and/or high-dependency units. If the pH is v7.25, NPPV should be administered in the ICU and intubation should be readily available. The combination of some CPAP (e.g. 4–8 cm H_2O) and PSV (e.g. 10–15 cm H_2O) provides the most effective mode of NPPV.

The NPPV can be considered successful when ABGs and pH improve, dyspnea is relieved, the acute episode resolves without the need of endotracheal intubation, mechanical ventilation can be discontinued and the patient is discharged from the hospital. One-year mortality was reported to be lower in patients receiving NPPV for exacerbations of COPD, as compared to both conventional mechanical ventilation and optimal medical therapy alone.

Flow chart for the use of noninvasive positive pressure ventilation (NPPV) during exacerbation of chronic obstructive pulmonary disease (COPD) complicated by acute respiratory failure.

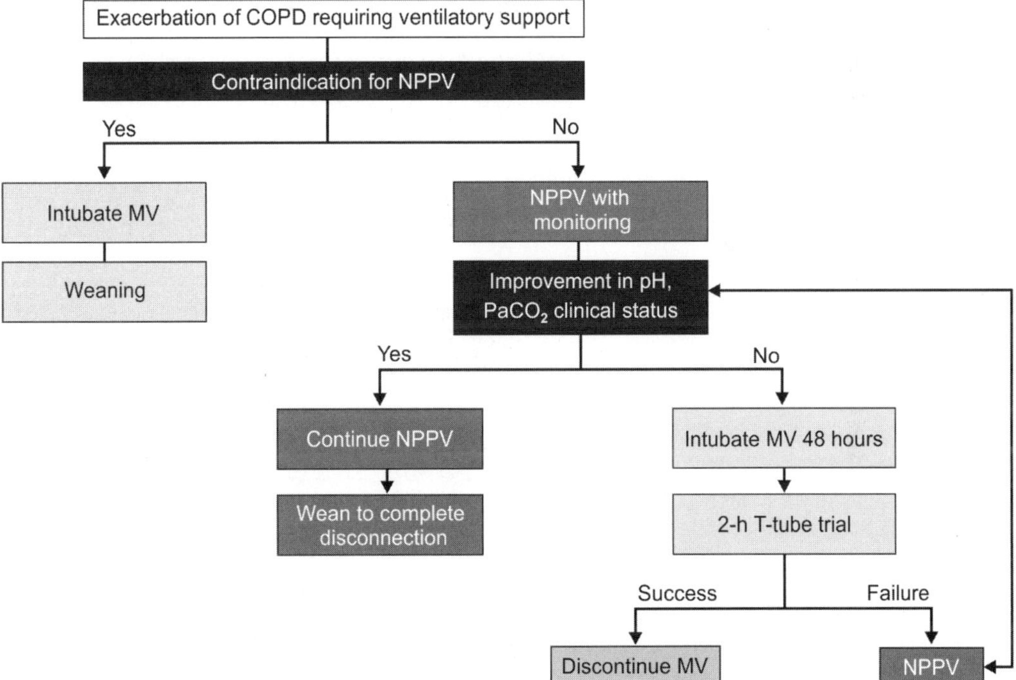

47. What are the indications for invasive mechanical ventilation?

Severe dyspnea with use of accessory muscles and paradoxical abdominal motion.

- Respiratory frequency > 35 breaths per minute.
- Life-threatening hypoxemia (PaO_2 < 5.3 kPa, 40 mm Hg or PaO_2/FiO_2 < 200 mm Hg).
- Severe acidosis (pH < 7.25) and hypercapnia ($PaCO_2$ > 8.0 kPa, 60 mm Hg).
- Respiratory arrest.
- Somnolence, impaired mental status.
- Cardiovascular complications (hypotension, shock, heart failure).
- Other complications (metabolic abnormalities, sepsis, pneumonia, pulmonary embolism, barotrauma, massive pleural effusion).
- NIPPV failure or exclusion criteria.

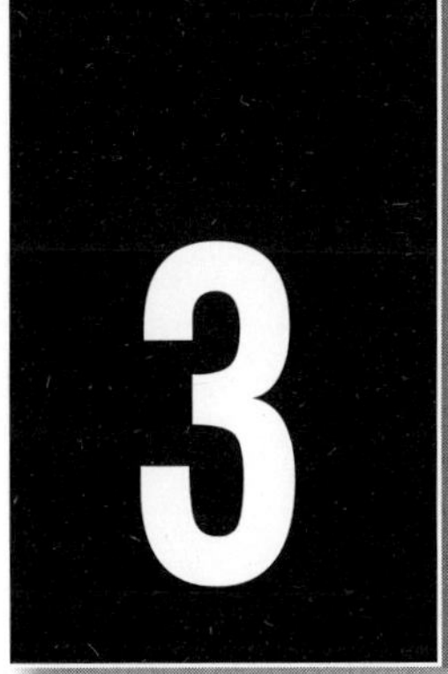

SHORT CASES

CHAPTERS

27

Hydrocephalus

LD Mishra, S Parashar

Many conditions exist where it is necessary to shunt cerebrospinal fluid (CSF) from the ventricles to another body cavity where it can be absorbed readily. The most common condition is hydrocephalus, which is a disorder of CSF accumulation that results in ventricular dilation resulting from increased intracranial pressure (ICP). This is a different entity from ventricular dilatation resulting from parenchymal loss (periventricular white matter atrophy) with passive filling by CSF. Accumulation of CSF in hydrocephalus is due to an imbalance between CSF production and absorption. Hydrocephalus has many causes and can be congenital or acquired.

CAUSES OF HYDROCEPHALUS

- *Excessive production of CSF:* Choroid plexus papilloma
- *Obstruction of CSF pathways:* Obstruction within the ventricular system
  - Lateral ventricular (atrium, body, foramen of Monro)
  - Third ventricular
  - Aqueductal (congenital stenosis, mass lesions)
  - Fourth ventricular (Dandy-Walker malformation)
  - Obstruction within the subarachnoid space
  - Basal cisterns (Chiari I malformation, infection)
  - Convexity
- *Decreased absorption of CSF:*
  - Arachnoid villi pathologic process (inflammation)
  - Dural venous sinus obstructions (thrombus, tumor, infection)
  - Extracranial venous sinus obstruction (achondroplasia).

PATHOGENESIS

Hydrocephalus results from overproduction, impaired circulation, or under absorption of CSF. CSF is produced by the choroid plexus, a collection of highly vascularized and epithelium-lined villous folds located in the lateral, third, and fourth ventricles. CSF flows from the lateral ventricles into the midline third ventricle via the interventricular foramen of Monro. From there, CSF drains through the aqueduct of Sylvius into the midline fourth ventricle, which is connected to the posterior fossa cisterns by a pair of laterally located foramina of Luschka and a midline foramen of Magendie.

Cisterns are focally enlarged intracranial subarachnoid spaces that channel CSF from the ventricular system and the spinal subarachnoid space up to the hemispheric convexity, where CSF is absorbed into the systemic circulation by the subarachnoid villi. Any disturbance in the normal production, flow, and absorption in the aforementioned pathway will lead to accumulation of CSF and increased ICP with resultant ventriculomegaly.

Although hydrocephalus is characterized by ventricular dilation, a significant rise in ICP usually occurs before demonstrable change in ventricular size. Hydrocephalus is rarely caused by CSF production but can be seen in choroid plexus disorders such as choroid plexus papillomas. The most common cause of congenital hydrocephalus is impaired circulation or obstruction of flow caused by structural abnormalities such as stenosis of the aqueduct of Sylvius, tumors, malformations (Chiari's malformation, Dandy-Walker malformation), and trauma-related defects. The most common genetic cause of congenital hydrocephalus is X-linked hydrocephalus due to aqueductal stenosis, which is associated with other CNS structural abnormalities as well as characteristic adducted thumbs. Hydrocephalus caused by decreased CSF absorption is infrequent and is seen mostly after CNS infections that cause inflammation of the subarachnoid villi. Intrauterine TORCHES infections (toxoplasmosis, rubella, cytomegalovirus infection, herpes simplex, syphilis) are classic examples.

SIGNS AND SYMPTOMS

Hydrocephalus can be acute, subacute, or chronic. The rate at CSF accumulation and the compliance of the CNS determines the clinical presentation. In general, symptoms are nonspecific and are independent of the underlying cause. If hydrocephalus occurs before the closure of cranial sutures (approximately 18–24 months of age), the rise in ICP is generally mitigated by expansion of the intracranial space. Once cranial sutures have closed the noncompliance of the system can lead to a rapid rise in ICP.

Newborns and Infants

Hydrocephalus most often manifests as an enlarged head resulting from separation of the cranial bone plates. The anterior fontanelle can be full or bulging, and the scalp veins may be prominent because of increased venous pressure. The infant may also display so-called sun-setting eyes, an impaired ability to gaze upward caused by compression of the midbrain. Other signs and symptoms of CNS parenchymal compression include third and sixth nerve palsy, papilledema, bradycardia, systemic hypertension, disturbances in respiratory pattern, endocrine abnormalities, and impaired fluid and electrolyte balance. Headaches along with nausea and vomiting result from stretching of the meninges and intracranial vessels. Infants may be irritable and then become progressively lethargic with increasing ICP. Stretching of the motor cortex can also occur if hydrocephalus is severe, resulting in spasticity. A continued rise in ICP that exhausts ventricular expansion capacity can cause disruption of the ventricular ependymal lining, which leads to parenchymal edema and necrosis with resultant white matter atrophy (periventricular leukomalacia).

Older Children and Adults

The presenting signs and symptoms include severe headache, seizures and emesis, deteriorating mental status, focal neurologic deficits, papilledema, pupillary abnormalities, autonomic dysfunction (Cushing triad).

Any newborn or infant with an enlarged head should undergo evaluation for hydrocephalus. Serial head circumference measurement is an easy and effective means of monitoring the progression of hydrocephalus. Most infants can be treated conservatively if head circumference increases at a slow and steady rate unless clinical symptoms are present. Rapid increase in size usually requires surgical intervention even if the child is relatively asymptomatic. Diagnosis is confirmed with neuroimaging (head ultrasonography for newborns, CT and MRI for infants and older children).

TREATMENT

Medical Therapy

It mainly consists of diuretic treatment (furosemide and acetazolamide decrease CSF production), although this remains controversial in children.

Surgical treatment:

- Serial lumbar punctures have also been tried, but are only a temporizing measure and do not significantly reduce the need for subsequent shunt surgery.
- Hydrocephalus associated with intracranial and intraventricular hemorrhage has been treated with fibrinolysis at some centers, but the benefits have not been shown to outweigh the potential risks.
- The majority of children require surgical treatment in the form of either shunt placement or shuntless endoscopic third ventriculostomy (ETV). The former consists of inserting a catheter into the lateral ventricle that is connected to a one way valved shunt system that drains into the right atrium (ventriculoatrial shunt) or the peritoneal space (ventriculoperitoneal shunt). In ETV, an endoscope is placed via a burr hole first into the lateral ventricle and then into the third ventricle, where a blunt perforation is made through its floor. This allows shuntless CSF drainage from the ventricular system into the cisterns beneath the third ventricle. Choroid plexectomy is sometimes performed at the same time to decrease overall CSF production. ETV is most successful in children older than 1 year of age. Finally, any structural cause of hydrocephalus such as tumor or Chiari's malformation must also be addressed.

ANESTHETIC MANAGEMENT

Preoperative assessment: In most cases, the raised ICP is reduced preoperatively by removing CSF via the access device. The child then comes to theater with a normal or near normal ICP. In this case, the procedure is usually scheduled to take place once the child is fasted. IV access will usually have been secured on the ward before the patient reaches theater. Rarely, a child with ↑ ICP must be anesthetized as an emergency.

Fasting: Fasting status should always be assessed before taking the child inside the OR. NPO for solid foods is for 6 hours and clear fluids are allowed till 2 hours.

Premedication: A delicate balance must be maintained between promoting calmness by pharmacologic means and minimizing the risk of hypoventilation. A careful preoperative assessment, consisting of history taking, review of current clinical symptoms, and physical examination, usually provides the most useful information about the severity of ICP and its impact on the child's neurologic status. Specifically, it is important to note the mental status (lethargy, drowsiness) as well as any focal neurologic deficits the child may have.

Induction: On theoretical grounds, an IV induction is preferable to minimize ↑ in ICP. But in reality, an IV or gaseous induction can be used depending on the circumstances. Many anaesthetists take the view that a gaseous induction is less detrimental to ICP than a difficult IV cannulation that causes crying and struggling. Volatile agents are potent cerebral vasodilators and increase ICP by increasing cerebral blood flow. This effect can be attenuated by preinduction hyperventilation, but this is not an easily accomplished or feasible task in most children. Children with significantly increased ICP are usually lethargic, which permits easier awake intravenous catheter placement. With the exception of ketamine, virtually all intravenous anesthetic agents lower ICP by decreasing cerebral blood volume and generally preserve cerebral perfusion pressure better than volatile agents. Ketamine is contraindicated because it can precipitate a sudden increase in ICP and rapid neurologic decompensation.

The neurophysiologic effects of dexmedetomidine, an $\alpha 2$-agonist, is not as well understood. Studies show that it generally decreases cerebral blood volume and cerebral blood flow and has minimal effect on the cerebral metabolic rate. Succinylcholine may be used if necessary. It can increase cerebral blood flow and ICP, but the effects are transient and can be attenuated by premedication with a "defasciculating" dose of a nondepolarizing muscle relaxant.

Maintenance: Anesthesia is maintained with oxygen mixed with air, fentanyl and either intravenous agent or inhalational agent. Nitrous oxide may be used safely with intravenous agent for maintenance.

Ventilation: Normocapnia should be maintained for patients with normal ICP, whereas mild hypocapnia is helpful to prevent further increases in ICP; severe hypocapnia can precipitate cerebral ischemia. Invasive blood pressure monitoring is not needed in most cases of shunt surgery or ETV, but may be useful to help guide anesthetic management to optimize cerebral perfusion pressure, particularly if an ICP monitor is in place (cerebral perfusion pressure = mean arterial pressure – ICP).

Monitoring: All standard monitors, such as, ECG, NIBP, SpO_2, temperature and $EtCO_2$ should be used.

Positioning: The patient is positioned with the head remote from the anesthetist and anesthetic machine to allow unrestricted surgical access. Connections between the ETT and circuit are checked and tightened before the head is draped. A warming mattress is used to maintain normothermia.

Finally, positional changes can have serious consequences. Extreme positioning of the head (flexion, lateral rotation) can cause further displacement of a structural abnormality (Chiari's malformation) and impair venous drainage, which leads to increased ICP.

Fluid management: Blood loss is minimal for this procedure. Fasting deficit and maintenance fluid requirements are given as isotonic crystalloid, e.g. Hartmann's during the procedure.

Extubation: Neuromuscular blockade reversed with inj neostigmine 0.05 mg/kg and injection glycopyrrolate 0.01 mg/kg on return of spontaneous respiration. Patient is usually extubated awake.

POSTOPERATIVE CARE

Neurological observations are made for the first postoperative 24 hours and medical staff informed if there is any deterioration in the patient's clinical state or a drop in the appropriate coma scale of two points or more. Maintenance fluids are prescribed until oral intake resumes.

1. What are the normal values of intracranial pressure?

Ans.

- *Neonates:* 3–6 mm Hg
- *Toddlers:* 6–11 mm Hg
- *Adolescents:* 13–15 mm Hg

2. What are the options for postoperative pain management?

Ans. Paracetamol 15 mg/kg oral 6-hourly and ibuprofen 10 mg/kg oral 6-hourly generally meet analgesic requirements, with codeine phosphate 1 mg/kg oral 4-hourly if required.

3. What is the management of blocked perioperative shunt?

Ans.

- The shunt drains excess CSF from a ventricle to the peritoneal cavity and keeps the ICP normal. Blockage or fracture of a V-P shunt is relatively common and requires either revision of one component or replacement of the whole thing.
- Shunts usually consist of three parts:
  1. A proximal end placed into the ventricle.
  2. A valve that allows unidirectional flow. This can have various opening pressures. It usually has a reservoir that allows for checking shunt pressure (indicative of ICP) and sampling of CSF.
  3. A distal end placed into the peritoneum by tracking the tubing subcutaneously.
- A separate intraventricular CSF access device is often in place. This is a dome-shaped, self-sealing reservoir attached to a catheter. The reservoir is implanted underneath the skin and the catheter is inserted into the ventricle to provide access to cerebrospinal fluid. The reservoir volume is usually 1.5–2.5 mL. These devices provide access for the measurement of intracranial pressure, sampling of CSF, and occasionally the administration of antibiotics or chemotherapy.
- The median survival of a shunt (before need for revision) in a child less than two years of age is 2 years; over two years of age it is 8–10 years.
- Signs and symptoms of blockage or fracture include:
  - Headache
  - Drowsiness
  - Malaise
  - Vomiting
  - Bulging fontanelle
  - Cranial nerve palsies (especially sixth)
  - ↑ in seizures.
- Most commonly, the proximal ventricular end is obstructed with cells, choroid plexus, or debris. There also may be kinking of the tubing, disconnection or fracture of components or migration of the distal end.
- Diagnosis is based on signs and symptoms and is confirmed by CT scan of the head or shunt tap.

4. What are the complications of shunt surgery?

Ans.

- Obstruction or over drainage
- Shunt failure
- Shunt infection
- Pneumocephalus
- Seizure
- Hemorrhage
- Allergy
- Shunt migration
- Herniation.

BIBLIOGRAPHY

1. Doyle. Pediatric anaesthesia, 1st edn, 2007.
2. El-Dawlatly AA, Murshid W, El-Khwsky F. Endoscopic third ventriculostomy: A study of intracranial pressure vs. haemodynamic changes. Minim Invasive Neurosurg; 1999;42:198.
3. Michelle W, Thomas J. Stoelting's anaesthesia and coexisting disease, 6th edn.
4. Motoyama, Davis: Smith's Anesthesia for Infants and Children, 7th edn.

28

Cleft Lip/Palate

Dilip K Pawar

1. What is the incidence of cleft lip and cleft palate ?

Ans. When considered together, this constitutes third most common congenital anomaly that requires surgical correction at an early age. Cleft lip or cleft palate may occur together or separately. A cleft lip with or without a cleft palate occurs in 1 in 1000 births and is more common in boys. A cleft palate alone occurs 1 in 2500 births and isolated cleft palate is more common in girls. Highest incidence occurs among Asians > Whites > African Americans.

Ref: Aston SJ, Beasley RW, Thorne CHM (Eds). Grabb and Smith's Plastic Surgery, 5th edn. Philadelphia: Lippincott Raven; 1997.pp.245-55.

2. What is the anatomical concept of a cleft lip and palate?

Ans. Congenital cleft lip occurs due to failure of fusion of the maxillary and the medial and lateral nasal processes. It may vary from a single notch in upper lip to complete cleft lip, unilateral or bilateral with protruding premaxilla. The cleft palate is divided into:

a. Prepalatal
b. Postpalatal
c. Submucosal

Prepalatal involves anterior palate, alveolus, lip, nostril floor and *alae nasi*. Postpalatal cleft may extend anywhere from soft and hard palate to incisive foramen. In submucosal cleft, only bony defect exists without mucosal defect.

Left complete cleft of prepalatal and palatal structures is the most common variety and midline cleft of all the soft palate and part of hard palate without a cleft in the prepalatal area is the second most common variety.

Ref: Aston SJ, Beasley RW, Thorne CHM (Eds). Grabb and Smith's plastic surgery, 5th edn. Philadelphia: Lippincott Raven; 1997.pp.245-63.

Ref: Gregory GA (Ed). Pediatric anesthesia, 4th edn. New York: Churchill Livingstone; 2002.p.731.

3. What is the cause of cleft lip or cleft palate?

Ans. Major components of face develops between 4 and 7 weeks of fetal life. There are three mesodermal islands, one central and two lateral. Prepalatal cleft is caused by failure of these elements to develop and fuse. Palatal cleft is caused by failure of the palatal ridges to migrate medially contact and fuse.

Ref: Aston SJ, Beasley RW, Thorne CHM (Eds). Grabb and Smith's plastic surgery, 5th edn. Philadelphia: Lippincott Raven; 1997.pp.230-4.

4. What are the other conditions which are associated with cleft lip and palate?

Ans. Associated anomalies are 30 times more common in patients with isolated cleft palate than in the noncleft population. Nonsyndrome-related abnormalities are umbilical hernia, clubfoot, limb or ear deformity. The most common syndromes associated with deformities are:

Pierre-Robin syndrome: Characterized by cleft palate with retrognathia/micrognathia, glossoptosis-resulting in airway obstruction in early infancy which may lead to death if left untreated.

Treacher-Collins syndrome: Characterized by high arched cleft palate, auricular and ocular defects, mandibular/zygomatic hypoplasia, small oral cavity and airway with normal sized tongue.

VSD is very commonly associated with cleft palate.

Goldenhar's syndrome: Characterized by, auricular defect, mandibular hypoplasia, occipitalization of atlas and cleft palate.

Down syndrome: Macroglossia, increased salivation.

Klippel-Feil syndrome: There is fusion of cervical vertebra resulting in restriction in neck movements.

In all these cases, patients very often present with difficult airway.

Ref: Sumner E, Hatch D (Eds). Pediatric anesthesia, 2nd edn, Arnold, London; 2000.pp.383-4.

5. What is the ideal age of surgery for cleft lip and cleft palate?

Ans. Functional goal of cleft palate repair is development of normal speech, hearing and maxillofacial growth for which the patient needs a specialized team care consisting of pediatrician, surgeon, anesthesiologist, speech therapist and orthodontist. This repair sequence provides total palatal closure before speech evolves.

Surgical repair of cleft lip is performed at 3–6 months of age and the repair of cleft palate at 9–12 months of age. Pharyngoplasty, performed for velopalatal insufficiency is usually performed later at 5–15 years.

Ref: Nelson WE, Behrman RE, et al. (Eds). Nelson textbook of pediatrics, 17th edn. Philadelphia: WB Saunders; 2004:1207-8.

Ref: Malek R (Ed). Cleft lip and palate, lesions, pathophysiology and primary treatment. London: Martin Dunitz; 2001.pp.197-205.

6. What laboratory investigations will you need before operation?

Ans. Following laboratory investigations will be required before operation:

- Blood for complete hemogram
- Hematocrit level
- Throat swab culture
- If VSD is suspected, then echocardiography may be done
- X-ray of mandible

As periosteoplasty and lip adhesions are carried out as soon as the segments are in alignment and the surgery is also less extensive, Rule of 10 can be used with moderate license:

- Weight approximately 10 pounds
- Hemoglobin 10 gm% or more
- WBC count less than 10,000/cmm
- Age can be less than 10 weeks

With open cleft palate, however, it is common to have crusting and low-grade infection of the nasopharynx because of food and fluid regurgitation through the cleft. Unless an acute inflammation is present, this usually does not lead to complications as it is sometimes not possible to eliminate this completely.

Ref: Barrett BM Jr (Ed). Patient care in plastic surgery. St Louis: Mosby; 1996.pp.343-4.

7. What information do you want to obtain during preoperative visit?

Ans. From parents:

- History of birth injury
- History of respiratory distress syndrome
- History of prematurity
- History of less than 60 weeks of postconceptual age—as there is increased risk of post-operative apnea and perioperative bradycardia.

But most important clinical examination during preoperative visit is—Airway anatomy and cardiorespiratory status.

8. How will you prepare the patient for surgery and what preoperative order will you follow?

Ans. As it is an elective operation, patient should be kept in fasting. The fasting guidelines are:

Formula or cow's milk and solid food	- 6 hours
Breast milk	- 4 hours
Clear fluid	- 2 hours

To reduce emotional trauma, premedication with oral midazolam (0.25–0.5 mg/kg) may be given. In case of anticipation of difficulty in intubation, it is always better to avoid premedication. Children less than 8 months of age rarely require premedication.

Ref: Cote CJ. Preparation, premedication and induction of anesthesia in children. ASA annual meeting refresher course lectures. Park Ridge: American Society of Anesthesiologists; 2001.p.243.

9. What will be the antibiotic prophylaxis protocol in a child with VSD posted for palatal surgery?

Ans. Nonventricular septal defect has a moderate risk of development of bacterial endocarditis. Amoxicillin or ampicillin is the first line of antibiotic, one dose prior to an hour of incision. Operated one does not need any prophylaxis. In a child with allergic to penicillin clindamycin or azithromycin may be administered.

10. What intraoperative monitoring do you need for this patient?

Ans. Heart rate, blood pressure, respiration, temperature and oxygen saturation are to be monitored. So, precordial stethoscope, ECG, pulse oximetry, end-tidal CO_2 and temperature probe are essential monitoring devices.

11. What are the different techniques for anticipated difficult intubation?

Ans. Whenever there is anticipated difficult intubation it is wise to withheld muscle relaxant and the child is anesthetized with inhalational anesthetic agent keeping spontaneous respiration intact.

12. What is the proper anesthetic management?

Ans. If an IV catheter is in place, anesthesia can be induced with thiopentione, otherwise with oxygen, nitrous oxide and either halothane or sevoflurane. In cleft lip/palate surgery, the surgeon infiltrates with bupivacaine with epinephrine (1 in 400.000/- dilution) to prevent excessive bleeding and to facilitate mucosal dissection. In children, 10 mcg/kg appears to be a safe maximal dosage of epinephrine for infiltration. Halothane sensitizes myocardium and decrease the arrhythmia threshold of exogenous epinephrine but sevoflurane does not. After the baby has been anesthetized, IV cannulation can be performed fluid initiated.

Airway management for most of these children is straight forward but when associated with alveolar margin defect and retrognathia intubation could be difficult. The laryngoscope blade tend to slip in to the alveolar margin gap leaving minimal space to manipulate the tube for manipulation. In the presence of macrognathia bougie-guided, retromandibular or fiberoptic intubation is performed.

A balanced anesthetic technique of inhalational agent (with or without nitrous oxide), an opioid, and a muscle relaxant (optional) is effective and safe. Muscle relaxation is achieved by atracurium and intubation is done by proper sized RAE preformed tube because the preformed bend in the tube facilitates the use of the mouth retractor. An arm or reinforced tube which do not kink with flexion can be used to secure the airway in some situations where there is a risk of main stem intubation in a smaller infant or if there is increased risk of extubation where an unexpectedly small endotracheal tube is required. Fixation of the tube is done in midline without facial distortion as symmetry is very much essential. Surgical preparation of the field can result in removal of the tape from the tube if it is not secured well. A pharyngeal pack with a moistened ribbon gauge is inserted in cleft lip surgery, because it helps to keep the endotracheal tube in proper place and it also prevents the blood to trickle into trachea by absorbing it intraoperatively.

In cleft palate, the surgeon will insert the pack if necessary after insertion of Dingman-Dott mouth retractor.

Ref: Gregory GA (Ed). Pediatric anesthesia, 4th edn. New York: Churchill Livingstone; 2002.p.731.

Child should be extubated in lateral position after through suction of the oropharynx under direct vision.

Insertion and removal of throat pack has to be documented including timing and name of person involved.

13. Is suxamethonium safe for use in children?

Ans. Suxamethonium is safe in girl child and boys beyond 6 years. As Duchenne muscle dystrophy does not affect girls and it get fully manifested by the age of six in boys, there is no fear of hyperkalemia.

14. What are the difficulties encountered during intubation?

Ans. In cleft lip, especially in bilateral cleft lip with protruded and hanging premaxilla, laryngoscopy and intubation becomes difficult. In such cases, a tooth guard made-up of several layers of sticking plaster or soft plastic is applied as a wedge in the gap to protect the gum from injury by the laryngoscope blade during laryngoscopy and intubation. In complete cleft palate, the blade of straight blade laryngoscope may be trapped and immobilized in the cleft. Then a gauge pack or dental roll is to be inserted in the gap before laryngoscopy. Some studies have described the incidence of difficult laryngoscopy (the laryngoscopic view of Cormack and Lehane laryngoscope view grades 3 and 4) to be as high as 4–7% (Xue et al 2006). Despite this high percentage of poor laryngoscopic view, only 1% of patients were difficult to intubate, and only one patient had a failed intubation (Gunawardana, 1996).

15. What should be the recommended position of the patient?

Ans. In cleft palate surgery, maximal extension of the head is necessary for better exposure of palate to aid in surgical activity. So whole body of the child is raised with a thick foam mat allowing head to drop back hyperextended into a stockinette head support. The advantage of this position is good exposure of the operating area for the surgeon, allows blood to flow away towards nasopharynx which is removed continuously by suction. But the disadvantage is, there may be inadvertent extubation. So, it is mandatory to auscultate both sides of the chest after positioning of the patient.

16. What precautions should be taken during placement of the mouth gag?

Ans. The surgeons apply the Dingman-Dott mouth retractor the bag should be manually ventilated and feel any rise in pressure to ventilate, which could be due to partial or complete occlusion of the tube by the retractor SpO_2 should be monitored closely.

17. What intraoperative problems may be encountered?

Ans. After placement of mouth retractor, ventilation should be re-evaluated because of possible compression of the endotracheal tube against mandible and because advancement may cause single-lung ventilation. Surgeon's tools and hands and anesthesiologist's endotracheal tube occupy the same very small space. So, there should be good communication and cooperation between the surgeon and anesthesiologist for better outcome of the patient. Look for blood loss in palate repair especially in older children.

Ref: Gregory GA (Ed). Pediatric anesthesia, 4th edn. New York: Churchill Livingstone; 2002.p.731.

18. What precautions are to be taken in cheiloplasty or palatoplasty operation?

Ans. Following precautions are to be taken in cheiloplasty and palatoplasty operation:

- During induction of anesthesia with oxygen, nitrous oxide and inhalational agents, respiratory obstruction may take place due to falling back of tongue due to presence of cleft palate.
- Throat packs can result in airway obstruction, if unintentionally left in place, and confirmation of their removal must take place before extubation. For protection of eye, ocular lubricants are to be placed in eye and upper eyelids are to be splinted with tape. Particular attention should be paid to protecting the infant's chest wall and extremities from the breathing circuit and the tight monitoring leads.
- Auscultation of both sides of lung is mandatory after insertion of tube, after placement of throat pack, after extension or positioning and after insertion of mouth pack in palatoplasty.

19. Is nasal airway indicated after cleft palate operation?

Ans. Nasal or oral airway is to be avoided as it may cause suture disruption. There may be postoperative problems like respiratory distress because the child does not learn the art of oral breathing in response to surgical closure of the cleft. If tongue falls back, tongue suture is given and child nursed in lateral position.

Logan's bow is applied to take the tension off the newly sutured lip.

Elbow restraints are essential and are to be placed on the infant before leaving the operating room.

Ref: Aston SJ, Beasley RW, Thorne CHM (Eds). Grabb and Smith's plastic surgery, 5th edn. Philadelphia: Lippincott-Raven; 1997.p.247.

20. What are the problems during feeding and what is the protocol of feeding?

Ans. These patients are unable to suck due to presence of cleft lip and cleft palate and may be unable to swallow leading to aspiration. So the protocol of feeding is, the child is to be held at 45 degrees during feeding. So, less milk is escaped into nasal passage. Use of a long soft nipple is recommended and more than usual amount of burping is required as increased amount of air is swallowed.

21. What will be the position of the child in postoperative period to protect the airway?

Ans. The child should be nursed in prone or lateral position, with the head dependant and turned to the side and hyperextended. This position can be achieved by placing a bulky bath blanket under the hip of the infant.

22. What is laryngospasm and how would you manage?

Ans. This is defined as glottic closure resulting from a reflex constriction of the laryngeal muscles.

It occurs usually at induction or recovery. The main cause is noxious stimuli at lighter plane of anesthesia. It is more often seen with sevoflurane or desflurane as compared to halothane. It can be treated by applying positive pressure to the airway, deepening anesthesia by a bolus of propofol, and administering muscle relaxant suxamethonium.

Ref: Sumner E, Hatch DJ (Eds). Pediatric anesthesia, 2nd edn Arnold, London; 2000.pp.205-6.

23. Is postoperative analgesia and sedation necessary?
Ans. Yes necessary.

24. What postoperative analgesia will you give?
Ans. No child should be discharged from the recovery, room with uncontrolled pain. As the children has been infiltrated with bupivacaine or lignocaine, they do not need any analgesic in the immediate postoperative period. Analgesics should be initiated as soon as possible. Paracetamol oral dose of 20 mg/kg, IV dose of 10–15 mg/kg slowly or rectal dosage of 40 mg/kg, followed -6 hourly is safe. Nonsteroidal anti-inflammatory agents may be used for postoperative analgesia after palatoplasty (Sylaidis and O'Neill 1998). Although some evidence suggests there may be no increased risk of bleeding, many surgeons and anesthesiologists choose not to use them routinely. The dosage of opioids, if administered, should be appropriate for body weight, to minimize the respiratory compromise in infants. For infants undergoing surgery, a safe starting dosage of morphine is 0.05 mg/kg every 3–4 hours, as needed. Infants undergoing cleft surgery and being given parenteral narcotics should be appropriately monitored (oxygen saturation and electrocardiography) in an well-equipped postanesthetic care room as there is increased chance of apnea, bradycardia, nausea and vomiting in these patients. Fentanyl 1 mcg/kg, pethidine 1 mg/kg can also be given, all through intravenous routes, but with proper monitoring.

Bilateral infraorbital nerve block can be used for pain control after cheiloplasty. The block, which can be performed by anesthesiologists or surgeons, provides better analgesia than peri-incisional infiltration or opioids alone (Pradeep et al. 1999; Rajamani et al. 2007). The infraorbital nerve block has been described for all age groups including neonates (Bosenberg and Kible, 1995). There are two approaches for infraorbital nerve block; extraoral (percutaneous) and intraoral. Infants scheduled for cleft lip repairs require 0.5–1 mL of local anesthetic solution on each side; for older children and adolescents, 1.5–2 mL can be used. Bupivacaine (0.125%, 0.25%, or 0.5%, with or without epinephrine [5 mcg/mL]) or ropivacaine (0.2% or 0.5%) can be used for the block.

Nasopalatine and palatine nerve block can be used to provide pain relief after palatoplasty.

Ref: Badgwell JM (Ed). Clinical pediatric anesthesia. Philadelphia: Lippincott-Raven. 1997.pp.229-35.
Ref: Motoyama EK, Davis PS (Eds). Smith's anesthesia for infants and children, 7th edn. St Louis: Mosby; 2006. pp.733-5.
Ref: Sumner E, Hatch DJ (Eds). Pediatric anesthesia, 2nd edn, Arnold, London; 2000.pp.272-8.

25. What are the complications seen in recovery room?
Ans. Following complications may be encountered in the recovery room:
Airway obstruction: The most important and grave complication. It is due to combination of closed palate, small mandible, large tongue, edema, blood and residual effects of anesthesia.

Blood loss: Hypothermia which delays emergence and produces metabolic acidosis and produces respiratory and myocardial depression.

Ref: Motoyama EK, Davis PS (Eds). Smith's anesthesia for infants and children, 7th edn. St Louis: Mosby; 2006. pp.733-5.

26. What are the problems of anesthesia in developing countries?
Ans.
1. Pathologies that occur in infants in developing countries are malnutrition, anemia, parasitic infestation. Many of these pathologies may not be identified. So thorough preoperative screening process is needed.
2. The availability of drugs and equipment are various lavel of care might be different. A well-trained anesthetist should be able to provide reasonable good care to these children.
3. Nonavailability of support service like high dependent care area or ICU in case of any complication.

BIBLIOGRAPHY

1. Aston SJ, Beasley RW, Thorne CHM (Eds). Grabb and Smith's Plastic Surgery, 5th edn. Philadelphia. Lippincott-Raven, 1997.
2. Barrett BM Jr (Ed). Patient care in plastic surgery. St Louis, MO: Mosby–Year book, 1996.
3. Cooper HK (Ed). Cleft palate and cleft lip: a team approach. Philadelphia: WB Saunders, 1979.
4. Gregory GA (Ed). Pediatric anaesthesia, 4th edn. New York: Churchill Livingstone, 2001.
5. Motoyama EK, Davis PS (Eds). Smith's anesthesia for infants and children, 6th edn. St Louis, MO: Mosby, 1996.
6. Nelson WE, Behrman RE, et al. (Eds). Nelson's textbook of pediatrics, 16th edn. Philadelphia: WB Saunders, 2000.
7. Sumner E, Hatch D (Eds). Pediatric anesthesia, 2nd edn, Arnold, London; 2000.
8. Yao FSF. Yao and Artusio's Anaesthesiology, 6th edn. Lippincott Williams & Wilkins: Philadelphia.

29

Role of Anesthesiologist in Acute Burn

Sudakshina Mukherji

1. Why burn injury is treated as an emergency?

Ans. Burn injury, however minor it may be, starting from erythema or scalds to major burns are everyday problems in emergency department which requires immediate treatment. Few areas of medicine are as challenging medically and surgically as burn care. Patient of any age group of either sex may become a victim of burn injury and the geriatric and pediatric age group requires special attention. The chance of survival depends not only on the treatment plan but also on the time spent from the rescue of the victim and initiation of proper treatment. All major burn cases are to be treated according to advance trauma life support (ATLS) protocol.

2. What is the definition of major burn?

Ans. According to the American Burn Association, a major burn is defined as follows:
- Full thickness burns more than 10% of total body surface area (TBSA)
- Partial-thickness burns more than 25% in adults or 20% at extremes of age
- Burns involving face, hands, feet, genitalia, perineum or major joints
- Inhalational, chemical or electrical burns
- Burns in patients with serious pre-existing medical disorders.

3. Is it mandatory to admit all burn patients to hospitals or burn care centers?

Ans. No, minor injury can easily be managed in emergency department or outpatient clinic, but extensive burn injury remains potentially fatal and requires immediate hospitalization and more aggressive treatment to prevent multiorgan system failure which increases not only mortality and morbidity but prolongs hospital stay also, thereby causing increased cost of treatment.

4. What is the incidence of burn and rate of survival after major burn injury?

Ans. According to National Institutes of General Medical Sciences, an estimated 1.1 million burn patients require medical attention annually in United States, out of which 50,000 require hospitalization and 4,500 die annually from burn injuries.

Previously mortality rate after major burn was very high. But survival rate has significantly been improved over the course of 20th century. The reasons are many-better understanding of the patient's status, and more aggressive treatment which includes improvement in resuscitation with appropriate fluids, the introduction of topical antimicrobial agents, use of broad spectrum antibiotics, nebulization and early intubation (in case of airway burns) and most importantly, the recent practice of early burn wound excision followed by skin grafting—all contribute to the better and improved outcome after severe burn injury. However, the mortality rate is still very high in third world countries after major burn injury.

5. Where burn patients are to be treated?

Ans. Except minor burns, all major burns according to American Burn Association, require referral to a burn center after initial assessment and initiation of treatment. Patients with suspected inhalational injury, circumpherential burns, burns with associated trauma are also to be referred to a burn center. Pediatric patients are to be transferred to a center capable of providing qualified personnel and equipment.

6. What are the criteria for admission to an intensive care unit (ICU)?

Ans.
- Adults with burn injuries greater than 15–20% for adequate monitoring and control of infection
- Infants and children and elderly with less extensive burns
- Patients with suspected inhalational injury for close airway monitoring
- Patients who require frequent neurovascular checks to assess the viability of a limb

These patients are to be admitted to an ICU for treatment with better outcome and survival rate.

7. What is a burn care team?

Ans. The essence of successful burn care is the team and is best delivered in a center where experienced physicians, surgeons, anesthesiologists, nurses, nutritionists, psychologists, physical and occupational therapists, and social workers all can participate in the care of the individual.

8. What are the causes of burn?

Ans. Burn injury results from a variey of causes.

Scald burn: The most common cause of civilian burn, depth is related to temperature and viscosity of the liquid, and duration of exposure with the liquid. Typically heal without skin grafting.

Grease burn: Tend to result in deeper burn and sometimes surgical intervention is required.

Flame burn: Next most common cause, result from house-fire, campfire, and burning of dry leaves and trashes. Usually full thickness if the clothes of the victim catches fire.

Flash burn: Quite common and result from ignition of propane and gasoline, usually result in partial thickness burns affecting exposed areas of skin (most commonly face and extremities).

Contact burn: Result from contact with woodstoves, hot metals, plastics, or coals, usually deep but limited in extent.

Blast burn: Caused by an explosion, producing direct injury, may be penetrating, or buildings falling on body, the heat producing direct thermal burns. The explosion produces high energy sound waves which tend to give up energy at the interface between body fluid and air, thereby causing injury to air containing organs like lungs and bowel.

Other than these burns injury can result from chemical and electric burn.

Electric burn: The high voltage supply will cause extensive and massive tissue destruction which is usually difficult to assess by looking at the entry and exit points of the current in body. The skin injury may look small but there is gross deep-tissue damage.

9. How a burn patient has been transported?

Ans. Prior to transfer of the patient, specific steps are to be followed to ensure safe transport.
- First rescue the patient from accident site.
- Intimate the burn care center.
- Look for cervical spine injury, if suspected, then put a cervical collar if available.

- Transport the patient in a warm and dry dressing to prevent hypothermia during transport.
- If suspect inhalational injury, secure the airway before transportation.
- If suspect carbon monoxide or cyanide poisoning, then give 100% oxygen through face mask
- Initiate fluid resuscitation after securing intravenous access
- Insert a Foley catheter in place.

10. What are the measures taken on arrival to a burn care center?

Ans. On arrival, a thorough evaluation is performed and a treatment plan is developed. The presence of other life-threatening injuries are to be excluded and a patent airway, breathing and circulation are to be ensured according to ATLS protocol. Then the extent and depth of burn are assessed after admission of the patient.

11. How extent of burn is calculated?

Ans. There are several techniques to calculate the total body surface area (TBSA). While calculating TBSA, only the areas of partial or full thickness burns are taken into account leaving the superficial areas of burn involving only the epidermis. The rule of nine is the best known method of estimating extent of burn, which is as follows in an adult is as follows:

Head and neck	9%
Right upper extremity	9%
Left upper extremity	9%
Right lower extremity	18%
Left lower extremity	18%
Anterior trunk	18%
Posterior trunk	18%
Perineum	1%

In infants and children, the heads tend to be proportionately greater than 9% and the lower extremities less than 18% of TBSA. Lund and Browder charts are a more accurate method of assessing extent of burn. They provide an age based diagram to assist in more precisely calculating the burn size.

12. How depth of injury is assessed?

Ans. After determination of extent, the depth of injury is to be assessed whether the epidermis or a portion or the entirety of dermis or the subcutaneous tissue or other deeper structures are involved, as the depth affects the healing of wound, assessment of depth is important for appropriate wound management and ultimately the decision for surgical intervention.

Superficial burn: Usually heals within 3–5 days by treating with topical agents and oral analgesics are used to alleviate pain.

Superficial partial thickness burn: Typically heals within 2 weeks by covering with greasy gauge coated with antibiotic ointments. They do not result in scarring but could result in alteration of pigmentation.

Deep partial thickness burn: Usually heal within 3–8 weeks if protected from infection, but heal with contraction, scarring and possible contracture, operative excision and skin grafting may be needed if do not heal within 3 weeks.

Full thickness burns are best treated by excision and skin grafting.

13. What initial management plan is usually undertaken?

Ans. *Initial management:* Intravenous access is very important and two peripheral lines are usually sufficient for less than 30% burns. Patients with more severe burns may require central line placement. If the patient remain intubated, placement of arterial line may be necessary. Though peripheral and central lines can be placed through burned tissue after proper preparation of skin with antimicrobial agents, arterial line placement should preferably be done through unburned tissue though sometimes not possible. The peripheral lines are used for fluid resuscitation as well as for intravenous medication. Central venous line and arterial line are to be removed as soon as possible regardless of location. As in all wounds, the tetanus immunization status of the patient is to be checked and prophylactic measures are to be taken.

History of any allergy and any medication are also to be noted.

14. How fluid resuscitation is instituted?

Ans. Vigorous fluid resuscitation should be instituted immediately to combat hypovolemic shock and to ensure good tissue perfusion and adequate urine output. Awake and alert patients should be encouraged to take adequate fluid through oral route but patients with more than 15–20% of TBSA, formal fluid resuscitation is required.

15. What are the guidelines for correct resuscitation?

Ans. *Guidelines for correct resuscitation:*

- Do not delay resuscitation
- Estimate burn size and calculate fluid requirements
- Fluid formulas are only a guideline; monitor urine output and tailor intravenous fluids to the response of the patient
- Monitor peripheral pulses, blood pressure, respiration rate, heart rate, urine output, oxygen saturation, and temperature
- Monitor central venous pressure and/or cardiac output and hemodynamic parameters in severe burns or patients at risk for complications
- Achieve a urine output of 0.5 mL/kg per hour in adults and 1 mL/kg per hour in children—no more, no less!
- Elevate the head, limbs, and genitalia; elevate all that can be elevated
- Maintain the core temperature of the patient over 37°C
- Start enteral feeding on admission
- The aim is to maintain an awake, alert, conscious and cooperative patient.

16. What fluid formula is usually used?

Ans. Though many fluid formulas are used, the Parkland formula popularized by Baxter has been adopted in most burn centers because of its simplicity, reduced cost and equivalent outcome.

Parkland formula:

First 24 hours: Electrolyte solution (lactated Ringer's) 4 mL/kg/percent of body area with second and third degree burn

Administration rate: 50% given in first 8 hours, 25% in next 8 hours and remaining 25% in the next 8 hours

Urine output: Maintain at 0.5–1 mL/kg/hour

Second 24 hours: Glucose in water—To replace evaporated water loss and maintain serum sodium concentration of 140 mEq/L.

Colloid solutions (e.g. albumin): Amount proportion to burn:

- *30–50% burn:* 0.3 mL/kg per percentage of burn
- *50–70% burn:* 0.4 mL/kg per percentage of burn
- *Larger than 70% burn:* 0.5 mL/kg per percentage of burn

Urine output to be maintained at 0.5–1 mL/kg/hour.

Children weighing less than 15 kg should also receive a maintenance intravenous rate with dextrose containing solution because they do not have adequate glycogen reserve.

In adult, an urine output of at least 0.5 mL/kg /hour and in children at least 1 mL/kg/hour indicates adequate resuscitation.

Use of colloid in early postburn period can lead to the leakage of colloid in the interstitial space, thereby aggrevating tissue edema. So its role is debatable in first 24 hours but after that period, capillary leak has started to seal and colloid can be used. Albumin is the most oncotically active solution, but fresh frozen plasma (FFP), and low molecular weight dextran (dextran 40) can also be used but with caution as there is risk of disease transmission with FFP and fatal allergic reaction with dextran in some patients.

17. What are the signs and symptoms of inhalational injury?

Ans.

- Diagnosis of inhalation injury is to be made by consideration of the circumstances surrounding burn injury and also findings on physical examination.

  The immediate cause of death in severe burn is asphyxia. So inhalational burn is suspected when one or more of the following signs are present:
- Presence of singed nasal or facial hair
- Presence of carbonaceous sputum, raw oral and nasal mucosa
- Soot on vocal cord on laryngoscopy
- Presence of cough, hoarseness of voice, difficulty in breathing.

18. How patients with inhalational injury are managed?

Ans. In suspected cases of airway burn, it is better to *intubate the patient in early postburn period because it may become difficult to intubate later due to rapid development of airway edema.* Management is usually supportive, aggressive pulmonary toilet, bronchodilators and clearing of secretions are essential components of patient management. Steroids are not beneficial and use of prophylactic antibiotics are to be avoided. Radiographs may be useful to evaluate possible pneumonia. Repeat broncoscopy may be needed if the patient cannot cough out the sloughed mucosa and the sputum is to be sent for culture. These patients are at increased risk of respiratory failure and subsequent infection. If patients show signs of adult respiratory distress syndrome (ARDS) which occurs secondary to the systemic inflammatory response triggered by the burn wound matrix, infection, and complications of burn therapy, should be placed on ventilatory support with low tidal volume to protect lung parenchyma from further damage.

19. What is carbon monoxide poisoning and how it is treated?

Ans. The inhalation of the product of combustion can lead to devastating pulmonary injury. Carbon monoxide inhalation is particularly injurious because it has a 200 times greater affinity for hemoglobin than oxygen. So, it displaces oxygen from its hemoglobin binding sites and interferes with the delivery of oxygen to tissues causing tissue hypoxia and metabolic acidosis. The usefulness of hyperbaric oxygen therapy for patients with elevated carboxyhemoglobin (HbCO) levels has long been debated. The potential benefit of hyperbaric oxygen (HBO) is the rapid reduction of carboxyhemoglobin level thereby minimizing the potential neurologic sequelae to carbon monoxide poisoning. Patients should be considered for HBO treatment if they are symptomatic and have an HbCO level >25%. However hyperbaric oxygen is not without risk. It cause pneumothorax and perforation of tympanic membrane and there are great technical difficulties also in the transfer and administration of HBO treatment in a severely burned patient. It is possible to effectively treat an elevated carboxyhemoglobin with 100% oxygen.

20. What are the problems associated with cyanide poisoning and how to manage it?

Ans. In cyanide poisoning, there is tissue hypoxia by inhibition of cytochrome oxidase which prevents mitochondrial oxygen consumption and arrests the tricarboxylic acid cycle. So for ATP production, anaerobic metabolism takes place leading to formation of metabolic acidosis. The clinical symptoms vary with the concentration:

50 ppm—headache, dizziness, tachycardia and tachypnea

100 ppm—lethargy, seizures and respiratory failure.

Treatment is usually conservative, but high cyanide levels and persisting metabolic acidosis should be treated with sodium thiosulfate, sodium nitrites and dicobalt edentate.

21. Why nutritional support is important in burn care and how it is maintained?

Ans. Nutritional support is a cornerstone of burn patient management. Hypermetabolism and hypercatabolism both occur after burn injury. The increase in basal metabolic rate is proportional to the size of the burn and the presence of infection, peaking at 7–10 days. Feeds whether oral or enteral should be initiated as soon as possible after admission. Most patients with burn injuries less than 20% TBSA can obtain enough calories of their own. But patients with major burn and patients who need intubation should have an enteral feeding tube on admission. Enteral feeding helps to maintain gut perfusion and intestinal mucosal integrity, helping to prevent bacterial translocation and has been shown to decrease weight loss and sepsis. Paralytic ileus commonly occurs after major burn injury which can be prevented by starting oral feeds immediately in the postinjury period. The nutritional needs are to be determined by the physician and dietician and appropriate adjustments to the patients nutrition plan, are to be made regularly. Burn patients usually receive high dose of narcotics for relief of pain so stool softeners are to be used routinely to prevent constipation and feed intolerance. There are several equations to estimate the caloric requirement. The Curreri formula differs for children and adults as follows:

- Adult 25 kcal × wt (kg) + 40 kcal × % TBSA
- Children 60 kcal × wt (kg) + 35 kcal × % TBSA

The Harris-Benedict formula provides an estimate of basal energy expenditure (BEE):

- Men—66.5 + 13.8 × wt (kg) + 5 × height (cm) - 6.76 × age (years)
- Women—65.5 + 9.6 × wt (kg) + 1.85 × height (cm) - 4.68 × age (years)

The calculated BEE is multiplied by an injury factor (typically 2.1 for patients with large burns). The Curreri formula generally overestimates caloric requirement and the Harris-Benedict formula underestimates caloric requirement, an average of the two is often used.

As burn patients catabolize significant amount of skeletal muscle, protein replacement is required to maintain muscle mass and wound healing. Patients with normal renal function require 2 gm of protein per kg per day. Supplemental vitamins, especially A, C, E and zinc, selenium and iron supplements are beneficial for wound healing. Regular nutrition monitoring should be performed weekly with C-reactive protein, albumin prealbumin and vitamin C levels, and 24 hours total urea nitrogen. Patient's blood glucose level is to be monitored closely because blood glucose level above 7.8 mmol/L increases mortality and benefits of tight glucose control in a critically ill patient is well-documented. Sliding scale insulin coverage is to be initiated in all major burn patients treated in the intensive care unit.

22. What gastrointestinal prophylaxis is given in burn patient?

Ans. Stress ulcers or Curling's ulcer were once a common complication following burn injury. But the development of prophylactic agents including histamine receptor blocker, sucralfate, and proton pump inhibitors have minimized the incidence of stress ulcer. Early feeding minimizes gastric atony. So oral feeding should be started as early as possible and stress ulcer prophylaxis should be limited to those patients who are unable to take oral feeds or patients with previous history of peptic ulcer.

23. How deep vein thrombosis has been prevented?

Ans. Patients who have burn injury on the extremities, thereby limiting their movement and intubated patients and presence of indwelling catheter, are at increased risk of venous thrombosis. The use of sequential compression devices and antiembolic stockings may not be feasible in patients with lower extremity burn. So these patients should receive subcutaneous heparin. If any patient develops sudden swelling of extremity or develops acute hypoxia, suspicion of deep vein thrombosis or pulmonary embolism should be kept in mind. In pediatric age group, if the patient is on prolonged bed rest, there is increased risk of deep vein thrombosis and pulmonary embolism, so deep vein thrombosis prophylaxis should be considered.

24. What measures are to be taken for infection control?

Ans. Down regulation of immune responses and loss of the skin barrier rendered burn patients highly susceptible to infection which remains a significant risk for burn patients. Burns are initially virtually free from bacteria but the dead and necrosed tissue soon becomes heavily colonized by bacteria. Prolonged intensive care unit stay, prolonged periods of intubation and ventilation, and potential colonization of burn eschar contribute to the risk of infection. Indwelling vascular and bladder catheters also provide another source of invasive infection. Due to loss of skin, mucous membrane, the barrier against infection is lost and as cellular and humoral portions of the immune response is compromised, the burn patients become immunocompromised. Previously, patients who survive the first week, frequently succumb to burn wound sepsis. Colonization of devitalized eschar would lead to bacterial invasion, ultimately to burn wound sepsis. The best treatment for burn wound sepsis is prevention. Nowadays, the practice of early burn wound excision has significantly decreased the incidence of burn wound sepsis and improved survival. Management of infection should be culture driven. Presumptive broad spectrum antibiotic coverage is not advised for fear of breeding resistant organisms and increasing the risk of fungal infections. So, selection of antibiotics should be based on culture results. Diagnosis of sepsis is difficult as leukocytosis, erythema, fever and a hyperdynamic state are all normal findings in a severely burned patient. Nearly all patients with more than 15% TBSA burn become febrile within the first 72 hours. So, following the initial 72–96 hours, periodic cultures are important in making a diagnosis of infection Any change in patient's status, including hypotension, altered mental status, intolerance to tube feeding, hyper or hypoglycemia, increasing base deficit or hypothermia should raise the suspicion of infection.

25. What is the regime for control of pain in burn?

Ans. *Pain management is important for burn patients who have two types of pain:* Background and procedural. Background pain is present on a daily basis with little variation. Many burns are extremely painful, but also many severe burns are relatively pain-free. Narcotics are the best analgesics and the best way to give pain relief is by small intravenous boluses of opioids. Non-steroidal medications are typically not used in patients who may have to undergo surgery because of increased risk of bleeding. Background pain is best treated with longer-acting agents like methadone initially, then the dose is tapered and discontinued and then oxycodone or morphine (0.1 mg/kg) can be used for breakthrough pain. However, this may need to be titrated to response as larger or smaller doses may be necessary.

Procedural pain occurs during daily wound care and therapy which are of short duration, so shorter acting agents are probably best. If the patient is tolerating oral feeding, oral analgesic is preferred. If oral analgesics proves to be inadequate then fentanyl can be used. Some patients may benefit from shorter acting benzodiazepines because wound care may be anxiety provoking in some patients. Intubated patients are usually treated with morphine and longer acting benzodiazepine.

26. How temperature is maintained and what derangements occur with hypothermia?

Ans. Massively burned patients with huge loss of skin have constant evaporation from open surfaces that will lead to development of hypothermia. So, patient should be placed on a clean sheet and wrap around and unburnt areas should be covered with a thermal blanket to avoid hypothermia because hypothermia causes many detrimental changes in patient's body physiology. It decreases metabolism, heart rate, cardiac output and blood pressure. Atrial pacing becomes irregular and ventricular ectopic increases at temperature less than 28°C. Ventricular fibrillation occurs between 25°C–30°C.

27. What is the management plan of anesthesia, if an emergency surgery has to be undertaken?
Ans. Emergency surgery which is usually undertaken in a severely burned patient is, early excision of wound followed by skin grafting. If the patient is already intubated, high dose narcotic-muscle relaxant technique is preferred as this technique gives good hemodynamic stability as well as excellent postoperative analgesia.

If the patient is not intubated and there is anticipated difficult intubation, the safest way to secure the airway is to perform an awake intubation with topical anesthesia and mild sedation. If there is no problem with the airway, then other techniques of anesthesia can be sought for with the help of intravenous or inhalational anesthetic agents.

It is recommended to avoid succinylcholine from 24–48 hours after burn injury up to about 2 years after complete healing of the wound because succinylcholine may cause a significant transient rise in serum potassium resulting in ventricular tachycardia, fibrillation, even cardiac arrest. Nondepolarizing muscle relaxant without histamine release should be preferred, though burn patients show increased resistance to nondepolarizers thereby increasing the dose requirement.It appears to be due to alteration in the number and affinity of the junctional receptors in burned patients though the alteration is quite variable.

In some patients, the leathery eschar of a full thickness burn form a constricting band that compromise limb perfusion or ventilation which may result in necrosis of limb or compromises thoracic cage excursion and thus ventilation, if not treated early. Escharotomy, even sometimes fasciotomy may have to be undertaken in the early postburn period on an emergency basis to save the life of the patient or to save the limbs from necrosis. But this increases the anesthetic risk as the patient is not optimally stabilized at that time and a major surgery is undertaken in the resuscitative phase of injury.

28. What is important to increase the survival rate in burn patients?
Ans. Despite all the advances in burn care over the past century, and the exciting prospects in the horizon, the core of burn care remains the burn team. As burn affects almost all the systems of human body, and each aspect of care becomes increasingly complex, the importance of a team of experts is very much needed for successful burn care and survival of the patient.

BIBLIOGRAPHY

1. Cole JK, Ergrav LH, Heimbach DM, et al. Early excision and grafting of face and neck burns in patients over 20 years. Plast Reconstr Surg. 2002;109:1266.
2. Colour Atlas of Burn Care edited by Jaun P Barret, David N Herndon, Saunders, 2004.
3. Course Manual of International Trauma Anaesthesia and Critical Care Society (Indian Chapter) 2008 Chapter X ;140-56.
4. Grab and Smith's plastic surgery, 6th edn by Lippincott Williams and Wilkins by (Lippincott-Raven Publishers) 2007.pp.132-49.
5. Heimbach D. Early burn excision and grafting. Surg Clin North Am. 1987;67:93.
6. Herndon D. Total Burn Care, New York: WB Saunders, 2002.
7. Janzekovic Z. A new concept in the early excision and immediate grafting of burns. J Burn Care Rehabil. 1970;10:1103.
8. Luce EA. Burn care and management, Clin Plast Surg. 2000;27:1.
9. Michael Tjeuw Burns Yao and Artusio's Anaesthesiology, 7th edn. 2011.pp.1200-20.

30

Postburn Contractures: Neck and Extremity

Anil Agarwal, Sujeet Kumar Singh Gautam

Must to know facts

1. What are the common issues associated with the anesthetic management of a case of postburn contracture neck and extremity?

Ans. The common issues associated with the anesthetic management of a case of postburn contracture neck and extremity include difficult airway, scarce venous access, no places available for monitoring, drug dependency, multiple anesthetics, tendency to hypothermia, difficult patient positioning, hyperkalemic response to suxamethonium and inaccurate estimation of blood loss. Difficult airway is the most critical and its consequences can be catastrophic. Hence, a meticulous airway examination is always a necessity.[1]

2. What are the key points which should be examined during preoperative assessment of these patients?

Ans. The anesthetic management of patients with severe postburn neck contracture presents many difficult problems. Difficult airway is the most challenging of these; hence it is imperative that a detailed airway assessment is carried out preoperatively to evaluate the degree of anticipated difficulty and to aid in planning strategies with alternatives. The history should seek to exclude previous problems of intubation during anesthesia. The most sensitive predictor of difficult intubation is however, a past history of airway problems during anesthesia.[2]

The history and physical examination may reveal fixed flexion deformity of the neck and cicatrized angles of the mouth, giving rise to reduced mouth opening and interincisor distance with Mallampati classification of higher grade. Usually it is difficult to assess sternomental and thyromental distances because of the contracture. The fixed flexion deformity make head extension impossible. Hence, the patient may present a multitude of difficulties in airway management.

The airway should be evaluated in sitting position, not in supine position. In addition to the routine assessment, the anesthesiologist should carefully examine the scar and contracture, paying special attention to the perinasal and circumoral regions and the size of the nasal and oral orifices. Mentosternal contractures may limit the mouth opening and cervical range of motion. Oro-maxillo-facial burn scars may also accompany skeletal deformities resulting in a small receding jaw.

Currently, there are no recommended guidelines for burn scar patients, so airway management of these patients relies on clinical judgment of the anesthesiologist entirely.

3. How would you manage difficult airway in patients with postburn mentosternal and circumoral scar contractures?

Ans. Because difficulty in managing the airway is one important cause of major anesthesia-related morbidity and mortality, preparations of many options for alternative to direct laryngoscopy must be made in advance. However, in patients with extreme contracture, the functional and anatomical distortion may lead to the failure of intubation. Hence, meticulous planning for airway management is essential.

Equipment check should be done prior to patient entry in the theater. Difficult intubation tray should be consisting of endotracheal tubes of different sizes, laryngeal mask airway of different sizes, gum elastic bougie, curved and straight blades of laryngoscope, intubating stylet or tube changer and different size facemasks. Resuscitative drugs including adrenaline, atropine, sodium bicarbonate and hydrocortisone should be available.

Few important points thought to be essential in airway management for scar contracture patients include through discussion and planning between anesthesiologists and surgeons. It is desirable that the operating surgeon should be present physically in the operating room at the time of induction of anesthesia, prepared for emergency release of contractures, tracheotomy, or both. Secondly we propose an awake fiber optic intubation under video laryngoscope guidance as an effective method in patients with anticipated difficult intubation. Nasal intubation using the fiber optic bronchoscope is of great value in many of these cases, but it relies greatly on the skill and experience of the operator and can be time consuming. The equipment is not only complex but also expensive and is not available in many developing countries.

Wong et al.[3] proposed several options for airway management with contractures involving the neck, face, and anterior chest. These are awake intubation with fiber optic bronchoscopy, face mask ventilation followed by surgical scar release then tracheal intubation, laryngeal mask airway anesthesia and scar release then intubation if needed, intubating laryngeal mask airway, tracheostomy or cricothyroidotomy, and surgical scar release under ketamine and local anesthesia followed by intubation.

4. How could mentosternal burn contractures affect the normal airway anatomy and airway management?

Ans. Contractures around the neck distort the normal anatomical pattern around the neck. Mandible may be distorted by underlying dense fibrous and hypertrophic sheets of scar. Cervical range of motion may be limited in all directions and the sniffing position may be unobtainable due to severe mentosternal contracture. The mandible may be displaced posteriorly with accompanying restrictions in mobility. Facial burns during early childhood can cause underdevelopment of the jaw (micrognathia), leading to further distortion of the upper airway. Finally, a history of inhalational injury may suggest tracheal stenosis which could hamper advance of endotracheal tube.

The directions and formations of scar patterns may determine the intubation route of choice. Finally, the epiglottis and vocal cords may be anteriorly placed and pulled toward the side of the scar. If a laryngoscope is used, it should be advanced ipsilaterally towards the direction of the scar. If muscle relaxants are given, the elasticity of scar tissue and loss of pulling action by the surrounding tissues will further aggravate scar retraction, making preoperative airway evaluation obsolete. Limited mouth opening may become so aggravated that neither oral airway nor laryngoscope blade can be passed through the mouth. The nasal orifices, as a potential alternative access, may also close down, leading to the inability to advance a nasal airway.[4]

5. What are the important pharmacokinetic changes seen in these patients?

Ans. Important pharmacokinetic changes seen in this group of patients include:

- Volume of distribution increases for water soluble drugs (resistance to non-depolarizing agents occurs)
- *Increased extracellular fluid:* Intracellular fluid ratio
- Albumin falls-less protein binding
- Increased metabolic rate/temperature leading to altered half life.

6. What precautions one should take during induction of anesthesia?

Ans. As already discussed induction of anesthesia and initial control of the airway are potentially hazardous; through discussion and planning between anesthesiologists and surgeons is a must. Ideally, the surgeon should be in the room at the time of induction of anesthesia, prepared for emergency release of contractures, tracheotomy, or both. If intubation proves difficult or impossible, rapid partial release of the contractures can greatly assist intubation.

7. Which anesthetic agents are preferred for the induction of anesthesia?

Ans.

- *Inhalational agents:* Inhalational induction is a good choice as it helps in preserving spontaneous ventilation; isoflurane and sevoflurane are good choices.
- *Muscle relaxant:*
  - Succinylcholine should be avoided because of the commonly seen hyperkalemic response in postburn patients:
    - The excessive potassium release associated with suxamethonium begins within three day after thermal injury[5] and may last up to ninety days.
    - The hyperkalemia (up to 10 mmol/L)[5] may cause severe arrhythmia and can progress to ventricular fibrillation and cardiac arrest.
    - Normal muscle releases enough potassium during succinylcholine induced depolarization to raise serum potassium by 0.5 mEq/L.[6] While this is usually insignificant in patients with normal baseline levels, a life threatening potassium elevation is possible in patients with burns injury.
  - Large doses of nondepolarizing muscle relaxants may be required due to altered protein binding and an increase extrajunctional acetylcholine receptor which bind nondepolarizing drug without causing neuromuscular effect.

8. How would you plan the postoperative management of these patients?

Ans. The following aspect should be taken care of in the postoperative period:

- Adequate postoperative analgesia
- Airway protection
- Oxygen therapy
- *Maintain body temperature:* Radiant heater, warming blanket; prevent shivering.
- Fluid and blood transfusion.

9. How would you manage postoperative pain in these patients?

Ans. A multimodal approach of pain management should be employed. In this approach, we use a combination of analgesics of different class having different mechanism of action; the advantage being that it provides superior pain relief with reduced analgesic related side effects:

- Paracetamol 1 gm IV QID (adult dose); it should always be a component because of its safety profile and good pain relief for mild to moderate pain intensity
- NSAIDs could be added to paracetamol if pain is of severe intensity; etoricoxib 120 mg OD (adult dose) or diclofenac 75 mg BD are useful options

- *Opioids:* Tramadol and Fentanyl are useful options
- *Patient control analgesia:* If facilities are available, this is definitely a very useful option
- *Pregabalin:* Once daily dosing helps in reducing pain and consumption of daily opioids.

Good to know facts

1. How would you position the patient in the operating table?

Ans. Positioning of patients with postburn neck contracture may be tricky in some situations; patients having mentosternal contractures could not lie supine, hence these patients require pillow of adequate size to support their head due to fixed flexion deformity owing to contractures.

2. How the neck contractures make the airway management challenging in these patients?

Ans. The traction forces caused by burn scar contracture may pull and cause insufficient neck extension, incomplete oral occlusion, cicatricial ectropion, and tracheal alterations affecting respiration. This results in difficult intubation that can be life threatening and can result in multiple serious complications and sequels.[7,8]

3. How does the release of neck contractures might help the anesthesiologist?

Ans. The traction forces caused by burn scar contracture may pull and cause insufficient neck extension. To circumvent these complications contracture is released initially under local anesthesia to allow sufficient neck extension and following which airway management becomes easy.

4. How would surgeons help in the management of difficult airway?

Ans. The main challenge to the anesthetist in this patent is control of airway. It is therefore important that the attending surgeon understands the complementary role he might have to play in maintaining the airway. These roles are already discussed in preoperative assessment and dialogue with the surgical team. It is also obvious that, there is limited role for surgical tracheostomy due to the presence of the midline mentosternal contracture. The ear, nose and throat surgeons are however in attendance. In contrast, the role of the anesthetist is that of resuscitation, respiratory care, and provision of analgesia in burns.

5. What is the role of tumescent local anesthesia? Describe the technique.

Ans. The technique of tumescent local anesthesia helps in release of neck contracture release without the requirement of difficult endotracheal intubation; thus it helps in reducing contractures around the neck which increases the neck movements and makes airway management for future surgeries somewhat simpler. Other advantages of tumescent local anesthesia includes hydro-dissection of the tissues, easy disperse ability into the scar tissue, painless injection, good anesthesia, less bleeding during and after surgery and good postoperative analgesia in all patients.

In this technique, skin incision is marked and tumescent local anesthesia infiltrated along with the incision line and in to the surrounding areas. Volume of tumescent local anesthesia ranges from 70–200 mL depending upon the extent of contracture. Tumescent local anesthesia consisted of 0.4% lidocaine, 1 : 500,000 epinephrine with sodium bicarbonate and injection Hyaluronidase. It is prepared by mixing 30 cc of 2% lidocaine, 20 cc of sodium bicarbonate, one ampoule of epinephrine and one ampoule of injection Hyaluronidase in 450 cc of Ringer lactate solution. After waiting for 20 minutes the neck contracture is released and hemostasis achieved, and amount of split skin graft required is estimated. An anesthetic dose of intravenous ketamine 1–2 mg/kg is given and split skin graft is harvested. This skin graft is sutured over the raw area. If required an analgesic dose of ketamine 0.5 mg/kg could be repeated.[9]

A safe upper limit for lidocaine dosage using the tumescent technique is estimated to be 35 mg/kg.[10] Infiltrating a large volume of dilute epinephrine assures diffusion throughout the entire targeted area while avoiding tachycardia and hypertension. The associated vasoconstriction was so complete that there was virtually no blood loss in surgery.

Nice to know facts

1. **How would you classify postburn contractures of neck? What is its relevance in airway management?**

Ans. There has been effort to classify burn scar patients according to the degree of contracture and evaluate airway based on previous studies. Onah[11] suggested a classification system with four major numeric categories, which is based on the extent of flexion or extension by the contracted neck and the anatomical position of the neck. Classification is as follows:

1. Type 1 is a mild anterior contracture. The patient is able to flex the neck and bring the neck and jaws to the anatomical position while erect.
2. Type 2 is a moderate anterior contracture. Patients with this type of contracture are able to flex the neck and bring the neck and jaws to the anatomical position while erect. Attempts at extension away from the anatomical position results in a significant pull at the (uninvolved) lower lip.
3. Type 3 is a severe anterior mentosternal contracture. The patient's neck is contracted in the flexed position and the chin (and less frequently the lower lip) is occasionally restrained down to the anterior trunk. The patient is unable to reach anatomical position of the neck and jaws.
4. Type 4 is a posteriorly located contracture. The contracting band at the back of the neck prevents full neck flexion and may hold the neck in some degree of extension.

Difficulty with intubation can be expected in type 2 and 3; especially in type 3, the distance between the chin and the thyroid prominence distance is shortened.

REFERENCES

1. de Campo T, Aldrete JA. The anesthetic management of the severely burned patient. Intensive Care Med. 1981;7:55–62.
2. Baxendale BR, Aitkenhead AR: Pre-operative assessment. In: Clinical Anesthesia, 1st edn. Jones RM, Aitkenhead AR (Eds). New York: Churchill Livingstone; 1996.pp.1-29.
3. Wong TE, Lim LH, Tan WJ, et al. Securing the airway in a child with extensive postburn contracture of the neck: a novel strategy. Burns. 2010;36:e78-e81.
4. Han TH, et al. Managing difficult airway in patients with postburn mentosternal and circumoral scar contractures. Int J Burn Trauma. 2012;2(2):80-5.
5. Gronert GA, Theye RA. Pathophysiology of hyperkalaemia induced by succinylcholine. Anesthesiology. 1975;43:89-99.
6. Morgan E, Mikhail MS. Muscle Relaxants. In: Clinical Anesthesiology, 1st edn. Reinhardt S, Langan C (Eds). Lange medical McGraw-Hill; 1995.pp.149-64.
7. Shiby Ninan, Gupta AK, Ramkumar G. A technique in positioning the neck during mentosternal contracture release. Burns. 2003;29:613-4.
8. Nath S, Erzingatsian K, Simond S. Management of postburn contracture of the neck. Burns. 1994;20:438-41.
9. Agarwal P. Safe method for release of severe postburn neck contracture under tumescent local anesthesia and ketamine. Indian J Plastic Surg. 2004;37:51-4.
10. Klein JA. Tumescent technique for regional anesthesia permits lidocaine doses of 35 mg/kg for liposuction. Dermatol Surg Oncol. 1990;16:248-63.
11. Onah II. A classification system for postburn mentosternal contractures. Arch Surg. 2005;140:671-5.

31

Meningocele and Meningomyelocele

Jatisankar Rudra

1. Definition of spina bifida cystica and spina bifida occulta.

Ans. *Spina bifida cystica:* Absence of vertebral column with outpouchings of meninges and neural tissues.

Types: (a) Meningocele—herniation of meninges

(b) Myelomeningocele (MMC)—herniation of meninges + neural tissue

Spina bifida occulta: Absence of spinal process with overlying normal skin, tuft of hair, cutaneous angiomas, lipomas and skin dimple.

2. What is Arnold-Chiari malformation? What is the association between myelomeningocele and Arnold-Chiari malformation?

Ans.

- Arnold-Chiari malformation (ACM) is an anomaly of the hindbrain.
- It is present in nearly all patients with thoracolumbar, lumbar, and lumbosacral myelomeningocele.
- The major features of the anomaly are inferior displacement of the medulla and fourth ventricle into the upper cervical canal and inferior displacement of the lower cerebellum through the foramen magnum in the upper cervical region.
- It has three types—type I, II and III.
- In type II, the fourth ventricle and lower medulla are displaced below the level of the foramen magnum. Type II is usually associated with myelomeningocele.

3. What is the embryological basis of myelomeningocele (MMC)?

Ans. MMC is a progressive neurological disease with multiple complications and anomalies. It is due to failure of closure of the posterior neural tube. This leads to malformation of the vertebral column and spinal cord usually with other CNS anomalies. The closure occurs between 25th and 28th day of fetal life.

4. Explain the epidemiology of myelomeningocele.

Ans.

- 1 in 10,000, female > male
- More common in caucasians
- Parental consanguinity increases incidence

- Higher prevalence in lower socioeconomic groups
- Incidence is greatest in lumbar spine (67%) followed by
- Lumbosacral spine (25%).

5. How can myelomeningocele be diagnosed prenatally?

Ans.

- USG abdomen
- Alpha-fetoprotein raised at 16th week of gestation
- Acetylcholine esterase levels raised.

6. What are the other anomalies associated with MMC?

Ans.

- Arnold-Chiari malformation with or without hydrocephalus
- Congenital heart disease (ASD, VSD)
- Renal anamolies (hydronephrosis, neurogenic bladder)
- Anorectal malformation—congenital scoliosis or kyphosis
- Congenital hip displacement—clubfoot
- Facial clefts—VATER-L anomalies.

  Case discussion: An infant presents within the first few years of life with a swelling in the occipital, lumbar or lumbosacral region. A progressive swelling is present which may be a meningocele or a myelomeningocele (differentiated by transillumination test).

Common clinical findings: Paraplegia, hydrocephalus, cranial nerve dysfunction, seizures, neurogenic bowel and bladder, renal failure, progressive bony deformities of spine and joint, pathological fracture.

7. What are the special features that you will check for in the history?

Ans.

- Age, weight, duration of swelling and progression of size of swelling, history of leakage, movement of limbs, dribbling or soiling, seizures, unconsciousness and altered sensation. Fever, vomiting, apneic spell
- Antenatal history—fever, rash (rubella), folic acid (deficiency), vitamin A (hypervitaminosis), alcohol consumption, and X-ray exposure of mother. History of prolonged labor
- Maternal IDDM
- Drug history—valproic acid and carbamazepine
- History of consanguinity, MMC in other siblings (increased incidence), immunization history, developmental milestones.

8. How will you assess the swelling?

Ans.

- Duration of swelling, progression of swelling
- *Local inspection*: Site, size, borders, location anatomical landmarks, skin over swelling, leak, thickening, scab
- *Palpation*: Pulsatility, fluctuation, transillumination test, mobility of skin with signs of infection, bruit, confirmation of spina bifida.

9. Mention the important findings in the systemic examination.

Ans.

- Sensorium, cranial nerve examination, sensory nervous system of both upper and lower limbs, involuntary movements and signs of meningeal irritation, weakness or wasting of limbs, tendon reflexes, power in all four limbs, hydration status

- Airway assessment—to exclude facial clefts
- Examine for increased ICP (ophthalmoscopy and raised fontanelle).

10. What investigations will you advice?

Ans.

- Hemogram, urea, creatinine, chest X-ray, if symptomatic
- Blood grouping and cross-matching
- 2D echo MRI if suspected cardiac anomaly
- CT or MRI—if possible, to ascertain raised ICP and susceptibility to postoperative herniation.

11. What are the anesthetic considerations in this case?

Ans.

Age specific: Whether the patient is a neonate or infant

Airway—Pediatric airway difficulties + large head, facial clefts, problems of positioning, small trachea, vocal cord mobility is abnormal.

Case specific: Precautions to be taken because of anomalies

- Hydrocephalus—careful positioning of head, if there is a large hydrocephalus with MMC—intubation and surgery is preferably done in lateral position
- Arnold-Chiari malformation—avoid extreme flexion of head—herniation
- Congenital heart disease
- Renal problems
- Musculoskeletal disorders—muscle relaxants should be used cautiously and judiciously
- Difficulties due to surgical manipulation—prone position
- Extreme head flexion—brainstem compression
- Improper positioning—venous congestion
- ↑ Abdominal pressure—venacaval compression
- Difficult dissection—due to tethering of the nerves
- Hypothermia and blood loss.

Postoperative complications:

- Apnic spells
- Nursing—in post-tonsillectomy position, legend up
- Acute hydrocephalus—due to closure or due to shunt malfunction
- Cardiovascular or respiratory complications following acute herniation of the brain.
- These patients have predilections for latex allergy. So, remain careful.

12. What are the essential monitoring to be done?

Ans.
- BP, pulse, ECG, temperature, $EtCO_2$
- Precordial stethoscope
- Urine output.

13. What is the cause of latex allergy?

Ans. Repeated exposure to latex containing gloves from early childhood for clean catheterization and multiple surgeries leads to latex sensitization.

Patients with myelomeningocele have a higher incidence of allergy at any point in the perioperative period. Preoperatively, there is itching, rashes, and wheezing. Intra- or postoperative manifestations include cardiovascular collapse and bronchospasm.

14. Outline the steps of conduction of anesthesia?

Ans.

- Select appropriate anesthetic agents and technique to prevent build-up of transtentorial pressure gradient
- Maintain OT temperature, difficult pediatric intubation trolley
- Monitors
- IV cannulation—EMLA or after inhalational induction.

Proper positioning for intubation:

- By using doughnut so that the swelling is accommodated into its hole. The rest of the body is lifted from the operating table using folded towels below the legs. The chest and the head to avoid injury to the swelling
- Injection glycopyrrolate in standard dosage may be used for premedication
- Induction may be inhalational or intravenous
- Preoxygenation
- In inhalational technique, sevoflurane is preferred—suspect a difficult airway
- *IV induction*: *Propofol*: 3 mg/kg IV (until 6 years of age)—if IV cannulation is done previously. Na-thiopentone may also be used.

Muscle relaxants:

- *Succinylcholine:* 2.0 mg/kg IV (controversial)—better avoided especially in the presence of neurological deficit
- If muscular dystrophy is suspected it should be avoided because of possibility of hyperkalemia.
  Analgesic: 1–2 mcg/kg IV fentanyl.

Intubation in supine position (swelling in doughnut) or if the swelling is very large, lateral position may also be adopted.

Preoperative care:

- Prevent infection, maintain ECF volume, careful handling of sacks as it is prone to trauma and leakage. Cover with saline soaked gauge.
- *Aspiration prophylaxis:*
  - Empty stomach as per fasting guidelines
  - Glycopyrrolate may be considered.

- Armoured tube is used if proper size is available and is connected to Jackson Rees modification of Ayre's T-piece or pediatric bain circuit whichever is applicable.
- Securing of the airway in a definitive position and gauge packing is essential as the patient is made prone for surgery.
  Positioning—Patient is turned into prone (or lateral/semi-prone) position for operative procedure. Care is taken to see that the abdomen is kept free, pressure points are well padded, peripheral nerves are not pressed upon and joints are not unduly stretched. Head is positioned and restrained properly as per requirement.
- Eyes are properly padded and protected.
- Double check all connection.

Maintenance

Oxygen + N_2O + inhalational (sevoflurane) in appropriate concentration fentanyl for analgesia as required.

NDMR (atracurium 0.5–0.8 mg/kg loading dose or vecuronium 0.1 mg/kg)
Ventilation: IPPV with PEEP (JRMATP or pediatric bain circuit)
IV fluids: As per guidelines keeping the age of the patient in mind. Proper hydration of the patient has to be maintained. Avoidance of sudden drop in CSF pressure from the sac by adopting the head-low position and slow drainage of fluid.

15. Is blood required? How will you determine it?
Ans.
- Need for blood depending of maximum allowable blood loss, if loss >10%, blood transfusion is required.
- Blood requirement is calculated as per usual practice:

$$\text{MABL} = \frac{\text{EBV (Starting Hct - target Hct)}}{\text{Starting Hct}}$$

16. What are the postoperative considerations?
Ans.
- Reversal—neostigmine 50–70 mcg/kg with atopine 10–20 mic/kg once patient is fully awake, and able to maintain airway patency
- Nurse—prone with head down or lateral position (tonsillar position)
- Analgesia—LA instillation + paracetamol suppositories, IV paracetamol
- Check for—↑ ICP.

17. Can any other mode of anesthesia be used?
Ans.
- Direct spinal anesthesia (LA directly injected into the sac)
- Local anesthesia with sedation

VP shunt may be inserted in the same procedure:
- Operation done in semilateral position
- Replace deficit + intraoperative loss
- Intraoperative brain herniation and cranial nerve injury may be a cause of delayed awakening.

- Fetal surgery for closure of MMC defect have been tried with beneficial effects.
- A recent report has shown that many leading pediatric neurosurgeons have expressed their reluctance to operate upon MMC because, inspite of successful operation in the first few days of life, MMC patients have a reduced lifespan and lifelong disabilities.

Acknowledgment: The author gratefully acknowledges the help rendered by Dr Sujata Ghose in preparing the manuscript.

BIBLIOGRAPHY

1. George A Gregory, Dean B Andropopoulous. Gregory Pediatric Anaesthesia. 2012.
2. James E Cottrell, William Young. Cottrell & Youngs Neuroanesthesia 2010.
3. Goldschneider Kenneth, Davidson Andrew. Clinical Pediatric Anesthesia-a case based handbook 2012.
4. Paul Mongan. A Practical Approach to Neuroanaesthesia 2013.
5. Robert S, Holzman, Thomas J Mancuso, David M Polander. A Practical Approach to Paediatric Anaesthesia 2008.

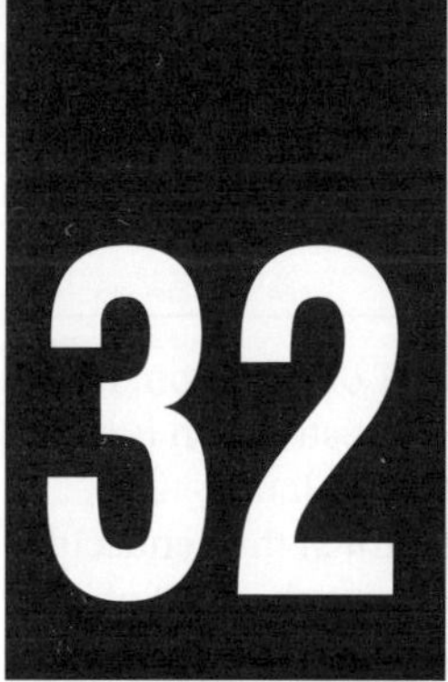

Cyanotic Congenital Heart Disease: Tetralogy of Fallot

Soumendu Pal

1. What is your case?

Ans. A 3-year-old, male child, admitted with history of bluish discoloration of lips, tongue and fingers. Parents had noted for the first time when the child was 6-month-old. The bluish discoloration increases with crying and exertion. There is also history of spells, when the child becomes very much blue and breathless after crying for a long time. The spells are terminated spontaneously after comforting the child. There is no history of frequent lower respiratory tract infections (LRTIs), sweating during feeding, frequent hospitalizations, swelling of feet, puffiness of eyes, decreased urine output [suggestive of congenital heart failure (CHF)], ear discharge, unconsciousness, fever, bleeding from nose or other mucosal regions.

On examination, child is awake and alert, with central cyanosis and grade II clubbing with grade II malnutrition (weight 10 kg, expected weight for age 14 kg). Cardiovascular examination showed heart rate 96/min, regular rhythm, a systolic thrill at the upper and mid-left sternal border, and a long, loud (grade 3/6) ejection-type systolic murmur, which is best heard at the middle and upper left sternal borders.

2. What is the provisional diagnosis?

Ans. This is a case of congenital cyanotic heart disease, probably tetralogy of Fallot (TOF).

3. Describe the pathophysiology of Tetralogy of Fallot. (Must know)

Ans. Tetralogy of Fallot was first described by the French physician Etienne Fallot, who published his findings in 1888. Fallot in 1888 correlated the pathologic and clinical manifestations of this cardiac malformation, and he termed it as "la maladie bleue".

Tetralogy of Fallot (TOF) comprises a constellation of cardiac findings that share the following common anatomic abnormalities:

- A large malaligned ventricular septal defect (VSD)
- Overriding of the aorta over the septal defect
- Right ventricular outflow obstruction
- Right ventricular hypertrophy (RVH).

Physiologically, TOF requires two major abnormalities—a VSD large enough to equalize systolic pressures in both ventricles and a stenosis of the right ventricular outflow tract (RVOT). The degree of aortic override is highly variable, while the RVH is as a consequence of RVOT obstruction. RVOT obstruction is most frequently in the form of infundibular stenosis (45%). The obstruction is rarely at the pulmonary valve level (10%). A combination of the two may also occur (30%).

The presence of severe pulmonary stenosis (PS) produces a right-to-left shunt at the ventricular level resulting in cyanosis, with decreased pulmonary blood flow (PBF). Because the VSD of TOF is large enough to equalize systolic pressures in both ventricles, the RV and LV may be viewed as a single chamber that ejects blood to the systemic and pulmonary circuits. The ratio of flows to the pulmonary and systemic circuits is related to the ratio of resistance offered by the right ventricular outflow obstruction and the systemic vascular resistance (SVR). Either an increase in the pulmonary resistance or a decrease in the SVR increases the degree of the right-to-left shunt, producing more severe arterial desaturation. On the contrary, more blood passes through the right ventricular outflow obstruction when the SVR increases or when the pulmonary resistance decreases.

4. Describe the pathophysiology of a *tet* spell. (Must know)

Ans. Hypoxemic episodes, also called hypercyanotic spells or '*tet*' spells, are characterized by a severe and often prolonged decrease in arterial saturation. Because the VSD of TOF is large enough to equalize systolic pressures in both ventricles, the RV and LV act as a single chamber that ejects blood to the systemic and pulmonary circuits. The ratio of flows to the pulmonary and systemic circuits is related to the ratio of resistance offered by the right ventricular outflow obstruction and the SVR. Either an increase in the pulmonary resistance or a decrease in the SVR increases the degree of the right-to-left shunt, producing more severe arterial desaturation. The cyanotic spell is a result of an acute increase in right-to-left shunting owing to a change in the ratio between pulmonary and systemic vascular impedance.

The hypoxemic episodes may be mediated by dynamic changes in the degree of subpulmonic obstruction due to changes in contractility owing to endogenous catecholamines or exacerbated by hypovolemia. Controversy exists over the role of the spasm of the RVOT as an initiating event for the hypoxic spell. Pulmonary valve stenosis has a fixed resistance and does not produce spasm. The infundibular stenosis, which consists of disorganized muscle fibers intermingled with fibrous tissue, is almost nonreactive to sympathetic stimulation or catecholamines. The hypoxic spell also occurs in patients with TOF with pulmonary atresia in which the presence or absence of spasm would have no role in the spell. Therefore, it is more likely that changes in the SVR play a primary role in controlling the degree of the right-to-left shunt and the amount of PBF.

Excessive tachycardia or hypovolemia can increase the right-to-left shunt through the VSD, resulting in a fall in the systemic arterial oxygen saturation. The resulting hypoxia can initiate the hypoxic spell. Tachycardia or hypovolemia may narrow down the RV outflow tract, and a reduction of blood pressure related to hypovolemia can initiate hypoxic spell by increasing right-to-left ventricular shunt. Slowing of the heart rate by β-adrenergic blockers, volume expansion, and interventions that increase the SVR have all been used to terminate the hypoxic spell.

Tet spell consists of hyperpnea (i.e. rapid and deep respiration), worsening cyanosis, and disappearance of the heart murmur. Any event such as crying, defecation, or increased physical activity that suddenly lowers the SVR or produces a large right-to-left ventricular shunt may initiate the spell and, if not corrected, establishes a vicious circle of hypoxic spells. The resulting fall in arterial PO_2, in addition to an increase in PCO_2 and a fall in pH, stimulates the respiratory center and produces hyperpnea. The hyperpnea, in turn, makes the negative thoracic pump more efficient and results in an increase in the systemic venous return to the RV. In the presence of fixed resistance at the RVOT, the increased systemic venous return to the RV must go out through the aorta. This leads to a further decrease in the arterial oxygen saturation, which establishes a vicious circle of hypoxic spells.

5. What are the long-term complications of TOF? (Must know)

Ans. The long-term complications of TOF are:

- Polycythemia secondary to chronic cyanosis
- Growth retardation
- Brain abscess and cerebrovascular accidents
- Bacterial endocarditis
- Severe TOF may develop AR
- Coagulopathy may develop as a late complication of a long-standing cyanosis.

6. What are the ECG findings of TOF? (Must know)

Ans. The electrocardiogram in children with uncorrected TOF typically demonstrates isolated right ventricular hypertrophy and right axis deviation. It becomes evident beyond 3 months of age, when the normal neonatal right ventricular predominance would have resolved. In older children and adult patients with TOF not treated surgically, ventricular ectopy and other arrhythmias may evolve as the long-term effects of right ventricular hypertension and myocardial fibrosis.

7. What are the X-ray findings of TOF? (Must know)

Ans. The overall heart size is normal and there is attenuation and concavity of the left heart border that results from the associated infundibular and pulmonary arterial hypoplasia. The cardiac apex often appears to be upturned. This creates a cardiac silhouette that resembles a boot-shaped heart, or 'coeur en sabot'. The pulmonary vascularity is diminished in proportion to the degree of cyanosis. The aortic arch is right sided in roughly 25% of patients.

8. What are the echocardiographic findings of TOF? What pathologic features should be investigated in the preoperative echocardiogram? (Must know)

Ans. Echocardiography can demonstrate the large ventricular septal defect and associated overriding of aorta. Significant override of >50% may suggest double-outlet right ventricle.

Doppler interrogation of the ventricular septal defect flow will demonstrate low-velocity flow that is primarily right to left when there is significant pulmonary obstruction. The location and degree of infundibular, valvular, and pulmonary arterial hypoplasia should be interrogated.

The origin and course of the left and right coronary arteries should be determined. In about 5% of TOF patients, abnormal coronary arteries are present. The most common abnormality is the left anterior descending branch arising from the right coronary artery and passing over the right ventricular outflow tract, which prohibits a surgical incision in the region.

Atrial septal defects, abnormalities of the systemic venous and pulmonary venous anatomy, the aorta, the additional mid-muscular ventricular septal defects should be excluded.

Size and continuity of the pulmonary arteries should be determined. Stenosis at the origin of the branch PAs, especially the left PA, is common. Additional sources of pulmonary blood flow should be sought as major aortopulmonary collaterals (MAPCAs) are seen in severe cases of TOF. The proximal descending aorta should be carefully scanned as distally as possible to rule out the origin of any collateral arteries.

9. What is the role of cardiac catheterization in preoperative evaluation of TOF? (Must know)

Ans. Preoperative echocardiography can identify most of the defects with certainty. Some of the unresolved issues are solved with the help of CT angiogram and MRI. Questions about preoperative pulmonary artery anatomy, coronary artery anatomy, and systemic or pulmonary venous anatomy can frequently be resolved with 64-slice high-resolution CT scans. These noninvasive techniques have diminished the indications for diagnostic cardiac catheterization substantially.

Cardiac catheterization is useful for clarification or better definition of anatomic characteristics, such as pulmonary arterial or coronary arterial anatomy. Hemodynamic data constitute important information that complement the clinical and noninvasive data. It is helpful for imaging of the infundibular anatomy and pulmonary artery anatomy, degree of subpulmonic obstruction and deviation of the outlet septum, the ventricular septal defect, the degree of aortic override and additional ventricular septal defects. Definition of pulmonary artery anatomy and pressures is important for patients who have undergone palliative aortopulmonary shunts. Angiography should be directed toward identifying any significant arterial stenosis, either native or as a result of surgical distortion (due to a previous modified Blalock Taussig shunt).

Definition of coronary artery anatomy may be approached either by aortic root angiography, selective coronary artery injection, or a combination of both.

Definition of any aortopulmonary collaterals also should be included as a routine goal of catheterization. Aortography should define any significant collateral vessels, which usually originate from the descending aorta. Coil embolization of aortopulmonary collateral arteries is also an appropriate intervention prior to surgical correction. Coiling of vessels that perfuse pulmonary segments already supplied by pulmonary arterial flow serves to reduce left ventricular volume loading as well as to eliminate run-off into the pulmonary arterial bed during cardiopulmonary bypass.

10. Describe the management of tet spells. (Must know)

Ans. Treatment of hypoxic spells is aimed at breaking the vicious by using one or more of the following maneuvers:

- Picking up the infant in the knee-chest position traps systemic venous blood in the legs, thereby temporarily decreasing systemic venous return and helping to calm the baby. The knee-chest position may also increase SVR.
- Volume expansion for correction of hypovolemia
- PRBC transfusion for correction of anemia
- *Morphine sulfate:* It suppresses the respiratory center and abolishes hyperpnea.
- Sodium bicarbonate ($NaHCO_3$) corrects acidosis and eliminates the respiratory center-stimulating effect of acidosis.
- Administration of oxygen may improve arterial oxygen saturation.
- Vasoconstrictors such as phenylephrine raise SVR and improve arterial oxygen saturation.
- Ketamine may be used as it simultaneously increases SVR and sedates the patient.
- Propranolol has been used successfully in hypoxic spells, both acute and for chronic prophylaxis to prevent spells. When administered for acute cases, propranolol may slow the heart rate and perhaps reduce the spasm of the RVOT. Propranolol may increase SVR by antagonizing the vasodilating effects of β-adrenergic stimulation.
- If medical intervention fails to adequately reverse the cyanosis, then emergent surgical palliation or repair are required.

11. Describe the surgical palliative procedures and discuss their indications. (Must know)

Ans. Several palliative procedures (Fig. 1) were performed in the past. The modified Blalock-Taussig (Gore-Tex interposition) shunt is the usual popular procedure performed at this time.

Classic Blalock-Taussig shunt, anastomosed between the subclavian artery and the ipsilateral PA, is usually performed for infants older than 3 months because the shunt is often thrombosed in younger infants with smaller arteries. It is usually performed opposite to the arch.

Modified Blalock-Taussig (BT) shunt: A Gore-Tex interposition shunt is placed between the subclavian artery and the ipsilateral PA. This is the most popular procedure for any age, especially for small infants younger than 3 months of age. It is usually done on the same side of the aortic arch. Advantages of the modified Blalock-Taussig shunt (MBTS) are:

- It preserves blood flow to the arm

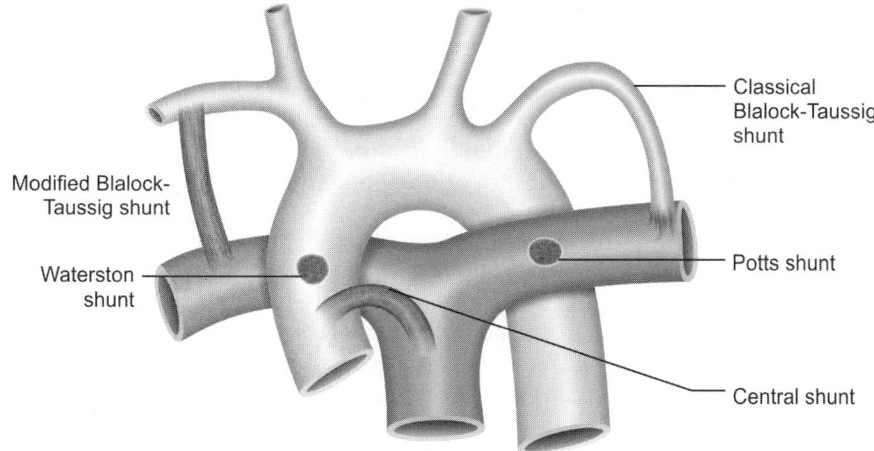

Fig. 1 Different surgical palliative procedures

- It can be used on either side, although most are done on the right side
- It avoids excessive PBF when appropriately sized.

The Waterston shunt, anastomosed between the ascending aorta and the right PA, is no longer performed because of a high incidence of surgical complications. Complications resulting from this procedure included too large a shunt leading to CHF or pulmonary hypertension, of both, and narrowing and kinking of the right PA at the site of the anastomosis.

The Potts operation, anastomosed between the descending aorta and the left PA, is no longer performed either. It may result in heart failure or pulmonary hypertension, as in the Waterston operation. A separate incision (i.e. left thoracotomy) is required to close the shunt during corrective surgery, which is performed through a midsternal incision.

A central shunt, between the ascending aorta and the MPA, using graft material is used as an alternative to the MBTS when the vascular anatomy precludes placement of the latter.

Indications

Shunt procedures are performed to increase PBF. Indications for shunt procedures vary from institution to institution.

- Neonates with TOF and pulmonary atresia
- Infants with hypoplastic pulmonary annulus, which requires a transannular patch for complete repair
- Children with hypoplastic PAs
- Unfavorable coronary artery anatomy
- Infants younger than 3–4 months old who have medically unmanageable hypoxic spells.

12. Describe the definitive surgical repair. (Must know)

Ans. The goals of total repair are threefold: (i) to close the VSD, (ii) to relieve right RVOT obstruction, and (iii) to repair associated anomalies.

Total repair of the defect is carried out under cardiopulmonary bypass. The procedure includes patch closure of the VSD, preferably through a transatrial and transpulmonary artery approach. Widening of the RVOT is accomplished by division and/or resection of the infundibular tissue and pulmonary valvotomy. If the pulmonary annulus and main PA are hypoplastic, transannular patching is done for widening the RVOT.

13. Describe the perioperative management of primary TOF repair. (Must know)

Ans. Patients are scheduled for operation early to avoid prolonged fasting. Light premedication is usually required as sedation is helpful during separation from parents. Excessive crying may precipitate spells in a vulnerable child. Oral or nasal midazolam or oral trichlophos are useful agents.

A complete review of previously derived history, physical, and laboratory data is required in order to comprehend the TOF pathophysiology of each individual patient. Children with minimal RVOT obstruction will have a predominately left-to-right shunt across a large VSD, pulmonary overcirculation, signs and symptoms of pulmonary congestion, and heart failure. Anesthetic management of patients should avoid interventions that decrease PVR and increase SVR. Excessive fluid administration may aggravate congestive heart failure.

On the other hand, severe outflow obstruction results in peripheral oxygen desaturation, intense cyanosis, polycythemia, and eventually clubbing. The goal in such children is to select agents that maintain or increase SVR relative to PVR in order to minimize right-to-left shunting. Volume loading may be useful in this situation.

Intraoperative Monitoring

ECG, SpO_2, $ETCO_2$, invasive blood pressure through radial or femoral arterial catheter, central venous pressure, and left atrial pressure monitoring are usually done for definitive repairs. Transesophageal (or epicardial) echocardiography is also done.

If intravenous access is available then anesthesia can be induced with a combination of ketamine and fentanyl and maintained with low concentrations of a volatile agent. It is important to maintain adequate SVR in order to limit right-to-left shunting through the VSD; sevoflurane is a good choice as this agent has the least effect on SVR.

The myocardial depressant effect of volatile agents is also useful in limiting infundibular spasm. Low SVR is treated with phenylephrine or norepinephrine; and preload is augmented with fluid boluses.

It is important to avoid most inotropes, as these will worsen infundibular spasm by increasing heart rate and contractility.

If there is no intravenous access, induction can be carried out rapidly and smoothly with sevoflurane. An alternative is to use intramuscular ketamine in unstable patients.

Anesthesia is maintained with fentanyl (10–20 μg/kg) supplemented with isoflurane as tolerated. Higher doses of fentanyl (20–50 μg/kg) minimize myocardial depression and curtail reactive pulmonary hypertension for patients undergoing prolonged, complicated repairs.

The finding of hypercyanotic spells as part of the patient's pathophysiology profoundly influences anesthetic management. Patients may be particularly vulnerable during induction and emergence of anesthesia, suggesting the need for increased preoperative sedation and postoperative analgesia to minimize catecholamine release. Anesthetic agents that increase sympathetic discharge, such as ketamine and pancuronium, should be used with caution in these children.

Treatment of intraoperative hypercyanotic episodes consists of:

- Fluid administration to reverse hypovolemia
- Increasing the depth of anesthesia with inhalation agents
- Esmolol or propranolol to attenuate myocardial hypercontractility
- Administration of fentanyl to slow heart rate and blunt catecholamine surges
- Administration of phenylephrine, abdominal compression, or flexion of legs to increase SVR
- Hyperventilation with 100% oxygen to lower PVR.

Pre-existing systemic pulmonary shunts are controlled prior to CPB to avoid pulmonary hyperperfusion. Hypothermic (28–32°C nasopharyngeal) CPB is established using a membrane oxygenator primed to provide a mixed machine/patient hematocrit of 22%.

Flow is maintained at 1.6–2.2 L/min/m^2. Perfusion pressure may be low despite adequate flow due to collaterals. Extensive collateral flow may necessitate multiple doses of cold blood cardioplegia to maintain myocardial hypothermia and electromechanical quiescence during aortic cross-clamping.

Most patients wean from CPB with minimal support. Pressure-controlled ventilation with 100% oxygen and the lowest possible airway pressure to maintain an arterial pCO_2 of 25 to 33 mm Hg and pH greater than 7.5 is used to minimize PVR.

14. Describe the postoperative complications and management. (Must know)

Ans. Right ventricle dysfunction is seen especially if the transannular incision was extended down the RV free wall. A ventricle compromised by surgical incisions and inadequate myocardial protection may not tolerate pressure loading from multiple etiologies like residual RVOT obstruction, increased PVR, excessive airway pressure, volume loading and pulmonary valve incompetence. The mainstays of treatment are fluid loading to higher filling pressures, inotropic support (Dopamine at 5 μg/kg/minute), and reduction of RV afterload. Nitroglycerin is also added at 2 μg/kg/minute to decrease RV afterload. Other acceptable alternatives for inotropic support are dobutamine or milrinone. Ventilation is adjusted to reduce PVR.

Arrhythmias and heart block: These are common after VSD repairs because of the close proximity of the conduction system. Epicardial pacing may be needed to accomplish weaning from CPB. In most instances heart block is a transient phenomenon due to the edema around the VSD patch. If it does not resolve after 7–10 days, permanent pacing may be required.

Junctional ectopic tachycardia (JET) is seen occasionally, although the onset is usually 12–24 hours later. This is characterized by AV dissociation and rapid junctional rates as high as 200–230 beats/minute. Treatment consists of cooling the patient to 34–35°C, and drug therapy with amiodarone or procainamide. Atrial overdrive pacing can also be used.

Post-CPB bleeding: Coagulopathy results from hemodilution of coagulation factors and the effects of CPB on platelet number and function, and may require transfusion of multiple component blood products. The use of antifibrinolytics such as ε-aminocaproic acid or tranexamic acid may reduce post-CPB bleeding and minimize the use of blood products.

Residual VSD: Leakage through or around the VSD patch or from a remote VSD can be detected by echocardiography. When the shunt is large and persists for more than a few days, reoperation may be necessary to revise the patch or close a remote VSD.

BIBLIOGRAPHY

1. Allen, Hugh D, Driscoll, David J, Shaddy, Robert E. Moss and Adams' Heart Disease in Infants, Children, and Adolescents: Including the Fetus and Young Adults.; Feltes, Timothy F (Eds), Lippincott Williams & Wilkins 7th edn, 2008.
2. Dean B Andropoulos, Stephen A Stayer, Isobel A Russell. Anesthesia for Congenital Heart Disease. Blackwell-Futura; 2005.
3. Lake Carol L, Booker Peter D (Eds). Pediatric Cardiac Anesthesia, 4th edn, Lippincott Williams & Wilkins; 2005.
4. Myung K Park. Pediatric Cardiology for Practitioners, Mosby Elsevier, 5th edn, 2008.

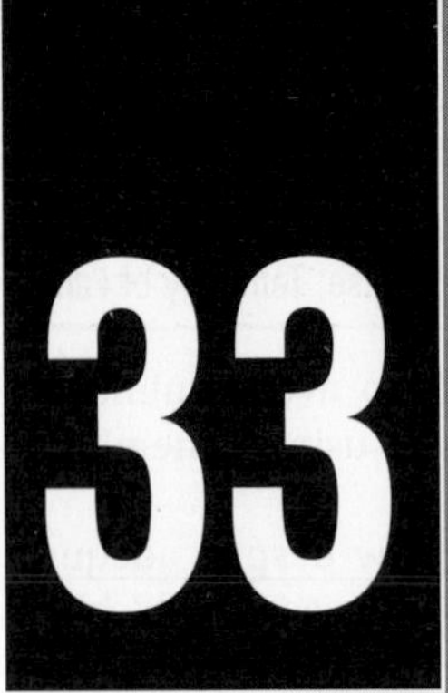

Patent Ductus Arteriosus

Mohona Mukherjee, Sudeshna Bhar (Kundu), Samarendra Pal

1. What is your case?

Ans. A one-year-old male child, admitted with history of recurrent chest infection since birth, and required frequent hospitalizations, mother complains of poor feeding since last 4 months, with gradual swelling of feet, puffiness of eyes, decreased urine output. Parents are worried also for increase precordial motion, distended and tender abdomen of child.

On examination, child is awake and alert, increased and tensed fontanel, grade II malnutrition, CVS examination showed with bounding pulse, heart rate 96/min. Apical impulse is localized and displaced downward and outward. Continuous but dominant systolic thrill at pulmonary area. Pulsation over suprasternal notch present. On auscultation, split second heart sound with continuous murmur covering second heart sound is heard. Cardiologist advised for routine hemogram, echocardiography, chest X-ray abdominal X-ray, urine exmination and USG of head and referred to preanesthetic clinic for preparation of catheterization laboratory interventions.

2. What is the provisional diagnosis?

Ans. This is a case of congenital acyanotic heart disease, probably patent ductus arteriosus (PDA).

3. What is patent ductus arteriosus?

Ans. Persistence of ductus arteriosus is known as patent ductus arteriosus (Fig. 1). It is derived from persistent distal portion of left 6th aortic arch. It forms a communication between descending aorta (just distal to the left subclavian artery) and pulmonary artery (usually left). In adult, it forms ligamentum arteriosum.

4. When does ductus arteriosus close? What are the initiating factors for ductus closure?

Ans. Ductus arteriosus functionally closes within 10–15 hours after birth. It permanently closes by thrombosis, intimal proliferation and fibrosis in 2–3 weeks after birth.

The initiating factors for functional closure of ductus arteriosus are:

- Aeration of the lungs
- Increased PaO_2
- Removal of prostaglandins produced in the placenta
- Release of vasoactive substances (bradykinin, thromboxanes and endogenous catecholamines).

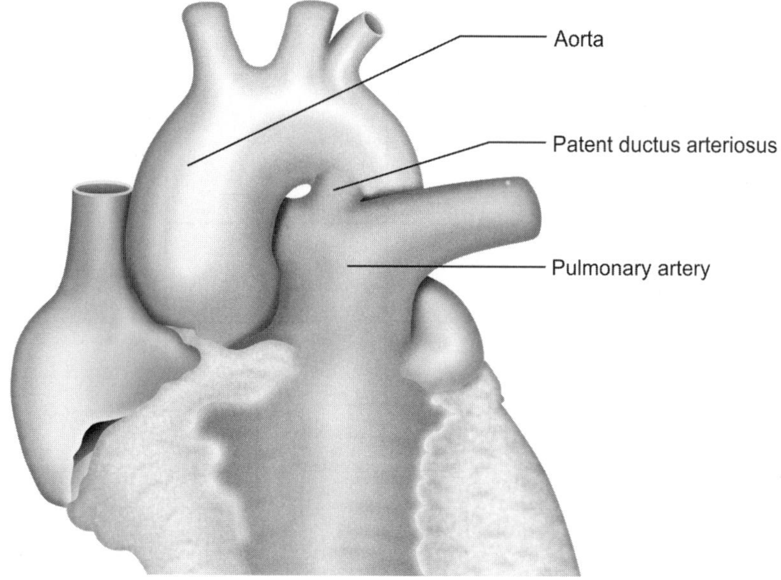

Fig. 1 Patent ductus arteriosus

5. What is the incidence of PDA?

Ans. Incidence varies from 1:2500–1:5000 live births.

Incidence is higher in:

- Premature babies
- Female sex (2–3 times higher)
- Down's syndrome
- History of rubella in mother during antenatal period.

6. Describe the pathophysiological changes in PDA.

Ans. The blood flow through a shunt depends on the size of the shunt orifice and the relative resistance on either side of the shunt. In PDA, the blood flow is primarily determined by the resistance of systemic and pulmonary vascular beds (The direction and magnitude of shunt at the atrial level are determined by the relative differences in ventricular compliance and respective atrioventricular valve function).

The pathophysiological changes in PDA (Fig. 2) are as follows:

- *Continuous murmur:* The PDA results in a left-to-right shunt from aorta to the pulmonary artery. The flow occurs both during systole and diastole as the pressure gradient is present throughout the cardiac cycle between the two great arteries, if the pulmonary artery pressure is normal. The flow of blood results in a murmur which starts in systole, after first heart sound, and reaches a peak at second heart sound. The murmur then diminishes in intensity and is audible during a part of the diastole. Thus it is a continuous murmur.
- *Left atrial enlargement:* The PDA results in systolic as well as diastolic overloading of the pulmonary artery. The increased blood flow after passing through the lungs reaches the left atrium. To accommodate the increased flow, left atrium enlarges in size.
- *Functional MS:* The increased volume of blood from the left atrium enters the left ventricle in diastole, across a normal mitral valve. The passage of this increased flow across the normal mitral valve results in functional MS characterized by an accentuated first heart sound and mitral delayed diastolic murmur.

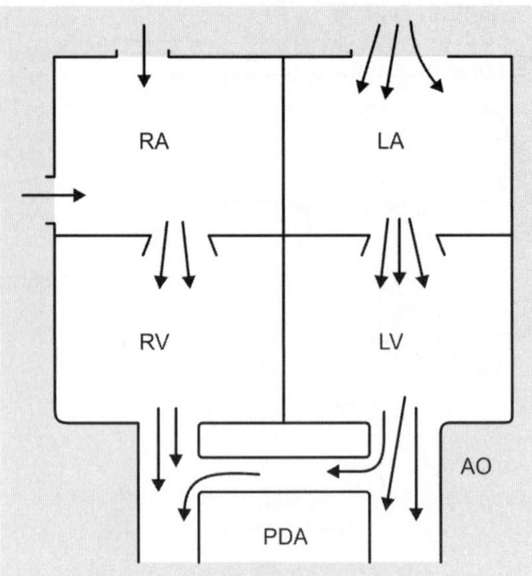

Fig. 2 Pathophysiology of patent ductus arteriosus (PDA)

- *Left ventricular enlargement:* The left ventricle receives the increased volume of blood during diastole leading to diastolic overloading of left ventricle. This causes left ventricular enlargement.
- *Delayed A_2, paradoxical split:* The large volume of blood in the left ventricle causes a prolongation of the left ventricular systole. The prolonged left ventricular systole results in delayed closure of the aortic valve and a late A_2. With large left to right shunts the S_2 may be paradoxically split.
- *Functional AS:* The large volume of blood from the left ventricle passing through a normal mitral valve results in an aortic ejection systolic murmur (functional AS). But on the bedside this murmur may be masked by the loud continuous murmur.

7. What is the difference between fetal and adult circulation?

Ans. Three channels characteristic of the circulation in utero allow preferential shunting of blood—ductus venosus, foramen ovale, and ductus arteriosus.

Ductus venosus: Well-oxygenated blood from the placenta (PaO_2= 33 mm Hg) travels through the umbilical vein to enter the liver. The ductus venosus allows one-half of this blood to be shunted from the liver directly to the inferior vena cava.

Foramen ovale: One-third of the blood entering the right atrium from the inferior vena cava is predominantly shunted across the foramen ovale into the left atrium. Superior vena cava blood (which is poorly oxygenated) primarily enters the right ventricle, with 2–3% shunting across the foramen ovale.

Ductus arteriosus: Right ventricular blood is largely shunted across the ductus arteriosus into the descending aorta, rather than perfusing the high resistance pulmonary circulation.

Implications: The structure of the fetal citculation allows the well-oxygenated blood from the inferior vena cava to perfuse the vital organs like the brain and coronary circulation, and in addition the upper extremities.

8. What is transitional circulation?

Ans. At birth significant changes occur in the circulation that allows the infant to adapt to the stresses of extrauterine life. A period of transition in the neonatal circulation occurs before permanent change to the adult pattern. Factors contributing to the instability of the transitional circulation are:

- The state of the ducus arteriosus, foramen ovale, pulmonary vascular bed
- Immaturity of the neonatal heart
- Hypoxia, hypercarbia, sepsis, prematurity and CHD.

Closure of the ductus arteriosus: Functional closure of the ductus arteriosus occurs within a few hours after birth but anatomic closure may occur after several weeks. During this period the resistance to ductus arteriosus blood flow responds to changes in arterial PaO_2. Prostaglandin (PGE_1) infusion relaxes the ductal musculature. Maintenance of the ductal patency may be important for the infant with cyanotic heart disease until surgery is performed.

Closure of the foramen ovale or ductus venosus: The foramen ovale functionally closes within a few hours after birth when the left atrial pressure exceeds the right atrial pressure. Anatomic closure does not occur for many months after birth and 30% of adults have a probe patency foramen ovale.

Intracardiac right to left shunting may occur across this ovale with coughing , Valsalva maneuver or if pulmonary hypertension develops. Umbilical arteries, umlical veins and ductus venosus close shortly after birth. The ductus venosus forms the ligamentum venosum.

Pulmonary vascular resistance (PVR): PVR is high in utero but falls rapidly to lower than systemic levels within 24 hrs after birth. Next the fall is moderate for 5–6 weeks and then more gradual for the next 2–3 years. Hypoxia, hypercarbia, acidosis or bronchospasm can result in an increase in PVR and shunting across the ductus arteriosus or foramen ovale or other cardiac defects.

9. Describe the natural history of PDA.

Ans. Table 1 shows the natural history of PDA.

Table 1 | Natural history of patent ductus arteriosus

Period of life	*Degree of pulmonary arterial hypertension*	*Amount of flow across the shunt*	*Manifestations*
At birth	Pulmonary artery pressure equals or slightly lower than systemic pressure	Minimum flow across shunt	No clinical manifestation
Mid to end of 1st week	Pulmonary artery pressure falls below systemic pressure	↑ Flow across the shunt	Murmur appears (ejection systolic)
6–10 weeks	Pulmonary vascular resistance reaches lowest value	Maximum flow across the shunt	Continuous murmur appears, patient may develop heart failure
Development of pulmonary hypertension	↑ Pulmonary vascular resistance	↓ Flow across the shunt or there may be reversal of blood flow across the shunt (Eisenmenger complex)	Ejection systolic murmur, normal splitting of S_2, differential cyanosis in Eisenmenger complex

10. What are the presenting symptoms of PDA?

Ans. History of repeated chest infections,

History suggestive of heart failure,

History suggestive of any other congenital anomaly,

Usually no history of bluish discoloration of the body (unless there is development of Eisenmenger complex),

In birth history, history of fever with skin rash in mother in the antenatal period (rubella).

11. Describe the clinical features of PDA.

Ans. A. General survey

Pulse—low volume

Blood pressure—low diastolic blood pressure. Diastolic runoff into the pulmonary artery results in lowered aortic diastolic pressure.

Signs of wide pulse pressure may be found:

Differential cyanosis: It is characteristic of PDA with pulmonary arterial hypertension (Eisenmenger complex) and right-to-left shunt. Since the right to left shunt through the PDA flows down the descending aorta, cyanosis is present in toes but not in the fingers. Thus it is called differential cyanosis.

B. Cardiovascular system

- Inspection
  - Visible apical impulse
  - Prominent carotid pulsation
- Palpation
  - *Apex beat:* Downward and outward displacement in left ventricular hypertrophy (LVH), hyperkinetic
  - Continuous thrill palpable at left 2nd intercostal space
- Auscultation
  - S_1—accentuated
  - S_2—masked by murmur (late A2, paradoxical split).

Murmur: (i) Continuous machinery murmur is heard at the left 2nd intercostal space and also below the left clavicle. (ii) Delayed diastolic murmur is heard over apical region. It is best heard at left lateral position with bell of the stethoscope at the height of expiration.

- Features of heart failure may be present.
- Features of pulmonary arterial hypertension may be present.

12. What do you mean by Nadas' criteria?

Ans. The assessment of a child for the presence or absence of heart disease can be done with the help of some guidelines suggested by Nadas and are called Nadas' criteria. The criteria are divided into major and minor criteria. Presence of one major or two minor criteria are essential for indicating the presence of heart disease.

Major criteria:

- Systolic murmur grade III
- Diastolic murmur
- Cyanosis—central cyanosis
- Congestive cardiac failure.

Minor criteria:

- Systolic murmur less than grade III
- Abnormal second heart sound
- Abnormal electrocardiogram
- Abnormal chest X-ray
- Abnormal blood pressure.

13. What are the important investigations needed in PDA?

Ans. *Complete hemogram:*
- Blood grouping
- Coagulation profile
- Urine examination
- Serum urea, creatinine, electrolytes
- Chest X-ray—cardiomegaly, prominent aortic knuckle, left atrial enlargement, plethoric lung fields
- Electrocardiogram—left atrial hypertrophy, left ventricular hypertrophy, deep Q wave with tall T wave in chest leads (suggestive of volume overloading of left ventricle)
- Echocardiogram with color doppler—identifies PDA, excludes other pathology
- Diagnostic cardiac catheterization, if needed.

14. How do you assess severity in a PDA patient?

Ans. The following features indicate the severity of PDA:
- Wide pulse pressure
- Third heart sound
- Delayed diastolic murmur over apex
- Enlarged heart size.

15. What are the treatment modalities in a PDA patient?

Ans. *A. Medical management:*
- Indomethacin
  - COX inhibitor, reduces prostaglandin synthesis
  - Can be given if diagnosis is made within first 2 weeks of life
  - Dose—0.1 mg/kg/dose orally 12 hourly for 3 doses
  - Side effects—decreases renal, cerebral and mesenteric blood flow
  - Contraindications—hepatic insufficiency, renal insufficiency, bleeding tendency
- Treat of heart failure
- Treat of infective endocarditis
- Treat of respiratory tract infection.

B. Surgical management:
- Transcatheter closure technique (coil embolization)
- Posterolateral thoracotomy with ligation or division of the PDA
- Video-assisted thoracoscopic surgery (VATS).

16. Enumerate the ductal dependant lesions.

Ans.
- *PDA provides systemic flow:*
  - Hypoplastic left heart syndrome
  - Coarctation of aorta
  - Interrupted aortic arch
  - Critical aortic stenosis
- *PDA provides pulmonary flow:*
  - Pulmonary atresia
  - Critical pulmonary stenosis
  - Severe subpulmonic stenosis with VSD
  - Tricuspid atresia with pulmonic stenosis

In the above cases, PDA should be maintained with PGE_1.

17. What should the anesthesiologist look for in the preoperative assessment in patients with congenital heart disease?

Ans.

- *Age of presentation:* Infants may present with persistent or intermittent cyanotic episodes associated with agitation, crying or exercise. In an older child, the cyanotic episodes may be associated with squatting (increases SVR and promotes increased pulmonary blood flow). This change in pulmonary dynamics may reduce the cyanosis. But severe episodes may result in unconsciousness or seizures.
- *Frequency of episodes:* If the cyanotic episodes are intermittent, the shunt is dynamic in nature, and meticulous balance between SVR and PVR is mandatory to reduce right to left shunting.
- *Cyanosis:* Clinical cyanosis depends on the absolute concentration of deoxygenated hemoglobin in blood. Central cyanosis is recognizable with more than 3 g/dL of deoxygenated arterial blood hemoglobin Or, an oxyhemoglobin saturation of approximately 62% (Hb level = 8 gm/dL), or 88% in a polycythemic infant (Hb level = 24 gm/dL). The newborn with a large proportion of fetal hemoglobin may have a large reduction of PO_2 before central cyanosis is clinically recognized.
- *Respiration:* Infants with cyanotic heart disease have an increased tidal volume, poor exercise tolerance, blunted response to hypoxia. Clubbing of fingers develops later.
- *Congestive heart failure (CHF):*
  - A history of feeding difficulties and failure to thrive characterize CHF. Tachypnea, tachycardia, irritability, inappropriate sweating, nasal flaring, sternal and intercostals retractions, cardiomegaly, hepatomegaly are the other features.
  - Wheezing, respiratory infections and pneumonia may be present.
  - Decreased pulses, pallor, and poor capillary refill can be encountered.
  - A severely compromised infant may be apathetic and have a poor cry.
- *Associated anomalies:* Other problems include difficulty with temperature regulation, coagulation abnormalities, susceptibility to dehydration and hypoglycemia and central nervous system disorders.

18. Which preoperative laboratory tests are helpful?

Ans.

- Hematocrit
- White cell count
- Coagulation studies
- Electrolytes
- Glucose
- Sickling test
- Electrocardiography
- Echocardiography and cardiac catheterization
- Chest X-ray
- Abdominal X-ray
- USG head.

19. When should oral intake be discontinued?

Ans. The NPO guidelines used for other infants and children can be used in patients with congenital heart disease. Clear liquids can be continued 2–4 hours before surgery. If uncertainty exists regarding the time of surgery, it is advisable to take an intravenous access and begin an infusion to prevent dehydration in patients with cyanotic heart disease.

20. Which sedation is considered appropriate?
Ans.
- Neonates and infants younger than 6 months rarely need any sedation as separation anxiety is not an issue.
- In older chidren, additional sedation may be unnecessary if the child's parents are allowed to accompany him to the preoperating holding area.
- Children between 1 and 5 years of age need meticulous sedation. Intravenous or oral midazolam is preferred to intramuscular injections. An oral dose of 0.5 mg/kg helps in easy separation from parents at 15–30 minutes. The intranasal dose of 0.2 mg/kg is helpful for separation after 10–15 minutes.
- The intravenous dose is titrated in 0.1–0.25 mg increments.
- Pulse oximetry and careful observation is mandatory after giving any kind of sedation.

21. When does a patient need intravenous infusion?
Ans.
- Children requiring vasoactive infusions preoperatively come to the operating room with an intravenous access.
- For others a gentle inhalational induction with subsequent venous catheter placement is practiced.
- If the time of surgery is uncertain, preoperative intravenous access is advisable to avoid dehydration.

22. What are the goals in anesthetic management of a PDA patient posted for ligation of PDA?
Ans. *Goals:*
- To prevent rise in systemic vascular resistance
- To maintain pulmonary vascular resistance
  - The anesthetic management for PDA ligation depends upon factors such as patient's clinical condition, prematurity, coexisting diseases, body weight and surgical technique. General anesthesia with positive pressure ventilation is the choice of anesthesia.

23. What are the anesthetic considerations in premature infants?
Ans. It is prudent to give attention to the respiratory care, temperature, and fluid management.
- These neonates generally come to the operation theater already intubated
- Continuous positive airway pressure helps to improve their oxygenation and manage excess lung water
- During the thoracotomy, the nondependent lung will be compressed and not ventilated and hypoxemia can occur
- It is important to balance the need to ventilate aggressively while avoiding high airway pressures that may injure the immature lungs
- These children must be kept warm
- Administration of fluids should be restricted as these neonates are fluid overloaded and in congestive heart failure.

  Management of the older child is straightforward: It is wise to ensure adequate venous access because there is chance of significant blood loss.

  Preoperative sedation helps in separating the patients from their parents. Any anesthetic technique is acceptable with an objective to extubate the patients at the end of the procedure.

24. How will you anesthetize such a patient for PDA ligation?

Ans.

- *Infective endocarditis prophylaxis:* Amoxicillin 25 mg/kg orally 1 hour before + gentamicin 2 mg/kg IM 30 minutes before surgery. Drugs should be repeated at least for 2 more doses after the surgery.
- Crossmatched blood should be kept ready
- Preoperative fasting
- Premedication, e.g. oral midazolam 0.5 mg/kg may be given 10–20 minutes before induction
- Monitoring
  - Pulse oximetry (Preductal—SpO_2 probe at right hand) and noninvasive blood pressure of both upper and lower extremities (to detect inadvertent ligation of the descending aorta), intra-arterial pressure monitoring (continuous)
  - Precordial stethoscope
  - Electrocardiogram
  - Temperature—hypothermia to be avoided
  - Capnograph—to maintain normocarbia
  - Urine output
  - Neuromuscular monitoring—adequate muscle relaxation
  - Bispectral index—adequate depth of anesthesia
  - Invasive blood pressure
  - Arterial blood gas analysis
- Wide bore venous access, avoid air bubble in intravenous line
- Forced air warmer
- *Induction:* Inhalational or intravenous (ketamine avoided). Choice of the induction agent depends on the patient's condition. Inhalational induction with halothane carries the risk of myocardial depression. The chance of myocardial depression is less with sevoflurane. Intravenous induction using opioids and benzodiazepine (e.g. midazolam) reduce the stress response and improve the postoperative outcome. The titration of induction agents is more important than the specific anesthetic technique.
- *Neuromuscular blocker:* Nondepolarizing agent (pancuronium avoided)
- *Endotracheal intubation:* Stress response should be minimized
- *Maintenance:* Inhalational agents, opioids, IPPV:
  - High FiO_2 is avoided (to maintain the pulmonary vascular tone and consequently to reduce the degree of left-to-right shunt).
  - Provide adequate anesthesia to prevent hypertension. Sudden ligation of PDA may result in acute rise in blood pressure leading to intraventricular hemorrhage. It may be prevented by gentle clamping of PDA, increased concentration of the volatile anesthetic agent or infusinn of vasodilators, e.g. sodium nitroprusside.
- Reversal and extubation.

Postoperative management: Close monitoring, intravenous fluids, adequate analgesia, maintenance of normothermia.

Oxygen supplement, postoperative mechanical ventilation, maintenance of normal blood gases level. SpO_2% may be needed to keep between 87 and 92% to reduce risk of retinopathy of prematurity.

25. What are the complications of the posterolateral thoracotomy with ligation or division of the PDA?

Ans.

- Bleeding (due to inadvertent rupture of the PDA)
- Intracranial hemorrhage
- Inadvertent ligation of the pulmonary artery or descending aorta
- Chylothorax, pneumothorax
- Vocal cord paralysis due to damage to recurrent laryngeal nerve
- Atelectasis
- Recurrence of patency
- Post-thoracotomy syndrome (rib fusion, chest wall deformities, scoliosis, and compromise of pulmonary function).

BIBLIOGRAPHY

1. Bent ST. Anesthesia for left-to-right shunt lesions, In: Andropoulos DB, Stayer SA, Russell IA (Eds). Anesthesia for Congenital Heart Disease, 1st edn, Blackwell Publishing; 2005.pp.297-317.
2. Frederick A Hensley Jr, Donald E Martin. A Practical Approach to Cardiac Anesthesia, 4th edn. Lippincott Williams and Wilkins. 2008;13:376-85.
3. Ghai OP. Essential Pediatrics, 4th edn. Interprint publication; 1996.pp.234-45.
4. Greeley WJ, Steven JM, Nicolson SC. Anesthesia for Pediatric Cardiac Surgery, Zn: Miller RD (Ed). Miller's Anesthesia, 6th edn, Elsevier Churchill Livingstone; 2005.pp.2005-50.
5. Laurie K Davies, Daniel G Knauf. Anesthetic management for patients with congenital heart disease.

Anesthetic Management of a Diabetic Patient Posted for Emergency Laparotomy

Ratul Kundu, Chiranjib Bhattacharyya, Rajib Samal

Case

A semi-comatose patient came to the emergency for emergency exploratory laparotomy. Surgeons suspected an intestinal perforation. Patient party revealed that, patient is on irregular treatment for diabetes and hypertension for last 7 years. Patient has not passed any urine for last 4 hours following catheterization before coming to this hospital and there is no rise of temperature. Capillary blood glucose level shows a value of 450 mg/dL. Urinary ketone strip shows ketone +++ve.

1. **What are the problems associated with this case?**

Ans. *Patient-related problems*

- Dehydration due to osmotic diuretic effect of glycosuria.
- Severe metabolic acidosis due to accumulation of ketoacids and lactic acids.
- Severe electrolyte imbalance mainly potassium and magnesium which may lead to intraoperative arrhythmia.
- Proteolysis and lipolysis with increased hospital stay in absolute insulin deficiency.
- Increased chance of postoperative infection and delayed wound healing.
- Increased risk of silent MI, cerebral infarct and renal ischemia due to greater incidence of coronary artery disease, arterial atheroma and renal parenchymal disease.

Anesthesia and surgery-related problems

Anesthesia and surgery cause catabolic stress response that could affect the homeostatic mechanisms relating to glucose metabolism. This stress response results in release of catabolic hormones-adrenaline, noradrenaline, cortisol, glucagon and growth hormones and inhibition of insulin secretion. These circulating stress hormones are anti-insulin and they have a deleterious effect on pancreatic B-cell function. Plasma insulin level falls and insulin response to glucose is impaired.

The anti-insulin effect of the metabolic stress response essentially reverses the physiological anabolic and anti-catabolic actions of insulin that are attenuate during surgery include stimulation of glucose uptake and glycogen storage, stimulation of amino acid uptake and protein synthesis by skeletal muscle, stimulation of fatty acid synthesis in the liver and storage in the adipocytes as well as renal sodium reabsorption and intravascular volume preservation.

The stress hormones released during surgery produces effect opposite to that of insulin. The net effect is severe hyperglycemia which is further exacerbated by increased glucagon secretion including hyperglycemia and ketoacidosis. The products of lipolysis and proteolysis provided substrates for increased gluconeogenesis by liver.

Thus, there is serious threat to glucose homeostasis in all diabetic patients especially if remain uncontrolled and that insulin therapy will be needed.

Complications

- Hyperglycemia producing osmotic dieresis and its consequences.
- Hyperosmotic state with hyperviscosity, thrombogenesis and cerebral edema.
- Ketoacidosis
- Proteolysis and decreased amino acid transport leading to delayed wound healing.
- Loss of polymorphonuclear cell phagocytic action and infection.

2. What is the provisional diagnosis?

Ans. This is probably a case of diabetic ketoacidosis.

3. How will you optimize and prepare this patient preoperatively?

Ans. *The diagnostic criteria for DKA include:*

- pH < 7.3
- $[HCO_3^-]$ < 15 mmol/L
- Blood glucose > 14 mmol/L (250 mg/dL)

Blood glucose *per se* is not a good determinant of severity, as euglycemic ketoacidosis is possible depending upon the hepatic glycogen stores prior to onset of diabetic ketoacidosis (DKA).

Assessment of a patient with DKA should include patency of airway, level of consciousness, cardiovascular and renal status, hydration status and possible source of infection.

Admission to intensive care unit (ICU), if indicated.

Correction of volume deficit

An infusion of isotonic saline is started at 15–20 mL/kg/hr initially over 1–3 hours and subsequently continued with 200–300 mL/hr of saline. The infusion is changed to 5% glucose with 0.45% saline at 100-200 mL/hr when plasma glucose decreases to 250 mg/dL. Avoid RL solution. Adequacy of replacement is monitored by urine output and CVP.

Correction of hypoglycemia

IV bolus of regular insulin 0.15 U/kg is followed by an infusion at 0.1 U/kg/hr, or, infusion rate of soluble insulin adjusted according to the following formula:

$$\text{Soluble insulin infusion rate} = \frac{\text{Blood glucose (mg/dL)}}{100\text{–}150}\ \text{units/hr}$$

This can be increased 2–10 fold, if no response is seen in 4–10 hours. Be wary of administering insulin as can lead to hypokalemia as well.

Serum potassium

Even though serum potassium level is increased, there is a deficit of total body potassium of about 3–10 mmol/kg. If potassium >5.0 mmol/L, do not administer potassium but check every 2nd hourly. Supplement with 20–30 mmol/L should serum potassium drop below 3.3 mmol/L.

Acid-base correction

Do ABG analysis. If pH >7.0, sodium bicarbonate is not indicated. If pH between 6.9 and 7.0, 50 mmol of sodium bicarbonate is diluted in 200 mL of sterile water (to reduce its osmolarity) is administered 200 mL/hr. If pH <6.9, give 100 mmol of sodium bicarbonate diluted in 400 mL of sterile water to be infused at 200 mL/hr.

Monitoring

Blood glucose is monitored hourly initially and then less frequently. Renal function test and serum sodium estimated initially and then less frequently. Serum potassium every hourly and then every 2–4 hourly.

Serum ketones (nitroprusside reaction) do not measure B hydroxybutyrate (main ketoacid present in DKA) and hence underestimates the degree of ketoacidosis.

4. When do you consider patient is adequately optimized in DKA?

Ans. Diabetic ketoacidosis (DKA) is considered to have resolved when the blood glucose is less than 200 mg/dL, serum bicarbonate is 18 mEq/L and venous pH >7.3.

In the event of a dire emergency, the patient can be taken up after partial correction of blood volume and blood sugar levels with frequent monitoring. For an elective procedure, full correction of the condition is advisable.

5. How will you differentiate between DKA and hyperglycemic hyperosmolar state (HHS)?

Ans. See Table 1.

Table 1 | Difference between DKA and hyperglycemic hyperosmolar state

Parameter	*DKA*	*HHS*
Glucose (mg/dL)	250–600	600–1200
Sodium (mEq/L)	125–135	135–145
Potassium	Normal to ↑	Normal
Magnesium	Normal	Normal
Chloride	Normal	Normal
Phosphate	↓	Normal
Creatinine	Slightly ↑	Moderately ↑
Osmolality (mOsm/mL)	300–320	330–380
Plasma ketones	++++	+/−
Sodium bicarbonate (mEq/L)	<15	Normal to slightly ↓
Arterial pH	6.8–7.3	7.3
Arterial PCO_2 (mm Hg)	20–30	Normal
Anion gap [Na-(Cl+HCO_3)]	↑	Normal to slightly ↓

6. How will you investigate and prepare a diabetic patient for elective surgery?

Ans. The management of diabetic patients who are to undergo surgery must take into account the type of diabetes, current treatment, metabolic status, pre-existing cardiac or renal problems, proposed surgery and anesthetic technique.

Whenever possible diabetic patients should be scheduled for surgery in the morning to reduce the period of preoperative fasting.

Frequent blood glucose monitoring with goal to maintain optimal blood glucose.

The aim of preoperative management should be to avoid—hypoglycemia, excessive hyperglycemia, loss of electrolytes (potassium, magnesium and phosphate) and to prevent lipolysis and proteolysis.

The diabetic status should be evaluated regarding type of diabetes, method of monitoring and usual metabolic control and details of antidiabetic therapy. The presence and severity of associated medical conditions, particularly, cardiovascular and renal diseases must be assessed.

Sensory and autonomic neuropathies are known complications of diabetes and must be sought. Any evidence of stiff joint syndrome due to glycosylation must warn the anesthesiologist about possible limitation in upper cervical spine mobility, consequent difficult laryngoscopy and tracheal intubation (Prayer sign positive).

Investigate the patients for:
- Fasting and postprandial (PP) blood sugar
- HbA_{1c}
- Complete hemogram
- Osmolality
- ABG and electrolytes
- Urine analysis
- Blood urea and creatinine, ketones, proteins
- Plasma lipid profile
- ECG, echocardiography
- Fundoscopy
- X-ray chest, PFT.

7. What are the various oral hypoglycemic agents available? How to optimize patients receiving these agents?

Ans. Sulfonylureas

Mechanism of action: Bind to sulfonylurea receptors on the B cells leading to closure of ATP dependent K channel. This leads to membrane depolarization, opening of voltage gated calcium channels and influx. Leading to insulin secretion.

First generation: Tolbutamide, Tolzamide

Second generation: Glibenclamide, glipizide, gliclazide, glimepiride

Contraindications to the use of sulfonylureas is Type I DM, pregnancy and lactation, hepatic and renal insufficiency.

Biguanides

Mechanism of action: Do not cause insulin release and hence do not produce hypoglycemia like sulfonylureas. Biguanides suppresses hepatic gluconeogenesis and glucose output, enhancing binding of insulin to its receptors and stimulate insulin mediated glucose disposal.

Drugs include phenformin and metformin. Lactic acidosis is more common with phenformin. It is recommended that metformin be stopped before major surgery and reintroduced only after the condition has stabilized and normal renal function has been documented.

Thiazolidinediones

Mechanism of action: Increase the sensitivity to insulin by decreasing the lipolysis and circulating free fatty acid levels, reduction in tumor necrosis factor and increased adiponectin levels.

Drugs are troglitazone, pioglitazone, rosiglitazone. These are slow acting drugs taking 6–12 weeks to reach full effect but do not have prolonged half-life.

Meglitinides: These drugs stimulate insulin secretion, partly in a manner similar to sulfonylureas, but are shorter acting with more rapid onset of action. For example, repaglinide.

α-glucosidase inhibitors: Alpha-glucosidase is an enzyme located on the intestinal brush border that breaks down oligosaccharides to monosaccharides so that they can be absorbed. Inhibition of these enzymes by drugs like acarbose slows carbohydrate absorption and lowers postprandial blood glucose.

8. What are the various types of insulin available? How to optimize these patients when they are posted for minor surgeries and major surgeries?

Ans. See Table 2.

Table 2 | Types of insulin

Insulin type	*Onset (hrs)*	*Peak (hrs)*	*Duration (hrs)*
Short-acting			
• Regular (soluble insulin)	0.5–1	2–4	6–8
• Prompt insulin zinc suspension	1.0	3–6	12–16
Intermediate-acting			
• Insulin zinc suspension (lente)	1–2	8–10	20–24
• Neutral protamine Hagedorn (NPH) or Isophane insulin	1–2	8–10	20–24
Long-acting			
• Extended insulin zinc suspension (crystalline)	4–6	14–18	24–36
• Ultralente protamine zinc insulin (PZI)	4–6	14–18	24–36

Diabetic patients are broadly categorized as:
Cat A: Blood sugar between 100 and 180 mg/dL
Cat B: Blood sugar >180 mg/dL

If the patient's sugar is controlled by diet:
- *For minor surgery:* Treat as normal patient
- *For major surgery:* As normal patient but blood sugar to be monitored perioperatively and injection insulin (soluble) as and when required.

If the patient is on the oral hypoglycemic agents:
- Long-acting sulfonylurea to be stopped 48 hours before and other OHA 24 hours before elective surgery.
- *For minor surgery:*
  - Measure fasting sugar on day of surgery
  - Omit OHA on morning of surgery
  - If blood sugar <180 mg/dL, no specific therapy
  - Check blood glucose postoperatively and OHA restarted with the first meal.
- *For major surgery:*
  - Check FBG in the morning of day of surgery
  - No OHA on the morning of the day of surgery
  - Treat patients as insulin dependent diabetes mellitus
  - On resumption of oral diet postoperatively, start injection soluble insulin 8–12 U SC 3 times daily before each meal
  - Taper insulin to less than 20 U and then start OHA.

If patients are on insulin:
- Patients receiving long or intermediate acting insulin if the total daily dose is less than 40 U or evening dose is less than 24 U, then continue the same.

- If the dose is more than 40 U or evening dose is more than 24 U, then change to soluble insulin SC 3 times daily before meal.
- For those on soluble insulin continue the regimen the day before surgery
- *For minor surgeries:* Non tight control regimen with no insulin no glucose regimen is preferred.
- *For major surgeries:* GLIK regimen, Alberti's regimen, sliding scale regimen, Vellore regimen or tight control regimen.

9. What are the different glycemic control regimens? What is tight control regimen?

Ans.

GLIK regimen

- Single combined infusion of soluble insulin and glucose with potassium added to avoid hypokalemia.
- Guided by BMI, preoperative insulin requirement, blood glucose and blood potassium levels.
- For BMI 20–30, 500 mL 10% glucose +10 U soluble insulin (Human SI) +10 mmol potassium at 1000 mL/hr to a maximum of 2–3 L/day.
- For BMI >30, 16 U of insulin added to the infusion bag.
- For BMI <20, 6–8 U of insulin added to infusion bag.
- *Blood glucose:* Maintain blood glucose between 5 and 12 mmol/L (90–220 mg/dL). If it falls below 5 mmol/L, change infusion bag with decreasing insulin by 4 U. If blood glucose rises above 12 mmol/L bag is changed with adding another 4 U insulin.
- *Plasma potassium:* Maintain between 3.5 and 5.0 mmol/L. If less then give 500 mL of 10% glucose with 20 mmol of potassium. If more than do not add potassium.

Sliding scale regimen

- Start 1 hour before surgery with a 50 mL syringe containing 50 U insulin (1U/mL of insulin)
- Also start IV 5% glucose with normal saline at 1.5 mL/kg/hr along with KCl as per plasma concentration of potassium.

Blood glucose (mmol)	*Blood glucose (mg/dL)*	*Insulin infusion rate (U/hr)*
< 4	<72	0
4.1–7	73–136	1.0
7.1–9	137–162	1.5
9.1–11	163–198	2.0
11.1–17	199–306	3.0
17.1–28	307–504	4.0
>28	>504	6.0

Classic nontight control regimen

- On day of surgery 5% dextrose at 125 mL/hr/70 kg BW to be started.
- Half the morning dose of insulin (which patient was receiving previously) by SC.
- 5% dextrose solution to be continued perioperative at same rate of 125 mL/hr/70 kg BW.
- Usually used for minor surgery and day care cases.
- Patient to be monitored closely.

Vellore regimen

- Advantage of combined glucose insulin infusion and variable insulin regimen.
- For every 1–50 mg/dL increase in blood glucose more than 100 mg/dL, 1 U of insulin is added to the infusion port of 100 mL measured volume set containing 5% dextrose.

Blood glucose (mg/dL)	*Regimen*
<70	Stop insulin and administer 100 mL 5% dextrose rapidly. Measure blood glucose every 15 minutes.
71–100	Stop insulin, infuse 5% dextrose at 100 mL/hr.
101–150	1 U insulin + 100 mL D5W/hr
151–200	2 U insulin + 100 mL D5W/hr
201–250	3 U insulin + 100 mL D5W/hr
251–300	4 U insulin + 100 mL D5W/hr
>300	1 U insulin for every 1–50 mg more than 100 mg/dL + 100 mL of NS/hr

Tight control regimen

- A tight control regimen is recommended to improve wound healing, prevent wound infection, fetal and maternal well being in obstetrics and weaning from cardiopulmonary bypass.
- Aim is to maintain blood glucose level between 70 and 120 mg/dL.
- Infusions
  - *Infusion 1:* 5% dextrose at 50 mL/hr/70 kg BW
  - *Infusion 2:* 50 U of soluble insulin in 250 mL normal saline through a pump piggy back to infusion 1.
  - *Infusion 3:* Other fluids required during and after surgery
- Adjust serum K^+ as per renal functions.
- Insulin infusion according to following formula,

$$\text{Soluble insulin infusion rate} = \frac{\text{Blood glucose level (mg/dL)}}{100\text{–}150} \text{ units/hr}$$

10. What are the diagnostic criteria of diabetes?

Ans. *American Diabetes Association (ADA) criteria:* Fasting blood glucose more than 110 mg/dL (6.1 mmol/L) on two separate occasions or an unequivocal hyperglycemia with acute metabolic decompensation or obvious symptoms.

WHO criteria: Blood glucose >180 mg/dL (10 mmol/L) on any occasion or more specifically, 2 hours after glucose load (75 g oral glucose).

Impaired fasting glucose: Fasting glucose above normal range but below diabetes mellitus diagnostic threshold.

11. What are the anesthetic implications of autonomic neuropathy in DM?

Ans. The presence of autonomic neuropathy has anesthetic implications. Bedside assessment in a patient with autonomic neuropathy may reveal resting tachycardia (earliest sign), lack of heart rate variability during deep breathing and orthostatic hypotension. Fall in systolic blood pressure in excess of 30 mm Hg after standing for 2 minutes is indicative of autonomic neuropathy.

Anesthetic implications of autonomic neuropathy are:

- *Gastroparesis:* These patients are at risk of aspiration and hence require aspiration prophylaxis and rapid sequence induction.
- *Orthostatic hypotension:* This may cause profound hypotension during anesthesia (especially during central neuraxial block).
- Arrhythmias are common.
- Silent ischemia is also well known and may be one of the reasons for sudden death in these patients.

BIBLIOGRAPHY

1. Harrison's Principles of Internal Medicine, 18th edn.
2. Miller RD. Miller's Anesthesia, 7th edn.
3. Miriam A. A simple glucose insulin regimen for perioperative blood glucose control: The Vellore Regimen. Anaes Analg. 2004.
4. Robertshaw HJ, McAnully GR. Anaesthetic management of patients with Diabetes Mellitus. Br J Anaesth. 2000.
5. Robertshaw HJ. Strategies of managing a diabetic patient. Best Pract Res Clin Anaesthesiol. 2004.
6. Stoelting's Anesthesia Co Existing disease, 5th edn.

4

MISCELLANEOUS

CHAPTERS

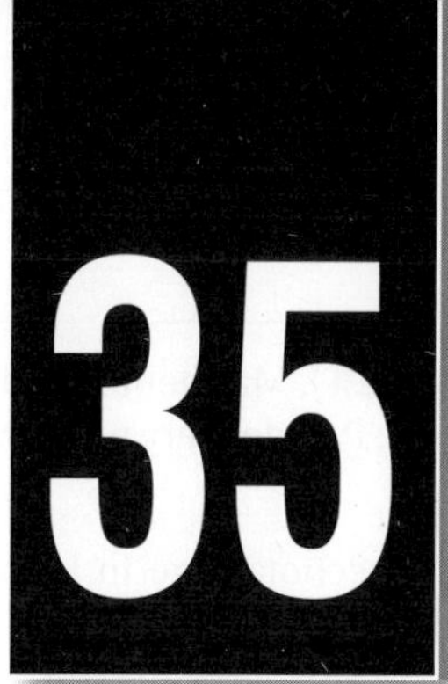

Inhaled Anesthetics

Mahendra Kumar

HALOTHANE

Amber colored bottle contains 250 mL halothane, an inhalational anesthetic agent. It is halogenated alkane derivative. It is clear liquid, nonflammable, nonirritant with pleasant odor. Boiling point is 50.2°C. Saturated vapor pressure: 244. Blood-gas partition coefficient: 2.5. Oil-gas partition coefficient: 224. MAC with 100% O_2: 0.75 and with O_2 and N_2O: 0.29. It is stored in amber colored bottles as it is susceptible to decompose to HCl, HBr, Br and phosgene. Thymol (0.01%) is preservative to prevent decomposition. Thymol left in vaporizers causes malfunctioning of vaporizers.

Metabolism

Fifteen to twenty percent of halothane gets metabolized in liver by cytochrome p-450 enzymes.

Effects on Various Systems

Cerebral metabolic rate and cerebral metabolic O_2 requirement (CMR O_2) is decreased.

But decrease is less than isoflurane. Cerebral blood flow increased. It is a very potent cerebral vasodilator. It increases in ICP due to increase in CBF. There is no neuroprotective effect. It is a potent anesthetic but not analgesic.

It decreases myocardial contractility, stroke volume and cardiac output, produces peripheral vasodilatation, decreases blood pressure and heart rate. It sensitizes the myocardium for catecholamines to produce arrhythmias in presence of catecholamines. There is increased risk of ventricular arrhythmias when adrenaline is used with it. It depresses the respiration, rate is increased but tidal volume is decreased with shallow breathing associated with increased $PaCO_2$ with dose dependent decreased ventilatory response to hypercarbia. It is a potent bronchodilator. It attenuates hypoxic pulmonary vasoconstriction. Repeat exposure to halothane may cause hepatotoxicity. Decreased renal blood flow, GFR and urine output. It is an excellent uterine relaxant, leads to uterine atony and postpartum hemorrhage. It is a good effect for removal of retained placenta.

Uses/indications: Induction of anesthesia particularly in pediatric patients (1–2%). Maintenance of anesthesia after IV induction (0.5–1). Useful in patients having bronchospasm. Postdelivery uterine manipulations.

Contraindications: In patients having arrhythmias, intraoperative use of catecholamine in high doses, uterine atony, hypotension, previous exposure to halothane, hepatitis.

Side effects: Hepatotoxicity, hypotension, bradycardia, arrhythmias, ectopics, malignant hyperthermia, PPH.

ISOFLURANE

Amber colored bottle contains 100/250 mL of 100% isoflurane, an inhalational anesthetic, colorless volatile liquid. It is halogenated methyl ethyl ether. Its molecular weight is 184.5 and boiling point is 48.5°C. Blood/gas partition coefficients is 1.43. Isoflurane is a clear, colorless, nonflammable, stable liquid, no effect of light or CO_2 absorbent, containing no additives or chemical stabilizers. It has a pungent, ethereal odor, MAC with 100% O_2 1.17 and with O_2 and N_2O 0.56. Only 0.2% of isoflurane gets metabolized in liver (cytochrome p-450 enzymes), so majority of the drug is exhaled unchanged.

Effects on Various Systems

Cerebral metabolic rate (CMR) and cerebral metabolic O_2 requirement (CMR O_2) is decreased more than halothane. There is minimal increase in CBF with mild increase in ICP that can be blunted by hyperventilation. There is no effect on CSF production or reabsorption. It is neuroprotective and can suppress the seizures activity. It causes minimal decrease in myocardial contractility and reduces systemic vascular resistance. It reduces blood pressure with 10–20% increase in heart rate. Cardiac output is maintained. There is no arrhythmogenic effect in presence of epinephrine. Respiratory effects are same as in case of halothane with more CO_2 retention than halothane. Dose-dependent respiratory depression occurs. It has a pungent smell so not good for induction of anesthesia although it is also a bronchodilator. It maintains the total hepatic blood flow but reduces renal blood flow, GFR and urine output in proportion to decrease in blood pressure. It is not nephrotoxic. Like halothane it is also uterine relaxant causes uterine atony but good for removal of retained products. It decreases uterine blood flow.

Dose: Depends on premedication, use of other induction agent and muscle relaxants. It may be used 1–2.5% for general anesthesia. Induction and recovery is slow as compare to sevoflurane and desflurane.

Uses/Indications

Induction of anesthesia: It is not suitable for it due to its pungent smell. It should be avoided for induction the anesthesia particularly in children.

It is good for smooth maintenance and recovery of general anesthesia. It has many advantages for nueoanesthesia.

Side effects: Induction of anesthesia may produce coughing, breath holding, or laryngospasm. It can react with desiccated carbon dioxide (CO_2) absorbents to produce carbon monoxide with carboxyhemoglobin in some patients. It may cause sensitivity hepatitis in patients who have been sensitized by previous exposure to halogenated anesthetics. It may also cause respiratory depression, hypotension and arrhythmias. Shivering, nausea, vomiting and ileus in the postoperative period.

Sevoflurane

Bottle contains 250 mL of sevoflurane (fluorinated methyl isopropyl ether), an inhalational general anesthetic, and clear, colorless, stable liquid containing no additives. It is noniflammable volatile with sweet smell. It has molecular weight 200.05D, boiling point 58.6°C, blood gas partition coefficient 0.63–0.69, MAC with 100% O_2 1.8 and with O_2 and N_2O 0.66 (varies with age also). It is poorly soluble in blood so induction and recovery is very fast, suitable for day care surgery. 3.5% is metabolized in liver by cytochrome p 450 by oxidative pathway only. Concentration of metabolites and fluoride ion is significantly low than recommended safe level.

Effects on Various Systems

Cerebral metabolic rate (CMR) and cerebral metabolic O_2 requirement (CMR O_2) is decreased similar to isoflurane. The CBF is minimally increased with mild increased in ICP and CPP. CSF production and reabsorption decreased. It does not provoke seizure activity. Myocardial contractility minimally decreased, blood pressure decreased, decrease in regional and systemic vascular resistance, heart rate and cardiac output maintained, blood flow to liver and kidney decreased but increased or maintained to brain. There is no increased risk of arrhythmia with adrenaline. Poor solubility causes abrupt increase in alveolar concentration of sevoflurane so it does not cause any significant neurocirculatory responses. Dose-dependent respiratory depression with reduction in tidal volume and increase in respiratory rate (rapid shallow breathing) occur. Increase in $PaCO_2$ is least with this among all agents. It is also potent bronchodilator. Hepatic blood flow is maintained and there is risk of hepatotoxicity. Renal blood flow, GFR and urine output are decreased (dose-related; similar in all agents) in proportion to reduction in blood pressure. Effect on gravid uterus is same as with other inhalational anesthetic agents.

Uses/indications: It is used for induction and maintenance of general anesthesia. Poor solubility and sweet smell make this agent suitable for rapid and smooth induction and recovery and quick change in depth of anesthesia.

Dose: For induction of anesthesia, it may be used up to 2MAC (4%) and anesthesia is maintained with 1–3% with or without nitrous oxide.

Side effects: Most adverse events reported were mild and transient bradycardia, tachycardia, hypotension, laryngospasm, breath holding, etc.

Desflurane

Desflurane (fluorinated methyl ethyl ether) is available in 250 mL bottle. It is colorless, noninflammable, stable, volatile inhalational anesthetic agent. Its odor is most pungent, not suitable for inhalational induction. Boiling point 22.8°C, boils at normal OT temperature, require power operated special vaporizer. Blood gas partition coefficient 0.42 indicates low solubility. Its MAC with 100% O_2 is 6.6 and with O_2 and N_2O, it is 2.38. It is less potent than other inhalational agents. Only 0.02% of desflurane gets metabolized in liver (cytochrome p-450 enzymes) by oxidative pathway. There is very less risk of nephro/hepatotoxicity due to minimal fluoride and toxic production.

Effects on Various Systems

Cerebral metabolic rate (CMR) and $CMRO_2$ is decreased similar to isoflurane. CBF is increased slightly with increase in ICP more than isoflurane and sevoflurane. Cerebral protective effect is doubtful as with sevoflurane. Abruptly increased inspired concentration of desflurane leads to progressive increase in sympathetic outflow which leads to hypertension and tachycardia for 4-5 minutes, due to stimulation of receptors in airway due to pungent smell. It causes minimum decrease in myocardial contractility and blood pressure. Heart rate is increased similar to isoflurane. Cardiac output is maintained while systemic vascular resistance is decreased. There is no risk of arrhythmias. Respiratory and $PaCO_2$ response to desflurane is same as with other inhalational agents (shallow respiration). It has pungent smell causes irritation to airway and bronchospasm with increased airway pressure. Like other agents it attenuates hypoxic pulmonary vasoconstriction leading to increase in V/Q mismatch. Hepatic blood flow and hence liver functions are well maintained. Renal blood flow and GFR are reduced due to reduction in cardiac output and blood pressure. Effect on gravid uterus is same as with other agents.

Dose: Induction, if done, start with 3% then increase with increment of 0.5–1% up to 4–11% end tidal desflurane.

Uses/indications: Induction of anesthesia should be avoided with this agent due to its pungent smell and consequent respiratory problems. Maintenance of anesthesia is well titrated with early recovery due to poor solubility.

Side effects: Bronchospasm, salivation, breath-holding, laryngospasm, tachycardia, hypertension, etc.

Ref: Ronald D. Miller. Miller's anesthesia, 7th edn. Churchill Livingstone, Elsevier; 2010.

Ref: Robert K Stoelting, Simon C Hiller. Pharmocology and physiology in anesthetic practice, 4th edn. Lippincott William & Wilkins, 2005.

Ref: Paul G Barash, Bruce F Cullen, Robert K Stoelting. Clinical anesthesia, 5th edn. Lippincott William & Wilkins, 2006.

OTHER DRUGS RELATED TO ANESTHESIA

Sodium Bicarbonate

Sodium bicarbonate 7.5% w/v solution is available in 10 mL and 25 mL ampoules.

It is hypertonic solution provides 0.9 mEq sodium ions and equal amount of bicarbonate ions per mL (90 mEq/100 mL). It is sterile, pyrogen-free to be used intravenously only.

Uses/indications: It is highly alkaline and mainly used to treat metabolic acidosis of various causes. In hyperkalemia, it is used to increase the pH (Alkaline) to shift the potassium from extracellular to intracellular space. It is hypertonic solution and containing good amount of sodium so may be used to treat the hyponatremia, particularly when large volume of water is not required. It reduces the serum calcium levels (related to pH) so may be used in patients of hypercalcemia. It is added to local anesthetic agents to enhance their onset of effect and potency. Earlier it was used for bronchial lavage and chest physiotherapy.

Contraindication: It is contraindicated in presence of metabolic or respiratory alkalosis, hypernatremia, CHF and volume overload. Its administration may worsen the hypocalcemia and patient may develop tetany.

Side effects: Excessive administration of sodium bicarbonate may lead to metabolic alkalosis, hypokalemia, hypocalcemia, hypernatremia, CHF, fluid overloading, respiratory depression. Oxygen dissociation curve may shift towards left side.

Doses: Dose of sodium bicarbonate may be calculated by a simple formula—body weight × base deficit × 0.3 or body weight × base deficit/3. Only 50% of the calculated value is given in mEq after converting it in mL (1 mL = 0.9 mEq, 7.5%) intravenously.

Potassium Chloride

Potassium chloride solution is available in ampoule of 10 mL, 15% weight/volume. Each mL contains 2 mEq potassium and 2 mEq chloride. It is a sterile, pyrogen-free, to be administered through intravenous infusion only after dilution in a good volume of fluid. Its average pH is 4.6-acidic.

Uses/indications: It is used in case of hypokalemia (Serum potassium level < 3 mEq/L), as a component of GKI (glucose, potassium and insulin) solution, with certain drug therapy like diuretic therapy and digitalis to prevent hypokalemia.

It is an important ion of intracellular fluid with a concentration of 150 mEq/L normal serum potassium level varies from 3.5–5.5 mEq/L.

In the body, it is essential for neural transmission and carbohydrate metabolism.

Daily normal requirement: It is 1–2 mEq/kg with a daily dietary intake 50–150 mEq of which 80–90% is lost through renal excretion.

There are certain factors which either decrease or increase the serum potassium level even without gain or loss of potassium. Acidosis increases and alkalosis decreases the serum potassium level by shifting the potassium from intra to extra and extra to intracellular fluid respectively. Glucose-insulin metabolism, adrenaline and β2 agonist shift the potassium from extra to intracellular fluid thus help in decreasing the serum levels so may be used to treat hyperkalemia. Aldosteron and diuretics promote the renal loss of potassium and decreasing potassium levels. Hyperventilation increases and hypoventilation decreases the potassium levels by shifting. Dietary intake also affects the potassium levels. Major causes of hypokalemia are gastrointestinal and renal losses of potassium without adequate replacement.

Contraindications: The absolute contraindication of potassium therapy is hyperkalemia of any cause. Other conditions where hyperkalemia may occur, it should be avoided, for example renal failure, metabolic acidosis, certain poisoning causing acidosis, massive burn and soft tissue injury, massive blood transfusion.

Side effects: The potassium therapy may results in certain complications/side effects like hyperkalemia and its consequences (arrhythmias, even cardiac arrest), acidosis, phlebitis and thrombophlebitis.

It should be administered diluted in IV fluid very slowly under ECG monitoring.

Doses: Maximum dose in 1st hour infusion should not be more than 40 mEq in severe hypokalemia and 10 mEq per hour thereafter. Total requirement or dose should be infused over a period of 24 hours.

Hyperkalemia is an acute and some times life-threatening condition must be diagnosed and treated immediately. Its presentation may have a reflexia, muscular or respiratory paralysis, mental confusion, weakness, hypotension, cardiac arrhythmia, heart block, electrographic abnormalities and cardiac arrest. In ECG it is characterized by tall and peaked T wave, small or absent P wave, prolonged P-R interval, wide QRS, finally ventricular tachycardia and fibrillation.

For treatment of hyperkalemia calcium gluconate 10%, 10–30 mL IV slowly given to control the effects of excess of potassium like arrhythmias. Acidosis is corrected by sodium bicarbonate. To promote the shifting of potassium to intracellular compartment glucose insulin solution and β_2-agonist may be used. For loss of potassium diuresis should be initiated, in case renal failure hemodialysis should be considered.

Calcium Gluconate and Calcium Chloride

Calcium gluconate: Ampoule contains 10 mL solution of 10% calcium gluconate. (1 gm calcium gluconate in 10 mL solution). It is a salt of gluconic acid and provides 9 mg Ca^{++}/mL (0.45 mEq/mL) which is about one-third of the calcium provided by calcium chloride.

Calcium chloride: Ampoule contains 10 mL solution of 10% calcium chloride. Each mL contains 100 mg calcium chloride that provides 27 mg Ca^{++}/mL (1.35 mEq/mL).

Both solutions are sterile, pyrogen-free and hypertonic for IV injection only.

Indications: Calcium gluconate is safer than calcium chloride as it is less potent. Ten percent calcium chloride injection is indicated for the treatment of severe hypocalcemia requiring urgent correction of low plasma calcium levels.

Generally, calcium gluconate is used to treat hypocalcemia and hypocalcemic tetany. Hyperkalemia is one of the prime indications of calcium to antagonize the effects of potassium so also indicated in massive blood transfusion. It is also used as 4th coagulation factor and positive ionotrope and to treat aminoglycoside induced neuromuscular block.

Contraindications: Ventricular fibrillation, asystole and digitalis toxicity, hypokalemia. It is not injected by intramuscular or subcutaneous or in other tissues as it may cause severe necrosis and sloughing of the tissue.

Normal concentration of calcium in serum is 8.5–10 mg/dL that is equal to 5 mEq/L or 2.5 mmol/L, out of which 50% is in an ionized form.

Side effects: Extravasation may cause necrosis. Rapid injection may cause bradycardia, dysrhythmias and cardiac arrest. Injections of calcium chloride are accompanied by peripheral vasodilatation and hot or burning sensation.

Drug interaction: Cardiac glycosides, ionotropes and calcium show synergistic effects and may develop cardiac arrhythmias when used together. So, intravenous use of calcium should be avoided in patients getting cardiac glycosides.

Magnesium Sulfate

Ampoule contains 2 mL solution of magnesium sulfate 50% weight/volume (0.5 gm in each mL). Each ampoule contains 1.0 gm (2 mL). It provides 8 mEq Mg^{++} /gm. Magnesium is a second most abundant cation of intracellular compartment after potassium. Its concentration inside the cell is 40 mEq/L while in serum it is 2 mEq/L. Its daily requirement is approximately 50 mEq.

Magnesium is very important as it is required in many physiological activities. It is required for more than 300 enzymatic reactions in side the cells. It is involved in energy production and synthesis of DNA, RNA and protein. It participates in skeletal muscle contraction.

Uses/indications: The main indication of magnesium is hypomagnesemia. Clinically, it is used as bronchodilator, vasodilator, tocolytic and antiarrhythmic agent. In obstetrical emergencies, it is used as anticonvulsant and vasodilator to control convulsions and blood pressure. As vasodilator, it improves cerebral circulation and perfusion. In premature labor, it is used as tocolytic agent to arrest the labor. In ICU, it has been used as anticonvulsant, bronchodilator and antiarrhythmic agent. Perioperatively, it has been used to control hemodynamic responses to laryngoscopy and intubation and to produce hypotensive anesthesia. As adjunct to analgesic and anesthetic, it has been used to reduce the requirement of analgesics and anesthetics.

Routes of administration: It has been IV, IM, intra-articular, epidurally and in subarachnoid space.

Doses: 2–4 gm IV very slow followed by 1 gm IV infusion/hr for eclampsia.

As antiarrhythmic: 2 gm (16 mEq) IV slowly over a period of 15–20 min.

Perioperatively as adjunct: 40–60 mg/kg over a period of 20 min under ECG monitoring followed by 10–15 mg/kg/hr infusion. Same dose is required for controlling hemodynamic parameters.

Side effects: Its infusion may leads to magnesium toxicity with muscular and respiratory paralysis, arrythmias, unconsciousness and cardiac arrest depending on serum level of magnesium.

Magnesium toxicity: Signs and symptoms of magnesium toxicity depends serum magnesium levels. At the level of 5 mEq/L, it causes hypotension and peripheral vasodilatation, at 7 mEq/L patient will have drowsiness and hypotonia with respiratory depression and depressed deep tendon reflexes. Respiratory and cardiac arrest occurs when it crosses 10 mEq/L and 15 mEq/L respectively.

Precautions during magnesium therapy: Magnesium is excreted through kidney, so assessment of renal functions prior and during therapy is essential. Urine out must monitored hourly during therapy. If urine out is inadequate, therapy must be withdrawn. Serial estimation of serum magnesium levels is desirable for early detection of toxicity.

Treatment of magnesium toxicity: Discontinue the therapy. Oxygen therapy for respiratory depression either by facemask or IPPV as case may be. IV fluids with ionotrops to manage hypotension, and antiarrhythmic drugs are to be given for dysarrhythmias. Diuresis or dialysis should be done for patients having compromised renal functions.

Adrenaline

Available in ampoules 0.5 mL 1:1000. 0.5 mg/ampoule 1 mg/mL.

It is a catecholamine, stimulates sympathetic nervous system (sympathomimetic). It directly acts on α and β receptors.

Stimulation of α_1 receptor causes vasoconstriction and α_2 receptor decreases insulin release and vasoconstriction. Stimulation of β_1 receptor causes positive ionotropic, chronotropic and dromotropic effecting the heart and β_2 receptor stimulation causes vasodilatation, intestinal relaxation, skeletal muscle vasodilatation, tremors, increased insulin and glucagon secretion and lipolysis.

Dose: 0.5–1 mg diluted in 10 mL normal saline (NS) given slowly IV or subcutaneous 0.5–1 mg.

Routes: It can be given subcutaneously, IV, fir infiltration in the tissue along with NS to get dry surgical field. It is also used along with local anesthetic agents to increase their safe dose and to prolong the duration of action.

Uses: It is used to resuscitate the patient having cardiac arrest, circulatory collapse, anaphylactic shock, bronchospasm, racemic form for nebulization, with local anesthetic agents.

Side effects: Tachycardia, hypertension, decreased renal blood flow, hyperglycemia, lipolysis, hypokalemia, dry mouth, mydriasis,

Contraindication: Significant tachycardia, hypertension, CAD, arrhythmias.

Vasopressin

It available in ampoules containing 10 U for IV, IM or subcutaneous injection.

It is a hormone (ADH) produced by posterior pituitary. It acts on V_1 and V_2 receptors.

V_1 receptors: All vasopressin receptors except those present on renal collecting ducts, and some blood vessels. It is responsible for vasoconstriction, visceral smooth muscle contraction, glycogenolysis, platelet aggregation and ACTH release

V_2 receptors: Present on renal collecting ducts and blood vessels responsible for regulation of water permeability of kidney. *Half time:*10–20 min.

Uses: In diabetes insipidus, vasopressin is used for treatment of central diabetes insipidus.

Esophageal varices are treated with IV infusion of 20 U of vasopressin over 5 minutes or direct infusion into superior mesenteric artery. In refractory cardiac arrest 40 U/IV single dose is used. It causes marked peripheral vasoconstriction increases venous return.

It is used as alternative to epinephrine for vasopressor therapy during CPR; found to be more effective than epinephrine in asystole and refractory cardiac arrest.

Side effects: Hypertension, increased pulmonary artery pressure, facial pallor, angina pectoris, ventricular dysrhythmias.

Amiodarone

Amiodarone HCl injection is a sterile clear, pale-yellow solution. Each mL contains 50 mg of amiodarone HCl, 20.2 mg of benzyl alcohol, 100 mg of polysorbate 80, and water for injection. It is an antiarrhythmic drug of class III, it prolongs effective refractory period in SA node, atrium, AV node, his purkinje system ventricle. It has antiadrenergic action and causes potent vasodilatation. Its elimination half is 29 hours, metabolized in liver. It has extensive protein binding so difficult to remove even by hemodialysis.

Uses: VT or VF resistant to electrical defibrillation 300 mg IV. For premedication, it is given orally. It decreases incidence of AF after surgery. Supraventricular and ventricular tachyarrhythmias are treated with 5 mg/kg IV over 5 min.

Doses: Initial dose (IV)—1000 mg over the first 24 hours, 150 mg over the first 10 minutes (15 mg/min), followed by 360 mg over the next 6 hours (1 mg/min). Maintenance infusion—540 mg over the remaining 18 hours (0.5 mg/min).

Side effects: Pulmonary toxicity is most serious side effect due to increased production of free oxygen radicals in lungs. Patient has progressive dyspnea, cough, weight loss, pulmonary infiltrates on chest X-rays and later on fever. In CVS toxicity tachyarrhythmias, AV heart block, bradycardia, hypotension, etc. Peripheral neuropathy, fatty liver, thyroid dysfunction are other side effects.

Drug interactions: It increases concentration of digoxin, procainamide. Quinidine, warfarin, cyclosporine and displaces digoxin from protein binding sites. Exaggerated negative inotropic effects in presence of beta-blockers and calcium-channel blockers.

BIBLIOGRAPHY

1. Paul G Barash, Bruce F Cullen, Robert K Stoelting. Clinical anesthesia, 5th edn. Lippincott William & Wilkins, 2006.
2. Robert K Stoelting, Simon C Hiller. Pharmocology and physiology in anesthetic pracice, 4th edn. Lippincott William & Wilkins, 2005.
3. Ronald D Miller. Miller's anesthesia, 7th edn. Churchill Livingstone, Elsevier; 2010.

36

Intravenous Fluids: Crystalloids and Colloids

Mahendra Kumar

GENERAL CONSIDERATION OF INTRAVENOUS FLUIDS

- Water is an important constituent of our body. It constitute about 60% of our body weight with few exceptions, e.g. fat, female (less than 60%) and infants (more than 60%). Out of 60%, 1/3rd is present in extracellular space while remaining 2/3rd is available in intracellular space. Water in extracellular space (1/3rd of total) is again distributed in intravascular and interstitial space in proportion of 1/3 and 2/3rd respectively.
- Hydrostatic, osmotic and oncotic pressures are the main factors to keep the total body water in various compartments in proportions mentioned above.
- Osmotic pressure depends on number of osmotically active particles, capable to hold some amount of water.
- Oncotic pressure is exerted by substances having high molecular weight, capable to hold the water more than osmotic pressure. Albumin is responsible for major fraction of total oncotic pressure.
- Normal value of osmotic and oncotic pressure is 285 ± 5 mOsmol/L and 25–32 mm Hg respectively.
- Whenever there is loss of water/blood (dehydration/hypovolemia) its replacement is essential to maintain the total body water and normovolemia for normal physiological activities of body.
- Replacement of body fluid is achieved by intravenous infusion of fluids and transfusion of blood and its product, type of IV fluid will depends on nature of fluid loss.
- Normal requirement of fluid is as follows:

  For 1st 10 kg—4 mL/kg/hr
  10–20 kg—2 mL/kg/hr
  >20 kg—1 mL/kg/hr.
- *Intraoperative requirement of fluid is managed as follows:*
  Fluid of fasting period (deficit) is replaced as per normal requirement of fluid, calculated for fasting hours. 50% of total volume of fasting deficit is given in first hour, remaining 50% of volume is given in next 2 hours (25% in each hour). In addition to this, maintenance fluid is also given as per normal requirement of fluid per hour. Only crystalloids fluids are used for these purposes.

Actual loss of blood and other fluids is replaced by crystalloid/colloids/blood/blood components as per the need. Third space loss is compensated for major surgery 6 mL/kg/hr, for moderate surgery 4 mL/kg/hr and for minor surgery 2 mL/kg/hr.

Intravenous (IV) fluids are the preparation of fluids having water, electrolytes and other substances as constituents which are to be administered through intravenous route. These are sterile, pyrogen free and clear fluids with limited life. They are mainly classified into two groups: (i) Crystalloid and (ii) Colloids.

1. How will you classify the IV fluids?

Ans. These are classified in many ways on the basis of:

(i) *Chemical composition:*
- Crystalloids, e.g. 5D, NS, DNS, RL, etc.
- Colloids, e.g. gelatin, dextran, HES, albumin, etc.

(ii) *Indication:*
- Maintenance fluids, e.g. 5D, DNS, RL, etc.
- Replacement fluids, e.g. NS, RL, colloids.

(iii) *Osmolarity:*
- Iso-osmotic/isotonic
- Hyper-osmotic/hypertonic, e.g. DNS, hypertonic saline
- Hypo-osmotic/hypotonic, e.g. N/2 or N/5 saline solutions.

Crystalloid IV fluids comprised of *water* and *electrolytes* or *simple crystal* compound only, e.g. dextrose, NS, RL, Isolyte-P, hypertonic saline solutions.

Colloids IV fluids have, in addition, substances of *high molecular weight* like *proteins, starch* or *gelatin* efficient to produce *oncotic pressure* like albumin, haemaccel, dextran, HES.

2. What are the differences between crystalloid and colloid solutions?

Ans. Crystalloid fluids are composed of water and electrolytes only and responsible to produce osmotic pressure, while colloid fluids, as they have high molecular weight substances, produce oncotic pressure. Colloids stay relatively for longer period in vascular compartment as compare to crystalloids. Crystalloids leave the vascular compartment and move into interstitial space within short period. For the replacement of blood crystalloids are required three times of blood loss whereas colloids are required in the volume equal to blood loss. Some colloids interfere with cross matching of the blood (dextran and degraded gelatin). Anaphylactic and allergic reactions may occur with colloids.

3. What are the types of colloids?

Ans. Colloids are of two types:

1. Natural, e.g. albumin, blood.
2. Synthetic, e.g. Dextran, gelatin.

Synthetic colloids are usually preferred as:
- These are easily available and economic
- There is no risk of transmission of diseases like HIV, Serum hepatitis
- There is low incidence of anaphylactic reaction as compared to natural colloids.

CRYSTALLOID INTRAVENOUS FLUIDS

5% DEXTROSE SOLUTION

- A bottle contains 500 mL solution of dextrose in the strength of 5% weight/volume
- It is sterile, pyrogen and preservative free for IV single infusion

- Each 100 mL contains dextrose—5 gm and water for injection
- It provides calorie—20 kcal /100 mL.

Type of Fluid

- It is crystalloid, maintenance and calorie providing fluid
- It is isotonic with osmotic pressure 278 mOsmol/L.

10% DEXTROSE SOLUTION

- A bottle contains 500 mL dextrose solution in the strength of 10% w/v
- It is sterile, pyrogen free, without preservative for IV single infusion
- Each 100 mL contains: Dextrose—10 gm and water for injection.
- It provides calorie—40 kcal /100 mL.

Type of Fluid

- It is crystalloid, maintenance and calorie providing fluid
- It is hypertonic having Osmolarity 556 mOsmol/L.

4. What are the uses of dextrose solution?

Ans. It is a source of water and carbohydrate. It is used to keep the IV line open for IV administration of drugs. In case of diabetes mellitus, it is used to avoid and to treat hypoglycemia. It is a major component of total parenteral nutrition and glucose potassium insulin (GKI) solution. It is also used when sodium containing fluids are contraindicated and restricted fluid is required, e.g. CHF, renal failure.

Contraindications: It should not be used in diabetic (mellitus) patients without insulin except in hypoglycemia. Simultaneous infusion of 5% D with blood transfusion is not recommended to avoid Rouleaux formation of RBCs. Cerebral edema and fluid overloading are contraindicated as carbohydrate gets metabolized and only water remains in the body that may further aggravate the condition.

Side effects: Febrile reaction, infection at the site if venous line, phlebitis and thrombophlebitis, overhydration, congestion of lungs, dilution of blood and hence electrolytes.

5. What precautions should be undertaken during infusion of a fluid?

Ans.
- Aseptic precaution is to be taken strictly
- There should not be any sign of contamination in the form of suspended particle
- There should not be any preexisting puncture or leakage from the container
- Expiry date is to be checked.

NORMAL SALINE (NS) SOLUTION

A bottle contains 500 mL solution of sodium chloride in the strength of 0.9% w/v (Sodium chloride-0.9 gm/100 mL). It is sterile, pyrogen free, without preservative for IV single use only.

It provides: Na^+ 154 mEq/L and Cl^- 154 mEq/L

It is a crystalloid, maintenance and replacement fluid with osmotic pressure 308 mOsmol/L.

6. What are the uses of NS?

Ans. NS is used to replace the body fluid (like in case of hypovolemia, dehydration) as a source of water and sodium and hence to treat the hyponatremia also. Hyperglycemia and hyperkalemia can also be treated by dilutional therapy with NS when good volume of NS is infused. Various drugs are dissolved and diluted in NS for IV administration in OR and ICU.

7. What are the side effects of NS?

Ans. When infused in excess it may cause:
- Hypernatremia/hyperchloremia.
- Overhydration
- CHF
- Pulmonary edema.
- Infection at venous site
- Febrile episode
- Phlebitis and thrombophlebitis.

DEXTROSE NORMAL SALINE (DNS) SOLUTION

- A bottle contains 500 mL solution of dextrose and saline. (5D+NS)
- Each 100 mL contain—Dextrose—5 gm, Sodium chloride—0.9 gm and water.
- It provides-Na^+ 154 mEq/L, Cl^- 154 mEq/L and Calorie—20 kcal/100 mL
- It provides dextrose (calories) and electrolytes for replacement and daily maintenance.

Type of Fluid

- It is a crystalloid and hypertonic solution with osmolarity 585 mOsmol/L.
- It is a maintenance as well as replacement fluid.
- Uses and other things are as in cases of Dextrose and NS.

RINGER LACTATE SOLUTION

A bottle contains 500 mL solution of ringer lactate. It is sterile, pyrogen free, without preservative for single IV use only.

It contains:
- Sodium—131 mEq/L
- Potassium—5 mEq/L
- Calcium—4 mEq/L
- Chloride—111 mEq/L
- Bicarbonate as lactate—29 mEq/L.

Type of Fluid

- It is crystalloid, replacement as well as maintenance fluid
- It is isotonic solution with osmotic pressure 280 mOsmol/L.

Uses

- It is an excellent replacement solution among the crystalloid
- It is a plasma expender, also known as poor man's white blood
- It is used intraoperatively, and in patients of burn, trauma and hypovolemic shock.

Contraindications

Hepatic failure and other conditions as in case of NS.

PEDIATRIC ELECTROLYTE SOLUTION (ISOLYTE P) MULTIELECTROLYTE SOLUTION IN 5% DEXTROSE

A bottle contains 500 mL solution of electrolytes and dextrose for pediatric use. It is sterile, pyrogen free, without preservative for IV single use.
It contains:

Dextrose	:	5 gm/100 mL (50 gm/L)	Sodium	:	25 mEq/L (N/6)
Potassium	:	20 mEq/L	Magnesium	:	6 mEq/L
Chloride	:	22 mEq/L	Acetate	:	23 mEq/L
Phosphate	:	3 mEq/L	Calorie	:	20 kcal/100 mL

Type of Fluid

- Crystalloid, maintenance, hypertonic solution. (Sod. N/5 or N/6 in 5% dextrose)
- It has osmolarity 340 mOsmol/L.

Uses

- It is used as maintenance fluid for pediatric age group
- It may be used in adults as a source of potassium.

Side Effects

It can cause hyperkalemia, should be used carefully in cases of renal failure.

COLLOID INTRAVENOUS FLUIDS

GELATIN SOLUTION (HAEMACCEL)

It contains 500 mL solution of degraded gelatin in the strength of 3.5% w/v and electrolytes. It is sterile, pyrogen free, without preservative for single IV infusion.

Each 100 mL contains:			
	Degraded gelatin		3.5 gm
	Sodium	:	145 mEq/L
	Chloride	:	145 mEq/L
	Potassium	:	5.1 mEq/L
	Calcium	:	12.5 mEq/L
	Water for injection.		

Type of Fluid

It is colloid, replacement, isotonic fluid.

- Osmotic pressure is 300 mOsmol/L
- Average molecular weight of gelatin is 30,000 dextrose.
- It stays in intravascular space for about 2–3 hours
- It exerts colloid osmotic pressure (*oncotic pressure*).

Indications/Uses of Gelatin Solution

- It is used as plasma expander in hypovolemic shock, burns, trauma and perioperatively to replace the blood loss

- As preloading fluid in spinal anesthesia
- Dose 20 mL/kg/day (1000 mL–50 kg).

Contraindications: It is contraindicated in the following conditions:

- Allergy to gelatin solution
- Over hydration, CHF, pulmonary edema, oliguria/anuria, cardiogenic shock, etc.

Side Effects/Demerits

- It may cause anaphylactic/allergic reactions
- Over hydration may lead to pulmonary edema/CHF following its use
- It has low water binding capacity
- It has relatively short stay period in the vascular compartment (2–3 hour)
- It may interfere in coagulation (particularly in high doses).

DEXTRAN 40 AND DEXTRAN 70

A bottle contains 500 mL solution of dextran 40 in the strength of 10% w/v in NS. It is sterile, pyrogen free for single IV infusion.

Each 100 mL contains:	Dextran 40	:	10 gm
	Sodium chloride	:	0.9 gm
	Water for injection.		

Type of Fluid

It colloid, replacement and isotonic fluid.

8. What are the preparations of dextran solution?

Ans. Dextran solution is available mainly in two preparations:

1. Dextran—40 (10%) and
2. Dextran—70 (6%).

Each is available with either NS or 5% dextrose.

9. What do you mean by number 40 and 70?

Ans. These numbers indicate their average molecular weight:
40 → 40,000 D and 70 → 70,000 D.

10. What is dextran?

Ans.

- Dextran is a polysaccharide (glucose polymer)
- It is synthesized by fermentation of sucrose
- It has water binding capacity
- *Dose:* 25 mL/kg/day
- Intravascular stay period of two preparations is different. For dextran 40 (10%) it is 2–4 hours while in case of dextran 70 (6%) it is 6 hours.

11. What are the indications and contraindications of dextran?

Ans. *Indications/uses of dextran solution:*

- It is used as plasma expander
- As an antithrombotic (anticoagulant) agent
- It improves perfusion (microcirculation) of the tissues
- It may be used in cerebrovascular insufficiency.

Contraindications

It is contraindicated in following conditions:
- Allergy to dextran
- Overhydration, CHF, pulmonary edema, renal failure anuria/oliguria
- Coagulation disorder, bleeding tendency.

Side Effects

- It may cause anaphylactic/anaphylactoid reaction
- It interferes in blood coagulation and cross matching
- It increases the bleeding time
- It decreases the platelets adhesiveness
- Its excessive infusion may cause overhydration—CHF, pulmonary edema.

HYDROXY ETHYL STARCH (HES)

A bottle contains 500 mL solution of HES-200 in the concentration of 10% w/v in NS. It is sterile, pyrogen free, for single IV infusion.

Each 100 mL contains: HES—10 gm and Sodium chloride—0.9% in water for injection.

Type of Fluid

It is a colloid, replacement and isotonic solution with osmotic pressure—308 mOsmol/L

12. What are the preparations of HES solution?

Ans.
- Following are the available preparations of HES 200, 450

	Molecular weight	*Concentration*
• HES-200	200,000	3%, 6%,10%.
• HES-450	450,000	--- 6% ---

- All preparations are in NS
- Water binding capacity is better than degraded gelatin and dextran.

13. What are the indications and contraindications of dextran?

Ans. *Indications/uses of HES solutions:*
- It is used as plasma expander in hypovolemic state in patients of burn, trauma, surgery, sepsis, etc.
- It is used for preloading and loading of fluid during spinal anesthesia
- It may be used for hemodilution during cardiac surgery and vascular surgery
- It improves *tissue perfusion, oxygen delivery and its utilization* at tissue level.

Contraindications

Same as in case of dextran solution.

Side Effects

Patient may develop after getting infusion of HES anaphylactic reaction, skin rashes, bronchospasm, thrombocytopenia, and bleeding disorder with low incidence.

Daily dose of different preparations of HES and their intravascular stay period is as follows:

	Dose	*IV stay period*
HES-200	3% 60 mL/kg/day	1–2 hours
	6% 30 mL/kg/day	3–4 hours
	10% 20 mL/kg/day	4–8 hours
HES-450	6% 20 mL/kg/day	6–8 hours

HUMAN ALBUMIN

A bottle contains 50 mL solution of (human) albumin 25% w/v, it is sterile, tested to be free of hepatitis and HIV antibodies. For IV single infusion.

Each 100 mL contains: Human albumin—25 gm (12.5 gm in 50 mL), Sodium—130–160 mEq/L and water for injection. Source of human albumin is FFP of blood.

Type of Fluid

- It is a natural colloid and used as isotonic replacement fluid
- It is available in the concentration of 5%, 20%, and 25%
- It produces colloid osmotic pressure higher than that of plasma in strength of 20 and 25%
- Water binding capacity of albumin is 17 mL/gm
- Molecular weight of albumin is 68000 D.

Indications/Uses

- It is used as plasma expander to restore/maintain blood volume as in cases of sepsis, burn, trauma, shock
- Hypoproteinemia due to any reason, e.g. dietary, renal.

Contraindications

- It should be avoided when history of allergy to albumin is positive
- In presence of hypervolemia associated with CHF, pulmonary edema, severe anemia with water retention and anuric renal failure, it should not be used.

Side Effects

- It may cause anaphylactic reactions
- Over-loading/retention of water may develop CHF, pulmonary edema
- Transmission of infectious diseases like HIV, serum hepatitis, etc. is a major problem with albumin infusion.

37

Surgical Airway

Sabyasachi Das

DEFINITION

The surgical airway includes the techniques by which a transcutaneous airway can be created which connects trachea and lower airway to the atmosphere or anesthetic circuit or other airway devices bypassing the larynx and the upper airway. It mainly includes tracheostomy and cricothyrotomy.

The rate of failed emergency department intubations and subsequent surgical airway management is lower than 0.6%. The success rates for intubations performed in emergencies are high and cricothyrotomy is required in very few cases (0.7% of adult and less than 1% of pediatric patients). In the emergency department, especially in trauma patients, cricothyrotomy has been used for 1.0–2.8% of all intubation.

INDICATIONS OF SURGICAL AIRWAYS

Any condition where noninvasive techniques fail to relieve CVCI scenario in which the patient is having on going or impending hypoxia such as:

- *Failure of oral or nasal endotracheal intubation as in conditions like:*
  - Massive oral, nasal, or pharyngeal hemorrhage, uncontrolled emesis, masseter spasm, clenched teeth
  - Structural deformities of oropharynx (congenital or acquired)
- *Traumatic injuries making oral or nasal endotracheal intubation difficult or potentially hazardous such as in:*
  - Maxillofacial injuries
  - Cervical spine instability
- *Need for prolonged intubation*
- *Need for definitive airway during procedures on face, neck, or upper airway such as in:*
  - Laryngeal surgery
  - Oral surgery
  - Maxillofacial surgery

The indications of surgical airways can be emergency or elective. The emergency indications include all CVCI scenarios and in these situations cricothyrotomy is the procedure of choice. Elective situations such as need for prolonged mechanical ventilation need tracheostomies.

Anatomical Considerations

To establish a surgical airway one needs to have some basic idea about the anatomy of the neck. The central structure of importance is the cricothyroid membrane which is an elastic membrane located in between the lower border of thyroid cartilage and the upper border of the cricoid cartilage. On average an adult cricothyroid membrane is 9 mm vertically and 30 mm horizontally. The lateral portion of the membrane is covered by the cricothyroid muscles but the central portion is subcutaneous. The thyroid cartilage consists of two laminae joining in the midline to form the laryngeal prominence. Superiorly, the thyroid cartilage is attached to the hyoid bone by the thyrohyoid membrane through which passes the superior laryngeal vessels and the internal laryngeal nerve. Cricoid cartilage forms the inferior border of the cricothyroid membrane and it is the only complete circular cartilage of the larynx with a broad posterior segment that tappers laterally to form a narrow anterior arch. Tracheal rings descend inferiorly to the cricoid cartilage. The area adjacent to the cricothyroid membrane is relatively avascular and devoid of other significant anatomical structures. Cricothyroid arteries; branches of the superior thyroid arteries may form anastomotic arch traversing the superior aspect of the membrane. The external laryngeal nerves runs along the lateral aspect of the larynx and innervates the cricothyroid muscles inferior to the membrane. The isthmus of the thyroid gland overlies the second and third tracheal rings. However, the pyramidal lobe of the thyroid gland may sometimes extend superiorly over the cricothyroid membrane (Figs 1A and B).

Locating of the cricothyroid membrane while establishing a surgical airway, may be difficult especially in female and obese patients. It is identified as a shallow depression between the thyroid cartilage and the cricoids cartilage. However, if the surface landmarks are less prominent, location can be estimated by four fingerbreadths above the sternal notch or 2–3 cm below the laryngeal prominence.

TECHNIQUES

Figure 2 shows technique of surgical cricothyrotomy.

Surgical Cricothyrotomy

Evidences from model lung studies have shown that surgical cricothyrotomy provides effective ventilation independent of the degree of upper airway obstruction. It is the ultimate attempt to make in CVCI scenarios.

1. Under emergent condition there may be no time to administer sedative or analgesic medications; however, if the patient is agitated a sedative or analgesic medication can be given to control the patient.
2. Place the patient in supine position and extend the neck (if cervical injury is known or suspected neck should be in neutral position). Patient is to be given high flow oxygen preferably by bag valve mask. Bag mask ventilation is to be discontinued once the incision is made to avoid insufflations of the soft tissues.
3. For right handed person proper position is the right side of the patient. Immobilize the larynx by the nondominant hand. Palpate the cricothyroid membrane in relation to the anatomical land marks mentioned. Proper stabilization and continuous palpation serves as the foundation of the procedure.
4. Make a midline vertical skin incision 3–5 cm long through the skin over laying the membrane. The midline skin incision avoids vascular structures located laterally and vertical orientation allows extending the incision according to the need.

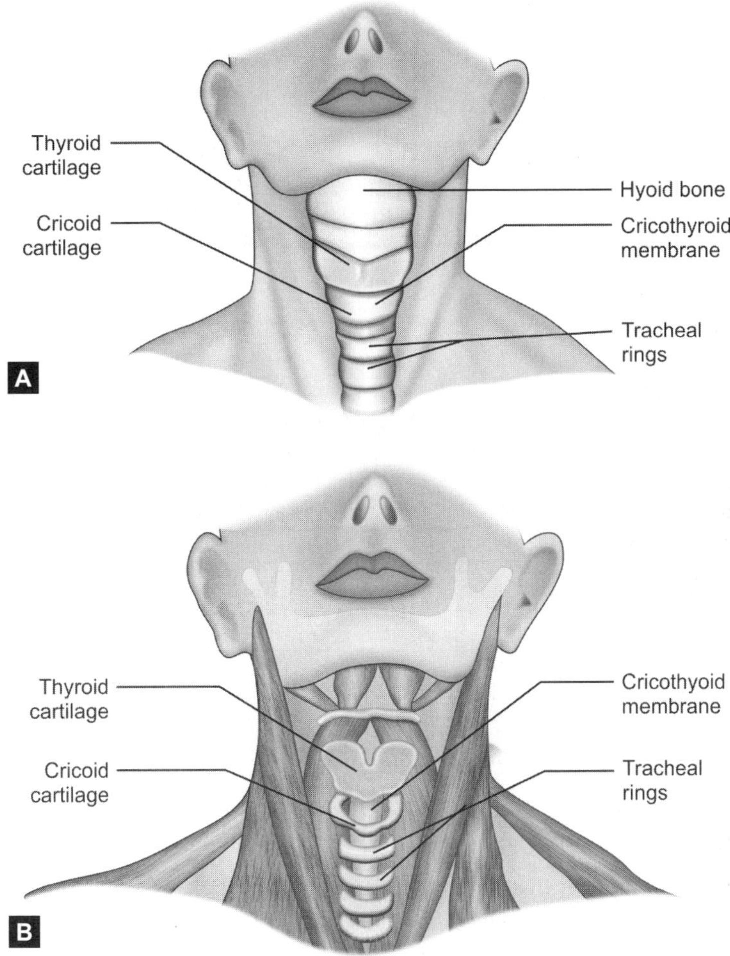

Figs 1A and B Surgical airway cricothyroid

5. Make 1 cm horizontal incision on the cricothyroid membrane. Aim the scalpel in caudal direction to avoid the vocal cords which are located 0.5–2 cm above the membrane. Once incision on the membrane is made keep the tip of the index finger in the entry to the incision so as not to lose the opening.
6. Insert the tracheal hook under the thyroid cartilage and ask the assistant to give upward traction.
7. Enter the trousseau dilator and open it to enlarge the incision vertically. Leave the dilator unless the tube is placed or the thyroid and cricoid cartilages will spring back into place and the opening will be obscured.
8. After dilating the opening rotate the dilator 90 degree so that the handle of the dilator faces towards the feet of the patient. Insert the tube in between the blades of the dilator. If the dilator remains in the previous position the inferior blade will itself prevent the insertion of the tube. After the tube has been advanced into the trachea tracheal hook and dilator is to be removed. Here one must be careful not to puncture the balloon of the tube while removing the tracheal hook.

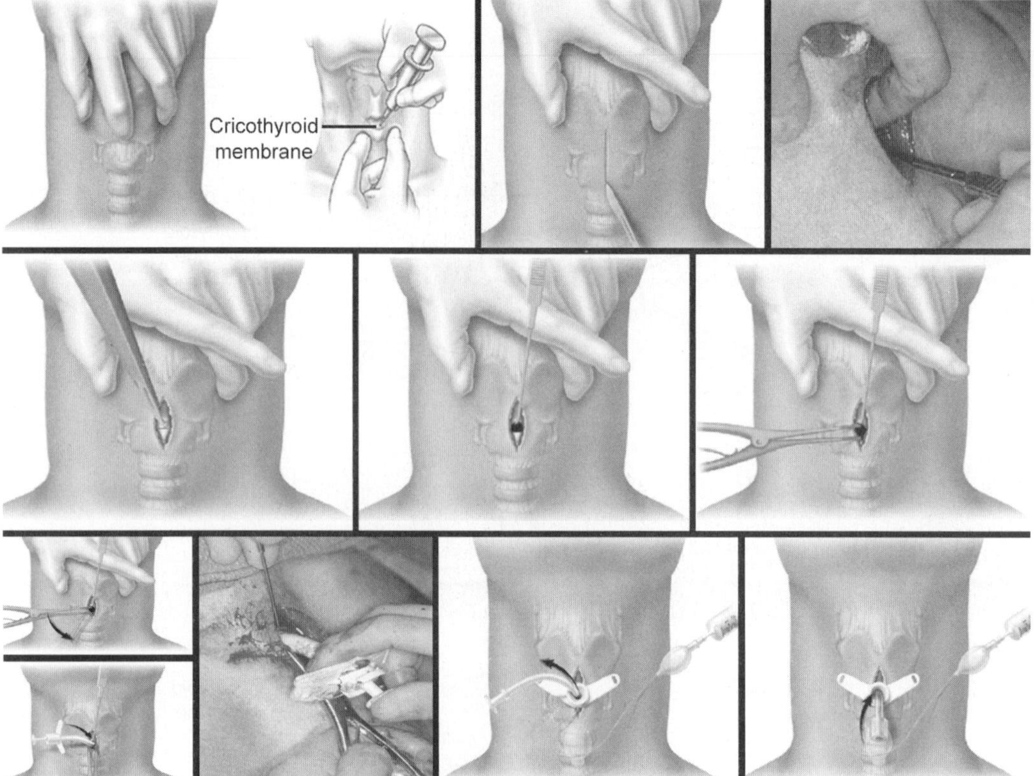

Fig. 2 Techniques of surgical cricothyrotomy *(For color version, see Plate 1)*

9. Remove the obturator, insert the inner cannula and inflate the cuff. While inflating, make sure that the cuff is full but not tense. Over inflation increases the risk of pressure related injury to tracheal mucosa.

Rapid Four Step Technique

It is an alternative way to do emergency cricothyroidotomy. The steps are:

1. Identify the cricothyroid membrane by palpation and stabilize the larynx (Fig. 3A).
2. Make a horizontal 2–3 cm stab incision through the skin, and cricothyroid membrane by scalpel (Fig. 3B).
3. Insert the tracheal hook and give downward traction on the cricoid cartilage (Fig. 3C).
4. Insert the tracheostomy tube (Fig. 3D).

A small modification sometimes makes the rapid four step technique easier. This can be done by introducing a tracheal tube introducer or bougie by the incision and then rail roading the tracheostomy tube by its guidance. Study has shown that this modification significantly increases the speed of performance. Bramwell et al. found that experienced clinicians took 23 secs and inexperienced clinicians 180 secs to complete cricothyrotomy by the standard technique. Brofeldt et al. found this time to be 46 secs of experienced clinicians. Holmes et al. showed that RFST was significantly faster than the standard surgical technique.

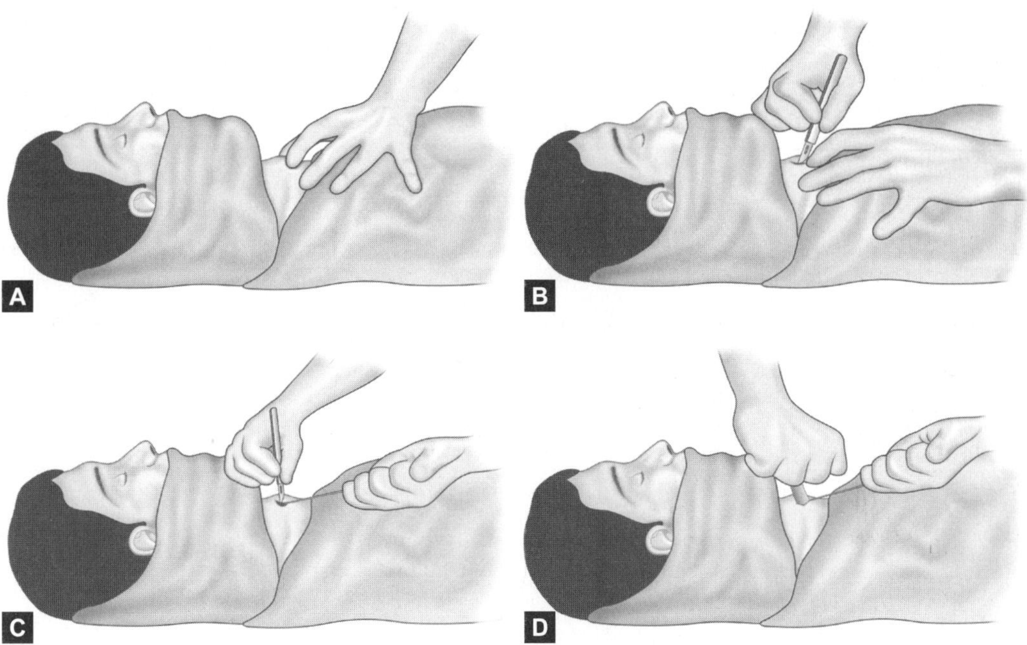

Figs 3A to D Rapid four step technique

PERCUTANEOUS CRICOTHYROTOMY

Studies have shown that although surgical cricothyrotomy is the ultimate measure in CVCI scenarios, anesthesiologists lack their confidence in performing these procedures as they perform surgical procedures less often. Here comes the importance of percutaneous cricothyrotomy devices which are less invasive and easier to insert. Most of the studies have shown that performance time is similar or better for percutaneous cricothyrotomy in comparison to the surgical techniques. In this chapter we are going to discuss about three large bore cuffed emergency cricothyrotomy devices as some of the previous studies have shown that earlier versions of these devices have performed rather poorly due to small diameter and lack of cuff.

Cook Melker Cricothyrotomy Kit

This is a preassembled kit that includes a scalpel, a 12 or 6 mL syringe, an 18 gauge catheter introducer needle, an 18 gauge catheter, a 0.038 inch guidewire and a tapered dilator nested in a 5 mm ID cuffed curved tube.

Technique

Figures 4A to E show cook Melker cricothyrotomy technique.

- Palpate the cricothyroid membrane and fix the larynx.
- Attach the needle to a saline filled syringe and insert it through the membrane pointing caudally at 45 degree to the skin and frontal plane.

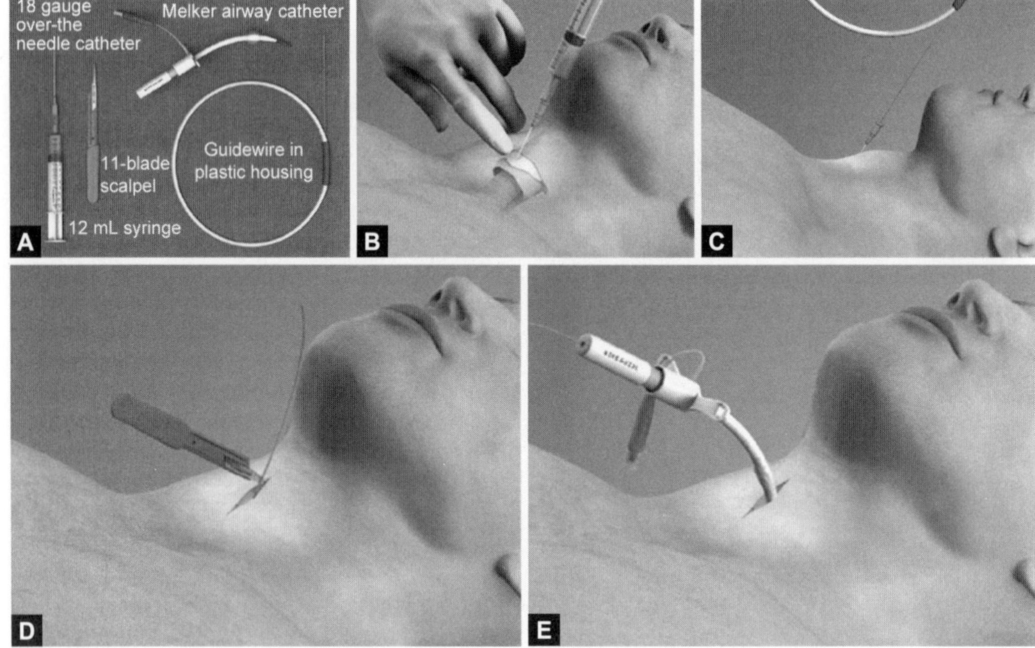

Figs 4A to E Cook Melker cricothyrotomy *(For color version, see Plate 1)*

- Aspirate for free air bubbles as a sign of entry in the trachea.
- Remove the syringe and thread the guidewire through the needle into the trachea approximately 15 cm.
- Remove the needle; make a small, vertical incision in the skin at the point at which the guidewire enters.
- Place the gray tipped dilator into the airway catheter and over the guidewire as a single unit. Advance the catheter till its hub is flushed to the skin.
- Remove the guidewire and the dilator; fix the catheter in place with circumferential neck tape.

Portex Cricothyrotomy Kit

It is a packaged preassembled kit (Fig. 5) in which a locator spring loaded needle is nested in a dilator, over which a 6 mm ID cuffed cricothyrotomy tube is snugly fitted. The tube has a 15 mm connector. The kit also includes a scalpel and a 10 mL syringe.

Technique

- Locate the cricothyroid membrane and fix the larynx with the non-dominant hand.
- Make a vertical skin incision with the scalpel.
- Insert the locator spring loaded needle; the tissue contact is indicated by the red flag. The needle is to be inserted perpendicularly to the skin and into the trachea. Once the needle goes into the tracheal lumen and the tissue contact is lost the red flag disappear into the needle hub.
- The needle is advanced further until the red flag reappears which indicate contact with the

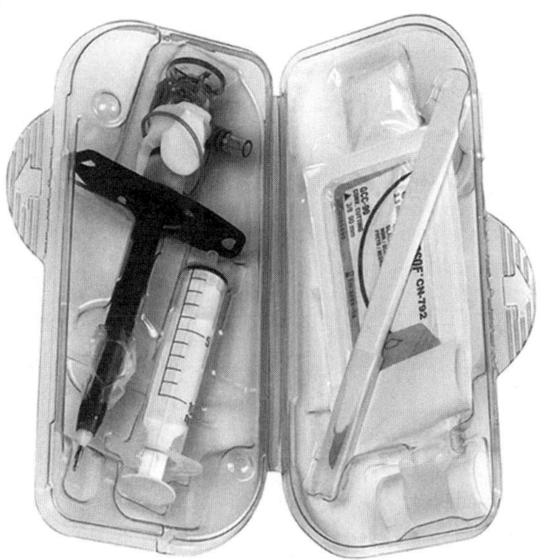

Fig. 5 Portex cricothyrotomy kit *(For color version, see Plate 2)*

posterior tracheal wall. At this point angle the device caudally unless the flag goes down and then advance the whole assembly a further 1–2 cm.

- Remove the needle, slide the cricothyrotomy tube over the dilator and then remove the dilator. Fix the tube by the circumferential neck tie.

Quick Trach 2 Device (Fig. 6)

It is also a preassembled device with a specially grinned needle tip, the tip of which cuts approximately 2 mm and dilates about 4 mm, a cuffed cricothyrotomy tube, a red stopper as a safety measure which prevents needle form being inserted too deep, a green colored safety clip. The metal cannula is fitted behind with a 5 mL syringe.

Technique (Figs 7A and B)

- Palpate and fix the cricothyroid membrane.
- Hold the entire assembly and puncture through the membrane keeping the device about 45 degree to the skin surface. Ensure proper position inside the trachea by aspirating for free flowing air bubbles.
- Proceed further till the red stopper flushes against the skin.
- Remove the red stopper and proceed further still the hub of the airway cannula flushes against the skin.
- Take out the large bore needle and fix the cannula to the skin by circumferential neck tape.

Studies have been done in the past comparing these three devices regarding the procedural time, success rate, incidence of airway injuries and results have been variable. Murphy et al. a study done on porcine model comparing all three devices to the surgical cricothyrotomy showed that Quick trach 2 had the fastest insertion time, highest success rate and least trauma followed by the Cook

Safety clip
The plastic cannula is pushed forward until the safety clip clicks into position

The safety clip is firmly fixed at the connector and therefore avoids that the metal needle is pushed out of the cannula again by mistake

Neck tape
- For safe fixation
- From soft foam material

Stopper
Prevents the needle from being inserted too deep and therefore reduces the risk of posterior tracheal wall perforation

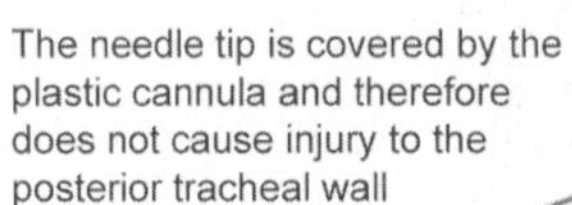

The needle tip is covered by the plastic cannula and therefore does not cause injury to the posterior tracheal wall

Cuff
- Allows sufficient ventilation with aspiration protection
- Cuff is made of ultra–thin material and is very robust

Memory effect
After complete removal of the metal needle the anatomically shaped cannula adjusts to the trachea due to the memory effect

Metal needle
- Specially grinded needle tip only cuts 2 mm and dilates to 4 mm (adult size)
- No scalpel incision necessary

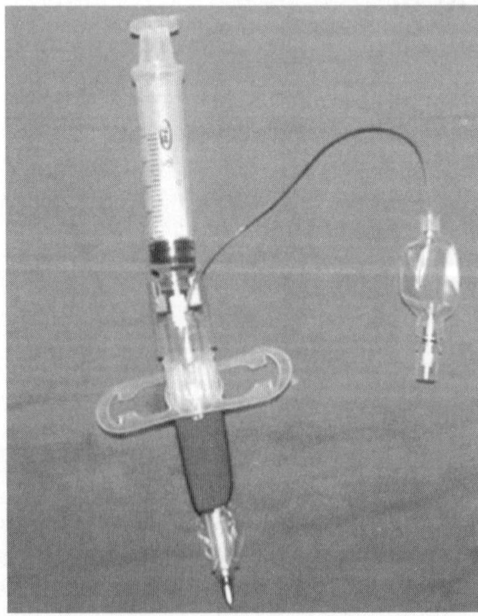

Fig. 6 Quick trach 2 device

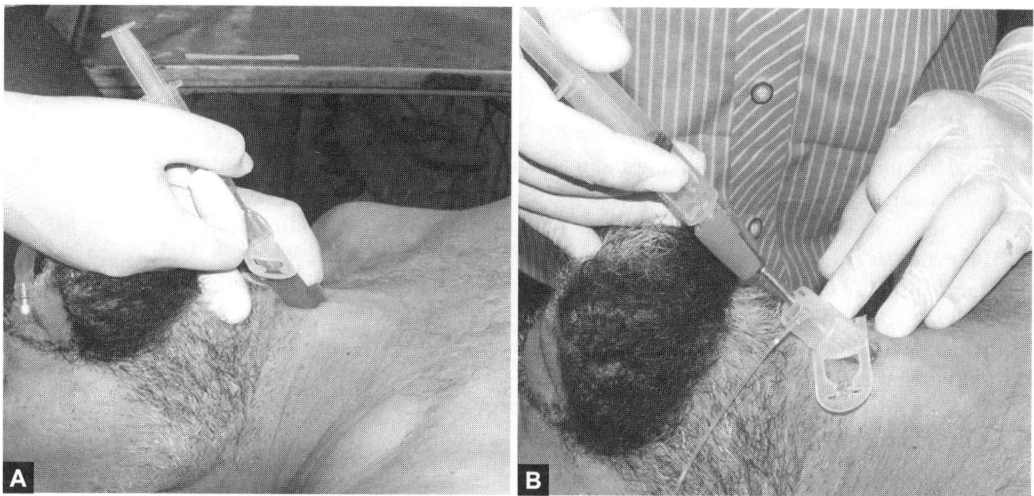

Figs 7A and B Cricothyrotomy using portex kit *(For color version, see Plate 2)*

Melker kit. Portex cricothyrotomy kit was associated with highest insertion time, lowest success rate and maximum incidence of airway trauma. Assman et al. done on mannequins compared between Cook Melker kit and Portex cricothyrotomy kit showed that insertion times were faster with the PCK than the other. However, the success rates were similar by both the devices. Benkhadra et al. done on human cadavers also compared between PCK and Cook Melker kit and showed that PCK was associated with shorter insertion time but with higher incidence of failure and airway injury. It is therefore not easy or possible rather to conclude which one is the better technique or safer technique. However, the choice of device has to be individualized based upon institutional practice and expertise of the person doing the procedure. We recommend Cook Melker kit because it seems to be associated with lesser incidence of airway injury and follows the basic principle of Seldinger technique which most of the anesthesiologists are already familiar with. Quick trach 2 although seems to be better than Cook Melker in some aspects (mentioned above), but the diameter of the cricothyrotomy tube of this device is lesser (4 mm) than the Cook Melker kit (5 mm) and lesser diameter requires more pressure to ventilate. The tidal volume delivered has also been seen to vary depending upon the device used and in this regard Cook Melker showed best performance. Regarding performance time the values have varied in different studies. But it has been shown in a study that after optimization of skill one can perform percutaneous cricothyrotomy in 40 secs or less in mannequins. However, an anesthesiologist with optimum skills should be able to perform these procedures within 120 secs. A permanent tracheostomy should be done within 24 hrs. Cricothyrotomy stomas maintained for more than 2 days have been seen to be associated with a higher glottic and subglottic stenosis.

PERCUTANEOUS TRACHEOSTOMY

Percutaneous dilatational tracheostomy was described by Ciaglia and colleagues in 1985 and it is a cost-effective alternative to the surgical tracheostomy. The safety of this procedure has been shown in a series of critically ill patients and it can be performed rapidly and early in the patient's ICU course. In this chapter we will describe the technique by using Ciaglia blue rhinopercutaneous tracheostomy kit which is used in our institution.

The Ciaglia blue rhinotracheostomy kit comes as a preassembled set containing. The contents of the set is shown in Figures 8A and B.

Technique

- Place the patient supine with hyperextension of the neck; if there is cervical injury, neck is kept in the neutral position (Fig. 9A)
- Give appropriate sedation and muscle relaxation, perform endotracheal intubation (Fig. 9B).
- Make a vertical 1.5 cm incision just inferior from the cricoid cartilage (Fig. 9C).

Under direct vision of laryngoscope, pull the endotracheal tube till the balloon reaches just beneath the vocal cords.

- Insert the Ciaglia kit needle in between the first and second tracheal rings (Fig. 9D).
- Aspirate for free flow of air bubbles (Fig. 9E).
- Advance the guidewire through the hollow bore needle into the tracheal lumen (Fig. 9F).
- By bronchoscope confirm that (Fig. 9G):
  - The wire is within the lumen down to the carina.
  - The wire has not passed through the Murphy eye of the endotracheal tube.
  - By digital palpation confirm that the wire goes into the anterior surface of trachea between the 11 o'clock and 1 o'clock positions and between the first and second or the second and third tracheal rings.
- Approximately, a finger should fit between the cricoid and the wire insertion point (Fig. 9H).

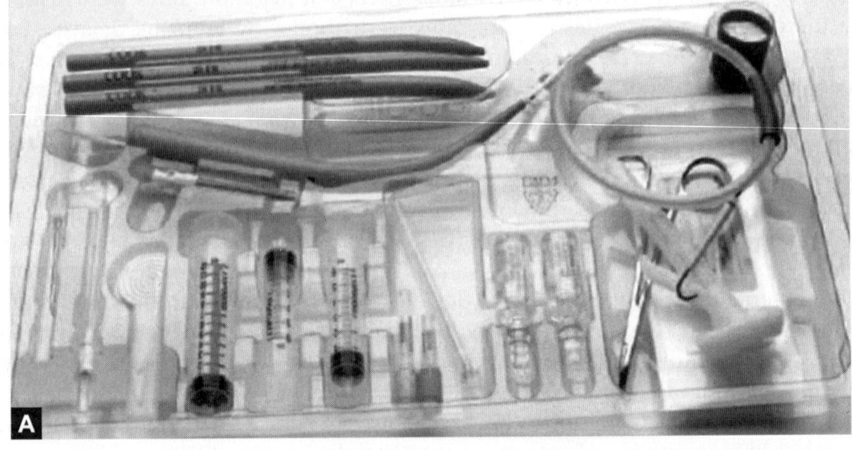

B

- Ciaglia blue rhino G2 percutaneous tracheostomy dilator with preloaded guiding catheter
- 0.052 inch diameter wire guide
- 15 gage, 5 cm introducer needle
- 15 gage, 7 cm introducer needle
- 15 gage, 7 cm FEP sheath needle
- 14 Fr, 4.5 cm dilator
- Tracheostomy tube loading dilator
- Disposable #15 scalpel
- Curved mosquito Damps
- 22 gage infiltration needle
- 25 gage infiltration needle
- Double-swivel connector
- Suture with needle
- Needle driver
- Dale® adjustable tracheostomy tube holder
- Needle holder cup
- Disposable syringes
- Fenestrated drape
- Kendall® Excilon® split tracheostomy dressing
- Lubricating jelly
- Gauze sponges

Figs 8A and B Percutaneous tracheostomy kit

- Next step is rhinodilation. Before doing that confirm that (Fig. 9I):
  a. Tip of the dilator is seated on the white inner cannula
  b. Sauter mark on the wire should be lined up with the distal portion of the white inner cannula.
  c. Skin mark of the dilator—the limit of insertion into the trachea.
- After rhinodilation load tracheostomy tube is appropriately on the blue dilator (Fig. 9J).
- By an overhand pass place the tube inside the airway, remove the introducer and the guidewire (Fig. 9K).
- Final confirmation of the tube placement is to be done by bronchoscopy and the tube is fixed by suturing (Fig. 9L).

Tracheostomy now a days is a standard and very commonly performed procedure specially in ICUs because, apart from protecting the airway it provides some added benefits such as decreased anatomical dead space, better oral care, early weaning, reduced sedation requirement, greater patient comfort, less incidence of ventilator-associated pneumonia and tracheobronchial pulmonary toilet. Percutaneous tracheostomy has been found to be as good as surgical tracheostomy or even better in the context of procedural time, simplicity of the procedure, associated morbidity, complications and cost-effectiveness in various studies. The procedure can be done in the bed side, and thus, the patient need not be shifted which decreases the risks associated with shifting. The stroma is formed in between the tracheal rings and so there is lesser chance of disruption of the blood vessels. The procedure is less invasive and therefore chances of infection are less. Small and neat stoma of percutaneous tracheostomy results in relatively neat scar. There are many devices and techniques to perform percutaneous tracheostomy.

1. *Rapitrach:* Developed by Schachner et al. in 1989, uses sharp, cutting tools to easily penetrate the pretracheal tissues as it is advanced over the guidewire.
2. *Ciaglia technique:* Developed in 1985, uses dilational Seldinger technique for 'Blind' insertion of cannula (air bubbles in syringe to verify tracheal placement), initially insertion was in between cricoid and first tracheal ring, later on the technique modified by changing the insertion point lower down from cricoid to prevent cartilage stenosis.
3. *Griggs technique:* Developed in 1990, uses Seldinger technique, and blunt forceps to dilate.
4. *Translaryngeal tracheostomy:* Described by Fanconi et al. 1993, in this technique the tracheostomy tube is passed through the larynx and upward through the anterior wall of the larynx. Its advantage is that it prevents pressure and damage to posterior wall, however, it is cumbersome.
5. *Blue rhino:* Single conical dilator.
6. *Percu twist:* Developed in 2002 based on single step screw dilator with Seldinger technique. It does not compress anterior tracheal wall, hence there is decreased risk for posterior wall injury.
7. *Ciaglia Blue Dolphin system:* A new balloon dilation percutaneous dilational tracheostomy.

Despite of the differences the devices of percutaneous tracheostomy follow the basic principle of needle puncture of the trachea and insertion of a guidewire. Bronchoscopy is suggested while doing the procedure to avoid misplacement of the guidewire in the Murphy eye of the endotracheal tube which will make decannulation of the endotracheal tube impossible after dilatation and placement of the endotracheal tube. This is also necessary to ensure that the guidewire has not been placed to the back wall of the trachea into the esophagus. A few important facts are to be kept in mind while doing percutaneous tracheostomy: Respiratory system mechanics rapidly change during the procedure when a bronchoscope is used. The resistance of the airway increases and if patient has been kept on a pressure controlled mode in ventilator, there remains every chance of under ventilation. After the procedure is done there is always small reduction of the dead space and if the patient is on volume controlled mode there remains every chance of hyperventilation if the minute volume is not changed accordingly. The bronchoscopy during percutaneous tracheostomy

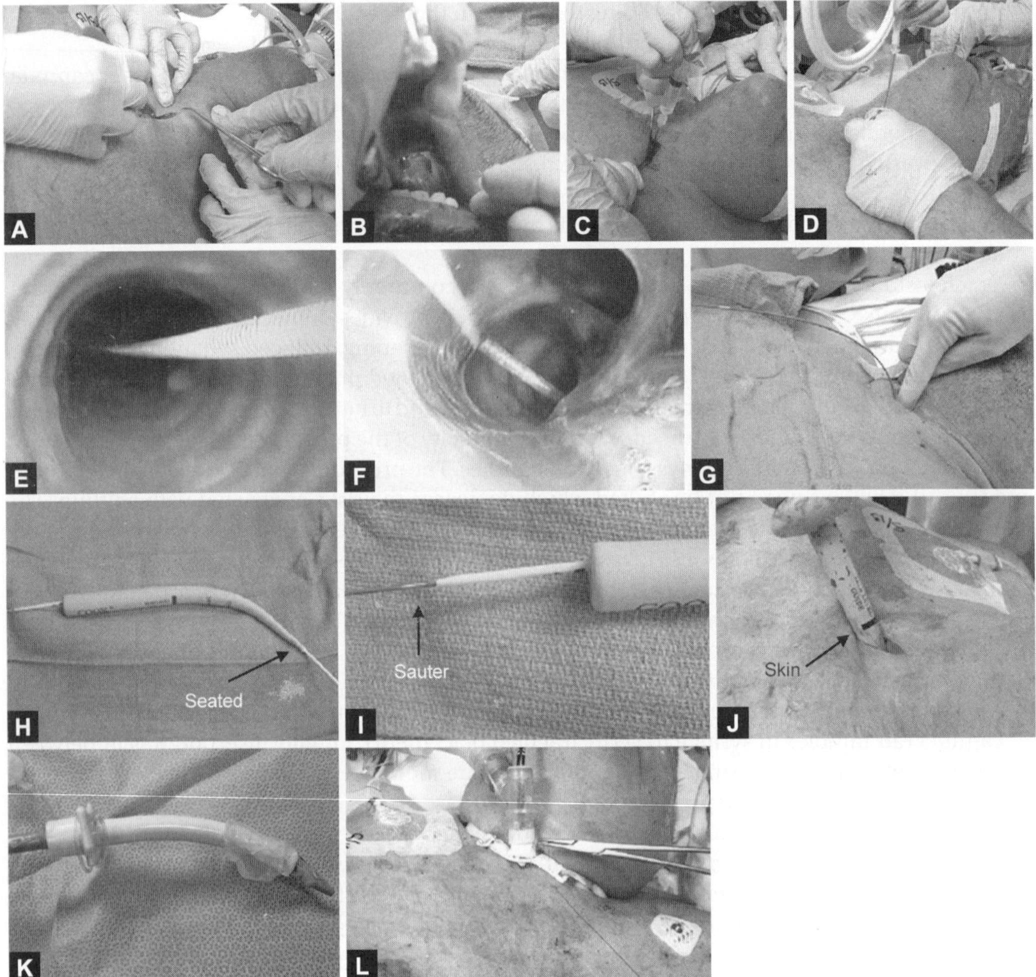

Figs 9A and L Techniques of percutaneous tracheostomy *(For color version, see Plate 3)*

is usually done through the endotracheal tube. For this purpose the cuff of the endotracheal tube is to be deflated and the tube is to be withdrawn until the cuff is located at the level of the vocal cords. Failure to position the endotracheal tube correctly can result in further complications during the course of the procedure, such as rupture of the tube cuff, transection of the tube with the needle, inability to ventilate, and accidental tracheal extubation. Any of these complications can result in life threatening hypoxia. Studies have shown that if LMA is used instead of the endotracheal tube for doing bronchoscopy avoids some of these risks and provide superior visualization of the larynx and trachea. However, this is applicable only for selective cases which do not present with contraindications of LMA insertion.

Contraindications

Absolute

- Emergency tracheostomy
- Pediatric patient
- Midline neck mass
- Nonintubated patient

Relative

- Peep > 20
- Coagulopathy
- Obesity
- Previous tracheostomy (although there is study that has concluded that repeat percutaneous tracheostomy is a safe procedure when performed by trained physicians)
- Cervical spine immobilization
- Tracheomalacia.

CRICOTHYROTOMY

The only absolute contraindication is age. The lower age limit ranges from 5–12 years according to various studies. The most conservative approach is to take 12 years as the lower limit. In emergency situations below this age group, transtracheal ventilation by a 14 gauge needle is preferred. Cricothyrotomy is to be done with jet ventilation.

Among the relative contraindications:

a. Possible or known transaction of the trachea
b. Laryngotracheal disruption with retraction of the distal end of trachea into the mediastinum
c. Fractured larynx.

In these situations, tracheostomy or stabilization of the proximal trachea followed by direct intubation is to be done. It is better to avoid surgical cricothyrotomy in patients with bleeding diathesis. However, in CVCI scenario with impending or ongoing hypoxia, need of an emergent airway supersedes the risk of bleeding.

Complications

Early

- Bleeding
- False passage through tissues
- Subcutaneous emphysema
- Posterior tracheal, mediastinal or esophageal perforation
- Laryngeal injury
- Injury to the vocal cords
- Pneumothorax
- Injury to the thyroid gland
- Hypercarbia (in needle cricothyrotomy)

Late

- Dysphonia
- Persistent stoma
- Glottic or subglottic stenosis
- Laryngeal stenosis
- Tracheoesophageal fistula
- Tracheomalacia.

Among the three major complications bleeding, esophageal perforation, and subcutaneous emphysema are very important. Bleeding is usually not very severe and can be controlled with direct pressure only. However, major bleeding may occur if superior thyroid arteries are injured. As mentioned before these arteries run along the lateral aspect of the membrane. So the chance of injury occurs when surgical cricothyrotomy is tried, and initial incision is extended laterally especially during RFST. So maintaining careful awareness about the land marks and using vertical, midline incision will prevent significant hemorrhage. Another source of bleeding is cricothyroid arteries. To avoid injury to these vessels the membrane must be incised or punctured in the inferior aspect. Esophageal perforation can occur during surgical cricothyrotomy if scalpel is introduced too deep inside the cricothyroid membrane or during percutaneous procedure if introducer needle is inserted too deep. So to prevent this complication allow only distal 1.3 cm of the blade to enter the trachea and while introducing the needle in percutaneous cricothyrotomy, fix the larynx properly; maintain 45° angulation to the frontal plane and continuously check for free air bubbles as sign of entry into the trachea. False passage through tissues occur when larynx is not fixed properly and thus during manipulation to introduce the tube, the larynx gets displaced. Early detection of this complication is very important; otherwise there will be hypoxia and subcutaneous emphysema. Once the false passage has occurred, the tube is to be removed and the procedure is to be done again.

Subglottic stenosis is one of the late complications which was detected in very early days of cricothyrotomy practice and the procedure was out of practice for some time. However, later it was found that chronic subglottic stenosis was not very frequent, and it was associated with laryngotracheal pathology, prolonged time to decannulation, old age and diabetes.

Tracheostomy

Minor

- Minor bleeding
- Subcutaneous emphysema
- Cuff puncture
- Anterior passage of tube
- Mild wound infection

Intermediate

- Desaturation
- Posterior tracheal wall injury
- Conversion to surgical tracheostomy
- Abandoning procedure
- Hemorrhage requiring surgical intervention, blood transfusion, causing fall in Hb by > 2 gm%

Major

- Death
- Posterior tracheal tear
- Tracheoesophageal fistula
- Pneumothorax
- Aspiration of blood
- Intratracheal hemorrhage
- Obstruction/displacement of tube
- Sepsis
- Tracheal stenosis

The most common perioperative complication is bleeding. Although a meta-analysis of surgical and percutaneous tracheostomy has shown that perioperative complications are more common with percutaneous than surgical tracheostomy, bleeding is more commonly associated with the surgical technique. The overall complication rate ranges between 12 and 15% and majority of these are minor complications. Major complications occur in 20%.[4] Minor peristomal bleeding can be managed with local compression. Lignocaine and epinephrine injection into the soft tissues of four corners of the stomal area. Erosion of the innominate artery may cause major bleeding. This can be prevented by low placement of the tube. Rest of the complications are similar to the cricothyrotomy and likewise the basic principle of preventing them is same. Careful maintaining of the anatomical landmarks, proper fixation of the larynx, avoiding too deep insertion of the locator needle usually prevents complications like posterior tracheal injury, tracheoesophageal fistula.

CONCLUSION

A well planned airway management minimizes the requirement of surgical airway. The most difficult part for an airway manager is to pick-up the scalpel. The surgical airway established by an experienced ENT surgeon has minimum complications. All providers of surgical airway should be cognizant of their ceiling of their expertise in emergency and elective situations. Cricothyrotomy as a rescue measure is hardly employed in children as chances of injury to the larynx is high. Fourth National Audit Project (NAP4) has witnessed high rate of failure (65%) of needle cricothyrotomy in adults. Paramount important is to continue training of staffs to get accustomed with it.

BIBLIOGRAPHY

1. Aslani A, Ng S, Hurley M, McCarthy KF, McNicholas M, McCaul CL. Accuracy of identification of the cricothyroid membrane in female subjects using palpation: An observational study. Anesth Analg. 2012;114:987-92.
2. Assman NM, Wong DT, Morales E. A comparison of new indicator guided with a conventional wire guided percutaneous cricothyroidotomy device in mannequins. Anesth Analg. 2007;105:148-54.
3. Bacchetta M, Girardi L, Southard E, et al. Comparison of open versus bedside percutaneous dilatational tracheostomy in the cardiothoracic surgical patient: Outcomes and financial analysis. Ann Thorac Surg. 2005;79:1879-85.
4. Bair AE, Filbin MR, Kulkarni RG, Walls RM. The failed intubation attempt in the emergency department: analysis of prevalence, rescue techniques and personnel. J Emerg Med. 2002;23:131-40.
5. Beltrame D, Zussino M, Martinez B, et al. Percutaneous versus surgical bedside tracheostomy in the intensive care unit: a cohort study. Anesthesia. 2008;74:529-35.
6. Benkhadra M, Lenfant F, Nemetz W, Anderhuber F, Feigl G, Fasel J. A comparison of two emergency cricothyroidotomy kits in human cadavers. Anesth Analg. 2008;106:182-5.
7. Bramwell KJ, Davis DP, Cardall TV, et al. Use of trousseau dilator in cricothyrotomy. J Emerg Med. 1999;17:433-6.

8. Brantigan CO, Grow JB. Cricothyroidotomy elective use in respiratory problems requiring tracheotomy. J Thorac Cardio Vasc Surg. 1976;71:72.
9. Brofeldt BT, Panacek EA, Richards JR. An easy cricothyrotomy approach: the rapid four-step technique. Acad Emerg Med. 1996;3:1060-3.
10. Bushra JS, McNeil B, Wald DA, Schwell A, Karras DJ. A comparison of trauma intubations managed by anaesthesiologists and emergency physicians. Acad Emerg Med. 2004;11:66-70.
11. Cattano D, Abramson S, Buzzigoli S, Zoppi C, Melai E, Ginnta F, Hagberg C. The use of the laryngeal mask airway during guide wire dilating forceps tracheostomy. Anesth Analg. 2006;103:453-7.
12. Chan TC, Vilke GM, Bramwell KJ, Davis DP, Hamilton RS, Rosen P. Comparison of wire guided cricothyrotomy versus standard surgical cricothrotomy technique. J Emerg Med. 1999;17:957-62.
13. Craven RM, Vanner RG. Ventilation of a model lung using various cricothyrotomy devices. Anesthesia. 2004;59:595-9.
14. Eisenburger P, Laczica K, List M, et al. Comparison of conventional surgical versus Seldinger technique emergency cricothyrotomy performed by in experienced clinicians. Anesthesiology. 2000;92:687-90.
15. Fikkers BJ, vanVugt S, vander Hoeven JG, vanden Hoogen FJ, Matrres HA. Emergency cricothyrotomy; a randomised cross over trial comparing the wire guided and catheter over-needle techniques. Anaesthesia. 2004;59:1008-11.
16. Golzari SE, Khan ZH, Ghabili K, Hossein H, Soleimanpour H, Azarfarin R, Mahmoodpoor A, Aslanbadi S, Ansarin K. Contributions of medieval Islamic physicians to the history of tracheostomy. Anesth Analg. 2013;116:1124-32.
17. Hasio J, Pacheco-Foeler V. Cricothyroidotomy. N Eng J Med; 2008.
18. Henderson JJ, Popat MT, Latto IP, Pearce AC. Difficult airway society guidelines for management of the unanticipated difficult intubation. Anaesthesia. 2004;59:675-94.
19. Higgins K, Punthakee X. Meta-analysis: comparison of open versus percutaneous tracheostomy. Laryngoscope. 2007;117:447-54.
20. Hill C, Reardon R, Joing S. Cricothyrotomy technique using gum elastic bougie is faster than standard technique: a study of emergency medicine residents and medical students in an animal lab. Acad Emerg Med. 2010;17:666.
21. Holcroft JW, Anderson JT, Sena MJ. Shock and acute pulmonary failure in surgical patients. In : Doherty GM (Ed). Current diagnosis and treatment surgery 13th edn. McGraw Hill Companies 2010: Chapter 12.
22. Holmes JF, Panacek EA, Sakles JC, Brofeldt BT. Comparison of two cricothyrotomy techniques: standard method versus rapid four step technique. Ann Emerg Med. 1998;32:442-5.
23. Jackson C. High tracheostomy and other errors the chief cause of chronic laryngeal stenosis. Surg Gyneco Obstet. 1921;32:392.
24. Khan H,Meyers AD. Cricothyroidotomy. Emedicine.medscape.com/article/1830008-overview.
25. Kornblith LZ, Burlew CC, Moore EE, Haenel JB, Kashuk JL, Biffl WL, Barneyy CC, Johnson JL. One thousand bedside percutaneous tracheostomies in the surgical intensive care unit: time to change the gold standard. J Am Coll Surg. 2011;212:163-70.
26. Marx JA, Hockberger RS, Walls RM. Airway In: Rosen's Emergency Medicine Concepts and Clinical practice. Vol 1; 6th edn. Philadelphia: Mosby Elseveir; 2006.
27. McClelland Rm. Tracheostomy: its management and alternative. Proc R Soc Med. 1972;65:401-4.
28. Meyer M, Critchlow J, Mansharamani N, Angel LF, Garland R, Ernst A. Repeat bedside percutaneous dilatational tracheostomy is a safe procedure. Crit Care Med. 2002;30:986-8.
29. Murphy C, Rooney SJ, Maharaj CH, Laffey JG, Hate BH. Comparison of three cuffed emergency percutaneous cricothyroidotomy devices to conventional surgical cricothyroidotomy in a porcine model. BJA. 2010;106:56-64.
30. Panel D, Claudine G, Thomas P, Jean-Claude C. Percutaneous or surgical tracheostomy: A meta analysis. Critical Care Medicine. 1999;27:1617-25.
31. Sagarin MJ, Barton ED, Chng YM, Walls RM. Airway management by US and Canadian emergency medicine residents: a multicenter analysis of more than 6000 endotracheal intubation attempts. Ann Emerg Med. 2005;46:328-36.
32. Sagarin MJ, Chiang V, Sakles JC, Barton ED, Wolfe RE, Vissers RJ, et al. Rapid sequence intubation for pediatric emergency airway management. Pediatr Emerg Care. 2002;18:417-23.

33. Schaumann N, Lorenz V, Schellongowski P, Staudinger T, Locker GJ, Burgmann H, Pikula B, Hofbauer R, Schuster E, Fass M. Evaluation l of seldinger technique emergency cricothyroidotomy versus standard surgical cricothyroidotomy in 200 cadavers. Anesthesiology. 2005;102:7-11.
34. Serletis D. Paul of Aegina and Tracheostomy In: Whitelaw WA (Ed). The proceedings of the 10th Annual History of Medicine days. Calgary, AB: The Universith of Calgary; 2001.pp.26-9.
35. Strange GR, Niederman LG, Henretig FM, King C. Surgical cricothyrotomy. In Text book of Paediatric Emergency Procedures. Baltimore: Willams and Wilkins; 1997.p.351.
36. Sucrase I, Wollard M. Needle Vs surgical cricothyroidotomy: a short cut to effective ventilation. Anaesthesia. 2006;61:962-74.
37. Tigue SQ, Staber M, Hardman JG, Hendeson JJ. Emergency airway access equipment. Anaesthesia. 20004;59:505-6.
38. Vadodaria BS, Gandhi SD, McIndoe AK. Comparison of four different emergency airway access equipment sets on a human patient simulator. Anaesthesia. 2004;59:73-9.
39. Veelo DP, Dongelmans DA, Middelhoek P, Korevaar JC, Schultz MJ. Adaptive support ventilation with percutaneous dilatational tracheostomy: A clinical study. Anesth Analg. 2008;107:938-40.
40. Wong DT, Prabhu AJ, Coloma M, Imasogie N, Chung FF. What is the minimum training required for successful cricothyroidotomy? Anesthesiology. 2003;98:349-53.

How to Prepare Chest X-rays for MD/DA/DNB Examinations?

Prithwis Bhattacharyya

OBJECTIVES

1. *Technique:*
   - Learn the difference between PA vs AP chest X-ray
   - Learn the utility of a lateral decubitus chest X-ray
   - Understand the terms inspiration, penetration, and rotation as they apply to determine a technically adequate film.
2. *Anatomy:*
   - Learn the basic anatomy of the fissures of the lungs, heart borders, bronchi, and vasculature that can be seen on a chest X-ray.
3. *Interpretation:*
   - Develop a consistent and thorough technique for reading images
   - Learn how the silhouette sign can help localize pathology.
4. *Pathology:*
   - Learn the concept of atelectasis and how to recognize it on an X-ray
   - Learn how to differentiate it from pneumonia
   - Recognize how pleural effusions and pneumonia appear on chest X-ray
   - Recognize other common conditions that one is expected to meet with in day-to-day work.

Initially check the name and the date. Do this even before you put it on the screen.

Always check the technical quality of any film before interpreting it. In order to do this, one needs to examine in turn the projection, orientation, rotation, penetration and degree of inspiration. Problems with any of these can make interpretation difficult and unless one checks the technical quality carefully, one may be liable to misinterpret the film.

If one is not sure as to whether the chest X-ray is PA or AP, then one should look at the scapulae. If the scapulae overlie the lung fields, then the film is AP. If they do not it is probably PA. Check the left/right markings. On must not assume that the heart is always on the left. Dextrocardia is a possibility. However, a more common cause is that the mediastinum could have been pushed or pulled to the right by lung pathology. If in any doubt, always re-examine the patient.

The lateral view is (Fig. 1A) obtained with the left chest against the cassette. This diminishes the effect of magnification on the heart. Looking carefully at the posterior aspect of the chest on the lateral view, which ribs are left and right? Which is the right/left hemidiaphragm?

LATERAL POSITIONING

The right ribs (dotted arrows) are larger due to magnification and usually projected posterior to the left ribs if the patient was examined in a true lateral position. This can be very helpful if there is a unilateral pleural effusion seen only on the lateral view (Fig. 1B).

The left hemidiaphragm is usually lower than the right. Also, since the heart lies predominantly on the left hemidiaphragm the result on a lateral film is silhouetting out of the anterior portion of the hemidiaphragm, whereas the anterior right hemidiaphragm remains visible.

Notice how the right diaphragm (dotted arrows) continues anteriorly, while the left diaphragm disappears (black arrow) because of the silhouetting caused by the heart. Also notice how the right diaphragm at the arrow heads continues *past* the smaller left ribs and ends at the larger and more posterior right ribs (Fig. 2).

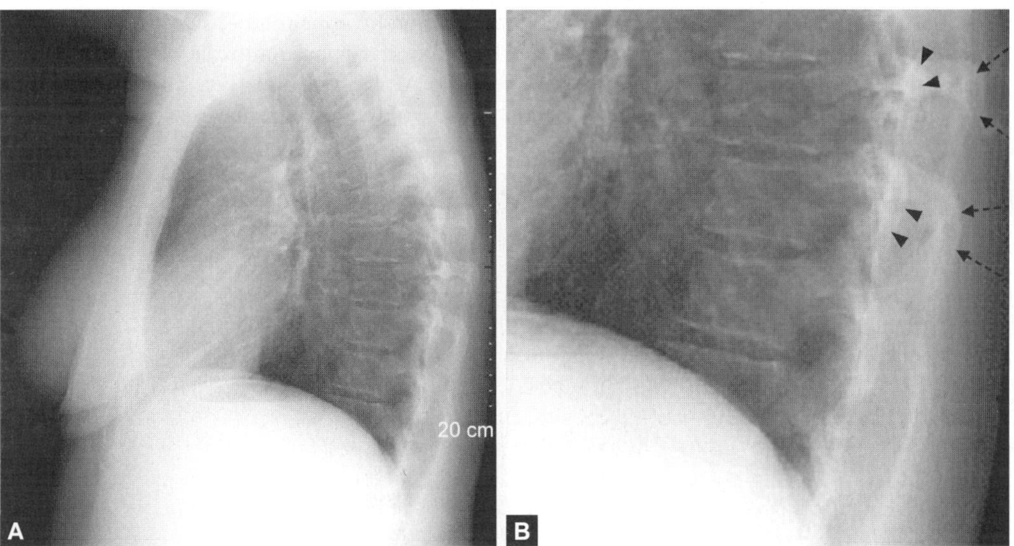

Figs 1A and B Lateral view of chest X-ray

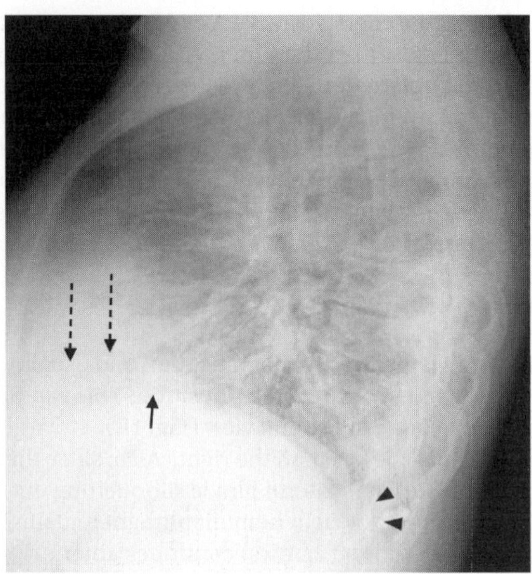

Fig. 2 The lateral view of chest X-ray to show right and left diaphragm

POSITIONING

The PA (posteroanterior) film (Fig. 3A) is obtained with the patient facing the cassette and the X-ray tube 6 feet away. This distance diminishes the effect of beam divergence and magnification of structures closer to the X-ray tube. On the film below the exam was obtained in an AP or anteroposterior position. Note that the chest has a different appearance. The heart shadow is magnified because it is an anterior structure. The pulmonary vasculature is also altered when patients are examined in the supine position. On the AP supine film (Fig. 3B), there is more equalization of the pulmonary vasculature when the size of the lower lobe vessels is compared to the upper.

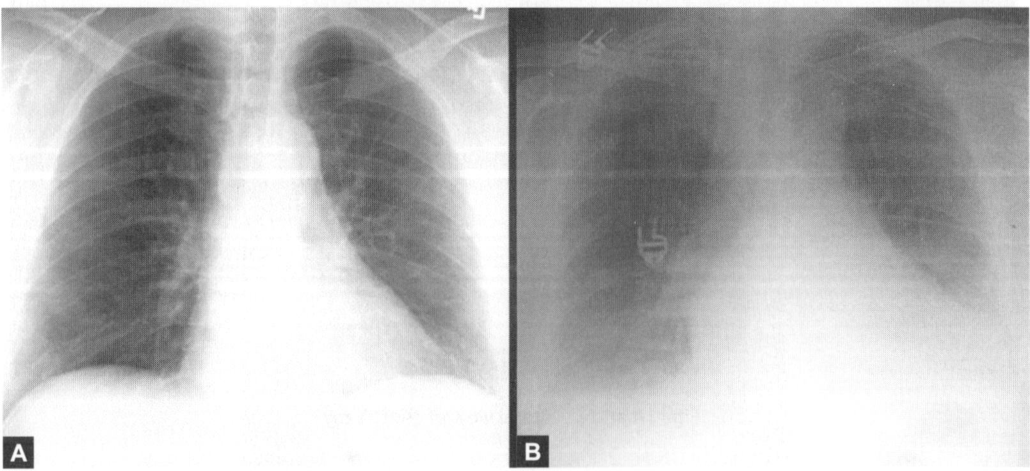

Figs 3A and B (A) PA view of chest X-ray; (B) AP view of chest X-ray

This is a PA film—the upper one compared with an AP supine film below. The AP shows magnification of the heart and widening of the mediastinum. Whenever possible the patient should be imaged in an upright PA position. AP views are less useful and should be reserved for very ill patients who cannot stand erect.

A patient can appear to have a very abnormal chest if the film is taken during expiration (Fig. 4A). The loss of the right heart border silhouette would lead one to the diagnosis of a possible pneumonia. However, the patient had taken a poor inspiration. On repeat exam with improved inspiration, the right heart border is normal (Fig. 4B).

Check that the film is technically adequate. It is very important to assess for the degree of penetration (Fig. 5).

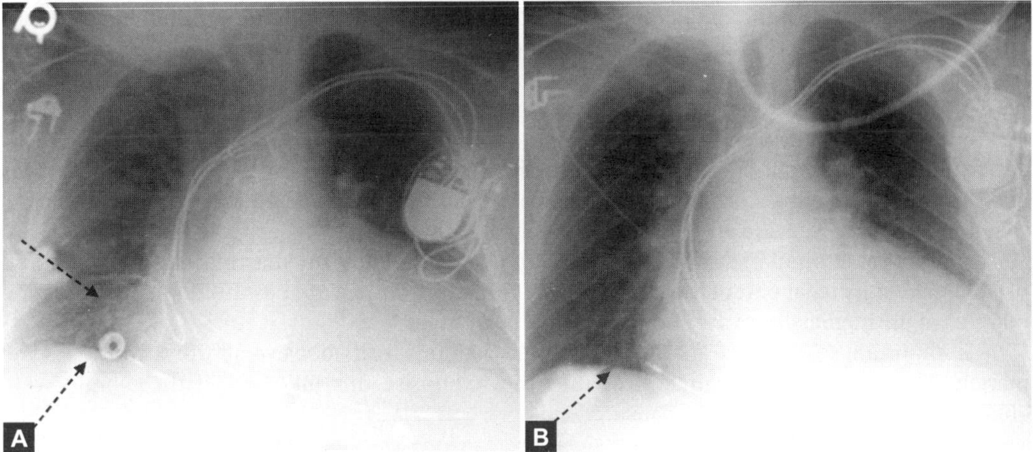

Figs 4A and B (A) Chest X-ray taken during expiration with adequate exposure of right border of heart; (B) Chest X-ray taken during inspiration showing prominent right border of heart

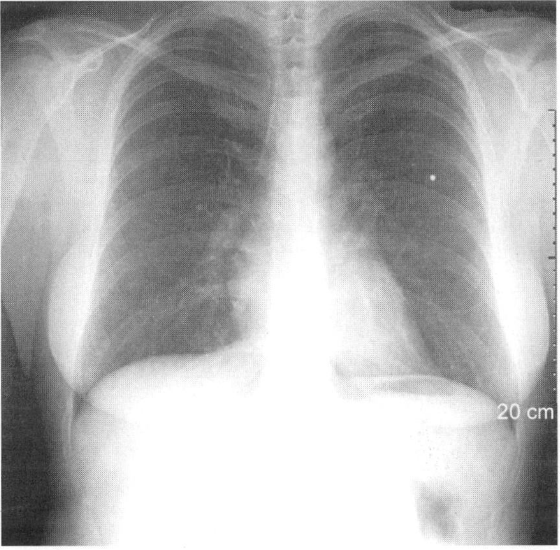

Fig. 5 PA view with sufficient penetration

Adequate penetration of the patient by radiation is also required for a good film. On a good PA film, the thoracic spine disc spaces should be barely visible through the heart but bony details of the spine are not usually seen. On the other hand penetration is sufficient that bronchovascular structures can usually be seen through the heart. If one cannot see the vertebral bodies at all, then the film is under penetrated and the lung fields will appear falsely white.

Rotation: If there is rotation of the patient, the mediastinum may look very unusual. Patient rotation can be evidenced by observing the clavicular heads and determining whether they are equal distance from the spinous processes of the thoracic vertebral bodies. If one clavicle is nearer than the other then the patient is rotated and the lung on that side will appear whiter.

To assess the film has been taken in full inspiration or not, count the number of ribs above the diaphragm. The midpoint of the right hemidiaphragm should be between the 5th and 7th ribs anteriorly. The anterior end of the 6th rib should be above the diaphragm as should the posterior end of the 10th rib. If more ribs are visible the patient is hyperinflated. If fewer are visible, the patient has not managed a full intake of breath (?due to pain/? exhaustion/?disease. This is important, as a poor inspiration will make the heart look larger, give the appearance of basal shadowing and cause the trachea to appear deviated to the right.

We need to know both the structures within the mediastinum forming the mediastinal margins and the lobes of the lungs forming the margins of the lungs along the mediastinum and chest wall (Figure 6 shows the specific anatomy of the PA chest X-ray).

If a mass or pneumonia 'silhouettes' (obscures) a part of the lung/mediastinal margin, we should be able to identify what part of the lung and what organ within the mediastinum are involved. The margins of the mediastinum are shown in Figure 7.

It is important to trace the margin of the mediastinum with your eye all the way around the margin. Think of the mediastinal structures that comprise this interface. If the margin were abnormal one could diagnose the cause.

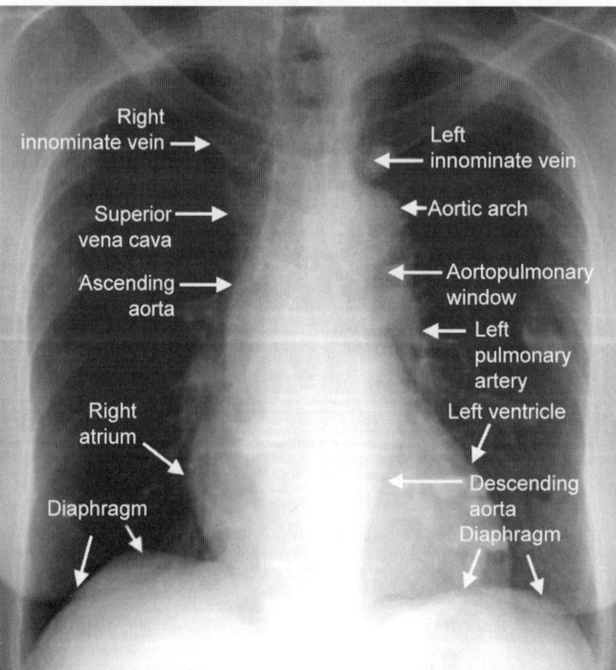

Fig. 6 The specific anatomy of the PA chest X-ray

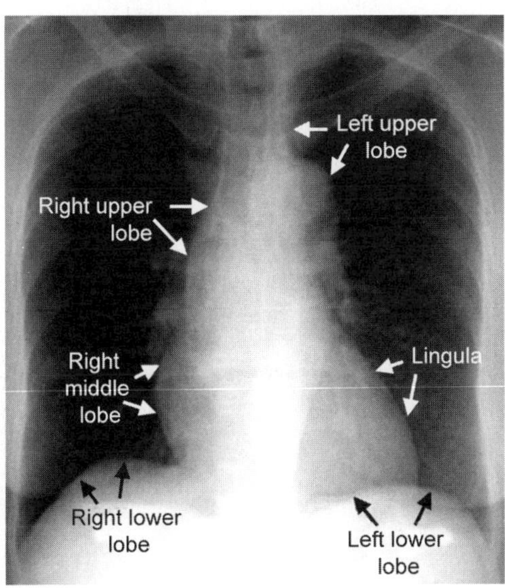

Fig. 7 The locations of each lung margin on chest X-ray

Reading the X-ray

- Turn off stray lights, optimize room lighting, view images in order
- Patient data (name, history of fracture, age, sex, old films)
- *Routine technique:* AP/PA, exposure, rotation, supine or erect
- *Trachea:* Midline or deviated, caliber, mass
- *Lungs:* Abnormal shadowing or lucency
- *Pulmonary vessels:* Artery or vein enlargement
- *Hila:* Masses, lymphadenopathy
- *Heart:* Thorax: heart width > 2:1 ? Cardiac configuration?
- *Mediastinal contour:* Width? mass?
- *Pleura:* Effusion, thickening, calcification
- *Bones:* Lesions or fractures
- *Soft tissues:* Do not miss a mastectomy
- *ICU films:* Identify tubes first and look for pneumothorax.

The silhouette sign: One of the most useful signs in chest radiology is the silhouette sign. This was described by Dr Ben Felson. The silhouette sign is in essence elimination of the silhouette or loss of lung/soft tissue interface caused by a mass or fluid in the normally air filled lung. In other words, if an intrathoracic opacity is in anatomic contact with, for example, the heart border, then the opacity will obscure that border. The sign is commonly applied to the heart, aorta, chest wall, and diaphragm. The location of this abnormality can help to determine the location anatomically.

For the heart, the silhouette sign can be caused by an opacity in the RML, lingula, anterior segment of the upper lobe, lower aspect of the oblique fissure, anterior mediastinum, and anterior portion of the pleural cavity. This contrasts with an opacity in the posterior pleural cavity, posterior mediastinum, of lower lobes which cause an overlap and not an obliteration of the heart border. Therefore, both the presence and absence of this sign is useful in the localization of pathology.

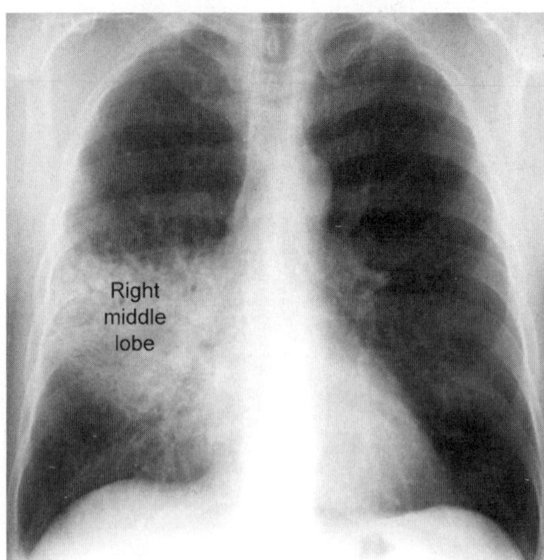

Fig. 8 Chest X-ray with silhouetted out the right border of heart

The right heart border is silhouetted out (Fig. 8).

This is caused by a pneumonia. Here we can determine which lobe the pneumonia affects.

Consolidation: Look first at the nature of the whiteness and its border. If it is univ\form with a well-demarcated border, one is more likely to be dealing with an area of collapse or a pleural effusion. If the shadowing is not uniform, and the border is not so well demarcated, the possiblilities are consolidation, fibrosis or some other infiltrative condition. It is apparent that it can be difficult to diagnose consolidation. It is important to remember the clinical history. In the presence of a temperature and signs of infection, consolidation is by far the most likely abnormality. If there is an old X-ray(s), and there is a similar whiteness, fibrosis is more likely (being a chronic condition) and, if it was not there earlier on, it might be consolidation (which is much more transient). The nature of shadowing—the alveolar spaces become filled with fluid making them appear white whereas the airways retain air (black). So, the area of consolidation, might show the small airways (black) against a white background—the 'air bronchogram'. One should also look at the distribution of the shadowing. Fluid sinks, so consolidation gets denser as one moves down the lung. Thus the shadowing in consolidation will often be denser and more clearly demarcated at its lower border.

Collapse of a lung: It is an important cause of a white lung on X-ray. When present, it indicates possible serious pathology—along with the fact that collapse of the lung leads to a loss of volume of that part of the lung and so the normal radiological landmarks will be distorted.

Right Lung Atelectasis

Right upper lobe atelectasis: Right upper lobe atelectasis (Fig. 9) is easily detected as the lobe migrates superomedially toward the apex and mediastinum. The minor fissure elevates and the inferior border of the collapsed lobe is a well demarcated curvilinear border arcing from the hilum towards the apex with inferior concavity. Due to reactive hyperaeration of the lower lobe, the lower lobe artery will often be displaced superiorly on a frontal view. Collapse of the right (or left) upper lobes will pull the trachea towards the area of collapse.

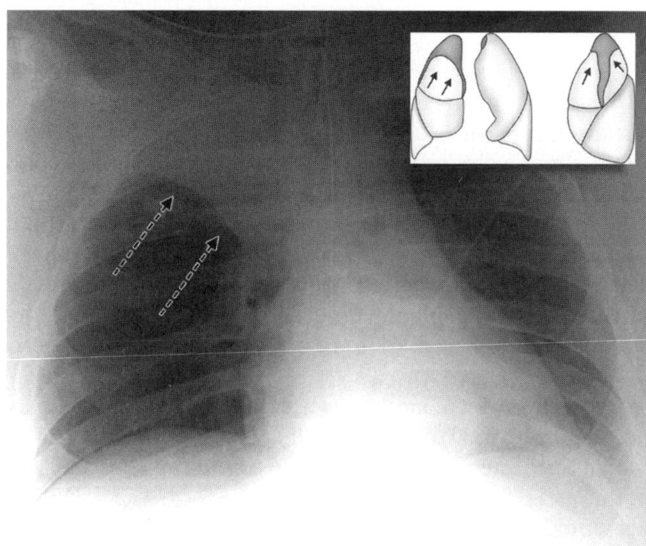

Fig. 9 The elevation of the horizontal fissure (arrows) caused by RUL atelectasis

Right middle lobe: Right middle lobe atelectasis (Figs 10A and B) may cause minimal changes on the frontal chest film. A loss of definition of the right heart border is the key finding (if the left heart border is blurred, lingular collapse is expected). Right middle lobe collapse is usually more easily seen in the lateral view. The horizontal and lower portions of the major fissures start to approximate with increasing opacity leading to a wedge of opacity pointing to the hilum. Like other cases of atelectasis, this collapse may confused with right middle lobe pneumonia.

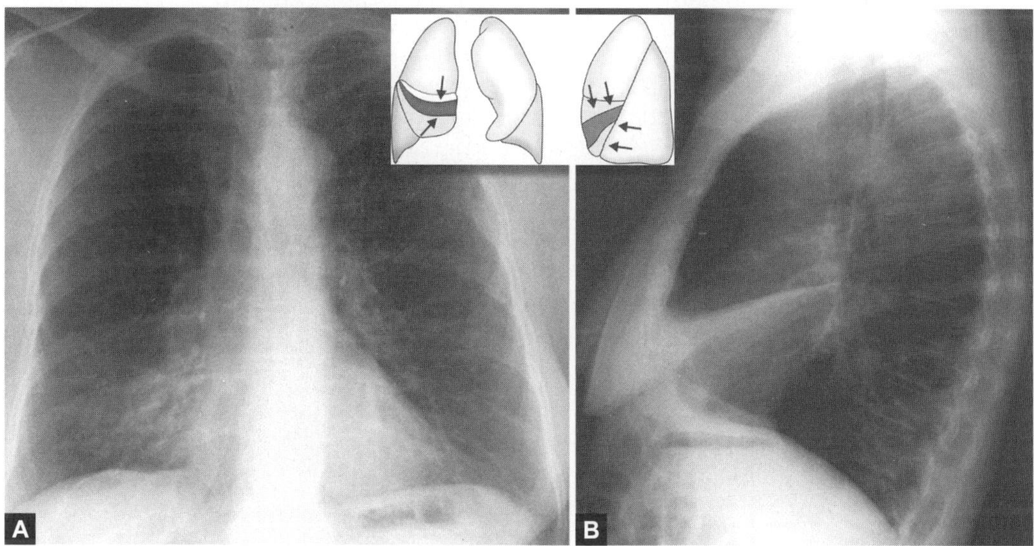

Figs 10A and B Right middle lobe atelectasis can be difficult to detect in the AP film. The right heart border is indistinct on the AP film. The lateral, though, shows a marked decrease in the distance between the horizontal and oblique fissures

Pleural Effusion

Common causes for a pleural effusion (Fig. 11) are CHF, infection (parapneumonic), trauma, PE, tumor, autoimmune disease, and renal failure.

On an upright film, an effusion will cause blunting on the lateral and if large enough, the posterior costophrenic sulci. Sometimes a depression of the involved diaphragm will occur. To differentiate an effusion from a raised hemidiaphragm, look again at the shape of the upper border of the effusion. The upper border, will peak much more laterally than one would expect the diaphragm to do. A large effusion can lead to a mediastinal shift away from the effusion and opacify the hemothorax. Approximately 200 mL of fluid are needed to detect an effusion in the frontal film vs approximately 75 mL for the lateral. About 5 liters of pleural fluid are present when there is total opacification of the hemithorax. Large effusions, especially if unilateral, are more likely to be caused by malignancy than smaller ones.

In the supine film, an effusion will appear as a graded haze that is denser at the base. The vascular shadows can usually be seen through the effusion. An effusion in the supine view can veil the lung tissue, thicken fissure lines, and if large, cause a fluid cap over the apex. There may be no apparent blunting of the lateral costophrenic sulci.

A lateral decubitis film is helpful in confirming an effusion in a bedridden patient as the fluid will layer out on the affected side (unless the fluid is loculated). Today, ultrasound is also a key component in the diagnosis. Ultrasound is also used to guide diagnostic aspiration of small effusions.

Once one has diagnosed an effusion, one should look at the X-ray for possible causes. Check the size of the heart (a large heart points to heart failure). Look at the hilum for possible enlargement. Look at the visible parts of the lung fields for obvious masses, and check the bones for signs of metastasis. Look very carefully at the apices of the lungs for tumors and tuberculosis (TB).

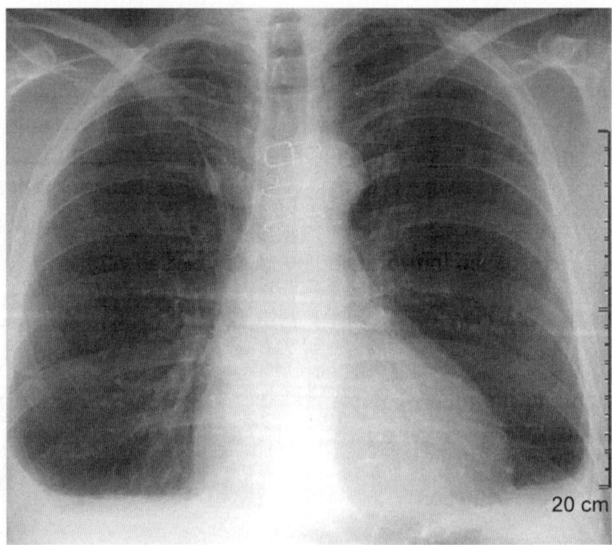

Fig. 11 Diagnosis of pleural effusion

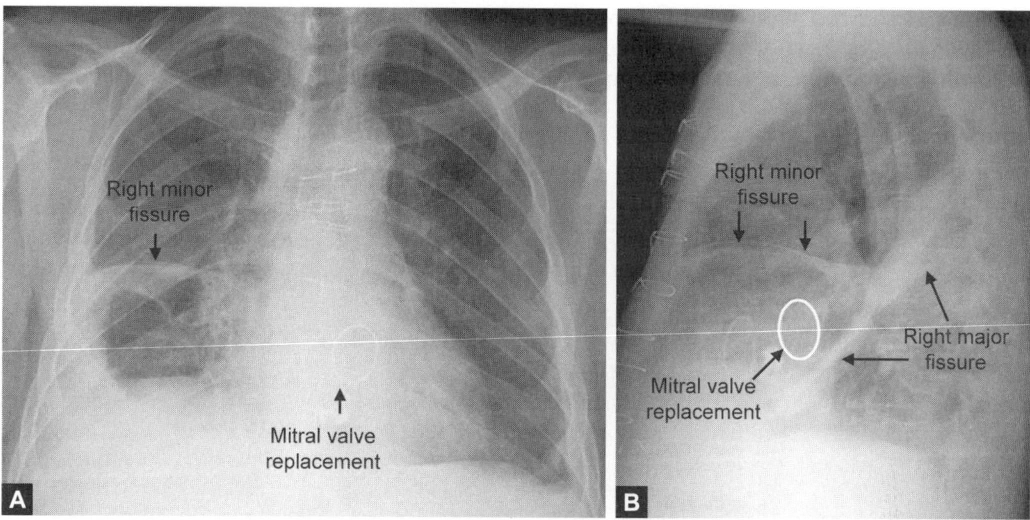

Figs 12A and B Chest X-ray showing pleural effusion expending into the fissure

The patient above has a pleural effusion extending into the fissure (Figs 12A and B). Which fissure is which?

Note: The bright loop near the center of the films.

Pneumothorax

A pneumothorax is defined as air inside the thoracic cavity but outside the lung. A spontaneous pneumothorax (PTX) is one that occurs without an obvious inciting incident. Some causes of spontaneous PTX are; idiopathic, asthma, COPD, pulmonary infection, neoplasm, Marfan's syndrome, and smoking cocaine. However, most pneumothoraces are iatrogenic and caused by a physician during surgery or central line placement. Trauma, such as a motor vehicle accident is another important cause. A tension PTX is a type of PTX in which air enters the pleural cavity and is trapped during expiration usually by some type of ball valve-like mechanism. This leads to a build-up of air increasing intrathoracic pressure. Eventually the pressure buildup is large enough to collapse the lung and shift the mediastinum away from the tension PTX. If it continues, it can compromise venous filling of the heart and even death.

On chest X-ray, a PTX appears as air without lung markings in the least dependent part of the chest. Generally, the air is found peripheral to the white line of the pleura. In an upright film this is most likely seen in the apices. A PTX is best demonstrated by an expiration film. It can be difficult to see when the patient is in a supine position. In this position, air rises to the medial aspect of the lung and may be seen as a lucency along the mediastinum. It may also collect in the inferior sulci causing a deep sulcus sign.

A hydropneumothorax is both air and fluid in the pleural space. It is characterized by an air-fluid level on an upright or decubitus film in a patient with a pneumothorax. Some causes of a hydropneumothorax are trauma, thoracentesis, surgery, ruptured esophagus, and empyema.

Figure 13 shows a right sided tension pneumothorax with right sided lucency and leftward mediastinal shift. This is a medical emergency. Failure to place a right chest tube immediately could allow venous return to diminish and lead to possible death. Chest X-ray with pneumothorax as shown in Figure 14.

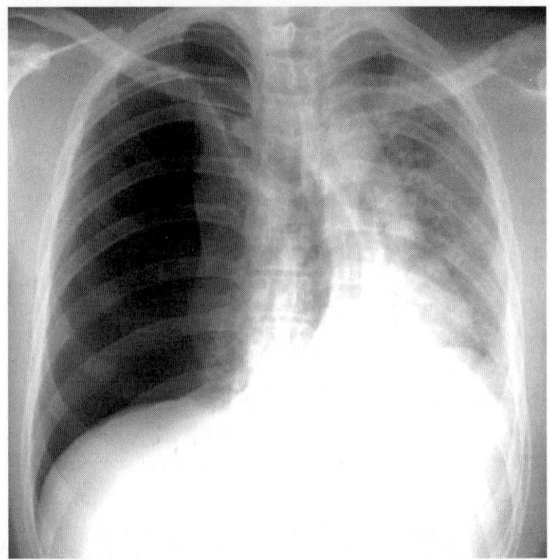

Fig. 13 Film X-ray showing right sided tension pneumothorax

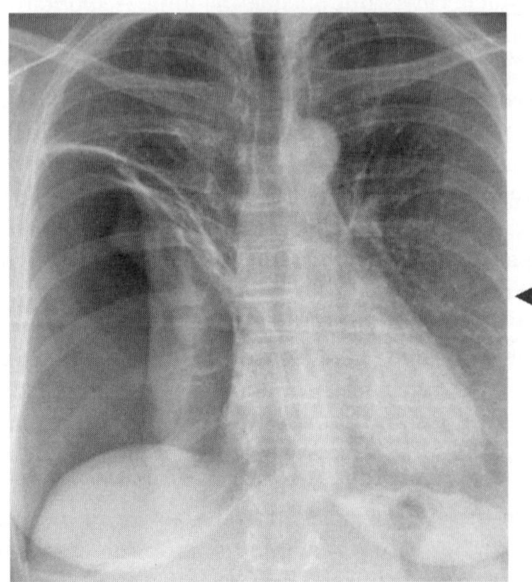

Study of the CXR

There are 3 important findings:

1. Notice that the mediastinum is slightly displaced to the left.
2. Does this mean that there is a tension pneumothorax?
3. Do you have an idea about the cause of the pneumothorax?

Fig. 14 Chest X-ray with pneumothorax

Pericardial Effusion (Fig. 15)

Pericardial effusion causes an enlarged heart shadow that is often globular shaped (transverse diameter is disproportionately increased). A 'fat pad' sign, a soft tissue stripe wider than 2 mm between the epicardial fat and the anterior mediastinal fat can be seen anterior to the heart on a lateral view. Serial films can be helpful in the diagnosis especially if rapid changes in the size of the heart shadow are observed. Approximately 400–500 mL of fluid must be in the pericardium to lead to a detectable change in the size of the heart shadow on PA chest X-ray. Pericardial effusion can be definitively diagnosed with either echocardiography or CT. It can be critical to diagnose pericardial effusion because if it is acute it may lead to cardiac tamponade, and poor cardiac filling. In the postoperative patient it could be a sign of bleeding, necessitating a return to the OR.

Patients in the ICU with bradyarrhythmias or heart block may require cardiac pacing. Transvenous pacers are introduced through the cephalic or subclavian vein into the apex of the right ventricle. Frontal and lateral projections are required to evaluate pacemaker placement. In the frontal view, the pacer tip should be at the apex with no sharp angulations throughout its length. On the lateral view, the tip should be imbedded within the cardiac trabeculae in such a way that it appears 3–4 mm beneath the epicardial fat stripe. A tip which appears beyond the epicardial fat stripe may have perforated the myocardium. Pacers placed within the coronary sinus will appear to be directed posteriorly on the lateral chest X-ray. The integrity of the pacer wire should be inspected along its entire length. Figure 16 shows single load pacer with tip in the right ventricle.

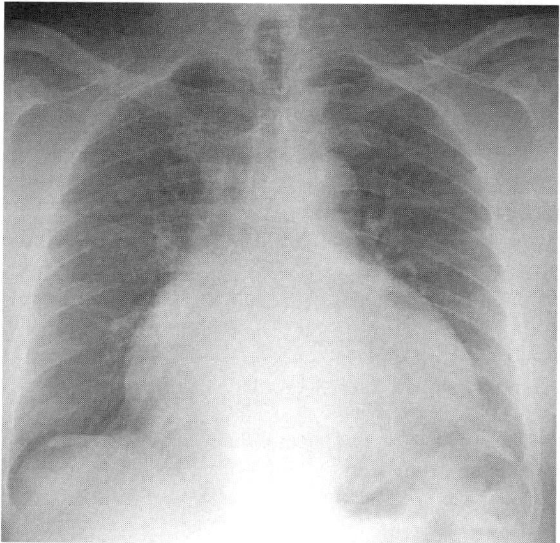

Fig. 15 PA view of a patient with a pericardial effusion

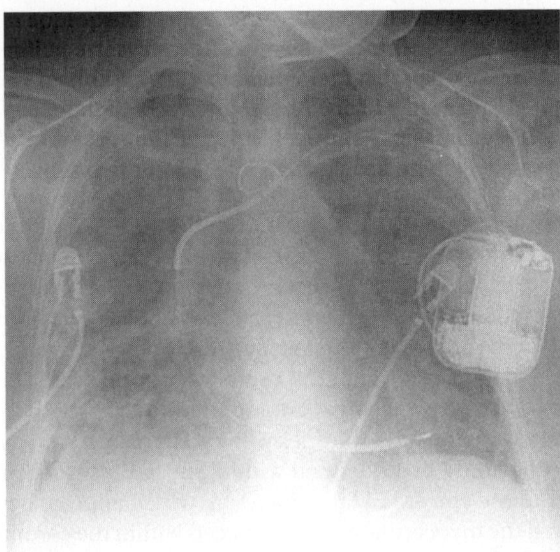

Fig. 16 Single lead pacer with tip in the right ventricle

Given that there will be many variations of the different examples given above, it important to remember the following points:

- Be aware there are many more detailed observations to learn in the future.
- Go through the various X-rays repeatedly until you understand the anatomy, and then start practicing a continuous review looking at a full frontal and lateral view.
- Many people find it helpful to talk their way through the film, the eye-brain-mouth loop does work.
- Finally look at films on a variety of normal people of all ages, sizes, and both sexes to develop a mental data base of normal references.

Practice the review sequence that works best for you until it is automatic, and then you can concentrate on the diagnostic findings.

BIBLIOGRAPHY

1. Corne J, Carroll M, Brown I, Delany D. Chest X-ray Made Easy. 1st edn. Churchill Livingstone, Singapore. 1997.
2. Spencer B Gay, Juan Olazagasti, Jack W Higginbotham, Atul Gupta, Alex Wurm, Jonathan Nguyen. Introduction to Chest Radiology. University of Virginia Health Sciences Center, Department of Radiology.

39

How to Prepare ECG for Examination of Postgraduate Students of Anesthesiology?

Sumanta Dasgupta

Must know for the students

NORMAL ECG AND THE 12-LEAD SYSTEM

The ECG is a surface recording of the electrical activity of the myocardium. It is recorded by connecting various electrodes through which electrical potentials are measured. It consists of recordings from each of the 12 electrodes on the body surface. ECG monitoring system consists of following three components:

1. Skin electrodes detect the electrical activity of the heart
2. An amplifier to boost the ECG signal
3. An oscilloscope displays the amplified signal.

BASIC ECG WAVEFORM

Figure 1 shows basic ECG

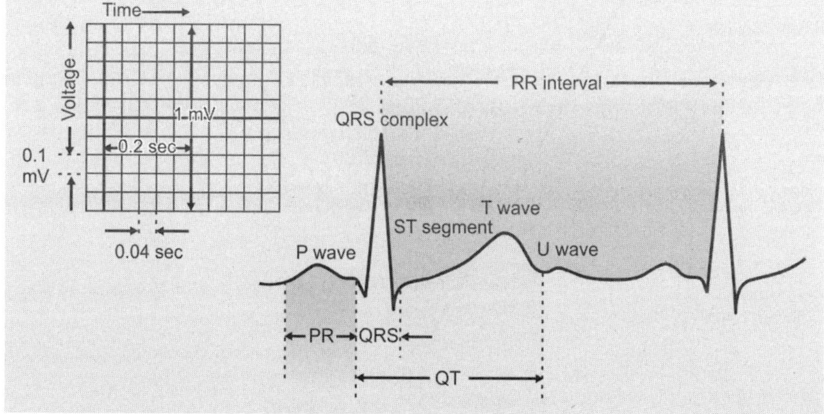

Fig. 1 Basic ECG waveform

The basic ECG waveform consists of three recognizable deflections. Einthoven named these as "P wave", "QRS complex" and "T wave". The **P wave** represents the spread of electrical activation (depolarization) through the atrial myocardium. Normally, it is a smooth, rounded deflection preceding the QRS complex.

The **QRS complex** represents the spread of electrical activation through the ventricular myocardium. The various components of the QRS complex are named on the basis of the following convention:

a. The first positive wave (above the baseline) is called r or R
b. Any second positive wave is called r' or R'
c. A negative wave that follows an r or R wave is called an s or S wave
d. A negative wave that precede an r or R wave is called a q or Q wave
e. An entirely negative wave is called a qs or QS wave
f. LARGE DEFLECTIONS are named with an appropriate CAPITAL letter and small waves with an appropriate small (lower case) letter.

The **T wave** represents electrical recovery (repolarization) of the ventricular myocardium. It is a broad, rounded wave following the QRS complex. The **U wave** may be due to slow repolarization of the papillary muscles. Some causes include: bradycardia, hypokalemia and digoxin.

DETERMINATION OF THE ELECTRICAL AXIS

The electrical axis of the heart can be derived from the six frontal plane, and leads to an accuracy of +/– 15°. The axis is measured by reference to the hexaxial reference system (Fig. 2).

Calculation of the axis requires determining the algebraic sum of the QRS deflections in each limb lead. This is done by adding the positive deflections and subtracting the negative deflections of the QRS complex in any given lead.

Follow these steps for calculating the QRS axis:

1. By inspection, find the frontal-plane lead in which the algebraic sum of the QRS complex deflections most closely approximates to zero (not necessarily the smallest QRS complex!).

   The axis will be approximately at right angles to this lead and must therefore lie in one of two approximate directions.

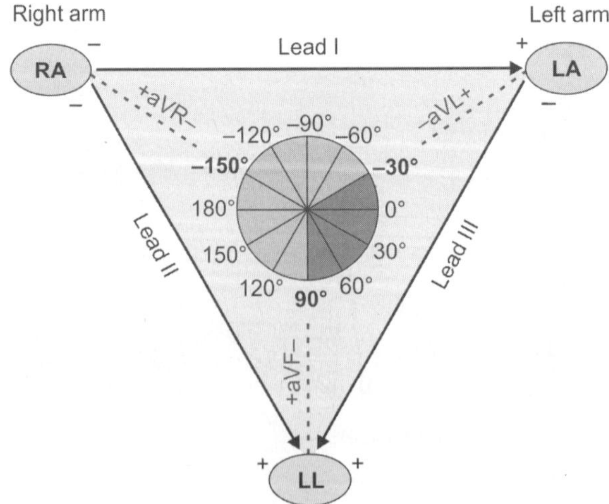

Fig. 2 Hexaxial reference system

For example, if the algebraic sum of the QRS complex deflections most closely approximates zero in lead I, then the axis must lie approximately at either –90° or +90°, which are the two directions perpendicular to lead I.

2. Now examine the QRS complex in that limb lead which occupies a position at right angles to the original lead (where the algebraic sum of the QRS deflections was close to zero), i.e. in lead aVF. If the QRS complex deflection in this lead is dominantly positive, then the QRS axis should be +90° (direction of aVF). But if predominantly negative, then the QRS axis will be –90°. The above calculation gives accuracy to the nearest 30°.
   Examples are as follows:
   a. *Normal axis: (Fig. 3)*
      - Lead aVF is the isoelectric lead
      - The two perpendiculars to aVF are 0° and 180°
      - Lead I is positive (i.e. orientated to the left)
      - Therefore, the axis has to be 0°.
   b. Axis in the left axis deviation (LAD) range (Fig. 4):
      - Lead aVR is the smallest and isoelectric lead
      - The two perpendiculars are –60° and +120°
      - Leads II and III are mostly negative (i.e. moving away from the + left leg)
      - The axis, therefore, is –60°.
   c. Axis in the right axis deviation (RAD) range (Fig. 5):
      - Lead aVR is closest to being isoelectric (slightly more positive than negative)
      - The two perpendiculars are –60° and +120°.
      - Lead I is mostly negative; lead III is mostly positive.
      - Therefore, the axis is close to +120°. Because aVR is slightly more positive, the axis is slightly beyond +120° (i.e. closer to the positive right arm for aVR).

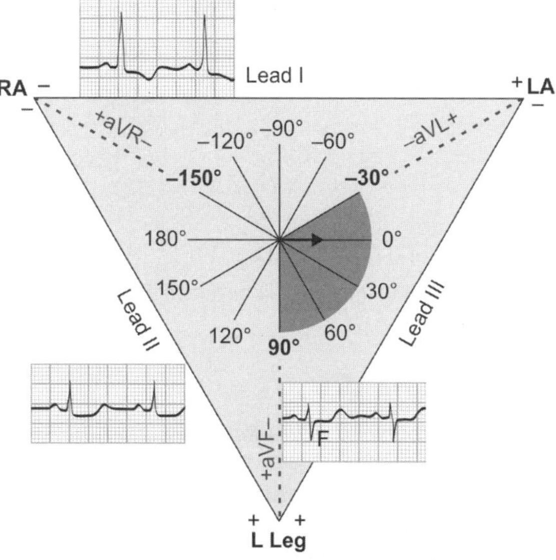

Fig. 3 Normal axis

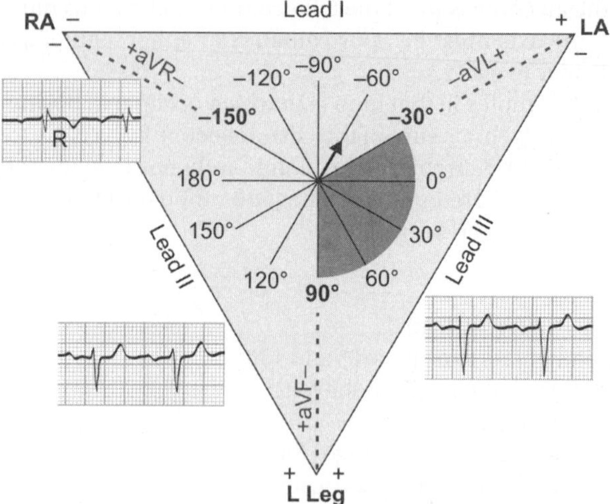

Fig. 4 Axis in the left axis deviation (LAD) range

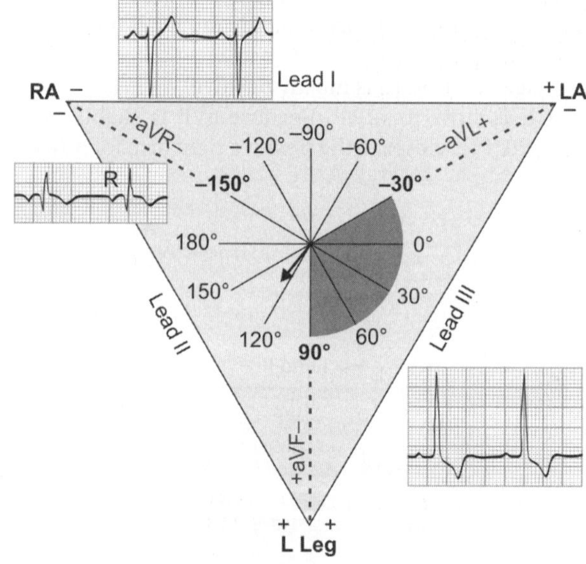

Fig. 5 Axis in the right axis deviation (RAD) range

NORMAL RHYTHM OF THE HEART

The heart is said to be in sinus rhythm based on the following criteria:

- P waves must be present and be regular
- P wave frequency should be within the range of 60–100 per min
- There must be one P wave for each QRS complex
- The P wave must precede each QRS complex
- The PR interval must be normal and constant.

Cardiac Dysrrhythmias

Dysrrhythmia is defined as abnormality of cardiac rate, rhythm or conduction which can be either lethal (sudden cardiac death), or symptomatic (syncope, near syncope, dizziness, or palpitations) or asymptomatic.[1] Cardiac arrhythmias are the most frequent perioperative cardiovascular abnormalities in patients undergoing both cardiac and noncardiac surgery. The occurrence of arrhythmias has been reported in 70.2% of patients subjected to general anesthesia for various surgical procedures.

Factors

1. *Patient specific*
   - *Pre-existing heart disease:* IHD, hypertensive heart disease, valvular heart disease, ventricular dilatation
   - *Old age:* Most common form of arrhythmia in perioperative setting is atrial fibrillation.
   - *Children:* Due to vagal predominance
   - Injury to cervical spine and upper dorsal spine, patient with subarachnoid hemorrhage.
2. *Anesthesia related factors:*
   - *General anesthesia:*
     - *Volatile anesthetics:* Halothane, enflurane may lead to increased chance of re-entrant tachyarrhythmia.
     - *Ketamine, pancuronium:* Tachycardia, increased sympathomimetic activities
     - *Opioids, vecuronium:* Bradycardia
   - *Local anesthesia:* Overdose and direct intravascular absorption
   - *Central neuraxis blockade:* Bradyarrhythmia
   - Hypoxia, hypercarbia, acidosis, hypothermia
   - Electrolyte imbalance
   - Inadequate depth of anesthesia, analgesia
   - Central venous cannulation, direct laryngoscopy may lead to both sympathetic and parasympathetic overactivity
   - *Drugs:* Adrenaline, atropine, neostigmine, β-blocker, vasoactives and inotropes.
3. *Surgery related:*
   - *Cardiac surgery:* Manipulation of heart
   - *Noncardiac surgery:* Traction of peritoneum, viscera, pneumoperitonium, thoracic surgery, carotid surgery, dental surgery.

MECHANISM OF GENESIS OF DYSRRHYTHMIA

Pathogenesis

1. Injury or damage to the cardiac conduction systems (various heart block and conduction defects)
2. *Re-entry:* Re-entry is a mechanism that may precipitate a wide variety of supraventricular and ventricular arrhythmias; even severe bradyarrhythmia may promote latent re-entrant tachyarrhythmia.
3. *Automaticity:* Abnormal depolarization of atrial or ventricular muscle cell during the periods of action potential can lead to arrhythmias (e.g. sinus tachyarrhythmia).
4. *Ectopic foci/irritable foci:* For exampe, JET, MET).

Action Plan—when Faced with an Abnormal Rhythm on the ECG Monitor

- Check the airway is patent
- Check the patient is breathing adequately or is being ventilated correctly
- Listen for equal air entry into both lungs
- Circulation—check pulse, blood pressure, and oxygen saturation. Is there any hemodynamic compromise?
- Does the abnormal rhythm on the monitor match the pulse that you can feel?
- Consider the following:
  - Increase the inspired oxygen concentration
  - Reduce the inspired volatile agent concentration
  - Ensure that ventilation is adequate to prevent CO_2 build up. Check end tidal CO_2 where this measurement is available
- Consider what the surgeon is doing—is this the cause of the problem? For example, traction on the peritoneum or eye causing a vagal response. If so ask them to stop while you treat the arrhythmia.

  If the arrhythmia is causing hemodynamic instability, rapid recognition and treatment is required. However, many abnormal rhythms encountered in everyday practice will respond to the above basic measures—sometimes even before identification of the exact rhythm abnormality is possible.

Practical Interpretation of Arrhythmias

When interpreting arrhythmias a paper strip is often easier to read than an ECG monitor. Where this is not possible from the theater monitor it may be possible to obtain a paper trace by connecting a defibrillator, most of which have a facility for printing a rhythm strip. The following basic points should be considered:

Examining an ECG strip:

1. *What is the ventricular rate? Arrhythmias may be classified as fast or slow:*
   - Tachyarrhythmias—rate greater than 100/min
   - Bradyarrhythmias—rate less than 60/min
   - Calculate approximate ventricular rate
2. *Is the QRS complex of normal duration or widened? Arrhythmias may be due to abnormal impulses arising from the:*
   - Atria = a supraventricular ryhthm
   - AV node = a nodal or junctional rhythm
   - Or the ventricles = a ventricular arrhythmia

   Supraventricular and nodal rhythms arise from a focus above the ventricles. Since the ventricles still depolarize via the normal His-Purkinje system the QRS complexes are of normal width (< 0.1 sec—2.5 small squares)—and are therefore termed 'narrow complex' rhythms. Arrhythmias arising from the ventricles will be 'broad complex' with a QRS width of >0.1sec. The QRS complexes are widened in these patients since depolarization is via the ventricular muscle rather than the His-Purkinje system and takes longer. In a few cases where there is an abnormal conduction pathway from atria to ventricles a supraventricular rhythm may have broad complexes. This is called 'aberrant conduction'.
3. *Is the QRS regular or irregular?*

   The presence of an irregular rhythm will tend to suggest ectopic beats (either atrial or ventricular), atrial fibrillation, atrial flutter with variable block or second degree heart block with variable block.

4. *Are there P waves present and are they normally shaped?*
   The presence of P waves indicates that the atria have depolarized and gives a clue to the likely origin of the rhythm. Absent P waves associated with an irregular ventricular rhythm suggest atrial fibrillation whilst a saw tooth pattern of P waves is characteristic of atrial flutter. If the P waves are upright in leads II and AVF they have originated from the sinoatrial node. However, if the P waves are inverted in these leads, it indicates that the atria are being activated in a retrograde direction, i.e. the rhythm is junctional or ventricular.
5. *How is atrial activity related to ventricular activity?*
   Normally, there will be one P wave per QRS complex. Any change in this ratio indicates a blockage to conduction at some point in the pathway from the atria to the ventricles.

A Systematic Approach to ECG Interpretation

Like the physical examination, it is desirable to follow a standardized sequence of steps in order to avoid missing subtle abnormalities in the ECG tracing, some of which may have clinical importance. The following order may be helpful:

1. *Documentation:* Any ECG record should include the name of the patient and the date and time it was recorded.
2. *Calibration signal:* The amplifier gain is normally adjusted so that a 1 millivolt signal through the ECG amplifier results in a vertical deflection of 10 mm (two large ECG squares). All voltage measurements on the ECG depend entirely on the accuracy of this calibration signal, (The paper speed is 25 mm/s, which amounts to 0.04 s per small box on the horizontal axis).
3. *Recording quality:* Look for any baseline drift (which makes ST segment analysis impossible), skeletal muscle interference (seen as sharp, irregular, spiky waves throughout the recording, e.g. during shivering) or mains frequency interference (seen as regular sine wave oscillation with a frequency of 50 Hz).
4. *Measurements:*
   a. *Heart rate:* Can be calculated easily from the ECG paper itself. Because ECG paper moves at a standardized rate of 25 mm/s, the vertical lines can be used to measure time. There is a 0.20 s interval between two of the large lines. Therefore, if you count the number of heart beats (QRS complexes) in between 30 large boxes (6 s) and multiply by 10, you have beats per minute. Conveniently, ECG paper usually has special markings every 3 s, so you do not have to count 30 large boxes.
      There is, however, an easier and quicker way to estimate the heart rate. As seen in the diagram below, when QRS complexes are one box apart, the rate is 300 bpm. Two boxes apart... 150 bpm, etc. So if you memorize these simple numbers, you can estimate the heart rate at a glance!
   b. *PR interval:* 0.12–0.20 s
   c. *QRS duration:* 0.06–0.10 s
   d. *Corrected QT interval (QTc):* Normal QTc = 0.40 s
      Bazett's formula: QTc = QT/RR1/2 (in seconds) $QTc = \frac{QT}{\sqrt{RR}}$
   e. *Frontal plane QRS Axis:* +90° to –30° (in the adult)
5. *Rhythm:* Normal sinus rhythm or any abnormalities present
6. *Morphological information:* It gives information about the physical condition of the heart. This information is contained in the P waves, QRS complexes, ST segments and T waves. The waves should be studied in both the limb and precordial leads, as discussed above.
7. *Comparison with previous ECG:* The present ECG should be compared with any previous ones in the patient's notes, to see if any significant changes have occurred. These changes may have important implications for clinical management decisions.

Note: Horizontal and vertical heart:

- Mean frontal plane QRS axis is between 0° to –30°, heart is said to be horizontal
- Mean frontal plane QRS axis is between +60° to +90°, the heart is said to be vertical.

Classification of Arrhythmias

Arrhythmias may be divided into narrow complex and broad complex for the purpose of rapid recognition and management.

Narrow Complex Rhythms

- Sinus arrhythmia
- Sinus tachycardia
- Sinus bradycardia
- Junctional/AV nodal tachycardia
- Atrial tachycardia, atrial flutter
- Atrial fibrillation
- Atrial ectopics.

Broad Complex Rhythms

- Ventricular ectopics
- Ventricular tachycardia
- Supraventricular tachycardia with aberrant conduction
- Ventricular fibrillation.

Narrow Complex Arrhythmias

1. *Sinus arrhythmia:* This is irregular spacing of normal complexes associated with respiration. There is a constant P-R interval with beat-to-beat change in the R-R interval. It is a normal finding especially in young people.
2. *Sinus tachycardia (Fig. 6):* There is a rate greater than 100/min in adults. Normal P-QRS-T complexes are evident. Causes include:
   Inadequate depth of anesthesia, pain/surgical stimulation, fever/sepsis, hypovolemia, anemia, heart failure, thyrotoxicosis, and drugs, e.g. atropine, ether, ketamine, catecholamines.
   Management: Correction of any underlying cause where possible. Beta-blockers may be useful if tachycardia causes myocardial ischemia in patients with ischemic heart disease, but should be avoided in asthma and used with caution in patients with heart failure.
3. *Sinus bradycardia (Fig. 7):* This is defined as a heart rate of less then 60 beats/minute in an adult. It may be normal in athletic patients and may also be due to vagal stimulation during surgery.

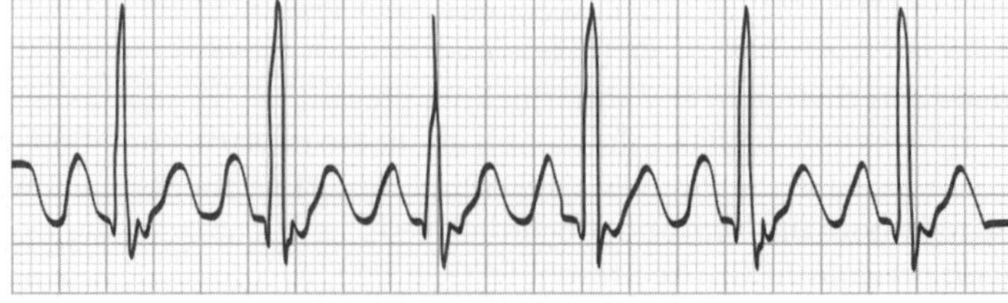

Fig. 6 Sinus tachycardia

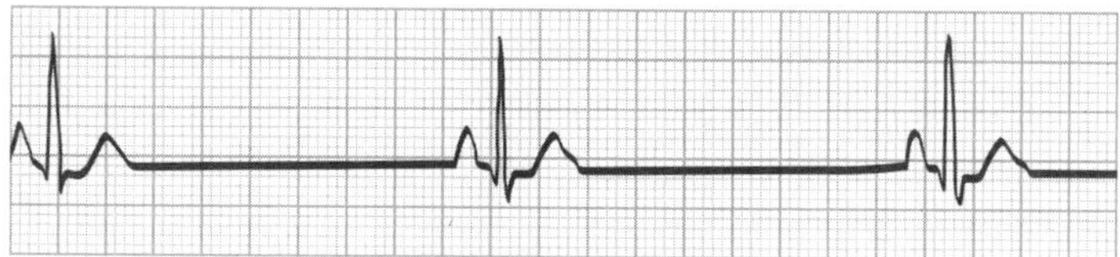

Fig. 7 Sinus bradycardia

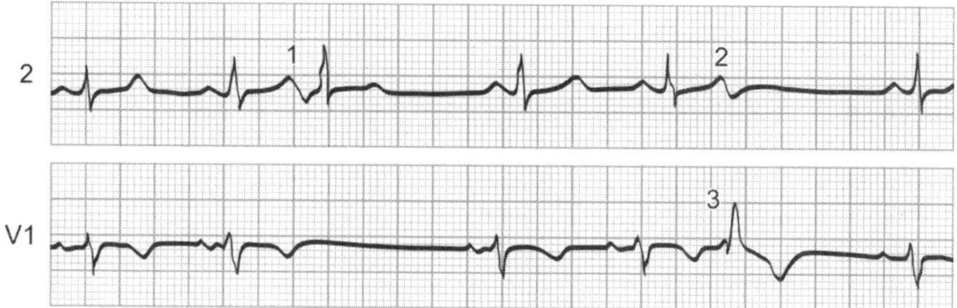

Fig. 8 Premature atrial complexes

Other causes include drugs, e.g. beta-blockers, digoxin, anticholinesterase drugs, halothane, second dose of suxamethonium (occasionally first dose in children), myocardial infarction, sick sinus syndrome, raised intracranial pressure, hypothyroidism and hypothermia.

Management: It is often not necessary to correct a sinus bradycardia in a fit young person, unless the rate is less than 45–50 beats per minute, and/or there is hemodynamic compromise. However consider:

- Correcting the underlying cause, e.g. stop the surgical stimulus
- Atropine up to 20 mcg/kg IV or glycopyrrolate 10 mcg/kg IV (Atropine works more rapidly and is usually given in doses of 300–400 mcg and repeated if required).
- Patients on beta-blockers may be resistant to atropine—occasionally an isoprenaline infusion may be required. Alternatively, glucagon (2–10 mg) can be used in addition to atropine.

4. *Premature atrial complexes (PACs) (Fig. 8):* These may occur as single or repetitive events and may be unifocal or multifocal in origin. The premature P wave (P' wave) differs in contour from the normal sinus wave, which is usually followed by a normal QRST sequence. The PR interval is normal or prolonged because the AV junction is often partially refractory when the premature impulse enters it.

PACs may have three different outcomes:

1. *Normal conduction:* Similar to normal QRS complexes in the ECG.
2. *Nonconducted:* No QRS complex because the PAC meets the AV node when still refractory.
3. *Conducted with aberration:* The PAC makes it into the ventricles but finds one or more of the conducting fascicles or bundle branches refractory, hence the resulting QRS is usually wide.

The pause after a PAC is usually incomplete, i.e. the PAC usually enters the sinus node and resets its timing, causing the next sinus P to appear earlier than expected (premature ventricular complexes, by contrast, are usually followed by a complete pause because they do not usually disturb the sinus node).

Clinical significance: PACs are commonly seen during anesthesia and during the postoperative period. Not uncommonly, they may be misdiagnosed as AV junctional premature beats, ventricular premature beats or sinus arrest.

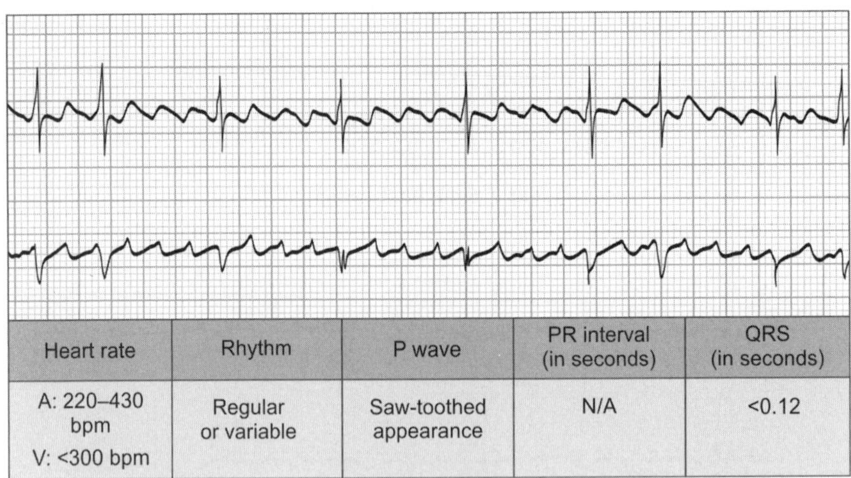

Heart rate	Rhythm	P wave	PR interval (in seconds)	QRS (in seconds)
A: 220–430 bpm V: <300 bpm	Regular or variable	Saw-toothed appearance	N/A	<0.12

Fig. 9 Atrial flutter

5. *Atrial flutter:* The ECG features of atrial flutter are (Fig. 9):
   - An atrial rate between 250-350 bpm
   - A saw-tooth appearance (F waves) is seen in leads II, III, aVF and V1. Variable degrees of AV block is seen (2:1 being more common).

Clinical Significance

- Atrial flutter usually results from a re-entrant circuit located totally within the atrial wall
- It is generally associated with heart disease, e.g. rheumatic heart disease (with mitral stenosis)
- 1:1 ventricular conduction may compromise cardiac output significantly
- Hemodynamic compromise may warrant electrical cardioversion
- Digitalis is very effective in slowing ventricular rate, while β-blockers or verapamil slow the ventricular rate and sometimes revert it to sinus rhythm.

Management

- This arrhythmia is very sensitive to synchronized direct current cardioversion—there is a nearly 100% success rate. Therefore in the anesthetized patient with any degree of cardiovascular compromise this should be the first line treatment
- Carotid sinus massage and adenosine will slow AV conduction and reveal the underlying rhythm and block where there is doubt
- Other drug treatment is as for atrial fibrillation.

6. *Atrial fibrillation (AF):* The ECG features of atrial fibrillation (Fig. 10) include:
   - Rapid, irregular fibrillating atrial waves (f waves) at a rate of 300–600 bpm, best seen in leads II, III, aVF and V1. Numerous microentry circuits within the atrial muscle probably cause the fibrillation
   - Ventricular rate is irregularly irregular, with a rate of 140–200 bpm due to a certain degree of AV block, which is always present
   - The differential diagnosis includes atrial flutter with an irregular ventricular response and multifocal atrial tachycardia, which is usually irregularly irregular.

Clinical Significance

- AF is usually associated with chronic heart disease (valvular, myocardial or pericardial)

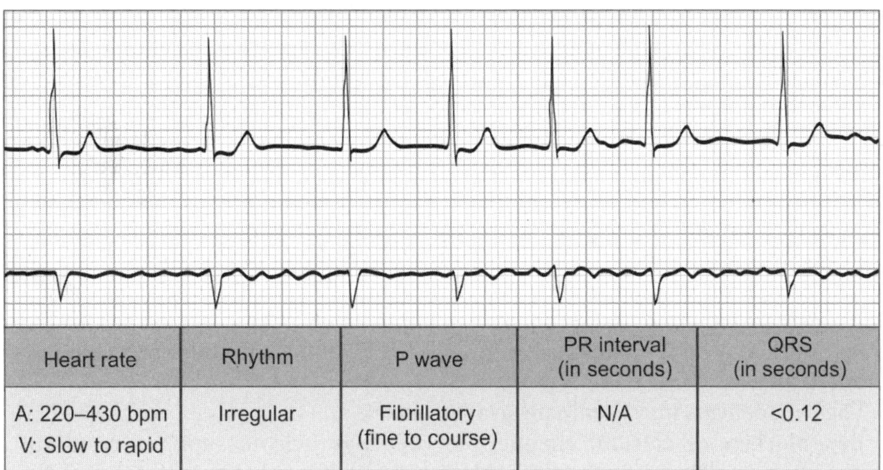

Heart rate	Rhythm	P wave	PR interval (in seconds)	QRS (in seconds)
A: 220–430 bpm V: Slow to rapid	Irregular	Fibrillatory (fine to course)	N/A	<0.12

Fig. 10 Atrial fibrillation

- Also seen in hyperthyroidism, pulmonary embolism and chronic lung disease
- Electrical cardioversion may be required in the acute setting with hemodynamic compromise.

Management

Acute AF—occuring in theater or of recent onset (less than 48 hours):

- Correction of precipitating factors where possible, especially correction of electrolyte disturbances.
- Synchronized DC cardioversion—for recent onset AF. If AF has been present for more than several hours there is a risk of arterial embolization unless the patient is anticoagulated. Shock at 200 J then at 360 J.
- Digoxin can be used acutely to slow the ventricular rate—in the presence of a normal plasma potassium concentration. An intravenous loading dose of 500 mcg in 100 mL of saline over 20 minutes may be given and repeated at intervals of 4–8 hours if necessary until a total of 1–1.5 mg has been given. This is contraindicated if the patient is already taking digoxin when lower doses are required. There is no evidence that digoxin is useful for converting AF to sinus rhythm or maintaining sinus rhythm once established.
- Amiodarone may be used to restore sinus rhythm—it is especially useful in paroxysmal atrial fibrillation associated with critical illness, and where digoxin or beta-blockers cannot be used. A loading dose of 300 mg IV via a central vein is given over 1 hour and then followed by 900 mg over 23 hours.
- Verapamil 5–10 mg slowly IV over 2 minutes can be used to control the ventricular rate. Where there is no impairment of left ventricular function or coronary artery disease, the subsequent administration of flecainide 50–100 mg slowly IV may restore sinus rhythm. However, flecainide should only be used where the arrhythmia is life-threatening and no other options are open. It should be avoided if left ventricular function is poor or there is evidence of ischemia.
- Beta-blockers are sometimes used to control the ventricular rate but may precipitate heart failure in the presence of an impaired myocardium, thyrotoxicosis or calcium channel blockers, and should be used with caution.

7. *Paroxysmal supraventricular tachycardia (PSVT):* These arrhythmias occur due to circus movements, thus utilizing the mechanism of re-entry. The onset and resolution are sudden and usually initiated by a premature beat, thus the term "paroxysmal." They are generally narrow-QRS tachycardias (unless there is pre-existing bundle branch block or aberrant ventricular conduction). There are several types of PSVT, depending on the location of the re-entry circuit.
   a. *AV nodal re-entrant tachycardia (AVNRT):* This is the most common form of PSVT accounting for approximately 50% of all symptomatic PSVTs. It is the most common cause of SVT in patients with structurally normal hearts (Fig. 11). The following features accompany it:
      - ECG shows normal regular QRS complexes with a rate of 140–240 bpm.
      - QRS complexes may sometimes show typical bundle branch block/aberration.
      - P waves are either not visible or are seen immediately before or after the QRS complex.
      - An attack may be spontaneously triggered but exertion, tea, coffee or alcohol may trigger an AVNRT.
      - Vagal maneuvers may terminate an acute attack.
      - Beta-blockers or calcium channel blockers may help to suppress recurrent attacks. The diagram illustrates the probable mechanism involving dual AV nodal pathways, alpha and beta, with different electrical properties. In the diagram, alpha is a fast AV nodal pathway with a long refractory period (RP), and beta is the slow pathway with a short RP. During sinus rhythm, alpha is always used because it conducts faster. An early PAC, however, finds alpha still refractory and must use the slower beta pathway to reach the ventricles. By the time it traverses beta, however, alpha has recovered, allowing retrograde conduction back to the atria. The retrograde P wave (called anatrial echo, for obvious reasons) is often simultaneous with the QRS and, therefore, not seen on the ECG, but it can re-enter the AV junction because of beta's short RP.
   b. *AV reciprocating tachycardia (extranodal bypass pathway):* This is the second most common form of PSVT and is seen in patients with Wolff-Parkinson-White (WPW) syndrome.

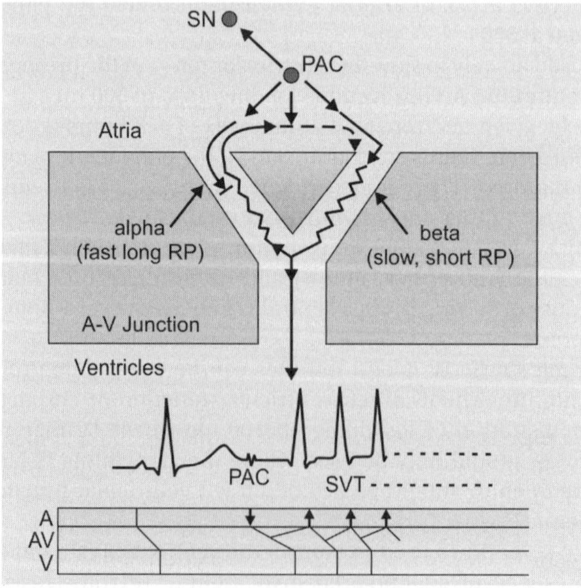

Fig. 11 AV nodal re-entrant tachycardia

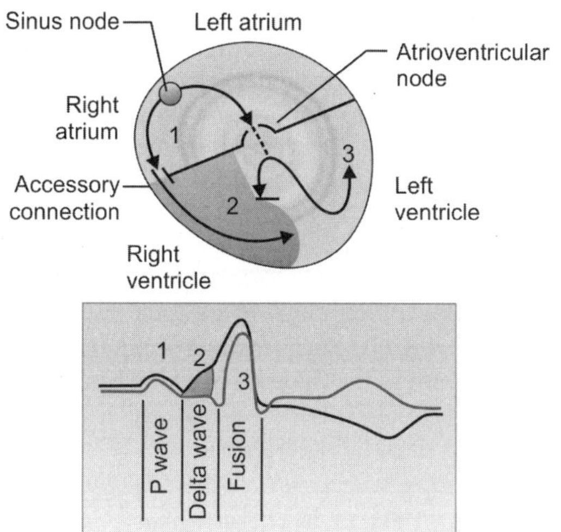

Fig. 12 AV reciprocating tachycardia

The WPW ECG, seen in the diagram, shows a short PR, delta wave and a somewhat widened QRS (Fig. 12).

8. *Junctional arrhythmias (Figs 13 and 14)*
   a. *Junctional rhythm:* This occurs when the sinus rate is slowed or when the junctional pacemaker increases its firing rate. The normal junctional pacemaker discharge rate is 40–60 bpm. Depending upon whether the conduction from the junctional pacemaker is anterograde or retrograde, inverted "P" waves (inferior leads) may be seen preceding, following or coinciding with the QRS complex. The QRS complex will be identical to that resulting from normal sinus conduction because the origin of firing is above the bundle branch divisions
   Clinical significance: Junctional rhythms occur commonly under anesthesia, especially using halogenated agents. This may cause a fall in cardiac output and blood pressure, and may need treatment with an anti-cholinergic agent or vasopressor.
   b. *AV nodal tachycardia:* This is manifested as a:
      - Passive escape rhythm with a rate of 70–140 bpm, or as a
      - Paroxysmal junctional tachycardia with a rate of 150–200 bpm
      - The P waves may occur before, within or after the QRS complexes, or be unrelated to it.
      - The QRS complex is usually narrow (may be wide with a bundle branch block).

Clinical significance: This arrhythmia is relatively common under halothane anesthesia. It rarely requires treatment. In patients receiving digitalis, this arrhythmia may represent digitalis toxicity.

Management: This arrhythmia may be associated with severe circulatory disturbance and needs to be managed as an emergency if it occurs during anesthesia.

- In the presence of hypotension, especially where the patient is anesthetized in theater, the first line treatment is synchronized direct current cardioversion with 200–360 joules.
- *Carotid Sinus Massage:* This rarely converts to sinus rhythm but slows the rate and will reveal the underlying rhythm if there is any doubt. It is helpful in differentiating it from atrial flutter and fast atrial fibrillation (The carotid sinus is a small dilatation of the proximal part of the internal carotid artery at the level of the superior border of the thyroid cartilage. It is vagally innervated and is involved in the control mechanism for causing a fall in heart rate and cardiac

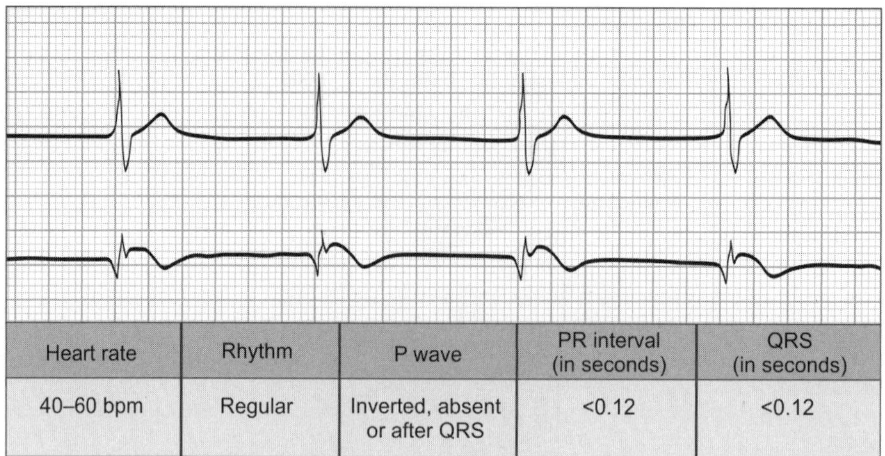

Heart rate	Rhythm	P wave	PR interval (in seconds)	QRS (in seconds)
40–60 bpm	Regular	Inverted, absent or after QRS	<0.12	<0.12

Fig. 13 Junctional rhythm

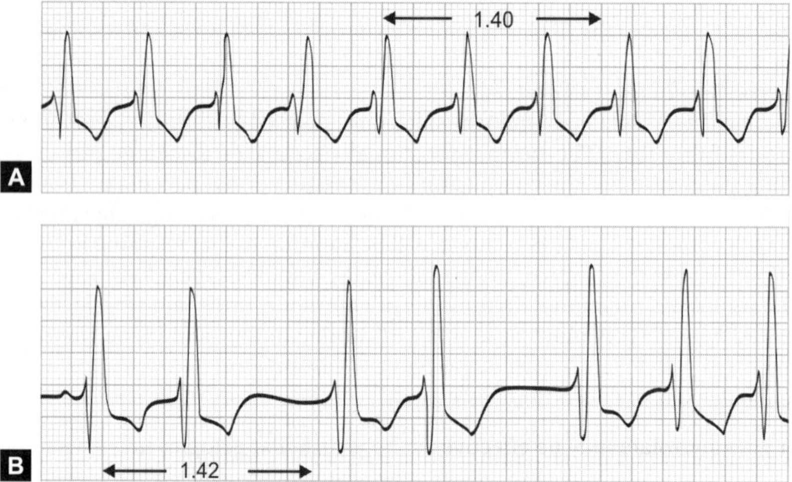

Figs 14A and B Diagnosis—digitalis intoxication: (A) Junctional tachycardia; (B) Junctional tachycardia with exit block

output in response to a rise in arterial pressure. Gentle pressure on the internal carotid artery at this level may result in a slowing of the heart rate and occasionally termination of a re-entry supraventricular tachycardia. It should never be attempted on both sides at once as this may result in asystole and occlusion of the main arterial blood supply to the brain.) It is contraindicated in patients with a history of cerebrovascular disease.

- *Adenosine:* This slows AV conduction and is especially useful for terminating re-entry SVTs of the Wolf Parkinson White type. Give 3 mg IV rapidly preferably via a central or large peripheral vein—followed by a saline flush. Further doses of 6 mg and then 12 mg may be given at 2 min intervals if there is no response to the first dose. The effects of adenosine last only 10–15 seconds.

It should be avoided in asthma.

- Verapamil, beta-blockers or other drugs such as amiodarone or flecainide may control the rate or convert to sinus rhythm.
  - Verapamil 5–10 mg IV slowly over 2 minutes. A further 5 mg may be given after 10 minutes if required. Avoid giving concurrently with beta-blockers as this may precipitate hypotension and asystole.
  - Beta-blockers, e.g. propranolol 1 mg over 1 minute repeated if necessary at 2 minute intervals (maximum 5 mg), or esmolol, a relatively cardioselective beta-blocker with a very short duration of action may be given by infusion at 50–200 mcg/kg/minute.

Digoxin should be avoided—it facilitates conduction through the AV accessory pathway in the Wolf-Parkinson-White syndrome and may worsen the tachycardia. Note that atrial fibrillation in the presence of an accessory pathway may allow very rapid conduction which can degenerate to ventricular fibrillation.

Broad Complex Arrhythmias

1. *Premature ventricular complexes (PVCs):* A premature ventricular contraction is an impulse that originates prematurely in the ventricles and perturbs the prevailing rhythm. The mechanism of PVCs may be either increased automaticity of ventricular foci or re-entry.

   ECG shows a premature wide, slurred, bizarre QRS complex followed by a T wave, usually in the opposite direction to the main QRS deflection. PVCs are usually followed by full compensatory pauses (Figs 15A and B).

   The events following PVC are of interest. Usually, PVC is followed by a complete compensatory pause because the sinus node timing is not interrupted; a sinus P wave is unable to reach the ventricles because they are still refractory from the PVC; the following sinus impulse occurs on time, the time course being dependent on the sinus rate. By contrast, PACs are usually followed by an incomplete pause because the PAC usually enters the sinus node and resets its timing; this enables the following sinus P wave to appear earlier than expected. These concepts are illustrated below.

Management:

- Correction of any contributing causes identified with the anesthetic ensuring adequate oxygenation, normocarbia and analgesia. A small dose of beta-blocker is worth trying as mentioned above.
- If the underlying sinus rhythm is slow <50 bpm, then increasing this rate using intravenous atropine or glycopyrrolate may be effective as the ventricular ectopics may be a form of escape rhythm.

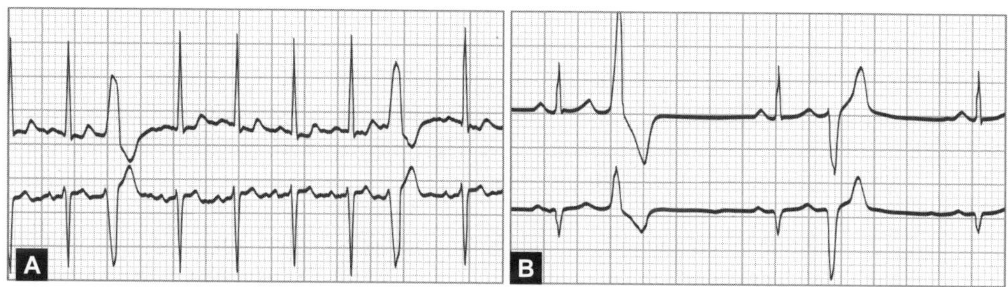

Figs 15A and B (A) Unifocal PVCs—identical shapes. *Note:* A single PVC is labeled isolated; (B) Multifocal PVCs—more than one shape

- Lignocaine is the drug of first choice. An initial loading dose of 50–100 mg IV over 2 minutes is given followed by infusion of: 4 mg/minute—for 30 minutes, then 2 mg/minute—for 2 hours and then 1 mg/minute. The dose should be reduced in the elderly, in liver disease and where there is bradycardia or hypotension.
- Alternatives include amiodarone 300 mg IV (preferably via a central venous catheter) overl hour, followed by infusion of 900 mg over 23 hours. Occasionally bretyllium or procainamide may be used (Fig. 16).

2. *Ventricular bigeminy* is said to occur when PVCs alternate with the normal beat. Causes may include electrolyte abnormalities, stimulants and digoxin toxicity (Fig. 17).

Multifocal PVCs are characterized by at least two abnormal QRS complexes of different configurations. Certain types of PVCs are potentially dangerous because they may deteriorate into a ventricular tachycardia. This is particularly true when PVCs occur in couplets or triplets, are multi-focal or there is an "R-on-T" falls on the T wave of the previous beat) (Figs 18A and B).

3. *Ventricular tachycardia:* This is defined as episodes of four or more consecutive PVCs. It arises in the specialized conduction system distal to the bundle of His bifurcation, the mechanism of VT being abnormal automaticity or re-entry. The ECG in VT shows a uniform series of widened QRS complexes, usually regular with a rate ranging from 70–250 bpm. The hallmark of VT is *AV dissociation (Fig. 19)*.

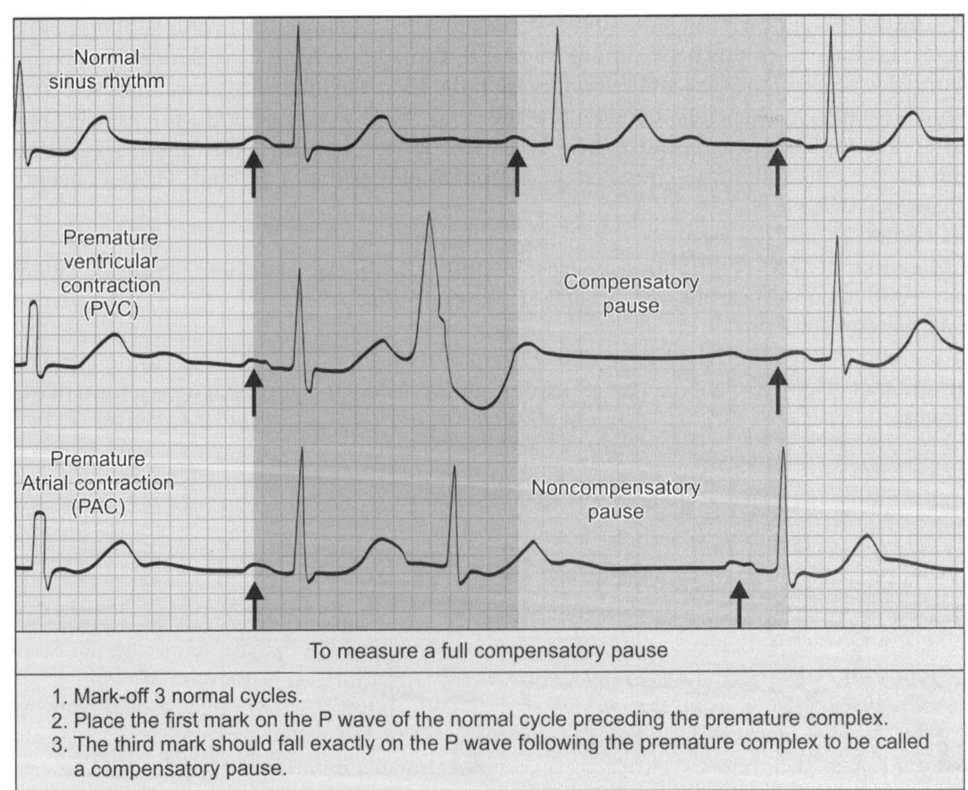

Fig. 16 Compensatory versus noncompensatory pauses

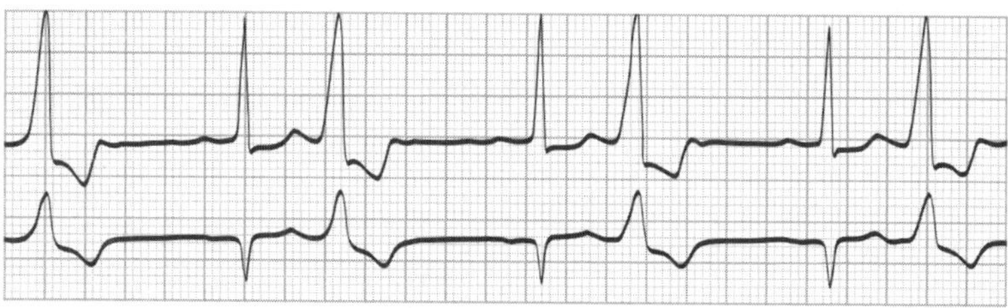

Fig. 17 Bigeminal PVCs—every other beat is a PVC

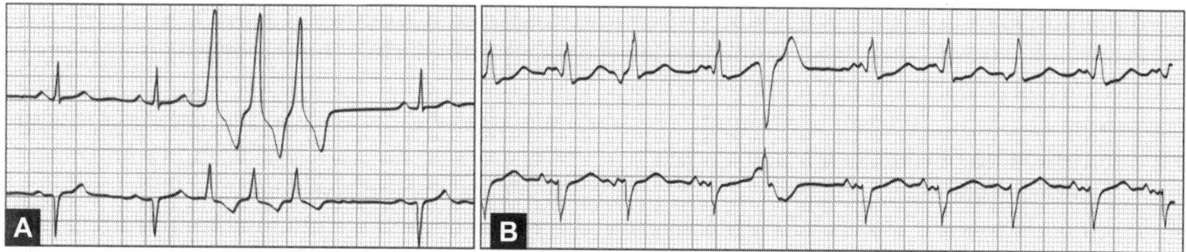

Figs 18A and B (A) Triplet PVCs—occur in groups of three; (B) R on T—occur on the peak of the T wave of the preceding beat

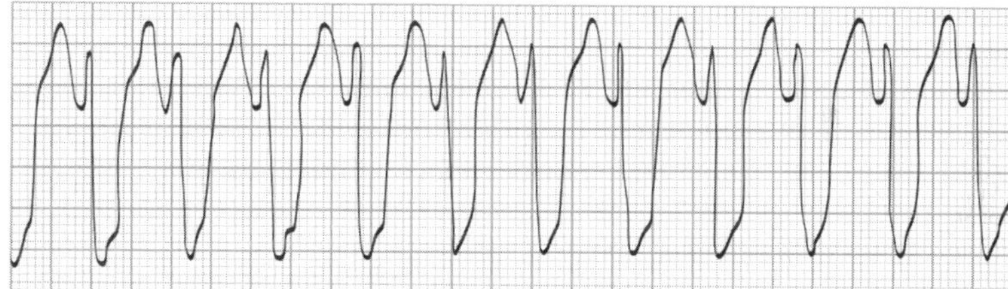

Fig. 19 Ventricular tachycardia

It is important to distinguish VT from a supraventricular tachycardia (SVT) with aberrant conduction. VT is diagnosed by the presence of *fusion and capture beats, AV dissociation, left axis deviation and compensatory pauses.* By contrast, an SVT with aberrant conduction is characterized by the *presence of P waves preceding the QRS complexes, the onset of the dysrhythmia with a premature P wave, an RSR' pattern in V1 and slowing/termination of the dysrhythmia by vagal stimulation.*

Management:

- Synchronized direct currentcardio version is the first line treatment if the patient is hemodynamically unstable. This is safe and effective and will restore sinus rhythm in virtually 100% of cases. If the VT is pulseless or very rapid, synchronization is unnecessary. But otherwise synchronization is used to avoid a 'shock on T' phenomenon, which may initiate VF. If the patient lapses back into VT, drugs such as lignocaine or amiodarone may be given to sustain sinus rhythm.

- Lignocaine given as a 100 mg bolus restores sinus rhythm in up to 60% and may be followed by a maintenance infusion as above.
- Verapamil is ineffective in ventricular tachycardia and may worsen hypotension and precipitate cardiac failure.

Other drugs which may be used if lignocaine fails:
- Amiodarone 300 mg IV—via a central venous catheter over 1 hour followed by infusion of 900 mg over 23 hours
- Procainamide 100 mg IV over 5 minutes followed by one or two further boluses before commencing infusion at 3 mg/min
- Mexiletine 100–250 mg IV at 25 mg/min followed by infusion 250 mg over 1 hour, 125 mg/hour for 2 hours, then 500 mcg/min
- Bretylium tosylate 400–500 mg diluted in 5% dextrose over 10 minutes
- Propranolol 0.5–1.0 mg IV and repeated if necessary particularly if the underlying pathology is myocardial ischemia or infarction.
  - Sotalol 100 mg IV over 5 minutes. This was shown to be better than lignocaine for acute termination of ventricular tachycardia.
  - Overdrive pacing can be used to suppress VT by increasing the heart rate.

4. *Torsade de pointes:* This is VT with a varying axis and is caused by anything that prolongs the QT (Fig. 20). Characterized by cyclical twisting of QRS axis and change in amplitude around baseline, occurring in setting of delayed ventricular repolarization evidenced by long QT interval or presence of u wave, and initiated by VPB that occurs near or T or U wave.

Causes include:
- Class Ia (quinidine, procainamide, flecanide) and III (amiadarone, sotalol, ibutilide) antiarrhythmic drugs
- *Psychotropic drugs:* Phenothiazines and TCA, haloperidol
- *Other drugs:* Erythromycin, levofloxacin, cisapride, droperidol
- *Electrolyte disturbance:* Hypokalemia, hypocalcemia, hypomagnesemia
- Complete heart block
- Hereditary long QT syndrome.

Management:
- Intravenous magnesium sulfate (2 gm bolus to repeat if necessary after 10 min)
- Correction of electrolyte abnormality
- Discontinuation of offending drugs
- Cardioversion.

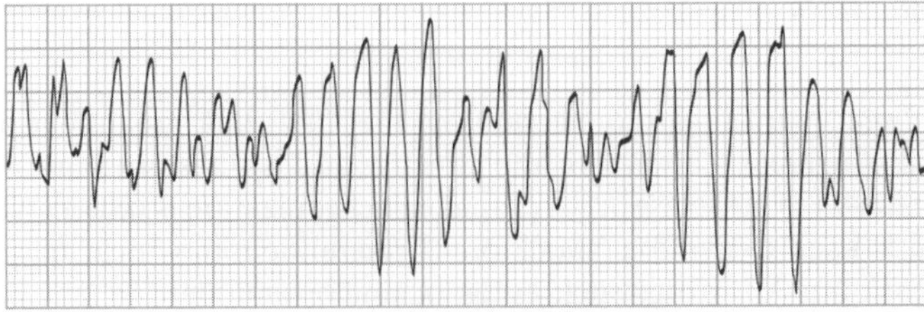

Fig. 20 Torsade de pointes

5. *Ventricular fibrillation (VF):* Ventricular fibrillation is an irregular rhythm resulting from a rapid discharge of impulses from one or more foci in the ventricles. The ventricular contractions are erratic and seen on the ECG as bizarre patterns of various sizes and configurations. No P waves are seen. Some causes of VF include myocardial ischemia, hypoxia, hypothermia, electrocution, electrolyte and acid-base imbalance, and drug effects. Due to the absence of any effective cardiac output, life must be sustained by artificial means, i.e. external cardiac massage and defibrillation is "the" treatment (Fig. 21).

Ventricular pre-excitation: WPW and LGL syndromes: The basic abnormality in ventricular pre-excitation is that the depolarization wave, after passing through the atrial myocardium, activates the ventricles earlier than would be expected if the impulse traveled normally from atria to ventricles via the AV node and the bundle of His. Hence, this is also known as accelerated AV conduction. In its most common form, there is the congenital presence of an "accessory" AV conduction pathway, which results in a rapid bypass of the normal slow route.

A. Wolff-Parkinson-White (WPW) syndrome: The ventricular pre-excitation syndrome, Wolff-Parkinson-White (WPW) syndrome, comprises two ECG criteria plus a clinical criterion:
- A short PR interval
- Widened QRS complex
- Episodes of paroxysmal tachycardia.

The PR interval is shortened by the rapid transmission of depolarization from atrial to ventricular myocardium. The accessory pathway passes first to the upper part of the right side of the interventricular septum, and this is the first part of the myocardium to be activated (normally, the left side of the upper part of the interventricular septum is the first part of the ventricles to be activated). This changes the initial direction of the QRS deflection. The initial part of the QRS complex is slurred and this premature, slurred initial portion is termed the delta wave. The normal pathways of intraventricular conduction are not followed and hence the QRS complex becomes distorted in shape and prolonged in duration. Since ventricular depolarization is abnormal, ventricular repolarization is also abnormal and ST-segment depression and/or T wave inversion may be seen. The presence of two pathways for AV conduction results in cyclical, repetitive entries of the depolarization wave between the atria and the ventricles, giving rise to paroxysmal tachycardia or atrial flutter.

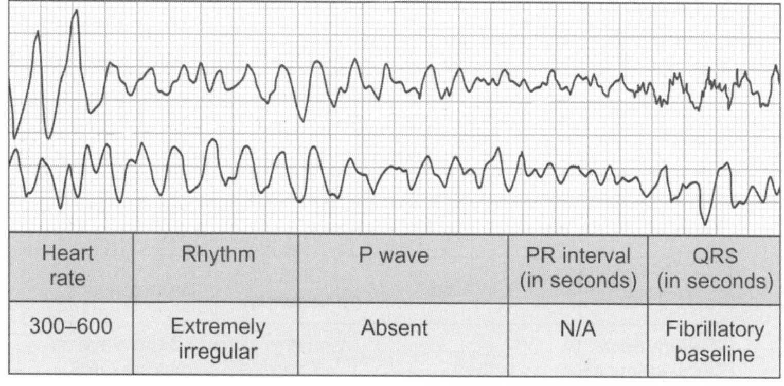

Heart rate	Rhythm	P wave	PR interval (in seconds)	QRS (in seconds)
300–600	Extremely irregular	Absent	N/A	Fibrillatory baseline

Fig. 21 Ventricular fibrillation

Diagnostic criteria for WPW-type pre-excitation: All of the following three criteria must be fulfilled for a diagnosis to be made:

- P-R interval <0.12 s (i.e. 0.11 s or less) in the presence of sinus rhythm
- Abnormally wide QRS complex >0.10 s (i.e. 0.11 s or more)
- Presence of initial slurring (in the first 0.03 to 0.05 s) of the QRS complex.

This ventricular pre-excitation syndrome must be distinguished from a complete left bundle branch block in which the P-R interval is normal, without any initial slurring of the QRS complex, but the similarity lies in the fact that the initial direction of QRS deflection is reversed and the total QRS duration is also prolonged (Fig. 22).

WPW syndrome can be of two types:

Type A: Dominantly upright QRS complex in right precordial leads. The bypass tract is usually situated in left ventricle.

Type B: Dominantly negative QRS deflection in right precordial leads. Here the bypass tract is usually located in right ventricle.

B. Lown-Ganong-Levine (LGL) syndrome: This is the next most common type of ventricular pre-excitation syndrome. Here, the accessory pathway is believed to run from the atrial myocardium to the distal part of the AV node or to the beginning of the His bundle, thus short-circuiting the normal AV nodal delay (short P-R interval). The intraventricular conduction (and hence the QRS complex) remains normal.

The ECG criteria for the LGL type of pre-excitation syndrome are:

1. PR interval <0.12 sec (i.e. 0.11 sec or less).
2. Normal QRS duration with no delta wave.

Patients having the above criteria fulfilled on their ECG in addition to the clinical criterion of having had episodes of paroxysmal tachycardia have the LGL syndrome.

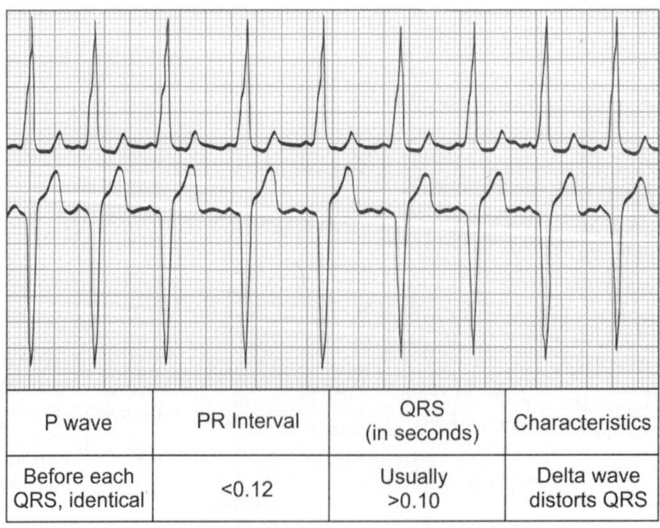

P wave	PR Interval	QRS (in seconds)	Characteristics
Before each QRS, identical	<0.12	Usually >0.10	Delta wave distorts QRS

Fig. 22 Pre-excitation syndrome (WPW-type)

Vaughan-Williams classification of antiarrhythmic drugs

Class	*Mechanism*	*Drugs*
1	Na^+ channel blockers	
A	Prolong action potential	Quinidine, procainamide
B	Shorten action potential	Lidocaine, mexiletine, phenytoin
C	No effect on action potential	Flecainide
II	Beta-blockers	Atenolol, esmolol, propranolol
III	K^+ channel blockers	Amiodarone, sotalol
IV	Ca^{++} channel blockers	Verapamil, diltiazem
V	Other mechanisms	Digoxin, adenosine

Conduction abnormalities

A. Sinus node block: This involves failure of the sinus node to depolarize or failure of impulse conduction from the sinus node to the atria. It may be seen during anesthesia (due to vagal reflexes); during drug therapy with digoxin, quinidine or phenylephrine; myocardial ischemia or infarction; and due to ischemia-induced fibrosis of the sinus node.

ECG changes: An absent P wave and often an absent QRS complex are seen. Manifested by a gradual shortening of the P-P intervals until a pause occurs (i.e. the blocked sinus impulse fails to reach the atria) (Fig. 23).

B. Sick sinus syndrome: It is a term used for a number of disorders that involve degenerative changes in the cardiac conduction system, resulting in sinus node dysfunction and, possibly, AV blocks too. Causes include myocardial ischemia or infarction, hypertension, electrolyte and endocrine abnormalities, cardiomyopathies, inflammatory diseases and drug effects.

C. Atrioventricular (AV) blocks: Possible sites of AV block include:
- AV node (most common)
- His bundle (uncommon)
- Bundle branch and fascicular divisions.

1st degree AV block: This may be seen in healthy individuals (Fig. 24). Features include:
- Prolonged PR interval, i.e. PR interval >0.20 sec
- All P waves are conducted to the ventricles.

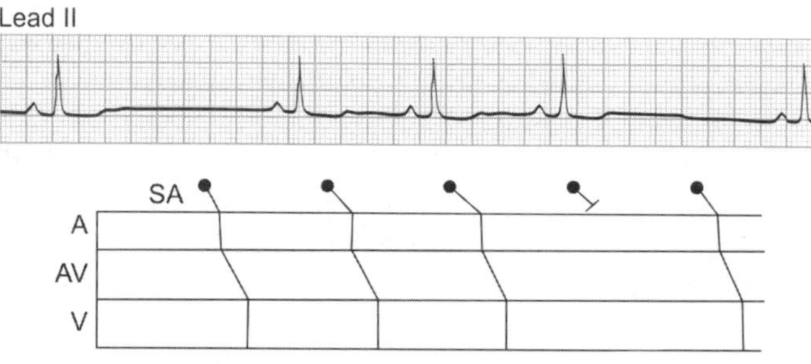

Fig. 23 Sinoatrial exit block (type I)

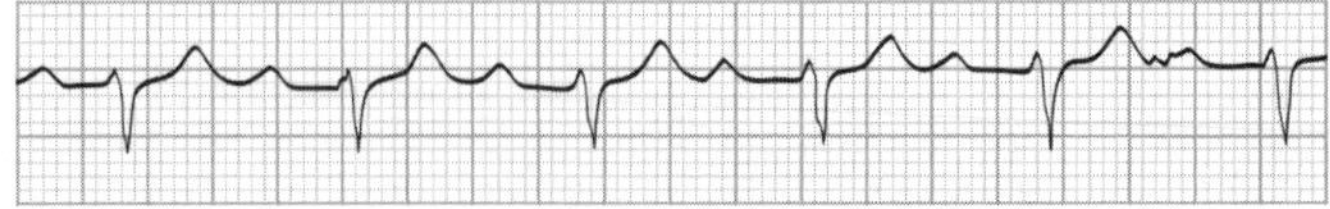

Fig. 24 1st degree AV block (PR = 280 ms)

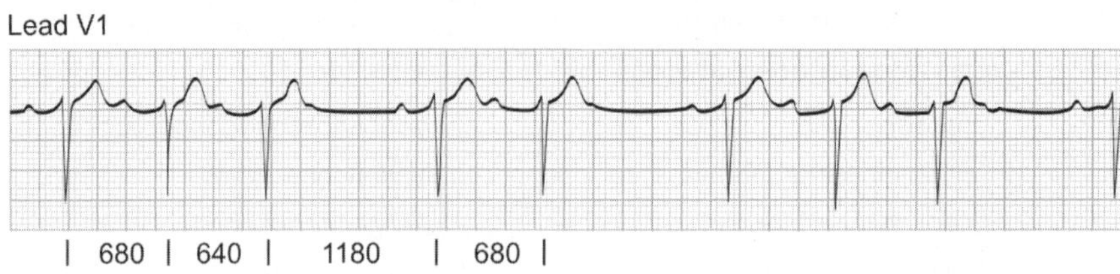

Fig. 25 Classic Wenckebach

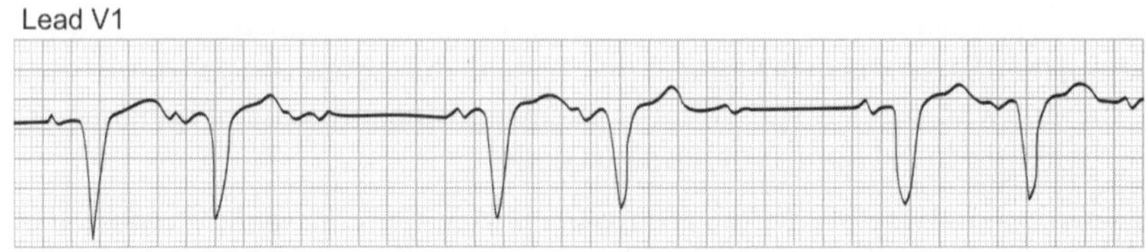

Fig. 26 Second degree AV block (type II) with LBBB

2nd degree AV block: All of the atrial impulses are not conducted to the ventricles. There may be, for example, a ventricular beat following every second or every third atrial beat (2:1 block, 3:1 block, etc.). 2nd degree AV block is subdivided into two classes as follows:

- *Mobitz type I (Wenckebach phenomenon):* The PR interval lengthens gradually until a P wave which fails to conduct to the ventricles occurs. The block in this case is almost always located in the AV node and may be caused by right coronary artery occlusion causing inferior wall infarctions (Fig. 25)
- *Mobitz type II:* This involves an intermittent block in conduction of the P wave into the ventricles, but the PR interval in surrounding beats is unaltered. Type II AV block is almost always located in the bundle branches. Type II block may result from anterior wall infarctions. These blocks are generally permanent, with a greater risk of progressing to complete heart block (Fig. 26).

3rd degree/complete heart block: This involves total disruption of conduction between the atria and ventricles. In this situation, life is maintained by a spontaneous escape rhythm (Figs 27A and B).

Narrow complex escape rhythm (<0.12 sec QRS complex): The escape rhythm originates in the His bundle and therefore the site of block lies more proximally in the AV node. The escape rhythm occurs at a rate of 50–60 bpm and is relatively reliable.

Treatment depends on etiology. But chronic symptomatic blockade requires permanent pacing.

Broad complex escape rhythm (>0.12 sec QRS complex): The escape rhythm originates below the His bundle and therefore the site of blockade lies more distally in the His-Purkinje system. The resulting rhythm is slow (15–40 bpm) and unreliable. Dizziness and blackouts (Stoke-Adams attacks) often occur. Temporary followed by permanent pacing may be required.

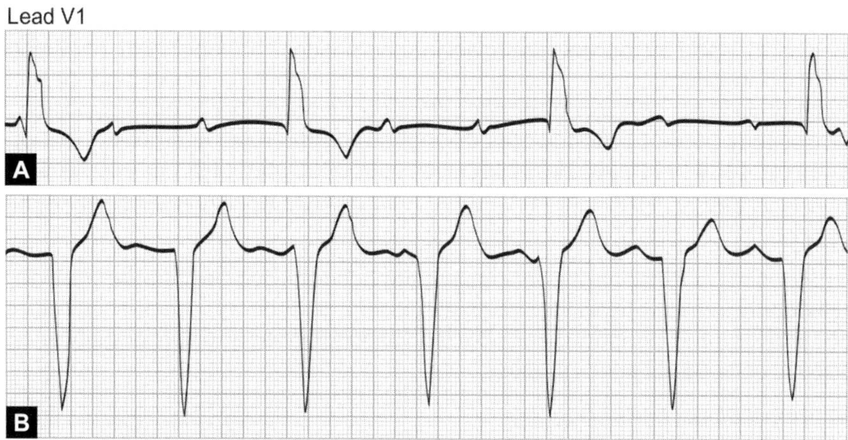

Figs 27A and B (A) Complete or 3rd degree AV block with a left ventricular escape rhythm, as evidenced by the upright QRS morphology; (B) The artificial right ventricular pacemaker rhythm

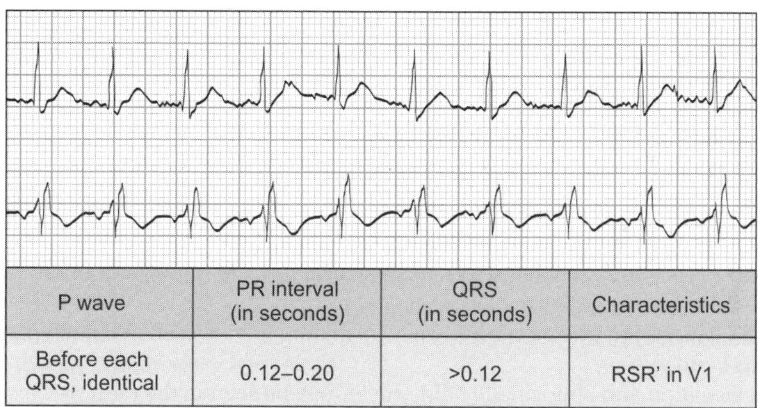

P wave	PR interval (in seconds)	QRS (in seconds)	Characteristics
Before each QRS, identical	0.12–0.20	>0.12	RSR' in V1

Fig. 28 Right bundle branch block

Right Bundle Branch Block

Intraventricular blocks Right bundle branch block (RBBB) (Fig. 28)
This involves:

- Total failure of conduction in the right bundle branch proximally
- No change in the direction of depolarization of the interventricular septum
- No change in the timing or direction of left ventricular depolarization

Diagnostic criteria for RBBB:

- 'Complete' RBBB has a QRS duration >0.12 sec
- A secondary R wave is seen in V1. The secondary wave is usually broad and slurred (the complex in V1 may be rsr', rSr', RSr', RSR' or M-shaped).

Additional features frequently seen in RBBB include:

- Deep, slurred S waves in left precordial leads (typically V4, V5, V6)
- Deep, slurred S waves usually seen in lead I and also aVL

- ST segment depression and T wave inversion are seen in the right precordial leads (typically in leads V1, V2, V3). This occurs due to secondary changes in ventricular repolarization (ST segment and T waves).

The mean frontal plane *QRS axis is usually within the normal range* in uncomplicated complete RBBB. The axis may move 15–30° towards the right, but abnormal right axis deviation is not a routine feature of RBBB. If left axis deviation is present, think about left anterior fascicular block, and if right axis deviation is present, think about left posterior fascicular block in addition to the RBBB.

Clinical significance: The RBBB may occur congenitally in normal hearts. It can be seen in a variety of disorders, including ischemic heart disease, hypertension, pulmonary embolism, cardiomyopathy, myocarditis, pericarditis, rheumatic heart disease, Chagas disease and congenitally in association with atrial septal defect and Fallot's tetralogy.

Left Bundle Branch Block (LBBB) (Fig. 29)
This involves:
- Total failure of conduction in the left bundle branch system
- Complete reversal of the direction of depolarization of the interventricular septum
- Delay in the initiation and velocity of depolarization of the free wall of the left ventricle.

Diagnostic Criteria for LBBB

- Total QRS duration >0.12 sec
- No secondary R wave in V1 to indicate RBBB
- No septal q wave in V5, V6 or in leads further to the left (lead I and aVL in horizontal hearts).

Additional features frequently seen in LBBB include:
- The QRS complexes in some leads may be notched (leads I, aVL, V5 and V6)
- The QRS complexes in V5, V6, I and aVL tend to have rsR', 'M' pattern or broad monophasic R waves
- Secondary ST depression and possibly T wave inversion may be seen in the left precordial leads (and in leads I and aVL)
- ST segment elevation and abnormally tall T waves may be seen in the right precordial leads
- Abnormally deep S waves in the right precordial leads

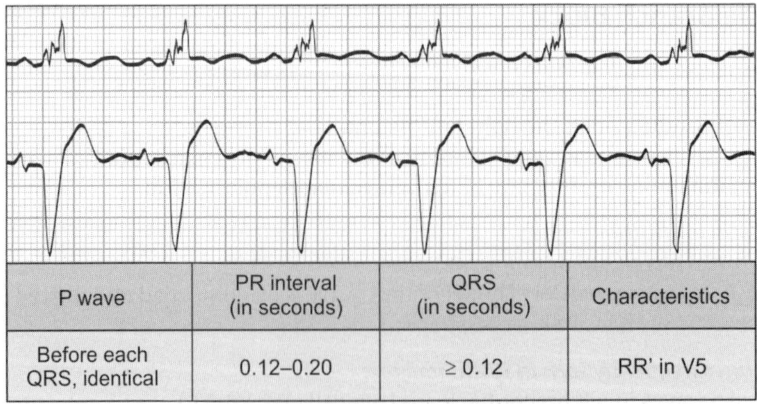

P wave	PR interval (in seconds)	QRS (in seconds)	Characteristics
Before each QRS, identical	0.12–0.20	≥ 0.12	RR' in V5

Fig. 29 Left bundle branch block

- Initial r waves in the right precordial leads may be very small or absent
- In the precordial leads, the dominant direction of the ST segments and the T waves tends to be opposite to the dominant direction of the QRS complexes in any given lead.

The mean frontal plane *QRS axis is usually within the normal range* in uncomplicated complete LBBB. The axis may move 15–30° towards the left when LBBB develops but abnormal left axis deviation is not a routine feature of LBBB. The axis may sometimes be indeterminate. When LBBB is combined with abnormal left axis deviation, extensive disease of the left ventricular conducting system is likely to be present.

Incomplete LBBB is diagnosed when:
- There is no septal q wave in V5, V6 or in leads further to the left (leads I and aVL)
- The total QRS duration is 0.10-0.11 sec.

Clinical significance: LBBB always indicates significant cardiac disease. It is seen most commonly in ischemic heart disease, hypertension, aortic stenosis and fibrous degeneration of the conducting tissue. It may also occur in congestive and hypertrophic cardiomyopathy, myocarditis, acute rheumatic fever, syphilis, cardiac tumors, postcardiac surgery and in congenital heart disease.

E. Fascicular blocks (Fig. 30): According to this concept, there are three fascicles of conduction:
1. Right bundle branch.
2. Anterior division of the left bundle branch.
3. Posterior division of the left bundle branch.

Normally, the left ventricle is depolarized simultaneously from two directions:
1. A depolarization wave spreading from below upwards and to the left as a result of transmission through the *posterior* (*inferior*) division.
2. A depolarization wave spreading from above downwards and to the left as a result of transmission through the *anterior* (*superior*) division.

Left Anterior Fascicular Block (LAFB)

In this abnormality, the anterosuperior division of the left bundle totally fails to conduct. Hence, the anterosuperior part of the left ventricle (LV) is activated in the opposite direction by the depolarization wave after it emerges from the posteroinferior part of the LV, which receives the wave in a normal manner through the posterior (inferior) division of the left bundle.

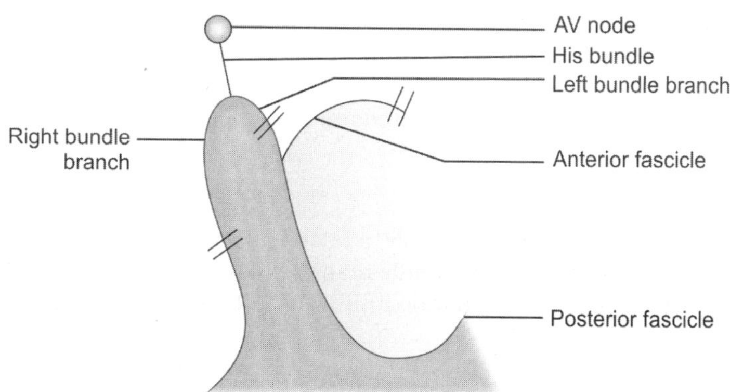

Fig. 30 Fascicular blocks (the conducting system)

Diagnostic criteria for LAFB are:

- Left axis deviation with QRS axis more negative than –30°
- Initial r waves in all inferior limb leads (leads II, III, aVF)
- Other recognized causes of left axis deviation must be absent.
- Total QRS duration is usually at the upper limit of normal (0.09–0.10 sec)

Other causes of abnormal left axis deviation include:

- Ventricular pre-excitations, e.g. Wolff-Parkinson-White syndrome
- Inferior myocardial infarction
- Tricuspid atresia and ostium primum atrial septal defect
- Hyperkalemia.

Clinical significance: Chronic LAFB may be a normal finding in the elderly without evidence of heart disease. It may be present after acute myocardial ischemia, hypertension, congestive and hypertrophic cardiomyopathy, myocarditis, calcific aortic stenosis and following aortic valve replacement.

Important differential diagnosis of LAFB: Abnormal left axis deviation is the most striking feature of LAFB. *The second most common cause of an abnormal left axis deviation is an inferior myocardial infarction.* The important difference in the ECG between the above two conditions is the presence of:

Initial r waves in all inferior limb leads (II, III, aVF) in LAFB, BUT there are *abnormal Q waves* in the inferior leads in *inferior myocardial infarction.*

Left Posterior Fascicular Block (LPFB)

This occurs less frequently than an LAFB. This is because the posterior division of the left bundle is thicker and shorter and has a much better blood supply than its counterpart. In this abnormality, the posteroinferior division of the left bundle fails to conduct. Hence, the posteroinferior part of the LV is activated in the opposite direction by the depolarization wave after it emerges from the anterosuperior part of the LV, which receives the depolarization wave in a normal manner through the anterosuperior division of the left bundle.

In left posterior fascicular block, the only ECG features seen are:

- A mild degree of right axis deviation (between +90° and +120°) and
- Total QRS duration is at the upper end of normal (0.09–0.10 s).

Due to only subtle changes brought about by a left posterior fascicular block on the ECG, it is impossible to be sure about a LPFB from the ECG alone. Other possible causes of right axis deviation should be excluded (e.g. emphysema, right ventricular hypertrophy, atrial septal defect and an extensive anterolateral myocardial infarction).

Bifascicular Blocks

When two fascicles are blocked simultaneously, a bifascicular block is said to exist. This includes the more common combination of right bundle branch block (RBBB) with left anterior fascicular block (manifest as LAD), and the less common RBBB with left posterior fascicular block.

Trifascicular Block

This is a combination of bifascicular block and 1st degree heart block (Fig. 31).

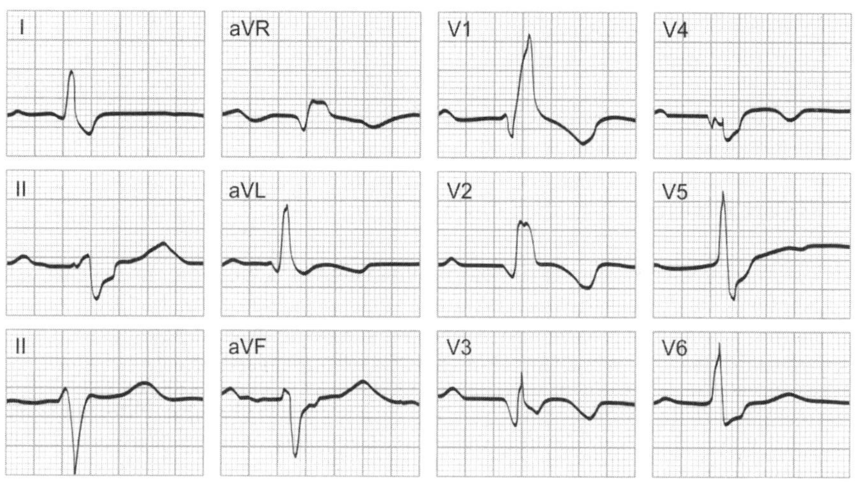

Fig. 31 Trifascicular blocks (bifascicular block with 1st degree heart block)

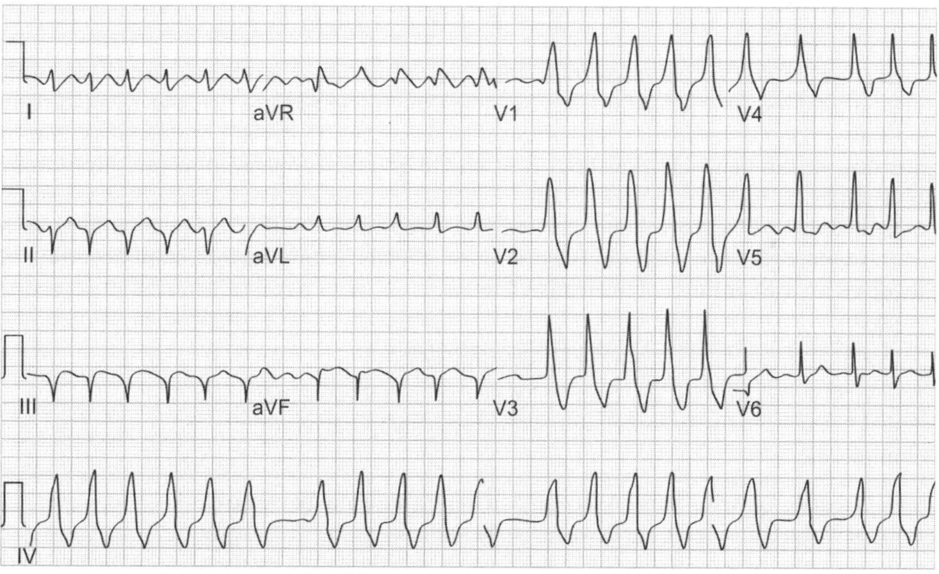

Fig. 32 RBBB with left anterior fascicular block

Diagnostic criteria for RBBB with left anterior fascicular block are:

- Total QRS duration = 0.12 sec
- A secondary R wave in V1
- Mean QRS axis is more negative than –30°
- An initial r wave is seen in the inferior limb leads (II, III and aVF).

In RBBB with left posterior fascicular block (Fig. 32), the ECG features are:

- Total QRS duration = 0.12 s
- A secondary R wave in V1
- Mean QRS axis is more positive than +90°.

Clinical significance: RBBB with LAFB is more common. But both of the above bifascicular blocks can occur in similar conditions. This includes conditions like atherosclerotic heart disease, calcific aortic stenosis, hypertrophic and congestive cardiomyopathy, and congenital endocardial cushion defects. Although an RBBB with LPFB is less common, 60–70% of those that do occur progress to a complete heart block.

Ischemic Heart Disease

The ECG is commonly used in the investigation of suspected ischemic heart disease (IHD). The ECG provides information about the myocardium and the specialized conducting tissues that have undergone ischemia. It should also be remembered that a percentage of patients with unequivocal angina pectoris may have normal resting 12-lead ECGs when first seen.

The ECG in acute myocardial infarction (MI): Acute MI may cause changes in the QRS complex, ST segment or the T wave. However, the only definitive diagnostic changes of myocardial infarction are changes in the QRS complex.

The QRS complex in infarction: Two types of QRS abnormalities may indicate infarction:
1. Inappropriately low R wave voltage in a local area and
2. Abnormal Q waves

Abnormal Q waves and QS complexes: In a *transmural infarction* (endocardium to epicardium), there will be *total loss of R waves* in leads overlying the infracted zone. This gives rise to entirely negative waves, i.e. *QS complexes.* These negative waves are the result of depolarization of the posterior wall of the ventricle traveling from endocardium to epicardium (i.e. away from the anterior leads).

The reduction in R wave voltage can only be confirmed if either a previous ECG shows a significantly greater R wave height in the appropriate leads before the infarction occurred, or the leads involved are two or more of the leads V2 to V5.

Therefore, the four possible QRS changes indicative of infarction are:
1. Reduced R wave voltage (confirmed by previous ECGs)
2. Abnormal Q waves without any conclusive evidence of R wave reduction
3. Reduced R wave voltage in association with abnormal Q waves and
4. QS complexes.

Abnormal Q waves: Q waves may be recognized to be abnormal because of:
- Abnormal width (duration), i.e. Q wave = 0.04 s or
- Abnormal depth (relative to the following R wave), i.e. depth of Q wave >25% of the height of the following R wave is abnormal.

ST segment changes in myocardial infarction: Dramatic ST segment changes occur in the early stages of myocardial infarction. Such changes indicate *myocardial injury rather than infarction.*

The injury state is unstable, and acute ST segment elevation *always* resolves to some extent and *usually* resolves completely. The resolution of the acute ST elevation is *usually* accompanied by development of the QRS changes of frank infarction, although *occasionally*, it may resolve without the development of diagnostic changes of infarction.

The ST segment shift is produced by myocardial injury, which causes a disturbance in the current flow across the cell membrane.

The essential change of myocardial injury is ST segment elevation above the isoelectric line.

The normal ST segment does not deviate by more than 1 mm above or below the isoelectric line. Abnormal ST segment elevation occurs in leads facing the infarction, both in transmural and subepicardial infarction. Reciprocal ST segment depression may be seen at the same time as the above primary changes in leads recording from positions opposite to the infarct.

Primary ST segment depression is seen in leads facing the infarct when a subendocardial infarction occurs.

T wave changes of infarction: The spectrum of changes in the T waves during infarction includes flattening of the T waves, bi-phasic T waves, inverted T waves and abnormally tall T waves.
The most typical T wave change in acute MI is deep, symmetrical T wave inversion.

Electrolyte disturbances and ECG changes: The normal state of cardiac cell membrane polarization is dependent upon the maintenance of a normal ionic balance across the membranes, with K^+ being the most important. Because changes in intracellular K^+ concentration are proportionately much smaller than changes in extracellular K^+ concentration, it follows that the *absolute level of extracellular K^+ concentration is the single most important factor* affecting the cell membranes.

Hyperkalemia

ECG changes: All of the ECG changes that occur with a raised K^+ concentration are nonspecific and may affect any part of the ECG (Fig. 33).

The typical progressive changes of hyperkalemia are as follows:

- Appearance of tall, pointed, narrow T waves.
- Decreased P wave amplitude, decreased R wave height, widening of QRS complexes, ST segment changes (elevation/depression), hemiblock (esp. left anterior) and 1st degree heart block.
- Advanced intraventricular block (very wide QRS with RBBB, LBBB, bi- or trifascicular blocks) and ventricular ectopics.
- Absent P waves, very broad, bizarre QRS complexes, AV block, VT, VF or ventricular asystole.

Advanced hyperkalemia: Marked widening of the QRS duration combined with tall, peaked T waves are suggestive of advanced hyperkalemia. Note the absence of P waves, suggesting a junctional rhythm, but in hyperkalemia the atrial muscle may be paralyzed while still in sinus rhythm. The sinus impulse conducts to the AV node through internodal tracts, without activating the atrial muscle.

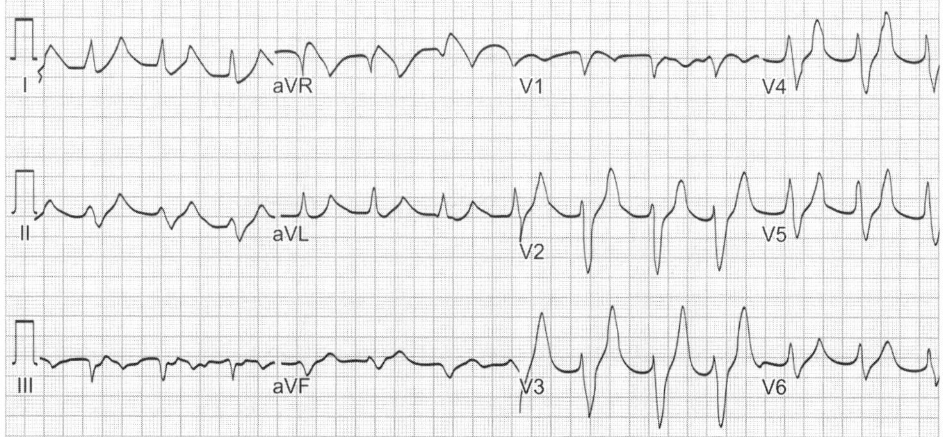

Fig. 33 Hyperkalemia ECG changes

Hypokalemia

ECG changes in decreasing order of frequency are:

- ST segment depression, decreased T wave amplitude, increased U wave height
- Cardiac arrhythmias
- Prolongation of the QRS duration, increased P wave amplitude and duration

Various types of arrhythmias may occur in hypokalemia. These may include atrial and ventricular ectopics, atrial tachycardia, heart blocks, VT and VF.

ECG changes of hypomagnesemia resemble that of hypokalemia
ECG changes of hypermagnesemia resemble that of hyperkalemia
Hypokalemia, hypomagnesemia and hypercalcemia aggravate digitalis toxicity

Hypothermia

A decrease in the body temperature is associated with the following ECG changes:

- Sinus bradycardia
- Prolonged P-R interval
- Prolonged Q-T interval.

J wave: This occurs when the body temperature falls below 25°C. It appears as an extra deflection at the end of the QRS complex just overlapping the beginning of the ST segment.

Hypothermia—J waves or Osborn waves (Fig. 34): In hypothermia, a small extra wave is seen immediately after the QRS complex (best seen in Lead I in this example). This extra wave is called a J wave or Osborne wave after the individual who first described it. This wave disappears with warming of body temperature. The mechanism is unknown.

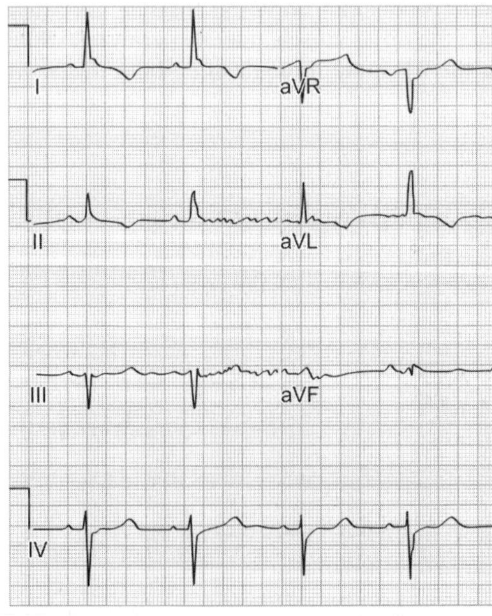

Fig. 34 Hypothermia (J waves or Osborn waves)

Good to know for the students

EINTHOVEN'S TRIANGLE HYPOTHESIS (FIG. 35)

Published in 1913, this hypothesis attempts to explain the principles of electrocardiography on a scientific basis. It is based on four assumptions which are not completely true, but do provide some basis. The four assumptions are as follows:

1. The trunk is a homogeneous volume conductor.
2. The mean of all the electrical forces generated during the cardiac cycle can be considered as originating from a dipole situated at the heart's center.
3. The limb leads pick-up voltage changes in the frontal plane only.
4. The attachments of the three extremities used in making the limb leads (R, L and F) form the apices of an equilateral triangle with the dipole at its center.

Lead System

There are 12 conventional leads, 6 in frontal plane (I, II, III, aVR, aVL, aVF) and 6 in horizontal plane (V1-V6). The heart is situated in the center of the electrical field which it generates. The electrical intensity diminishes as the distance increases from the center. The lead axes from three standard leads (lead I, II and III) form a triangle known as an Einthoven triangle. In routine practice, monitors with three limb leads are used. Three electrodes are placed as follows:

- One on the left arm (LA), usually color coded as yellow
- One on the right arm (RA), usually color coded as red
- One on the left leg (LL), usually color coded as green or black.

For convenience, during intraoperative monitoring left leg electrode is often placed over the left side of chest, near the apex beat. Lead I measures the potential difference between the right arm electrode and the left arm electrode. Lead II is derived from negative electrode on the right arm and positive electrode on the left leg, measures the potential difference between right arm and left leg electrode. It is usually the best lead for detecting rhythm disturbances. Lead III measures the potential difference between the left arm and left leg. For detecting ischemic changes, ST segment

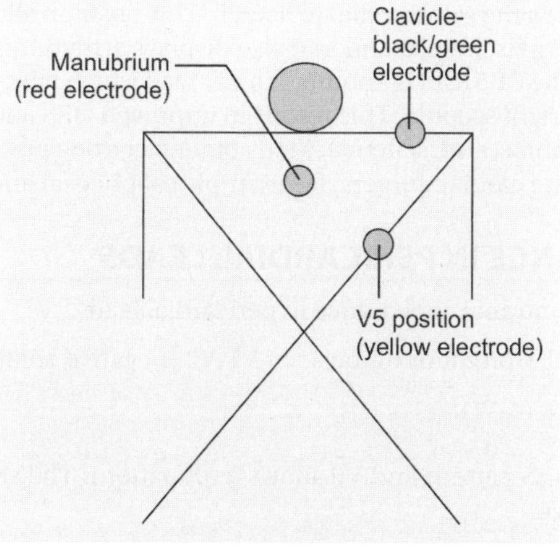

Fig. 35 V5—electrode connections

should be monitored in appropriate leads. The ST segment changes in lead V1-V4 usually monitor the left anterior descending artery territory, V4-V6 circumflex artery and lead II, III, aVF monitor the right coronary artery territory. When only bipolar leads are used then a modified V5 lead may be used for detecting ischemia. CM5 is a modified V5 lead where the right arm electrode of lead I is placed over the manubrium sternum, left arm electrode is placed over the left anterior axillary line in the 5th intercostal space and ground electrode is placed on the left shoulder.

Lead	*RA*	*LA*	*LL*
I	RA (negative)	LA (positive)	Ground
II	RA (negative)	Ground	LL (positive)
III	Ground	LA (negative)	LL (positive)
aVR	RA	Ground	Ground
aVL	Ground	LA	Ground
aVF	Ground	Ground	LL
CM5	Manubrium	V5	Ground

Lead I—measures the potential difference between the right arm electrode and the left arm electrode. The third electrode (left leg) acts as neutral.

Lead II—measures the potential difference between the right arm and left leg electrode.

Lead III—measures the potential difference between the left arm and left leg electrode.

Most monitors can only show one lead at a time and therefore the lead that gives as much information as possible should be chosen. The most commonly used lead is lead II—a bipolar lead with electrodes on the right arm and left leg as above. This is the most useful lead for detecting cardiac arrhythmias as it lies close to the cardiac axis (the overall direction of electrical movement) and allows the best view of P and R waves.

For detection of myocardial ischemia the V5 lead is useful. This is a bipolar lead with the right arm electrode placed on the manubrium and left arm electrode placed at the surface marking of the V5 position (just above the 5th interspace in the anterior axillary line). The left leg lead acts as a neutral and may be placed anywhere—the C refers to 'clavicle' where it is often placed. To select the V5 lead on the monitor, turn the selector dial to 'lead I'. This position allows detection of up to 80% of left ventricular episodes of ischemia, and as it also displays arrhythmias it can be recommended for use in most patients. The CB5 lead is another bipolar lead which has one electrode positioned at V5 and the other over the right scapula. This results in improved QRS and P wave voltages allowing easier detection of arrhythmias and ischemia. Many other electrode positions have been described including some used during cardiac surgery, for example esophageal and intracardiac ECGs.

NORMAL APPEARANCE IN PERICARDIAL LEADS

Figures 36 ECG shows the normal appearance in pericardial leads.

P waves: Upright in V4-V6. Upright or biphasic in V1-V2 (negative component should be smaller, if biphasic)

QRS complexes:
Morphology: V1 shows an rS pattern and V6 shows a qR pattern. The size of the r-wave increases progressively from V1 to V6.

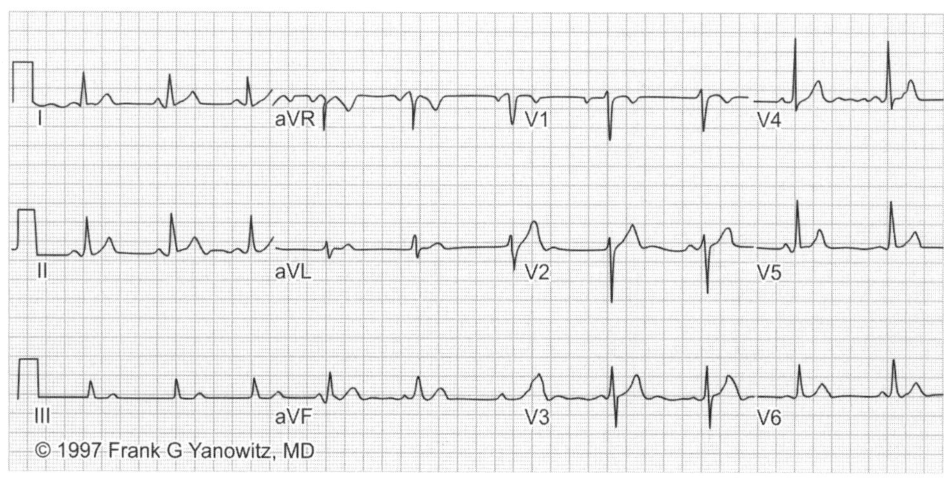

Fig. 36 Normal ECG appearances in precordial leads

Transition zone: The initial part of the QRS deflection is positive in the right precordial leads. The transition zone is the point between V1 and V6, where the initial deflection ceases to be positive and becomes negative.

Dimensions:
- QRS duration < 0.12 s
- Atleast one R wave in the precordial leads must exceed 8 mm
- The tallest R wave in the precordial leads must not exceed 27 mm
- The deepest S wave in the precordial leads must not exceed 30 mm
- The sum of the tallest R wave in the left precordial leads and the deepest S wave in the right precordial leads must not exceed 40 mm
- Precordial q waves must not equal/exceed 0.04 sec in duration
- Precordial q waves must never have a depth greater than one quarter of the height of the R wave, which follows them.

ST segments: Must not deviate above or below the isoelectric line by more than 1 mm. Normal ST segment elevation occurs in leads with large S waves (e.g. V1-3), and the normal configuration is concave upward (Fig. 37).

T waves: Upright in V4-V6. Often inverted in V1, may be inverted in V2 (provided already inverted in V1). The T wave height should not be more than two-thirds and not less than one-eighth of the height of the preceding R wave in any of the leads V3-V6.

Normal Appearances in Limb Leads (Fig. 38)

P waves: Best seen in lead II (Small-rounded waves)
- P wave height = 2.5 mm
- P wave duration = 0.12 s

QRS complexes: Mean frontal plane QRS axis range is between +90°and –30°; this implies that the QRS is mostly positive (upright) in leads I and II. R wave in aVL must not exceed 13 mm and R wave in aVF must not exceed 20 mm. Normal q waves reflect normal septal activation (beginning on the

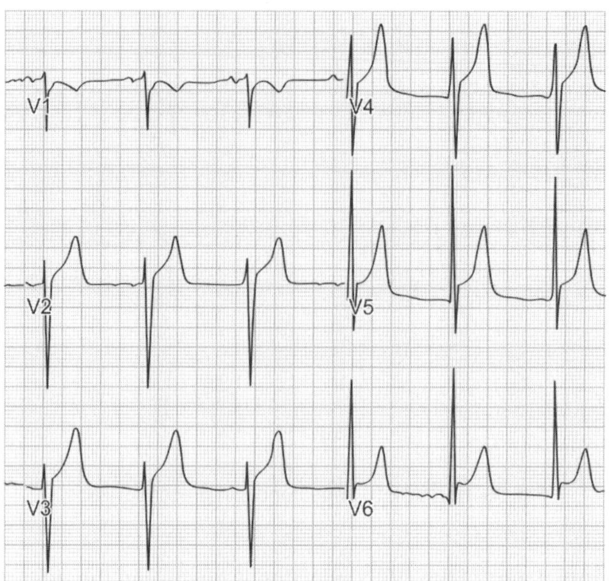

Fig. 37 Concave upward (ST segments)

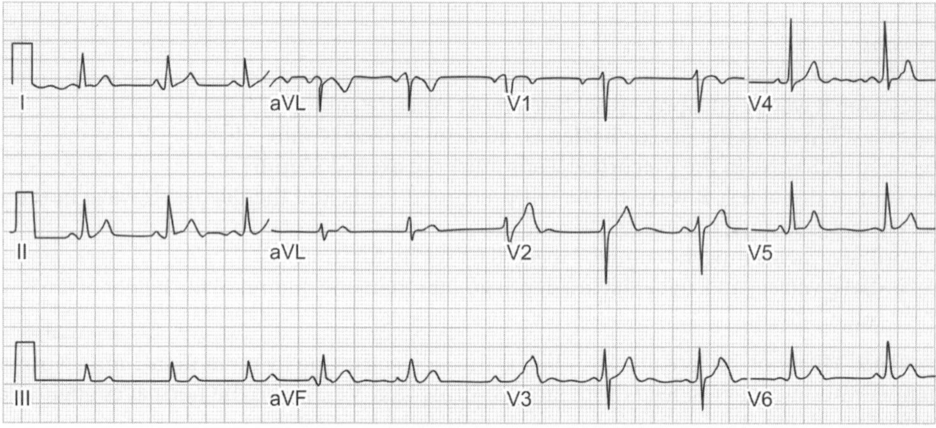

Fig. 38 Normal ECG appearances in limb leads

LV septum); they are narrow (<0.04 sec duration) and small (<25% the amplitude of the following R wave). They are often seen in leads I and aVL when the QRS axis is to the left of +60°, and in leads II, III, aVF when the QRS axis is to the right of +60°. Septal q waves should not be confused with the pathological Q waves of myocardial infarction.

Types of tachyarrhythnies is shown in Figure 39.

ST segments: Must not deviate above or below the isoelectric line by more than 1 mm. *T waves:* In the normal ECG, the T wave is always upright in leads I, II, V3-6, and always inverted in lead aVR.

U wave:

- U wave amplitude is usually < one-third T wave amplitude in same lead
- U wave direction is the same as T wave direction in that lead

U waves are more prominent at slow heart rates and usually best seen in the right precordial leads.

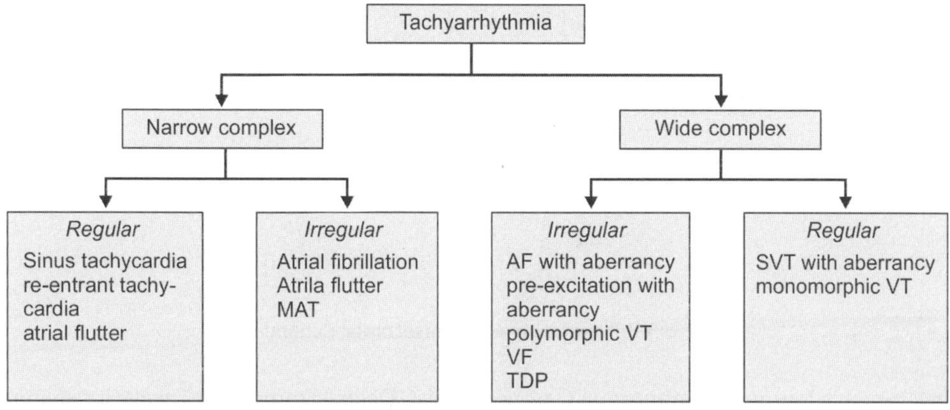

Fig. 39 Types of tachyarrhythmia

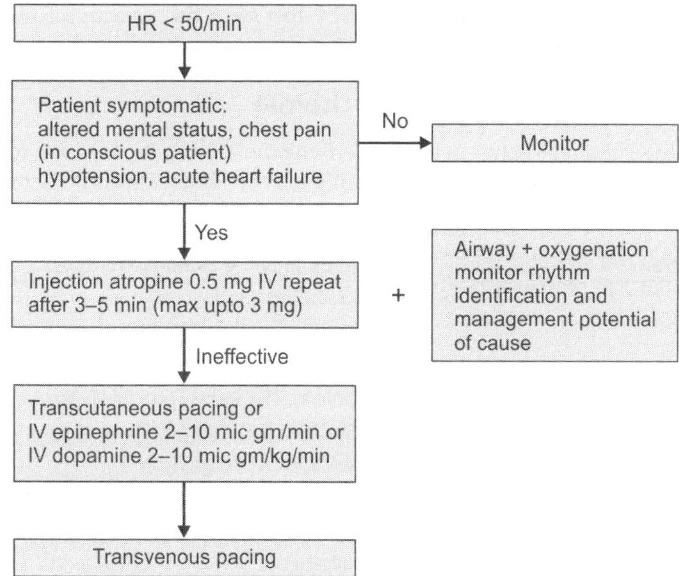

Fig. 40 Symptomatic brabycardia

Treatment of Symptomatic Brady Cardia

Figure 40 shows treatment of symptomatic bradycardia.

Sequence of Changes in Acute Myocordial Ischemia (Fig. 41)

(A) Shows the normal QRS complex in a lead; (B and C) Within hours of the clinical onset of an MI, there is ST segment elevation. At this stage, no QRS or T wave changes have occurred. This indicates myocardial damage only, not definitive evidence of infarction; (D) Within days, the R wave voltage falls and abnormal Q waves appear. This is sufficient evidence of an infarction. In addition, T wave inversion will also have appeared but the ST segment elevation may be less obvious than before; (E) Within one or more weeks, the ST segment changes revert completely to normal. The R wave

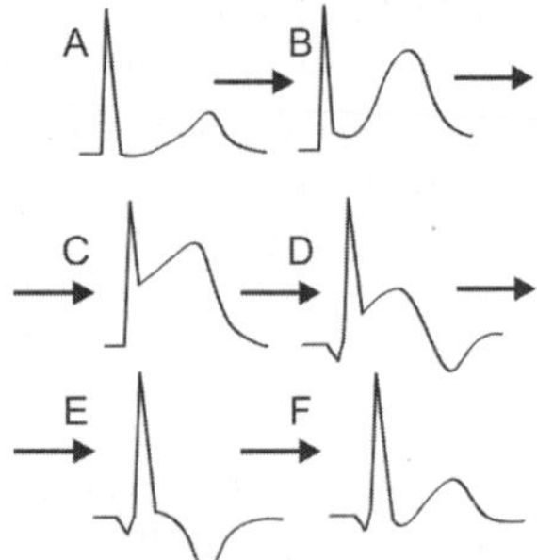

Fig. 41 Evolution of acute miyocordial ischemia

voltage remains low and the abnormal Q waves persist. Deep, symmetrical T wave inversion may develop at this stage; (F) Months after the MI, the T waves may gradually return to normal. The abnormal Q waves and reduced R wave voltage persist.

Occasionally, all evidence of infarction may be lost with the passing of time; this is due to shrinkage of scar tissue.

Location of Changes in Myocardial Ischemia

Because primary ECG changes occur in leads overlying the infarct, the location of an infarct can be derived by looking at the primary changes occurring in such leads. This is depicted in the following table:

Location of infarction	Leads showing primary changes
	Typical changes
Anterior infarction	
Anteroseptal	V1, V2, V3
Anterior	Some of V1-V3 plus some of V4-V6
Anterior extensive	V1, V2, V3, V4, V5, V6, I, aVL
Anterolateral	V4, V5, V6, I, aVL, possibly II
High lateral	aVL and/or I
Inferior infarction	
Inferior	II, III, aVF
Inferolateral (= apical)	II, III, aVF, V5, V6 and sometimes also I, aVL
Inferoseptal	II, III, aVF, V1, V2, V3
	Other changes
Posterior infarction	V1, V2 (inverse of usual changes elsewhere)
Subendocardial infarction	Any lead (usually multiple leads)

Diagnostic Criteria for Myocardial Ischemia

A definitive diagnosis of MI from the ECG can only be made on the basis of abnormalities in the QRS complex. The following changes are seen:

- q waves which are either 0.04 s or longer in duration (excluding aVR and lead III) or have a depth which is more than 25% of the height of the following R wave (excluding aVR and lead III).
- qs or QS complexes (excluding aVR and lead III).
- Local area of inappropriately low R wave voltage.

Additional changes frequently associated with MI are:

- ST segment elevation (convex upwards) in leads facing the infarcted zone.
- ST segment depression occurs as a reciprocal change in leads mutually opposite to the primary leads showing evidence of infarction.
- Horizontal ST segment depression may occur as a primary change in subendocardial infarction.

Reciprocal Changes

In addition to the primary changes that occur in the ECG leads facing the infarcted myocardium, "reciprocal changes" may occur in leads opposite to the site of infarction. The changes are just the inverse of the primary changes. Thus, "ST segment elevation and T wave inversion" will appear as "ST segment depression and tall pointed T waves", respectively. The inferior limb leads on the one hand and the precordial leads, together with leads I and aVL, on the other hand are "mutually opposite". Thus, primary changes in one of the above groups will usually be accompanied by reciprocal changes in the other group. It will be safe to assume that if on the ECG there is ST segment elevation in one group (as above) and ST segment depression in the other group, the elevation is the primary change and the ST segment depression is the secondary change.

True Posterior Myocardial Ischemia

Infarction evident in the inferior leads (II, III and aVF) was previously called posterior infarction (now called inferior infarction). However, true posterior infarction is quite rare and is not easily recognized, as none of the ECG leads are actually situated posteriorly. Hence, it is only recognizable by looking for "reciprocal" changes in the anterior leads. Primary changes are not seen, as there are no actual posterior leads.

The changes in the ECG of a true posterior infarction are:

1. Abnormally tall and broad "R" waves in V1 (reciprocal to abnormally deep and wide q waves in a posterior lead, if there were any)
2. ST segment depression in V1 in recent infarcts; in infarcts of intermediate age, tall T waves may be present in V1, V2 and V3.

Right-sided chest leads, V1R - V6R, are shown in Figure 42. The true posterior MI is evidenced by the marked ST segment elevation in V1R (actual V2) and V2R (actual V1). The RV MI is evidenced by the ST elevation in V3R to V6R.

Subendocardial Infarction

Infarcts are most commonly intramural infarcts (transmural or subepicardial). Subendocardial infarcts are relatively rare and may encircle the interior of the left ventricle.

The ECG shows primary ST segment depression or deep symmetrical T wave inversion without any changes in the QRS complexes. Since these changes can also be produced by myocardial ischemia without infarction, the diagnosis of a subendocardial infarction cannot be made with a single ECG (unless correlated with clinical or enzyme evidence of infarction). When ST depression is the primary change, it will be seen in all or most leads except the cavity leads (aVR always a cavity lead, aVL a cavity lead in a vertical heart and aVF: a cavity lead in a horizontal heart). By definition, cavity leads inevitably show QS complexes.

Changes in Myocardial Ischemia

Hypoxia of the myocardium may occur in the absence of infarction and necrosis. The changes may occur following stress (physical or emotional) or even spontaneously. Significant degrees

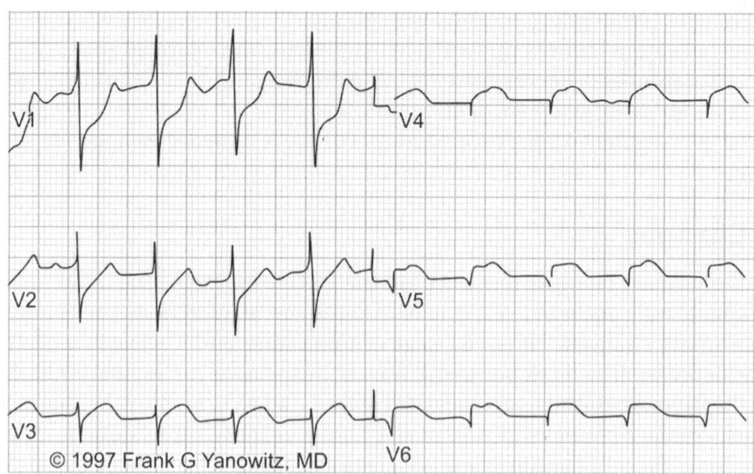

Fig. 42 Right side chest leads V1R-V6R

of ischemia may exist with no evidence of ECG abnormalities. The changes, when present, are confined to the ST segment and T waves. There will be *no change in the QRS complexes.*

The following ECG changes may accompany myocardial ischemia:

- Flattening of T waves
- Inverted T waves
- Abnormally tall T waves
- "Normalization" of primarily abnormal T waves
- Sloping ST segment depression
- Horizontal ST segment depression
- ST segment elevation
- Any combination of the above changes.

Nice to know for the students

ELECTROPHYSIOLOGY OF THE HEART

The myocardium can conduct an electrical impulse in any direction. The actual direction of spread will thus depend on where the activation was initiated. Conduction must occur in all directions from this point. But the predominant direction of spread will be in that direction in which the greatest mass of myocardium is available from the point of initiation.

The sinoatrial or SA node is situated in the right atrium at its junction with the superior vena cava. Normally, the SA node initiates activation of the atria, which causes a wave of contraction to pass across the atria. Following atrial contraction, the impulse is delayed at the atrioventricular (AV) node, located in the septal wall of the right atrium.

At rest the potential difference across the membrane of a myocardial cell is -90 mv (Fig. 43). This is due to a high intracellular potassium concentration which is maintained by the sodium/potassium pump. Depolarization of a cardiac cell occurs when there is a sudden change in the permeability of the membrane to sodium. Sodium floods into the cell and the negative resting voltage is lost (stage 0). Calcium follows the sodium through the slower calcium channels resulting in binding between the intracellular proteins actin and myosin which results in contraction of the muscle fiber (stage 2). The depolarization of a myocardial cell causes the depolarization of adjacent cells and in the normal heart the depolarization of the entire myocardium follows in a co-ordinated fashion. During repolarization potassium moves out of the cells (stage 3) and the resting negative membrane potential is restored.

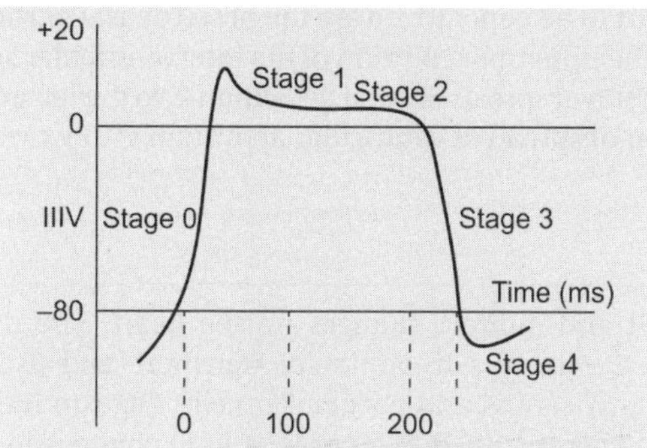

Fig. 43 The cardiac muscle action potential. Stage 0 = Depolarization, opening of voltage gated sodium channels; Stage 1 = Initial rapid repolarization, closure of sodium channels and chloride influx; Stage 2 = Plateau—opening of voltage gated calcium channels; Stage 3 = Repolarization, potassium efflux; Stage 4 = Diastolic prepotential drift

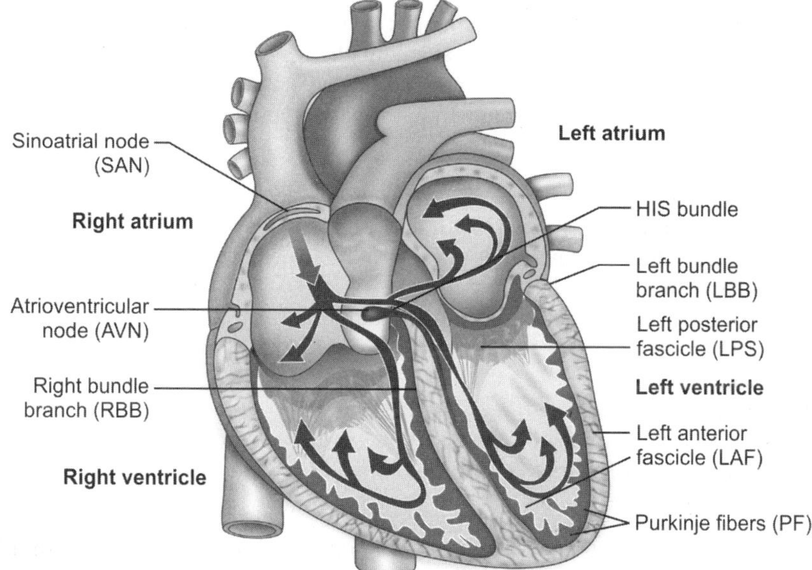

Fig. 44 Cardiac conduction system

Spread of electrical activation (Fig. 44)

- Activation of the atrial myocardium begins in the SA node. The radial spread of depolarization then converges on the AV node, where there is a delay for about 0.1 seconds (AV nodal delay).
- From here, His-Purkinje fibers allow rapid conduction of the electrical impulse via right and left branches, causing almost simultaneous depolarization of both ventricles, approximately 0.2 sec after the initial impulse has arisen in the SA node
- In humans, the ventricular depolarization starts at the left side of the interventricular septum and moves first to the right across the mid-portion of the septum
- It then spreads down the septum to the apex of the heart
- It then returns along the ventricular walls to the AV groove, proceeding from the endocardial to the epicardial surface

- The last parts of the heart to be depolarized are the posterobasal portion of the left ventricle, the pulmonary conus and the uppermost portion of the interventricular septum.

The predominant direction of spread of atrial activation is to the left and somewhat downwards. The predominant direction of spread of ventricular activation is downwards and somewhat to the left.

DIGOXIN

Digoxin can induce direct and indirect changes on the heart. The direct changes are due to inhibition of the normal active process of sodium ion transport (and also potassium ion transport) across the membranes of myocardial and pacemaker cells. Digoxin induces indirect changes by increasing the vagal tone. Therapeutic doses produce ECG changes in a patient taking digitalis. These changes are referred to as the "digoxin effect". These changes are:

- Decreased T wave amplitude
- ST segment depression
- Increase in U wave amplitude
- Shortening of the Q-T interval.

One of the earliest and most common changes is reduction in T wave voltage. Occasionally, biphasic or inverted T waves may be seen. ST segment changes are seen as a downward sloping ST segment depression, which is often associated with T wave flattening. This is called the "reversed tick" phenomenon (resembles the tick made by a left-handed person).

DIGOXIN TOXICITY

Toxicity due to digoxin presents clinically with anorexia, nausea and vomiting and, rarely, visual disturbances. Digoxin-induced arrhythmias are always a sign of toxicity, not just a therapeutic effect.

The following arrhythmias are seen commonly:

- Ventricular premature beats (including coupled and multifocal VPCs)
- Junctional tachycardia
- Sinus bradycardia
- Atrial tachycardia with A-V block
- Heart blocks (1st degree, 2nd degree Mobitz Type I and 3rd degree)
- Multifocal atrial premature beats
- Atrial fibrillation and flutter
- SA block and sinus arrest
- VF and VT.

ICD THERAPY

- Terminate abrupt onset life-threatening ventricular fibrillation often preceded by a run of ventricular tachycardia
- Component: a lead system. That senses electrical activity of ventricle and also delivers shock produced by pulse generator.

The ICD generator inserted in the area of pectoral muscle of left collar bone. Figure 45 shows development of a rapid polymorphic tachycardia later strips on ICD senses the rhythm and delivers a shock and word converts it in sinus rhythm.

- In tired or staged therapy, whenever it detects tachyarrhythmia, it perform anti-tachycardia (overdrive) pacing to convert it into sinus rhythm, if it persists or degenerates into VF, actual shocks are delivered at increasing intensities
- Also function as pacemaker in case of bradyarrhythmia.

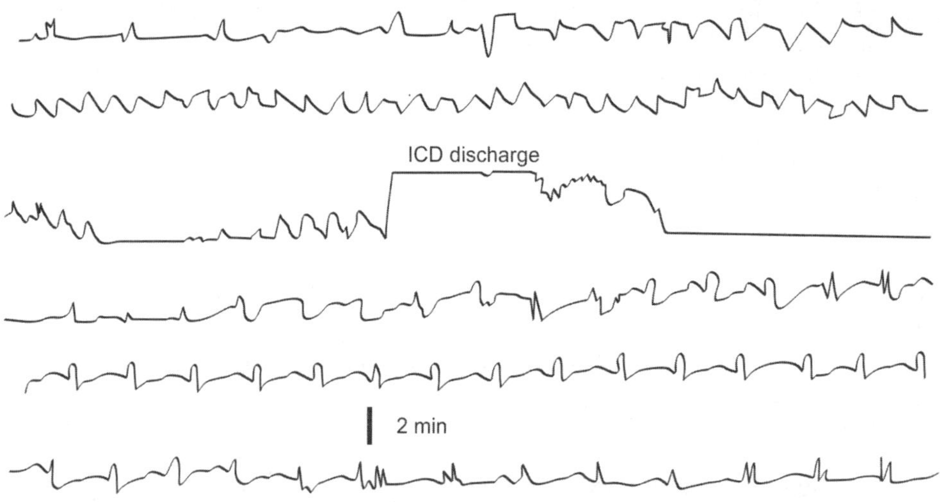

Fig. 45 Development of a rapid polymorphic tachycardia an ICD senses the rhythm and delivers a shock, and converts it in sinus rhythm

Class I indications for ICD therapy (ACC/AHA guidelines):

- Cardiac arrest caused by VF or VT not resulting from a transient or reversible cause
- Spontaneous sustained VT associated with structural heart disease
- Nonsustained VT in patients with coronary disease, prior MI, LV dysfunction, and inducible VF or sustained VT at EP study not suppressible by an NYHA Class I antiarrhythmic drug
- Spontaneous sustained VT in patients without structural heart disease not amenable to other treatments.

BIBLIOGRAPHY

1. Ary L Goldberger. Clinical Electrocardiography, 7th edn, 2006.
2. Dua N, Kumra VP. Management of perioperative arrhythmias. Indian J Anaesth. 2007;51:310-23.
3. Ganong WF. A review of medical physiology. McGraw-Hill Publishing Co, 2005.
4. Gregoratos G, et al. ACC/AHA guidelines for implantation of cardiac pacemakers and antiarrhythmia devices. Executive summary. Circulation. 1998;97:1325-35.
5. Hampton J. The ECG made easy. London: Churchill Livingstone, 1986.
6. Harrison's Principles of Internal Medicine, Goldberger's 17th edn.
7. Hinds CJ, Watson D. Intensive Care: A concise textbook. London: WB Saunders Company Ltd, 1996.
8. Hutton P, Prys-Roberts C. Monitoring in Anesthesia and Intensive care. London: WB Saunders Company Ltd,1994.
9. Mangano DT. Perioperative Cardiac Morbidity. Anaesthesiology 1990; 72:153-84.
10. Miller's Anesthesia, 7th edn.
11. Nathanson MH, Gajraj NM. The perioperative management of atrial fibrillation. Anesthesia. 1998;53:665-76.
12. Neumar RW, Otto CW, Link MS, Kronick SL, Shuster M, Callaway CW, et al. Part 8: Adult advanced cardiovascular life support: American Heart Association Guidelines for Cardiopulmonary Resuscitation and Emergency Cardiovascular Care. Circulation. 2010;122(18 Suppl 3):S729-67.
13. The Alan E Lindsay ECG Learning Centre. http://medlib.med.utah.edu/kw/ecg/index.html "Understanding the Electrocardiogram: a new approach Sections I and II by Derek J Rowlands. Imperial Chemical Industries Pharmaceuticals Division, 1981. The ECG in anesthesia and Critical Care by Daniel M. Thys and Joel A. Kaplan. Churchill Livingstone, 1987.

Cardiopulmonary Resuscitation Guidelines—the Science Behind Applications: What We Need to Know?

Saikat Sengupta, Simantika Ghosh

1. What are the phases of cardiac arrest?

Ans. Three phase model (Fig. 1):

1. *Electrical phase:* From the time of cardiac arrest to approximately 4 minutes following the arrest.
2. *Circulatory phase:* From approximately 4–10 minutes after cardiac arrest.
3. *Metabolic phase:* Extending beyond 10 minutes after cardiac arrest.

The three phases form a continuum in which each phase describes the predominant dysfunction and thus indicates the most suitable therapy. Phase 1 is treated most effectively with rapid defibrillation whereas in the phase 2 outcomes may be improved by delaying defibrillation to perform CPR because CPR may 'prime' the heart for defibrillation by restoring some measure

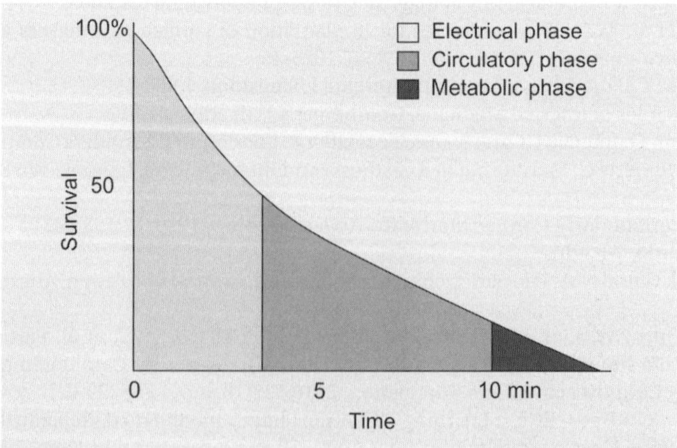

Fig. 1 This model predicts 50% survival rate for defibrillation provided in the electrical phase where electrical phase = 0–4 minutes, circulatory phase = 4–10 minutes, and metabolic phase 7–10 minutes (*Source:* Based on the model described by Weisfeldt and Becker. JAMA. 2002).

of oxygenated blood. During phase 3, advanced brain and cardiac cell injury may attenuate the survival benefit of CPR.

2. What is CPR?

Ans. Cardiopulmonary resuscitation (CPR) consists of a series of lifesaving actions that improve the chance of survival following cardiac arrest. Includes the use of chest compressions and artificial ventilation to maintain circulatory flow and oxygenation during cardiac arrest until the return of spontaneous circulation.

3. What is the exact physiology involved?

Ans. *Two components of CPR:* Chest compressions and ventilation.

Chest compressions have 2 phases: Active and passive

1. *Active phase:* Force applied downwards on the chest squeezes the heart between the sternum and spine. Ventricular compression causes blood to be pumped out to the lungs and body.
2. *Passive phase:* Venous blood returns to the heart and coronary arteries are perfused.

It takes 5-10 efficient chest compressions to achieve adequate coronary perfusion pressure. Stopping chest compressions > 10s causes drop in coronary perfusion pressure.

4. What are the hypotheses related to CPR physiology?

Ans. Two main hypotheses:

1. *External cardiac massage:* Chest compressions directly compress the heart between the depressed sternum and thoracic spine to eject blood into the systemic and pulmonary circulation. The cardiac valves limit backward flow during decompression.
2. *Thoracic pump:* Chest compressions intermittently ↑ global intrathoracic pressures with equivalent pressure exerted on vena cavae, aorta and heart. Blood is ejected retrograde from intrathoracic venous vasculature as well as antegrade from intrathoracic arterial vasculature—both arterial and venous pressures rise concomitantly.

5. What is 'chain of survival'?

Ans. Heterogeneity in the etiology of sudden cardiac arrest suggests that a single approach to resuscitation is not practical, but a core set of actions provides an universal strategy for achieving successful resuscitation. An useful metaphor for the elements of the emergency cardiovascular care (ECC) systems concept:

- *Adult (Fig. 2):*
  - Immediate recognition of cardiac arrest and activation of emergency response system
  - Early CPR with an emphasis on chest compressions
  - Rapid defibrillation
  - Effective advanced life support
  - Integrated postcardiac arrest care.
- *Pediatric (Fig. 3):* Cardiac arrest in children is often secondary to respiratory failure, which can be prevented by early identification.
  - Prevention of arrest
  - Early high-quality bystander CPR

Fig. 2 Chain of survival (adult)

Fig. 3 Chain of survival (pediatric)

- Rapid activation of emergency response system
- Effective advanced life support
- Integrated postcardiac arrest care.

6. What are the latest basic life support (BLS) guidelines across all groups of patients?

Ans. 2010 American Heart Association (AHA) Guidelines for CPR can be summarized as in Table 1:

Table 1 | Summary of key BLS components for adults, children and infants

	Recommendations		
Component	*Adults*	*Children*	*Infants*
Recognition	Unresponsive (for all ages)		
	No breathing or no normal breathing (i.e. only gasping)	No breathing or only gasping	
	No pulse palpated within 10 seconds for all ages (HCP only)		
CPR sequence	C-A-B		
Compression rate	At least 100/min		
Compression depth	At least 2 inches (5 cm)	At least ½ AP diameter About 2 inches (5 cm)	At least ½ AP diameter About 1½ inches (4 cm)
Chest wall recoil	Allow complete recoil between compressions HCPs rotate compressors every 2 minutes		
Compression interruptions	Minimize interruptions in chest compressions Attempt to limit interruptions to <10 seconds		
Airway	Head tilt-chin lift (HCP suspected trauma: jaw thrust)		
Compression-to-ventilation ratio (until advanced airway placed)	30:2 1 or 2 rescuers	30:2 Single rescuer 15:2 2 HCP rescuers	
Ventilations: when rescuer untrained or trained and not proficient	Compressions only		
Ventilations with advanced airway (HCP)	1 breath every 6–8 seconds (8–10 breaths/min) Asynchronous with chest compressions About 1 second per breath Visible chest rise		
Defibrillation	Attach and use AED as soon as available. Minimize interruptions in chest compressions before and after shock; resume CPR beginning with compressions immediately after each shock.		

7. Why was the CPR sequence changed?

Ans. In the majority of cardiac arrests, the critical initial elements of CPR are chest compressions and early defibrillation. In the C-A-B sequence, chest compressions will be initiated sooner and ventilation only minimally delayed until completion of the first cycle of chest compressions. The A-B-C sequence could be a reason why less than a third of people in cardiac arrest receive bystander CPR. A-B-C starts with the most difficult procedures: opening the airway and delivering rescue breaths.

8. Why was 'Look, Listen and Feel' removed from the BLS algorithm?

Ans. Because it was found to be inconsistent and time consuming.

9. Why was compression rate changed from 'at least 100/min' to 'approximately 100/min'?

Ans. The number of chest compressions delivered per minute during CPR is an important determinant of return of spontaneous circulation (ROSC) and survival with good neurologic function. In most studies, delivery of more compressions during resuscitation is associated with better survival, and delivery of fewer compressions is associated with lower survival.

10. Why was compression depth changed from 'approximately 5 cm' to 'at least 5 cm'?

Ans. Compressions generate critical blood flow and oxygen and energy delivery to the heart and brain. Rescuers often do not push the chest hard enough.

11. What is 'high quality' CPR?

Ans. It includes:

- Start compressions within 10 seconds of recognition of cardiac arrest.
- Push hard, push fast @ at least 100/min and at least 5 cm depth in adults and children (4 cm in infants).
- Allow complete chest recoil after each compression.
- Minimize interruptions in compressions (< 10s).
- Give effective breaths that make the chest rise.
- Avoid excessive ventilation.
- Switch providers every 2 minutes to avoid fatigue.

12. Cricoid pressure—is it recommended routinely in cardiac arrest?

Ans. No. Evidence shows that cricoid pressure can delay or prevent the placement of an advanced airway and does not nullify the chances of aspiration. Also, it is difficult to train rescuers in this skill.

13. What is 'Hands-only CPR'?

Ans. Hands-only (compression-only) CPR is easier for an untrained rescuer to perform and can be more readily guided by dispatchers over the telephone. In addition, survival rates from cardiac arrests of cardiac etiology are similar with either hands-only CPR or CPR with both compressions and rescue breaths.

14. Bag-valve-mask ventilation in CPR—what are the guidelines?

Ans. Recommended only in 2 rescuer scenarios. The rescuer should use an adult (1–2 L) bag to deliver approximately 600 mL tidal volume for adult victims. This amount is usually sufficient to produce visible chest rise and maintain oxygenation and normocarbia in apneic patients. If the airway is open and a good, tight seal is established between face and mask, this volume can be delivered by squeezing a 1 L adult bag about two-thirds of its volume or a 2 L adult bag about one-third of its volume. The health care provider should use supplementary oxygen (O_2 concentration >40%, at a minimum flow rate of 10–12 L/min) whenever available.

15. What is the simplified BLS algorithm?

Ans. Figure 4 shows simplified BLS algorithm.

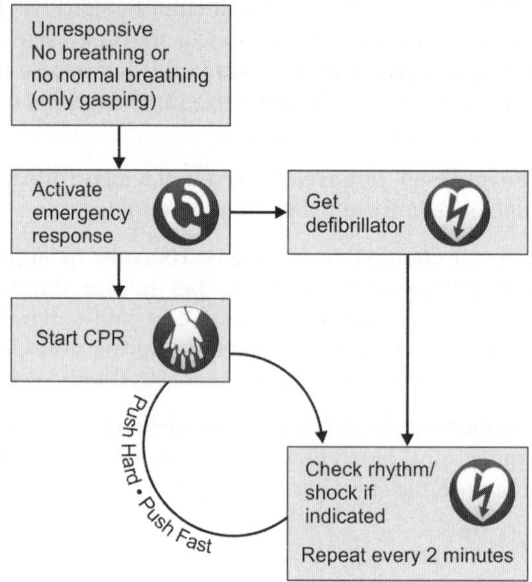

Fig. 4 Simplified BLS algorithm

16. What is the circular ACLS algorithm?

Ans. Figure 5 shows circular ACLS algorithm.

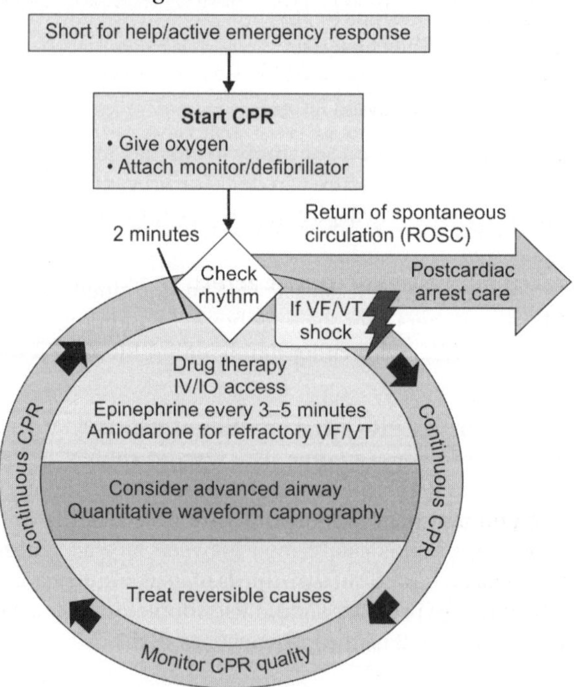

Fig. 5 Circular ACLS algorithm

17. Name the advanced airway devices included in the ACLS guidelines.

Ans. Laryngeal mask airway, laryngeal tube, esophageal-tracheal tube and endotracheal tube.

18. What is the rationale for resuming CPR after defibrillation?

Ans. Defibrillation does not restart the heart. It stuns the heart and briefly terminates all electrical activity, including VF and VT. If the heart is still viable, its normal pacemakers may resume electrical activity that ultimately results in a perfusing rhythm. However, any spontaneous rhythm after successful defibrillation is typically slow and does not create pulses or adequate perfusion. Thus, the patient needs high-quality CPR (beginning with chest compressions) for several minutes until adequate heart function resumes.

19. Why is early defibrillation critical?

Ans. The interval from collapse to defibrillation is one of the most important determinants of survival from cardiac arrest. For every minute that passes between collapse and defibrillation, the chance of survival from a witnessed VF sudden cardiac arrest declines by 7–10% per minute if no CPR is provided. CPR provided early can double or triple survival from witnessed sudden cardiac arrest.

20. What is ROSC?

Ans. Return of spontaneous circulation is heralded by

- Recordable pulse and blood pressure
- Abrupt sustained increase in P_{EtCO_2} (typically ≥ 40 mm Hg)
- Spontaneous arterial pressure waves with intra-arterial monitoring.

21. What comprises physiologic monitoring during CPR?

Ans. P_{EtCO_2}, CPP and S_{CVO_2} correlate with cardiac output and myocardial blood flow during CPR.

- End-tidal CO_2 — The main determinant of P_{EtCO_2} during CPR is blood delivery to the lungs. Persistently low values (< 10 mm Hg) suggest that ROSC is unlikely. Abrupt increases to normal values of 35–40 mm Hg indicate ROSC.
- Coronary perfusion pressure/arterial relaxation pressure—CPP is aortic relaxation (diastolic) pressure minus right atrial relaxation (diastolic) pressure. CPP < 20 mm Hg decreases likelihood of ROSC.
- Central venous oxygen saturation—values < 30% decreases likelihood of ROSC.

22. Enumerate the reversible causes of cardiac arrest.

Ans. Ready reckoner-5H+5T

1. Hypovolemia
2. Hypoxia
3. Hydrogen ion (acidosis)
4. Hypo-/hyperkalemia
5. Hypothermia

1. Tension pneumothorax
2. Tamponade, cardiac
3. Toxins
4. Thrombosis, pulmonary
5. Thrombosis, coronary

23. Why is atropine no longer recommended for treatment of pulseless electrical activity (PEA)/Asystole?

Ans. Evidence suggests that routine use of atropine in PEA/asystole is unlikely to have a therapeutic benefit.

24. Regarding neonatal resuscitation, should all newborns be subjected to endotracheal suctioning?

Ans. Suctioning immediately after birth should be reserved for babies who have an obvious obstruction to spontaneous breathing or require positive pressure ventilation. There is no evidence that active babies benefit from airway suctioning, even in the presence of meconium, and there is evidence of risk associated with this suctioning. The available evidence does not support or refute the routine endotracheal suctioning of depressed infants born through meconium stained amniotic fluid.

25. What is postcardiac arrest care?

Ans. Most deaths occur during the first 24 hours after cardiac arrest. Postcardiac arrest care has significant potential to reduce early mortality caused by hemodynamic instability and morbidity and mortality from multiorgan failure and brain injury. To improve survival for victims of cardiac arrest who are admitted to a hospital after return of spontaneous circulation, a comprehensive, structured, integrated, multidisciplinary system of postcardiac arrest care should be implemented in a consistent manner (Flow chart 1).

Flow chart 1 Adult immediate postcardiac arrest care

Return of spontaneous circulation (ROSC)

↓

Optimize ventilation and oxygenation
- Maintain oxygen saturation ≥94%
- Consider advanced airway and waveform capnography
- Do not hyperventilate

↓

Treat hypotension (SBP <90 mm Hg)
- IV/IO bolus
- Vasopressor infusion
- Consider treatable causes
- 12-Lead ECG

↓

Follow commands? — No → Consider induced hypothermia → STEMI OR high suspicion of AMI

Follow commands? — Yes → STEMI OR high suspicion of AMI

STEMI OR high suspicion of AMI — Yes → Coronary reperfusion → Advanced critical care

STEMI OR high suspicion of AMI — No → Advanced critical care

Doses/Details

Ventilation/Oxygenation
Avoid excessive ventilation, Start at 10–12 breaths/min and titrate to target P_{ETCO_2} of 35–40 mm Hg
When feasible, titrate FiO_2 to minimum necessary to achieve SpO_2 ≥94%

IV bolus
1–2 L normal saline or lactated Ringer's. If inducing hypothermia may use 4'C fluid

Epinephrine IV infusion
0.1–0.5 mcg/kg per minute (in 70 kg adult: 7–35 mcg per minute)

Norepinephrine IV infusion
5–10 mcg/kg per minute

Dopamine IV infusion
0.1–0.5 mcg/kg per minute (in 70 kg adult: 7–35 mcg per minute)

Reversible causes
– Hypovolemia
– Hypoxia
– Hydrogen ion (acidosis)
– Hypo-/hyperkalemia
– Tension pneumothorax
– Tamponade, cardiac
– Toxins
– Thrombosis, pulmonary
– Thrombosis, coronary

26. What are the recommendations for termination of resuscitative efforts?

Ans. The decision rests with the treating physician and is based on consideration of:

- Time from collapse to CPR
- Time from collapse to 1st defibrillation attempt
- Comorbid disease
- Prearrest state
- Initial arrest rhythm
- Response to resuscitative measures.

The duration of resuscitative efforts is an important factor associated with poor outcome. The chance that the patient will survive to hospital discharge and be neurologically intact diminishes as resuscitation time increases.

27. What are the recommendations regarding withdrawal of life support?

Ans. In adult postcardiac arrest patients treated with therapeutic hypothermia, it is recommended that clinical neurologic signs, electrophysiologic studies, biomarkers, and imaging be performed where available at 3 days after cardiac arrest. Currently, there is limited evidence to guide decisions regarding withdrawal of life support. The clinician should document all available prognostic testing 72 hours after cardiac arrest treated with therapeutic hypothermia and use best clinical judgment based on this testing to make a decision to withdraw life support when appropriate.

Good to know

1. Describe the approach to CPR in a pregnant woman.

Ans. Maternal cardiac arrest (Flow chart 2)

2. Enumerate some unconventional CPR techniques.

Ans.

- High-frequency chest compressions
- Open-chest CPR
- Interposed abdominal compression-CPR (IAC-CPR)
- 'Cough' CPR
- Prone CPR
- Precordial thump
- Percussion pacing.

3. Name few CPR devices.

Ans.

- Devices to assist ventilation:
  - Automatic transport ventilators (ATVs)
  - Manually-triggered, oxygen-powered, flow-limited resuscitators
- Devices to support circulation:
  - Active compression-decompression CPR (ACD-CPR)
  - Phased thoracic-abdominal compression-decompression CPR (PTACD-CPR)
  - Impedance threshold device (ITD)
  - Mechanical Piston Devices—LUCAS
  - Load-distributing band (LDB) CPR or vest CPR—autopulse device
  - Extracorporeal techniques and invasive perfusion devices.

Flow chart 2 Cardiopulmonary resuscitation (CPR) in a pregnant woman

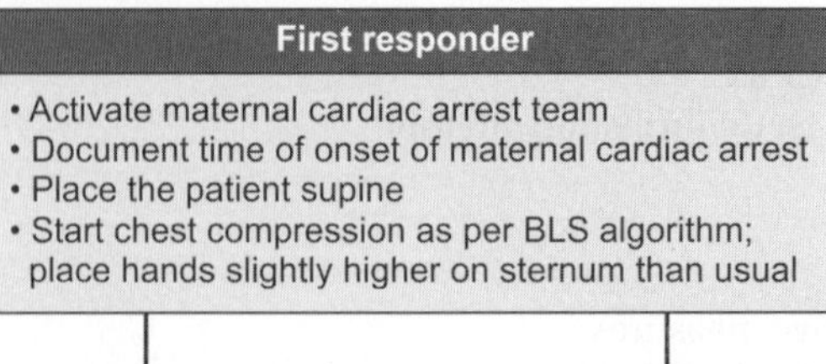

First responder

- Activate maternal cardiac arrest team
- Document time of onset of maternal cardiac arrest
- Place the patient supine
- Start chest compression as per BLS algorithm; place hands slightly higher on sternum than usual

↓

Subsequent responders

Maternal interventions

Treat per BLS and ACLS algorithms

- Do not delay defibrillation
- Give typical ACLS drugs and doses
- Ventilate with 100% oxygen
- Monitor waveform capnography and CPR quality
- Provide postcardiac arrest care as appropriate

Maternal modification

- Start IV above the diaphragm
- Assess for hypovolemia and give fluid bolus when required
- Anticipate difficult airway; experienced provider preferred for advanced airway placement
- If patient receiving IV/IO magnesium prearrest, stop magnesium and give IV/IO calcium chloride 10 mL in 10% solution, or calcium gluconate 30 mL in 10% solution
- Continue all maternal resuscitative interventions (CPR, positioning, defibrillation, drugs and fluids) during and after cesarean section.

Obstetric interventions for patient with an obviously gravid uterus*

- Perform manual left uterine displacement (LUD)—displace uterus to the patient's left to relieve aortocaval compression
- Remove both internal and external fetal monitors if present

Obstetric and neonatal teams should immediately prepare for possible emergency cesarean section

- If no ROSC by 4 minutes of resuscitative efforts, consider performing immediate emergency cesarean section
- Aim for delivery within 5 minutes of onset of resuscitative efforts

* An obviously gravid uterus is a uterus that is deemed clinically to be sufficiently large to cause aortocaval compression

Search for and treat possible contributing factors (BEAU-CHOPS)

Bleeding DIC
Embolism—Coronary/pulmonary/amniotic fluid embolism
Anesthetic complication
Uterine atony
Cardiac diseases (MI/ischemia/aortic dissection/cardiomyopathy)
Hypertension pre-eclampsia/eclampsia
Other—Differential diagnosis of standard ACLS guidelines
Placenta abruptio/previa
Sepsis

Nice to know

1. Enumerate the elements of effective resuscitation team dynamics.

Ans.

- Closed-loop communications
- Clear messages
- Clear roles and responsibilities
- Knowing one's limitations
- Knowledge sharing
- Constructive intervention
- Re-evaluation and summarizing
- Mutual respect.

BIBLIOGRAPHY

1. Circulation 2010. Vol 122, Issue 18 suppl 3.
2. Gilmore CM, et al. Three-phase model of cardiac arrest: time-dependent benefit of Bystander Cardiopulmonary Resuscitation. Am J Cardiol 2006;98:497-9.

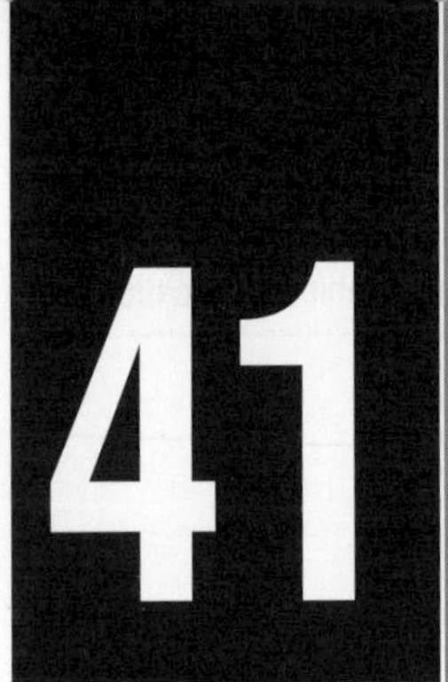

Neonatal Resuscitation

Rajat Choudhuri

Must know

- Approximately, 10% of newborns require some assistance to begin breathing at birth and less than 1% require extensive resuscitative measures.
- For the purpose of these guidelines the term newborn and neonate are intended to apply to any infant during the initial hospitalization and newly born specifically to an infant at the time of birth.
- Unlike adults hypoxia is the predominant cause of cardiac arrest.
- Term babies, having good muscle tone and crying are candidates not requiring CPCR.
- Sixty seconds is the golden minute and heart rate is a major monitoring parameter.
- Assessment should consist of simultaneous evaluation of 3 vital characteristics: Heart rate, respirations and the state of oxygenation.
- The most sensitive indicator of a successful response to each step of resuscitation is an increase in heart rate.

STEPS OF RESUSCITATION

1. Initial steps (with simultaneous assessment)
    - Provide warmth
    - Clear airway if necessary
    - Dry
    - Stimulate
2. Ventilation
3. Chest compression
4. Administration of drugs and/or volume expansion

Anticipation: From history and documentation, identify/anticipate which newborns shall definitely require resuscitation and recruit additional skilled personnel.

Initial Steps

Warmth

- Radiant heat source
- Plastic wrapping
- Exothermic mattress
  Goal is to achieve normothermia and avoid iatrogenic hyperthermia.

Dry, Stimulate Breathing, Clear Airway

- Avoid unnecessary suctioning.
- Suctioning immediately following birth should be reserved for babies who have obvious obstruction to spontaneous breathing or who require positive pressure ventilation.
- Nonvigorous babies with meconium stained amniotic fluid may require suctioning, bag mask ventilation and endotracheal intubation.
- Lack of cyanosis is a very poor indicator of the status of oxygenation.

Oximetry

- If resuscitation can be anticipated.
- When positive pressure ventilation administered.
- In persistent cyanosis.
- During oxygen administration.

Supplementary Oxygen

- Preferred (AIR +/– Blended oxygen)
- If heart rate < 60/minute after 90 seconds of resuscitation provide 100% oxygen.

Ventilation

Positive Pressure Ventilation

- Apneic
- Gasping
- HR < 100/minute after initial steps.
- Ventilatory assistance required around 40–60 bpm to maintain HR >100/min.

CPAP/PEEP

Better.

Assisted Ventilation Device

LMA → 2000 gm; > 34 weeks gestation.

Endotracheal Intubation

- Nonvigorous meconium stained newborn
- Ineffective/prolonged bag mask ventilation
- When chest compressions are performed
- Congenital diaphragmatic hernia
- Extremely LBW.

Chest Compressions

Assessment of heart rate is by auscultating the precordial pulse or palpation of umbilical pulse.
- When HR < 60/min despite 30 seconds of adequate oxygenation.
- Lower 1/3rd of sternum compress to 1/3rd AP diameter.
- 3:1 = C:V unless cardiac arrest of cardiac origin in which case 15:2 is the recommendation.
- Two finger technique/2 thumb encircling technique.

Drugs/Volume Expansion

Medications

- Rarely required, e.g. epinephrine 0.01–0.03 mg/Kg.
- Naloxone better avoided.
- No glycemic targets

Volume Resuscitation

Blood @10 mL/Kg.

Postresuscitation Care

- HR, oxygenation and ventilation maintenance.
- Induced therapeutic hypothermia (33.5–34.5°C) for 72 hours and to be started within 6 hours, slow rewarming over >/=4 hours for newborns >36 weeks gestational age.

Withholding and Discontinuation of Resuscitation

Withholding resuscitation:
- < 23 weeks
- < 400 gm
- Anencephaly
- Chromosomal anomalies, e.g. trisomy 13
- Parental desires if anticipated burden high.

Discontinuing resuscitation: If heart rate not detected for 10 mins.

Educational Programs to Teach Neonatal Resuscitation

Educational programs:
- Simulation based learning methodologies
- Briefing and debriefing techniques in designing an education program for the acquisition and maintenance of the skills necessary for effective neonatal resuscitation.

Flow chart 1 shows newborn resuscitation.

Flow chart 1 Newborn resuscitation algorithm

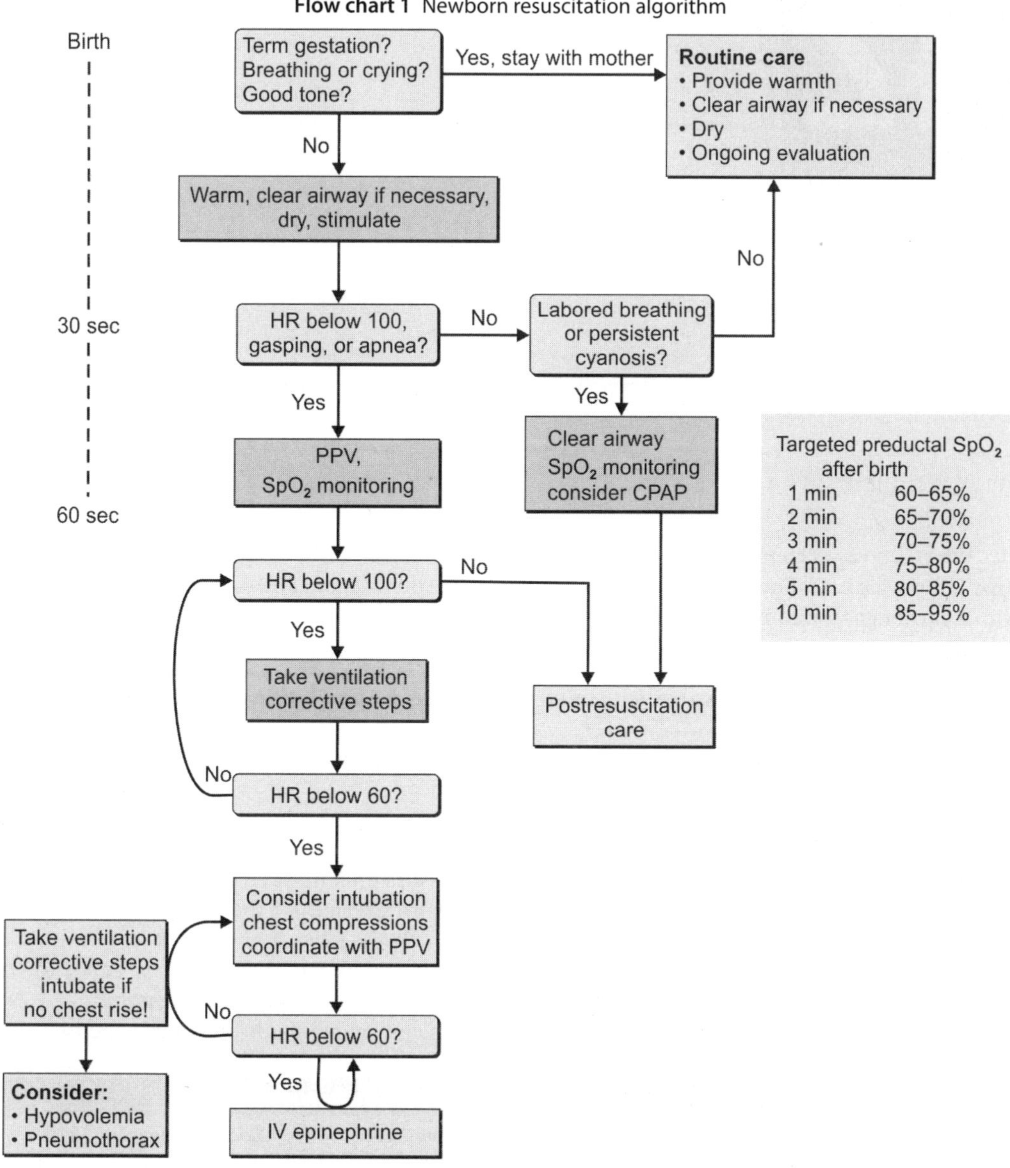

BIBLIOGRAPHY

1. Circulation. 2010;122(suppl 3):S909 –S919.
   *Co-chairs and equal first co-authors.
   (Circulation. 2010;122[suppl 3]:S909 –S919.)
   © 2010 American Heart Association, Inc.
   Circulation is available at http://circ.ahajournals.org DOI: 10.1161/CIRCULATIONAHA.110.971119
2. J Hazinski MF, Halamek LP, Kumar P, Little G, McGowan JE, Nightengale B, Ramirez MM, Ringer S, Simon WM, Weiner GM, Wyckoff M, Zaichkin
3. J. Part 15: neonatal resuscitation: 2010 American Heart Association Guidelines for Cardiopulmonary Resuscitation and Emergency Cardiovascular Care.
4. Kattwinkel J, Perlman JM, Aziz K, Colby C, Fairchild K, Gallagher.

42

Vaporizers

Sudeshna Bhar (Kundu)

1. What is a vaporizer?

Ans. The device that allows vaporization of the liquid anesthetic agent and its subsequent admixture with a carrier gas for administration to a patient is called a vaporizer.

Ref: Davey JA, Diba A. Ward's Anaesthetic Equipment, 5th edn. Elsevier Saunders; 2005.pp.65-90.

2. Define vapor, vapor pressure, saturated vapor pressure and boiling point of a liquid.

Ans.

- *Vapor:* It is the gaseous phase of a substance that is liquid at room temperature and atmospheric pressure.
- *Vapor pressure:* It is the pressure exerted by the vapor molecules bombarding per unit area of their surroundings. It depends only on the liquid and the temperature. It does not depend on ambient pressure within the range of barometric pressure encountered in anesthesia.
- *Saturated vapor pressure:* It is the maximum pressure exerted by the vapor molecules at a particular temperature.
- *Boiling point:* It is the temperature of a liquid at which its vapor pressure is equal to the atmospheric pressure. The lower atmospheric pressure, the lower is the boiling point.

  Table 1 shows the boiling point and vapor pressure of common volatile anesthetic agents.

Table 1 | Boiling point and vapor pressure of common volatile anesthetic agents

Anesthetic agent	*Boiling point (°C, 760 mm Hg)*	*Vapor pressure (torr, 20°C)*
Halothane	50.2	243
Enflurane	56.5	175
Isoflurane	48.5	238
Desflurane	22.8	669
Sevoflurane	58.6	157

Ref: Dorsch JA, Dorsch SE. Understanding Anesthesia Equipment, 5th edn. Lippincott Williams & Wilkins; 2008.pp.121-189.

3. Define partial pressure, volume percent, heat of vaporization, specific heat, thermal capacity and thermal conductivity.

Ans.

- *Partial pressure:* The part of the total pressure that results from any one gas in the mixture is called partial pressure of that gas. The total pressure of the mixture is the sum of the partial pressures of the constituent gases. It depends only on the temperature of the liquid agent and is unaffected by the total pressure above the liquid. The highest partial pressure exerted by a gas at a given temperature is its vapor pressure.
- *Volumes percent:* It is the number of units of volume of a gas in relation to a total of 100 units of volume for the total gas mixture.
  Volumes percent expresses the relative ratio of gas molecules in a mixture, whereas partial pressure expresses an absolute value.
  Partial pressure/Total pressure = Volumes percent
  Although vapor concentration delivered by a vaporizer is usually expressed in volumes percent, patient uptake and anesthetic depth are directly related to partial pressure but only indirectly to volumes percent.
- *Heat of vaporization:* It is the number of calories necessary to convert 1gm of liquid into a vapor.
- *Specific heat:* It is the quantity of heat required to raise the temperature of 1gm of the substance by 1°C. Water is the standard with a specific heat of 1 cal/gm/°C. Specific heat of an anesthetic agent should be low to facilitate vaporization.
- *Thermal capacity:* It is the product of specific heat and mass and represents the amount of heat stored in the vaporizer body. A vaporizer constructed from a substance with a high thermal capacity will change temperature more slowly than one with a low thermal capacity.
- *Thermal conductivity:* It is the measure of speed with which heat flows through a substance. The material for vaporizer should have high specific heat and high thermal conductivity.

Ref: Dorsch JA, Dorsch SE. Understanding Anesthesia Equipment, 5th edn. Lippincott Williams & Wilkins; 2008.pp.121-189.

4. What are the factors that can affect vaporization?

Ans. The molecules of liquid possess varying degrees of kinetic energy and are in constant motion. If the liquid has a surface exposed to any gas or vacuum, some molecules with high kinetic energy will escape from the surface resulting in vaporization.

The degree of vaporization depends on the following factors:

- *Temperature:* Vaporization is increased if the temperature of the liquid is raised, since more molecules will be given sufficient kinetic energy to escape.
- *Volatility:* A more volatile liquid has weaker cohesive forces. So they require less energy to vaporize.
- *Surface area of the liquid:* Greater the surface area, more space is available for the molecules to leave the liquid. Vaporization is directly proportional to the surface area of the liquid. Wicks or baffles may be used to increase the surface area.
- *Removal of the vapor from the vicinity of liquid:* Vaporization is proportional to the gas flow across the surface of the liquid as the gas will remove the vapor more quickly allowing fresh vapor to form.

Ref: Davey JA, Diba A. Ward's Anaesthetic Equipment, 5th edn. Elsevier Saunders; 2005.pp.65-90.

5. What do you mean by temperature compensated vaporizer?

Ans. As vaporization progresses, the vaporizing liquid as well as the vaporizer cools and the quantity of vapor produced decreases. This fall in vapor output is minimized in temperature compensated vaporizer by the following means:

- By supplying a finite quantity of heat with the help of a heat source, e.g. water bath, heating element or metal jacket.
- *By temperature compensating devices:* A greater proportion of the carrier gas is allowed to pass through the vaporizing chamber by altering the splitting ratio. Two types of temperature compensating devices are commonly used.
  - The first type (Figs 1A and B) consists of a bi-metallic strip. Two metals have different rates of expansion and contraction. So with change in temperature, it can bend and can vary the degree of occlusion in the aperture of a gas channel (usually the bypass).
  - The second type (Figs 2A and B) is a bi-metallic arrangement which consists of an inner rod made of invar, a relatively non-expansile metal. The outer jacket, made of an expansile metal (brass), comes in contact with the vaporizing liquid. When this contracts (with cooling) it drags the choke on the inner rod into the bypass, increasing the resistance to flow through it.

Ref: Davey JA, Diba A. Ward's Anaesthetic Equipment, 5th edn. Elsevier Saunders; 2005.pp.65-90.

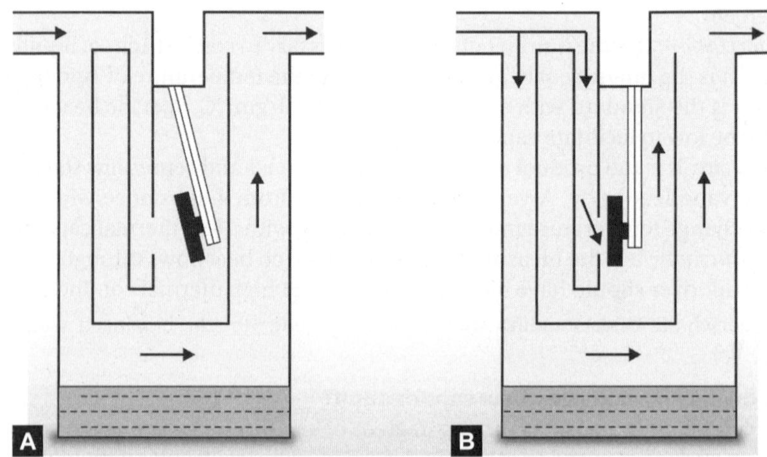

Figs 1A and B Bi-metallic strip, temperature compensating device

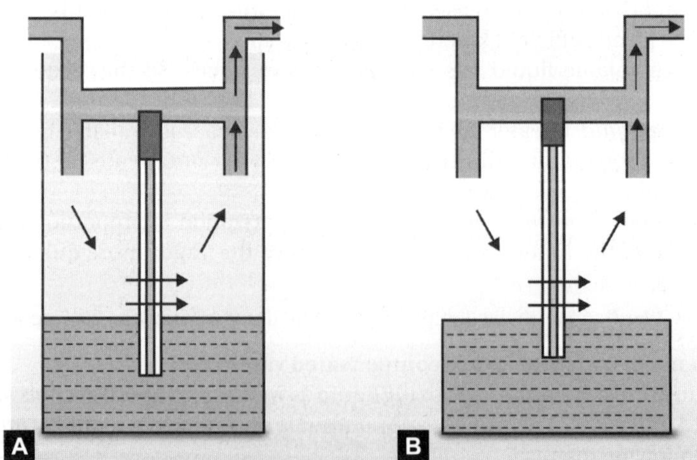

Figs 2A and B Bi-metallic arrangement, temperature compensating device

6. Classify vaporizer.

Ans. Vaporizers can be classified in several ways:

- Depending on the method of regulating output concentration
  - *Concentration calibrated/Variable bypass:* In OFF position, gas flows through the bypass channel. In ON position, the gas flow is divided into two portions. On part goes through the bypass and the other flows to the vaporizing chamber. Both gas flows rejoin downstream. The final vapor concentration may be changed by adjusting the splitting ratio (ratio of bypass gas to gas going to the vaporizing chamber is called the splitting ratio. It depends on the resistances in the two pathways)
  - *Measured flow:* It uses a measured flow of carrier gas, usually oxygen, to pick up anesthetic vapor. Example is copper kettle vaporizer.
- Depending on the method of vaporization
  - *Flow-over:* Carrier gas passes over the surface of the anesthetic liquid. The vaporization can be enhanced by increasing the area of carrier gas-liquid interface (using baffles, wicks or spiral tracks).
  - *Bubble-through:* Carrier gas is allowed to bubble through the anesthetic liquid. Vaporization is enhanced if bubble size is small as it provides larger surface area for contact.
  - *Injection:* Controls the vapor concentration by injecting a known amount of liquid anesthetic agent into a known volume of gas.
- Depending on the temperature compensation
  - Thermocompensation
  - Supplied heat
- Depending on the agent specificity
  - *Agent specific:* It is used for a particular agent
  - *Multiple agent:* It may be used with various anesthetic agents (universal/all-purpose vaporizer)
- Depending on the location
  - *Vaporizer outside the breathing circuit (VOC):* Vaporizer is placed between the flowmeter and machine outlet or between machine outlet and breathing circuit.
  - *Vaporizer inside the breathing circuit (VIC):* Vaporizer is placed inside the circle system.

Ref: Dorsch JA, Dorsch SE. Understanding Anesthesia Equipment, 5th edn. Lippincott Williams & Wilkins; 2008.pp.121-89.

7. What do mean by plenum vaporizer?

Ans. In plenum vaporizer, the carrier gas is pressurized to make it as dense as the vapor. So at lower flow rates, carrier gas would more readily mix with the vapor rather than tend to pass above it in the vaporizing chamber. It makes a vaporizer more accurate. The vaporizers are meant for unidirectional gas flow and have a relatively high resistance to gas flow. Thus they are not suitable for use as draw-over vaporizers or in the circle system.

Ref: Davey JA, Diba A. Ward's Anaesthetic Equipment, 5th edn. Elsevier Saunders; 2005.pp.65-90.
Ref: Paul AK. Drugs and Equipment in Anesthetic Practice, 5th edn. Elsevier; 2005.pp.287-300.

8. What is pumping effect?

Ans. When resistance is applied to the outlet of the anesthesia machine as occurs while using oxygen flush or controlled ventilation, there is an increase in the anesthetic gas pressure which is transmitted back to the vaporizer. The carrier gas in the vaporizer is compressed due to this back pressure. When the back pressure is released, the expanding carrier gas surges out through both the inlet and outlet of the vaporizing chamber. The gas that leaves the inlet enters into the bypass channel resulting in an increase in the final vapor output (Figs 3A to D).

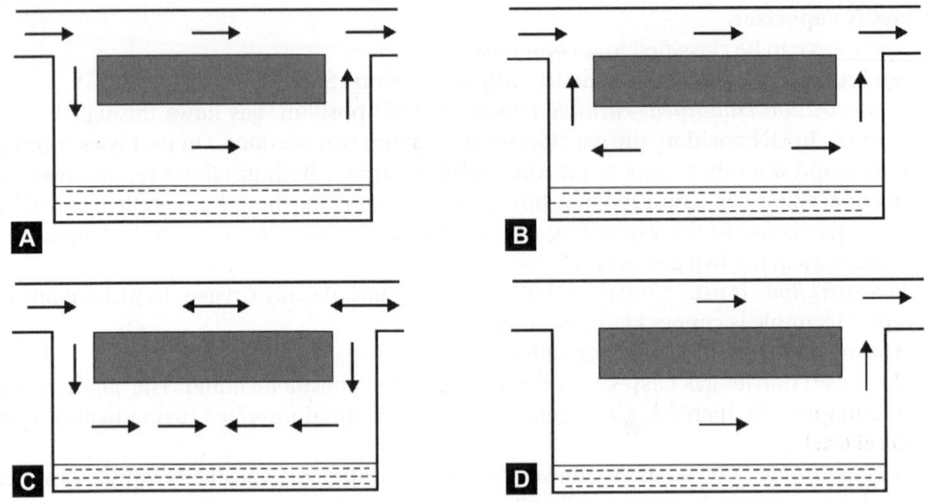

Figs 3A to D Pumping effect

This effect can be minimized by:

- Increasing the flow through the vaporizing channel and the bypass
- Elongating the flow passage into either the inlet or the outlet of the vaporizer
- Placing a nonreturn valve.

Ref: Davey JA, Diba A. Ward's Anaesthetic Equipment, 5th edn. Elsevier Saunders; 2005.pp.65-90.

9. What is pressurizing effect?

Ans. Increased pressure at the vaporizer outlet compresses the carrier gas. But the number of molecules of the vapor in the vaporizing chamber will not increase as the vapor pressure depends only on temperature and not on the ambient pressure. So the net result is decreased concentration of the anesthetic agent at the vaporizer outlet. The pressurizing effect is prominent at high gas flow and the pumping effect is prominent at low gas flow (Fig. 4).

Ref: Dorsch JA, Dorsch SE. Understanding Anesthesia Equipment, 5th edn. Lippincott Williams & Wilkins; 2008.pp.121-89.

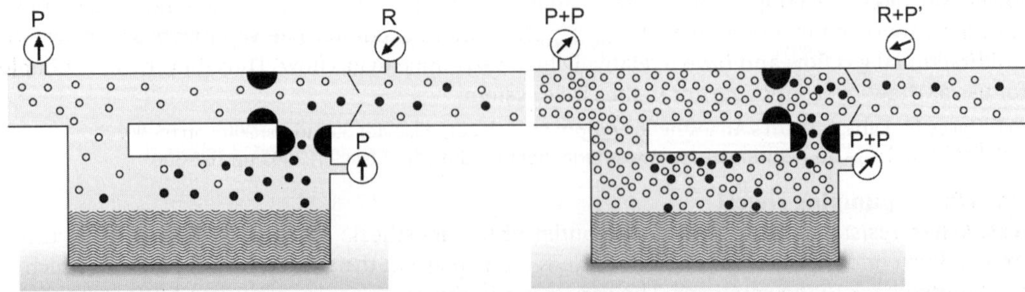

Fig. 4 Pressurizing effect

10. What are the criteria of an ideal vaporizer?

Ans.

- Simple, safe, light weight
- Low resistance
- Agent specific, temperature compensated
- Accurate and predictable delivery of the vapor
- No change in vapor output at different flow rates of the carrier gas
- No effect of back pressure
- Small liquid requirement
- Corrosion and solvent resistant.

Ref: Paul AK. Drugs and Equipment in Anaesthetic Practice, 5th edn. Elsevier; 2005.pp.287-300.

11. Mention the ASTM anesthesia workstation standard for vaporizer.

Ans. The ASTM anesthesia workstation standard includes the followings:

- The effects of variations in ambient temperature and pressure, tilting, back pressure, and input flow rate and gas mixture composition on vaporizer performance must be stated in the accompanying documents.
- The average delivered concentration from the vaporizer shall not deviate from the set value by more than ±20% or ±5% of the maximum setting, whichever is greater, without back pressure.
- The average delivered concentration from the vaporizer shall not deviate from the set value by more than +30% or -20% or by more than +7.5% or -5% of the maximum setting, whichever is greater, with pressure fluctuations at the common gas outlet of 2 kPa with a total gas flow of 2 L/minute or 5 kPa with a total gas flow of 8 L/minute.
- A system that prevents gas from passing through the vaporizing chamber or reservoir of one vaporizer and then through that of another must be provided.
- The output of the vaporizer shall be less than 0.05% in the 'OFF' or 'zero' position.
- All vaporizer control knobs must open counterclockwise.
- Either the maximum and minimum filling levels or the actual usable volume and capacity shall be displayed.
- The vaporizer must be designed so that it cannot be overfilled when in the normal operating position.
- Vaporizers unsuitable for use in the breathing system must have noninterchangeable proprietary or 23 mm fittings. Conical fittings of 15-mm and 22-mm cannot be used. When 23-mm fittings are used, the inlet of the vaporizer must be male and the outlet female. The direction of gas flow must be marked.
- Vaporizers suitable for use in the breathing system must have standard 22-mm fittings or screw-threaded, weight-bearing fittings with the inlet female and the outlet male. The direction of gas flow must be indicated by arrows and the vaporizer marked "for use in the breathing system."

Ref: Dorsch JA, Dorsch SE. Understanding Anesthesia Equipment, 5th edn. Lippincott Williams & Wilkins; 2008.pp.121-89.

12. What are the various types of vaporizer filling devices available?

Ans. There are several filling systems available.

- *Funnel fill system:* The vaporizer filling components include a funnel and a cap. When the cap is removed, liquid can be poured into the vaporizing chamber through a funnel. Agent is poured into the filling port until the level reaches the full mark. The filler cap is then securely placed.
- *Keyed fill system:* They are agent specific being geometrically coded (keyed) to fit the safety filling port of the vaporizer and anesthetic agent supply bottle. These devices minimize the chance of filling the vaporizer with the wrong agent and reduce the incidence of spillage. The fillers are

color coded (Red-halothane, orange-enflurane, purple-isoflurane, yellow-sevoflurane, blue-desflurane).

- *Quick fill system:* It is only used for sevoflurane. To fill the vaporizer, the filler cap and the bottle cap are removed. The bottle is inserted so that the projections fit into the corresponding grooves in the filler neck. The bottle is pushed into the vaporizer components far as it will go and is held firmly in place. This will open a valve and allow the liquid agent to flow into the vaporizer.
- *Easy fill system:* It is used on all four TEC 7 vaporizers. To fill the vaporizer, the bottle adaptor is attached securely to the bottle and the filler cap on the vaporizer is removed. The bottle nozzle is inserted into the filler block, aligning the adaptor grooves with projections in the filler block. When the bottle is fully inserted, liquid will flow into the vaporizer.

Ref: Dorsch JA, Dorsch SE. Understanding Anesthesia Equipment, 5th edn. Lippincott Williams & Wilkins; 2008.pp.121-89.

13. Describe the vaporizer mounting devices.

Ans.

- *Permanent mounting:* Tools are needed to remove or install a vaporizer on the anesthesia machine.
  Advantage: Less damage to the vaporizer, fewer leaks.
  Disadvantages: Machine may not have enough mounting locations to accommodate all the vaporizers that are likely to be needed. A malfunctioning vaporizer cannot easily be exchanged.
- *Detachable mounting:* These are standard on most new anesthesia machine. They allow the vaporizer to be mounted or removed without the use of tools. The advantage is that anesthesia machine can have fewer mounting locations allowing a more compact machine. Vaporizers can be easily replaced. If malignant hyperthermia is a potential problem, vaporizers can be removed. Disadvantages include obstruction to gas flow and leak.

Ref: Dorsch JA, Dorsch SE. Understanding Anesthesia Equipment, 5th edn. Lippincott Williams & Wilkins; 2008.pp.121-89.

14. What are the hazards associated with vaporizers?

Ans.

- *Incorrect agent:* It can result in inaccurate vapor output. If an agent of high potency or volatility is placed in a vaporizer designed for an agent of low potency or volatility, a dangerously high concentration may be delivered. It can also lead to mixture of agents. If a vaporizer is filled with a wrong agent, it must be completely drained and all liquid discarded. Gas should be allowed to flow through it until no agent can be detected in the outflow.
- *Tipping:* Liquid from the vaporizing chamber enters into the bypass or outlet. A high concentration of the anesthetic agent will be delivered. If tipping occurs, a high flow of gas should be run through the vaporizer with the concentration dial set at a low concentration until the output shows no excessive agent.
- *Overfilling:* Liquid may enter the fresh gas line and lethal concentration of the anesthetic agent may be delivered. Complete vaporizer failure may also occur so that no vapor output is seen. It is prevented by filling only to the top line on the liquid level indicator glass and filling only when the vaporizer is turned off and is in the vertical position.
- *Reversed flow:* In most cases, there will be an increased output.
- Control dial in wrong position.
- *Leaks:* It affects fresh gas composition and flow. Leak may pollute the operating room air. Leak can be detected by pre-use check with the vaporizer turned ON. Vapor leak into fresh gas line: Some vaporizers leak small amounts of vapor into the bypass even when the vaporizer is turned OFF. Although the amounts delivered are usually too small to produce a clinical effect, it might

cause a sensitized individual to react to a halogenated agent or trigger an episode of malignant hyperthermia. These leaks can be reduced by not turning a vaporizer from the OFF to the '0' setting unless it is to be used.

- *Contaminants in the vaporizing chamber:* These may be water, cleaning agents or other foreign substances. If foreign substances are known to have entered the vaporizer, the manufacturer should be contacted to determine what measures need to be taken.
- *Physical damage:* Chance of damage is less in case of permanently mounted vaporizers.
- *No vapor output:* Common cause is empty vaporizer. Other causes include incorrect mounting, overfilling, control dial in wrong position, improper vaporizer mounting. Failure to deliver adequate amount of vapor may be detected by an anesthetic gas monitor.

Ref: Dorsch JA, Dorsch SE. Understanding Anesthesia Equipment, 5th edn. Lippincott Williams & Wilkins; 2008.pp.121-89.

15. Describe the interlock system.

Ans. Interlock (vaporizer exclusion) system prevents more than one vaporizer from being turned on at a time. When the vaporizer of choice is turned on, a pin is forced into the notch on the concentration control knob of each of the other vaporizers. These vaporizers are then locked in the 'off' position. This mechanism is incorporated in North American Drager interlock system. For Datex Ohmeda vaporizers, operating the dial release activates two extension rods that prevent operation of any other vaporizer installed on the manifold.

Ref: Dorsch JA, Dorsch SE. Understanding Anesthesia Equipment, 5th edn. Lippincott Williams & Wilkins; 2008.pp.121-89.

SALIENT FEATURES OF SOME VAPORIZERS

EMO vaporizer (Epstein Macintosh Oxford vaporizer): It is a variable bypass, draw-over temperature compensated vaporizer with wicks. It is mainly used for ether. It may be used for chloroform, halothane and trichloroethylene. No compressed gas cylinder is required as air acts as a carrier gas.

Ref: Paul AK. Drugs and Equipment in Anaesthetic Practice, 5th edn. Elsevier; 2005.pp.287-300.

Goldman vaporizer: It is a variable bypass, flow-over vaporizer without wick, used in or out of the system. It has no temperature compensation and may be used for multiple agents. It is not accurately calibrated.

Ref: Paul AK. Drugs and Equipment in Anesthetic Practice, 5th edn. Elsevier; 2005.pp.287-300.

TEC 2 vaporizer: It is a variable bypass, flow-over vaporizer with wick, used out of the circuit. It is temperature compensated and agent specific (used only for halothane).

Ref: Paul AK. Drugs and Equipment in Anesthetic Practice, 5th edn. Elsevier; 2005.pp.287-300.

TEC 3 vaporizer: It is a variable bypass, flow-over vaporizer with wick, used out of the breathing circuit. It is temperature compensated and agent specific (used only for halothane). It has two bypass channels. Effect of back pressure is negligible. It is less affected by change in fresh gas flow.

Ref: Paul AK. Drugs and Equipment in Anesthetic Practice, 5th edn. Elsevier; 2005.pp.287-300.

TEC 4 vaporizer: It is a variable bypass, flow-over vaporizer with wick, used out of the circuit. It is temperature compensated and agent specific. It is used for halothane, enflurane and isoflurane. It has some significant design features. If it is accidentally inverted, liquid does not spill into the bypass channel. It also incorporates an interlock facility. The vaporizer dial cannot be turned on if the vaporizer is improperly mounted on the anesthesia machine.

Ref: Davey JA, Diba A. Ward's Anesthetic Equipment, 5th edn. Elsevier Saunders; 2005.pp.65-90.

TEC 5 vaporizer: It is a variable bypass, flow-over vaporizer with wick, used out of the circuit. It is temperature compensated and agent specific. They are designed for use with halothane, enflurane, isoflurane and sevoflurane. A schematic diagram of TEC 5 vaporizer is shown in Figure 5.

When the concentration dial is in the zero position, all of the gas from the flowmeter bypasses the vaporizer through the select-a-tec bar. When the dial is turned past zero, inflowing gas is split into two streams by the rotary valve. One stream is directed to the vaporizing chamber, the other through the bypass. Gas passing through the bypass flows down one side of the vaporizer and past the thermostat which is a bi-metallic strip in the base. As the temperature in the vaporizer decreases, thermostat permits less gas flow through the bypass so that more gas passes through the vaporizing chamber. From the thermostat, gas flows up the other side of the vaporizer and near the outlet joins the gas that has passed through the vaporizing chamber. The gas flowing to the vaporizing chamber first passes through the central part of the rotary valve, after which it is directed through a helical channel then past a spiral wick (increases the surface area of contact with the liquid agent) that is in contact with the wick skirt which dips into the liquid agent. Gas with vapor leaves the vaporizing chamber via a channel in the concentration dial rotary valve and flows to the outlet.

Greatest accuracy is at a fresh gas flow of less than 5 L/min and dial setting less than 3%. At higher flows and higher dial settings, there is a decrease in output. The greatest accuracy is between 15°C and 35°C. The thermostat does not respond to the temperature below 15°C and the output will be less than indicated on the dial. If the temperature is above 35°C, the output will be unpredictably high. It is prone to increase in output from the pumping effect. Carrier gas composition affects the output. At low flows, the output is less when air or nitrous oxide is used than when oxygen is used as the carrier gas.

Maintenance: The exterior of the vaporizer may be wiped with a damp cloth. No other cleaning or disinfection should be attempted. If the anesthetic agent contains additives or stabilizing agents, the vaporizer should be drained every 2 weeks or when the level is low. If there are no additives or stabilizing agents, the vaporizer can be drained at less frequent intervals. The vaporizer should be returned to the service center every 3 years.

Two additional features are the improved filling action for the key fill system and an easier mechanism than the TEC 4 for switching on the vaporizer dial and disengaging the dial lock (single handed action).

Ref: Dorsch JA, Dorsch SE. Understanding Anesthesia Equipment, 5th edn. Lippincott Williams & Wilkins; 2008.pp.121-89.

Ref: Davey JA, Diba A. Ward's Anaesthetic Equipment, 5th edn. Elsevier Saunders; 2005.pp.65-90.

TEC 6 vaporizer: It is designed for use only with desflurane. It is somewhat longer than TEC 5 vaporizers. The concentration dial at the top is calibrated from 1% to 18% in graduation of 1% up to 10% and 2% between 10% and 18%. The filler port is at the front on the left. The power cord attachment and the battery case are on the bottom.

The amber warm up LED indicates an initial warm up period after the vaporizer is first connected to the main power. Once warm up is complete, the green operational LED is illuminated; indicating that the vaporizer has reached its operating temperature and the concentration dial can be turned on. The red no output LED flashes and an auditory alarm of repetitive tones sounds if the vaporizer is not able to deliver vapor. The amber low agent LED accompanied by an audible alarm is illuminated if there is less than 50 mL of agent in the vaporizer. If less than 20 mL of the agent remains in the vaporizer, the no output alarm is activated. The amber battery low LED indicates that a new battery is required.

It has a capacity of 425 mL. Desflurane is heated to 39°C (102°F) by two heater at its base. Pure vapor is injected into the fresh gas flow. It requires electrical power and has alarms; two unusual aspects compared to other contemporary vaporizers.

The vaporizer is calibrated for flows from 0.2 to 10 L/min. The vaporizer is designed to be used at ambient temperature between 18°C and 30°C. Output is within ± 15% of dial setting. Tilting does not render the vaporizer inoperative or dangerous to operate. Fluctuating back pressure does not significantly affect the TEC 6 vaporizer. Carrier gas composition affects vaporizer output. The output is decreased with air or nitrous oxide as the carrier gas.

Ref: Dorsch JA, Dorsch SE. Understanding Anesthesia Equipment, 5th edn. Lippincott Williams & Wilkins; 2008.pp.121-89.

TEC 7 vaporizer: There are TEC 7 vaporizers for halothane, enflurane, isoflurane and sevoflurane. Although there are a number of improvements in this vaporizer compared to TEC 5, the schematic diagram of TEC 7 vaporizer is essentially the same as for the TEC 5. It is available with three filling devices: funnel fill, quick fill, and easy fill system. Approximately 300 mL of liquid is needed to fill a vaporizer with dry wicks. Approximately 75 mL is retained in the wicks when the vaporizer is drained.

Performance curves are similar to those of TEC 5. Greatest accuracy is at a fresh gas flow of 5 L/min and dial setting less than 3%. The greatest accuracy is between 15°C and 35°C. Fluctuating back pressure can affect the vaporizer and increase the delivered concentration.

Hazards: Intended to be operated in upright position. If a vaporizer is inverted, it should be connected to a scavenging system, the dial set to 5% and the vaporizer purged with carrier gas at 5 L/min for 5 minutes.

Maintenance: The external surfaces can be cleaned with a moist cloth and neutral detergent. Halothane vaporizer should be drained every 2 weeks. Other vaporizers should be drained once a year. Three years from the date of purchase and every 6 months thereafter, the vaporizers should undergo a safety inspection and the output checked.

Ref: Dorsch JA, Dorsch SE. Understanding Anesthesia Equipment, 5th edn. Lippincott Williams & Wilkins; 2008.pp.121-89.

Vapor 2000: It is a tippable vaporizer. The dial must first be rotated to a "T" setting ("transport" or "tip") which is beyond zero (clockwise).

Ref: Dorsch JA, Dorsch SE. Understanding Anesthesia Equipment, 5th edn. Lippincott Williams & Wilkins; 2008.pp.121-89.

Aladin cassette vaporizer: It is associated with anesthesia delivery unit (ADU). It is electronically controlled by a CPU. The device is free from the hazards of tipping, overfilling and incorrect filling.

Ref: Dorsch JA, Dorsch SE. Understanding Anesthesia Equipment, 5th edn. Lippincott Williams & Wilkins; 2008.pp.121-89.

Boyle vaporizer: It is variable bypass, flow-over or bubble through type with no temperature compensation, used for ether and trichloroethylene. It consists of a glass bottle which is calibrated up to 300 mL. It is dark brown colored to prevent the decomposition of ether. When the plunger is up, the gas passes over the surface of the liquid (flow-over type) and when the plunger is down, the gas flows through the liquid (bubble through type). Metal parts of U tube and the hood of plunger are made of copper which acts as anticatalyst and thus prevents decomposition of ether.

The volatile liquid with a lower boiling point should be placed first following rotameter, otherwise condensation of the same may be recovered from the second vaporizing bottle. That is why the ether vaporizer is placed first and the trichloroethylene vaporizer next.

Ref: Paul AK. Drugs and Equipment in Anesthetic Practice, 5th edn. Elsevier; 2005.pp.287-300.

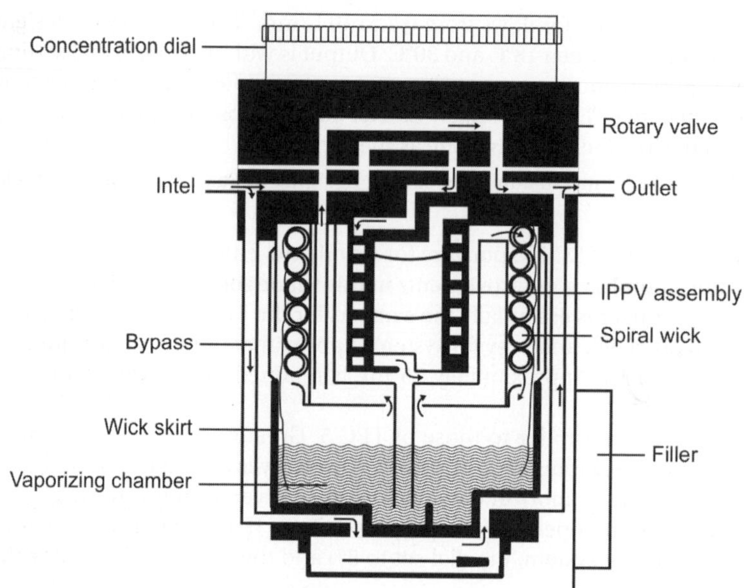

Fig. 5 Diagram of TEC 5 vaporizer in the on position

16. Give an example of a tippable vaporizer.

Ans. Vapor 2000.

Ref: Dorsch JA, Dorsch SE. Understanding Anesthesia Equipment, 5th edn. Lippincott Williams & Wilkins; 2008.pp.121-89.

17. Give an example of an electronic vaporizer.

Ans. Aladin cassette vaporizer (Fig. 5).

Ref: Dorsch JA, Dorsch SE. Understanding Anesthesia Equipment, 5th edn. Lippincott Williams & Wilkins; 2008.pp.121-89.

BIBLIOGRAPHY

1. Davey JA, Diba A. Ward's Anaesthetic Equipment, 5th edn. Elsevier Saunders; 2005.pp.65-90.
2. Dorsch JA, Dorsch SE. Understanding Anesthesia Equipment, 5th edn. Lippincott Williams & Wilkins; 2008.pp.121-189.
3. Paul AK. Drugs and Equipment in Anaesthetic Practice, 5th edn. Elsevier; 2005.pp.287-300.

Index

Page numbers followed by *f* refer to figure and *t* refer to table

F

G

H

I

P

T